WL 724 WIN

Foundations of Psychiatric Sleep Medicine

Foundations of Psychiatric Sleep Medicine

Edited by

John W. Winkelman MD, PhD
Associate Professor of Psychiatry, Brigham and Women's Hospital, Harvard Medical School, Boston, MA, USA

David T. Plante MD
Assistant Professor of Psychiatry, University of Wisconsin School of Medicine and Public Health, Madison, WI, USA

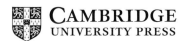

CAMBRIDGE
UNIVERSITY PRESS

CAMBRIDGE UNIVERSITY PRESS
Cambridge, New York, Melbourne, Madrid, Cape Town, Singapore,
São Paulo, Delhi, Dubai, Tokyo, Mexico City

Cambridge University Press
The Edinburgh Building, Cambridge CB2 8RU, UK

Published in the United States of America by
Cambridge University Press, New York

www.cambridge.org
Information on this title: www.cambridge.org/9780521515115

First published 2010

Printed in the United Kingdom at the University Press, Cambridge

A catalog record for this publication is available from the British Library

Library of Congress Cataloging-in-Publication Data

Foundations of psychiatric sleep medicine / editors, John W. Winkelman,
David T. Plante.
    p. ; cm.
  Includes bibliographical references and index.
  ISBN 978-0-521-51511-5 (Hardback)
1. Sleep disorders.   2. Sleep disorders–Psychological aspects.
3. Psychiatry.   4. Mental illness–Complications.   I. Winkelman, John W.
II. Plante, David T.   III. Title.
  [DNLM: 1. Sleep Disorders–diagnosis.   2. Sleep Disorders–
physiopathology.   3. Sleep Disorders–therapy. WM 188]
  RC547.F68 2010
  616.8′498–dc22

                                                    2010028666

ISBN 978-0-521-51511-5 Hardback

Contents

Section VII – Future Directions

Contributors

Candice A. Alfano PhD
Assistant Professor of Psychiatry and Behavioral
Sciences, Center for Neuroscience Research,
The Children's National Medical Center,
The George Washington
University School of Medicine,
Washington, DC, USA

J. Todd Arnedt PhD
Assistant Professor,
Departments of Psychiatry and Neurology,
Director, Behavioral Sleep Medicine Program,
University of Michigan Medical School,
Ann Arbor, MI, USA

Alon Y. Avidan MD, MPH
Associate Director,
UCLA Sleep Disorders Center; Director, UCLA
Neurology Clinic and
Neurology Residency Program;
Director, UCLA Department of Neurology,
Los Angeles, CA, USA

Ruth M. Benca MD, PhD
Director, Center for Sleep Medicine
and Sleep Research;
Professor, Department of Psychiatry,
University of Wisconsin–Madison,
Madison, WI, USA

Jed E. Black MD
Director, Stanford Sleep Disorders Center;
Associate Professor,
Center for Sleep Medicine,
Stanford University,
Stanford, CA, USA

Katy Borodkin MA
Department of Psychology,
Bar Ilan University,
Ramat Gan, Israel

Kirk J. Brower MD
Executive Director,
University of Michigan Addiction
Treatment Services;
Professor, Department of Psychiatry,
University of Michigan Medical School,
Ann Arbor, MI, USA

Ritchie E. Brown PhD
Department of Psychiatry,
VA Boston Healthcare System and
Harvard Medical School,
Brockton, MA, USA

Daniel J. Buysse MD
Department of Psychiatry,
University of Pittsburgh,
Pittsburgh, PA, USA

Dani Choufani MD
Assistant Professor of Medicine,
Thomas Jefferson University,
Philadelphia, PA, USA

Deirdre A. Conroy PhD
Clinical Assistant Professor,
Department of Psychiatry;
Clinical Director,
Behavioral Sleep Medicine Program,
University of Michigan Medical School,
Ann Arbor, MI, USA

Samuele Cortese MD, PhD
Child & Adolescent Psychopathology Unit,
Robert Debré Hospital,
Paris VII University,
Paris, France;
Child Neuropsychiatry Unit,
G. B. Rossi Hospital,
Department of Mother–Child and Biology-Genetics,
Verona University, Verona, Italy

Yaron Dagan
Medical Education Department,
Sackler School of Medicine,
Tel Aviv University,
Tel Aviv, Israel;
Institute for Sleep Medicine,
Assuta Medical Center, Tel Aviv, Israel

Joel E. Dimsdale MD
Professor, Department of Psychiatry,
School of Medicine,
University of California, San Diego,
La Jolla, CA, USA

Karl Doghramji MD
Professor of Psychiatry and Human Behavior;
Associate Professor of Neurology;
Medical Director,
Jefferson Sleep Disorders Center; Program Director,
Fellowship in Sleep Medicine, Thomas Jefferson
University,
Philadelphia, PA, USA

Fabio Ferrarelli MD, PhD
Assistant Researcher, Department of Psychiatry,
University of Wisconsin–Madison,
Madison, WI, USA

Marcos G. Frank PhD
Associate Professor of Neuroscience,
Department of Neuroscience,
School of Medicine, University of Pennsylvania,
Philadelphia, PA, USA

Philip R. Gehrman PhD, CBSM
Behavioral Sleep Medicine Program,
Department of Psychiatry,
University of Pennsylvania School of Medicine,
Philadelphia, PA, USA

Chad C. Hagen MD
Affiliate Faculty,
Sleep Disorders Program,
Department of Psychiatry,
Oregon Health and Science University,
Portland, OR, USA

J. Allan Hobson MD
Professor of Psychiatry,
Harvard Medical School,
Boston, MA, USA

Magdolna Hornyak MD, PhD
Associate Professor, Interdisciplinary Pain Center
and Department of Psychiatry and Psychotherapy,
University Medical Center,
Freiburg, Germany

Thomas D. Hurwitz MD
Department of Psychiatry,
Minneapolis VA Medical Center;
Assistant Professor of Psychiatry,
University of Minnesota Medical School,
Minneapolis, MN, USA

Anna Ivanenko MD, PhD
Department of Psychiatry and Behavioral Sciences,
Feinberg School of Medicine,
Northwestern University;
Division of Child and Adolescent Psychiatry,
Children's Memorial Hospital,
Chicago, IL, USA

Andrew D. Krystal MD, MS
Director, Insomnia and Sleep Research Program;
Professor of Psychiatry and Behavioral Sciences,
Duke University School of Medicine,
Duke University Medical Center,
Durham, NC, USA

Michel Lecendreux MD
Pediatric Sleep Disorders Center and Reference
Center for Pediatric Narcolepsy and Rare
Hypersomnias, and Child and
Adolescent Psychopathology Unit,
Robert Debré Hospital,
Paris VII University, Paris, France

In-Soo Lee MD
Postdoctoral Fellow, Department of Psychiatry,
University of California, San Diego,
La Jolla, CA, USA

Robert W. McCarley MD
Department of Psychiatry,
VA Boston Healthcare System and
Harvard Medical School,
Brockton, MA, USA

James T. McKenna PhD
Department of Psychiatry,
VA Boston Healthcare System and
Harvard Medical School,
Brockton, MA, USA

Valerie McLaughlin Crabtree PhD
Department of Behavioral Medicine,
St. Jude Children's Research Hospital,
Memphis, TN, USA

Thomas A. Mellman MD
Professor, Howard University Department of
Psychiatry and Behavioral Sciences,
Howard University College of Medicine,
Washington, DC, USA

Marta Novak MD, PhD
Head, Sleep Medicine Group,
Associate Professor of Psychiatry,
Institute of Behavioral Sciences,
Semmelweis University,
Budapest, Hungary;
Assistant Professor of Psychiatry,
Department of Psychiatry,
University Health Network,
University of Toronto,
Toronto, Canada

Michael Perlis PhD
Behavioral Sleep Medicine Program,
Department of Psychiatry,
University of Pennsylvania School of Medicine,
Philadelphia, PA, USA

Aimee L. Pierce MD
Fellow in Geriatric Neurology,
University of California,
Veterans Affairs San Diego Medical Center,
San Diego, CA, USA

David T. Plante MD
Assistant Professor of Psychiatry,
University of Wisconsin School of Medicine and
Public Health, Madison, WI, USA

Donn Posner PhD, CBSM
Clinical Associate Professor of Psychiatry and
Human Behavior,
The Warren Alpert Medical School of
Brown University,
Providence, RI, USA

Allen C. Richert MD
Associate Professor and Vice Chair for Education,
Sleep Medicine Division,
Department of Psychiatry and Human Behavior,

University of Mississippi Medical Center,
Jackson, MS, USA

Dieter Riemann PhD
Center for Sleep Research and Sleep Medicine,
Department of Psychiatry and Psychotherapy,
Freiburg University Medical Center,
Freiburg, Germany

Carlos H. Schenck MD
Department of Psychiatry,
Minnesota Regional Sleep Disorders Center,
Hennepin County Medical Center;
Professor of Psychiatry,
University of Minnesota Medical School,
Minneapolis, MN, USA

Michael Schredl PhD
Researcher, Sleep Laboratory,
Central Institute of Mental Health,
Mannheim, Germany

Gregory Stores MA, MD, DPM, FRCPsych, FRCP
Emeritus Professor of Developmental
Neuropsychiatry, Department of Psychiatry,
University of Oxford, Oxford, UK

Andras Szentkiralyi MD
Sleep Medicine Group, Institute of
Behavioral Sciences,
Semmelweis University,
Budapest, Hungary

Michael E. Thase MD
Mood and Anxiety Disorders Program,
Department of Psychiatry,
University of Pennsylvania School of Medicine,
Philadelphia, PA, USA

Wendy M. Troxel PhD
Department of Psychiatry,
University of Pittsburgh,
Pittsburgh, PA, USA

John W. Winkelman MD, PhD
Division of Sleep Medicine,
Department of Medicine,
Brigham and Women's Hospital;
Associate Professor of Psychiatry,
Harvard Medical School,
Boston, MA, USA

Preface

Sleep complaints are extraordinarily common among patients with psychiatric illness. Determining all the contributing causes of a sleep disturbance so that appropriate management can be implemented is a significant clinical challenge. Unfortunately, the majority of practicing clinicians are not given adequate training regarding sleep and its disorders, and thus optimal diagnosis and treatment are too often delayed or ignored.

Foundations of Psychiatric Sleep Medicine (FPSM) is a clinically accessible and academically rigorous primer designed to bridge the gap between the burgeoning field of sleep medicine and those who care for patients with psychiatric illness. Composed of 24 chapters divided into 7 sections, *FPSM* is a comprehensive resource with contributions from leaders in both fields detailing diagnostic and management issues at the nexus of sleep medicine and psychiatry. The first section discusses the history of the two fields, demonstrating the mutual influences and parallel development of the disciplines. The second section builds a foundation for the reader by detailing molecular and physiological mechanisms underlying sleep and wakefulness, methods used to characterize and stage sleep, as well as theoretical discussions of dreams and the functions of sleep.

The third section outlines sleep history-taking, with particular emphasis on the psychiatric patient. The fourth section details primary sleep disorders including sleep disordered breathing, sleep-related movement disorders, narcolepsy, parasomnias, and circadian rhythm disorders, with a particular focus on how these illnesses may present in psychiatric contexts. The fifth section focuses on insomnia, the most common sleep complaint in psychiatric practice, with separate chapters focusing on epidemiology and the role of insomnia in psychiatric illness, as well as pharmacological and psychotherapeutic treatments. The sixth section details the nature of sleep disturbance across the psychiatric disease spectrum including mood, anxiety, psychotic, substance use, and cognitive disorders. Also included are chapters devoted to disorders primarily occurring in children such as attention-deficit/hyperactivity disorder, pediatric mood and anxiety disorders, and developmental disorders. The book concludes with a discussion of future directions at the interface of sleep medicine and psychiatry. *FPSM* is an invaluable resource for the practicing mental health clinician, and more broadly for any practitioner who manages patients with co-occurring sleep and psychiatric complaints.

Editors' introduction

It is clear to any clinician who cares for those with psychiatric illness that disturbed sleep is a significant problem and great source of distress for patients. Long regarded as an epiphenomenon of the mental illness itself, it has previously been assumed that treatment of an underlying psychiatric disorder would result in resolution of the sleep disturbance. This paradigm has been called into question in recent years by growing evidence that sleep disturbance itself may play a vital role in the presentation, management, and course of many psychiatric disorders.

Sleep and psychiatric illnesses are powerfully linked in numerous ways. This is likely because, at both the observable and neurobiological levels, what and how we think and behave influences our sleep, and conversely, how we sleep influences our thinking and behavior. The most prevalent sleep complaint, insomnia, is frequently co-morbid with mental illness and is linked to a host of neuropsychiatric symptoms. In fact, insomnia may be present across the entire history of psychiatric disorders: as a risk factor for the development of incident mood, anxiety, and substance use disorders, as well as a symptom of active illness, an iatrogenic response to psychotropic medications, and risk factor for symptomatic relapse in a number of psychiatric disorders.

The value to psychiatrists of understanding sleep medicine has become increasingly evident over the past 20 years. The neuropsychiatric sequelae of primary sleep disorders such as sleep-related breathing disorders, sleep-related movement disorders, and circadian rhythm sleep disorders are increasingly recognized. In addition, psychotropic medications prescribed to treat psychiatric illness may inadvertently induce or exacerbate primary sleep disorders such as REM behavior disorder, obstructive sleep apnea, and restless legs syndrome, leading to unsuccessful treatments, paradoxical responses, or unwanted/unintended side-effects. Furthermore, psychotropic medications prescribed for the management of sleep-related symptoms presumed to be inherent to psychiatric illness, such as stimulants used to treat hypersomnia in atypical depression, may mask a primary sleep disorder (e.g. obstructive sleep apnea or narcolepsy) that may be the true underlying cause of the sleep-related complaint.

Due to the interrelationship between sleep and psychiatric illness, and psychiatrists' expertise in psychopharmacological and behavioral treatments, patients with sleep disturbance are often referred to mental health providers for evaluation and management. As a result, it has become increasingly important for the practicing mental health clinician to have a firm grasp of diagnostic and therapeutic techniques for patients with sleep complaints. To do so requires an understanding of the basic mechanisms of sleep and wakefulness, the pathophysiology of primary sleep disorders, the effects of psychiatric and psychological treatments on sleep, and the nature of sleep disturbance inherent to mental illness.

With the rise of sleep medicine as a specialty over the last half-century, our scientific understanding of sleep and its disorders has grown exponentially. The history and development of psychiatry and sleep medicine have been intimately intertwined, with psychiatrists and psychologists contributing significantly to this burgeoning field. Unfortunately, despite the contributions of these pioneering individuals, many of whom we are delighted to have as contributors to this book, there continues to be a chasm between sleep medicine and psychiatry. Few trainees (at any level of training or in any specialty) receive formal instruction on sleep and its disorders. Without such a knowledge base, patients with sleep-related complaints often do not receive optimal care because appropriate clinical questions are not asked, informed differential diagnoses are not developed, diagnostic tests are not pursued, and treatment plans are not thoughtfully composed.

Thus, the primary impetus for the development of *Foundations of Psychiatric Sleep Medicine (FPSM)* was to bridge the gap between sleep medicine and psychiatry, and to translate the findings from sleep and neuroscience into the clinical practice of caring for patients with psychiatric illness. As such, our goal was to develop *FPSM* to serve as a clinically useful, but academically rigorous, primer on sleep medicine for those who treat patients with mental illness. In addition, *FPSM* is a highly useful resource for sleep medicine clinicians with non-psychiatric backgrounds, who have not had formal training in managing patients with mental illness, as sleep medicine specialists are often asked to serve as consultants for patients with psychiatric disorders. Thus, this text is not an attempt to emphasize divisions within sleep medicine, but rather to highlight advances in sleep science and disorders to those in psychiatric and psychological professions. Furthermore, we hope it will simultaneously foster understanding within the interdisciplinary community of sleep medicine regarding the management of sleep disturbance in psychiatric populations.

The overall design of *FPSM* is straightforward and is comprised of seven sections. The first section reviews the history of sleep medicine and psychiatry, emphasizing the inter-related developments of both fields over the last century. The second section (Chapters 2–5) focuses on normal sleep, from molecular mechanisms of the circadian clock to the neurophysiology of sleep, including sleep staging and neuroimaging research. Other chapters discuss the theoretical functions of sleep and our current scientific understanding of dreams. The third section details clinical sleep history-taking, with a particular emphasis on psychiatric patients. Included are signs and symptoms that suggest referral for diagnostic studies and/or consultation with a sleep medicine specialist may be indicated. Section 4 of the book (Chapters 7–11) discusses primary sleep disorders including sleep disordered breathing, sleep-related movement disorders, narcolepsy, parasomnias, and circadian rhythm disturbances, with a particular focus on how these illnesses may present in psychiatric settings. This is particularly relevant to the practicing mental health clinician as many primary sleep disorders may present with neuropsychiatric symptoms, and several psychotropic medications can induce or exacerbate primary sleep disorders. Section 5 focuses specifically on insomnia, the most common sleep complaint in psychiatric practice. The principles of insomnia in psychiatric contexts, including the epidemiology and role of insomnia in the risk for development of and relapse to psychiatric illness are discussed. Additionally, separate chapters address pharmacological and psychotherapeutic treatments of insomnia. Section 6 (Chapters 15–23) details the nature of sleep disturbance in psychiatric illnesses across all major classes of psychiatric disorders including: mood, anxiety, psychotic, cognitive, and addictive disorders. Additionally, chapters devoted to disorders primarily occurring in childhood, including attention-deficit/hyperactivity disorder, pediatric mood and anxiety disorders, and developmental disorders, are provided. The book concludes with a discussion of the future directions of discovery and treatment at the nexus of sleep medicine and psychiatry.

We would like to take this opportunity to thank the authors who have so graciously contributed to this work, without whom such an endeavor would not have been possible. We also thank our families, whose patience and support have been invaluable throughout the process of developing this textbook. Finally we thank our teachers and mentors who have provided, and continue to provide, support for our growth and development. We hope that our efforts on this volume reflect their generosity and may spur the interest of future trainees to pursue clinical work and research at the interface of sleep medicine and psychiatry, in the hope of advancing both fields.

This material is based upon work supported by the American Sleep Medicine Foundation. Any opinions, findings, and conclusions or recommendations expressed in this publication are those of the author(s), and do not necessarily reflect the views of the American Sleep Medicine Foundation.

Sleep medicine and psychiatry: history and significance

J. Allan Hobson

Introduction

Psychiatry has not yet come fully to grips with sleep and dream research because it is not yet clear if or how the new science can replace the existing theoretical structures of the field. In terms of psychology, many psychiatrists still prefer psychoanalysis (despite its shortcomings) to the nascent cognitive psychiatry because psychoanalysis is more comprehensive and more hopeful. Sleep medicine has attracted some psychiatrists and provided the vast and reassuring data base of scientific medicine, but even that progressive move does not solve the mind–body problem that underlies psychiatry.

Initially posited by René Descartes in the seventeenth century, the notion of dualism of the mind and brain has been a central theme as psychiatry has developed. For much of its history, psychiatry has been polarized around the mind–brain dilemma, with major paradigm shifts pushing the field towards psychological versus biological trajectories. More recently, disenchantment with psychoanalysis and the growth of neurobiology and psychopharmacology have led many to proclaim themselves biological psychiatrists, and for them, sleep and dream research has provided some useful support. This belief, however, does little to solve the mind–brain problem that still fractures the field.

Sleep and dream research are truly foundational to psychiatry, and history reflects how psychiatry has struggled to come to terms with mind versus brain dualism. In the future, psychiatry may be advanced by taking advantage of the dramatic interaction between brain physiology, as it changes in sleep, and mental state. In reconstructing our notions of dreaming as an altered state of consciousness, rather than an unconscious mental state, we may begin to integrate the mind and brain in a more unified psychiatry.

Early history

In the late nineteenth and early twentieth century, medically oriented psychiatrists in Europe like Emil Kraepelin [1] and Eugen Bleuler [2] managed huge warehouses of deranged human beings. Their impact on the field of psychiatry is now widely acknowledged: Kraepelin for differentiating dementia praecox from manic depression; Bleuler for recognizing the former was not a true dementia, and subsequently coining the term "schizophrenia." Both were neurologically oriented and were masters of description and classification. Although they were hopeful the neurological basis for the mental illnesses they observed could be found, their work offered little insight into how the brain might mediate the horrendous symptoms of their patients. They ultimately had little to offer their patients in the way of treatment; in their time, a mentally ill person was sick for life.

Enter Sigmund Freud

Stimulated by speculative dynamic neurologists like Pierre Janet and Jean-Marie Charcot, Sigmund Freud created psychoanalysis in the same period Kraepelin and Bleuler labored. In so doing he turned away from both descriptive psychiatry and from brain science. He wanted to free his new theory of the mind from the shackles of medical science, especially neurology. This bold and rash revolt followed Freud's failure to produce a psychology based upon brain science of the time [3].

Of central importance to Freud's theory was his view of dreaming as an unconscious mental process by which dreamers could bowdlerize unacceptable unconscious wishes that threatened to invade consciousness and awaken them [4]. Freud's view was that dreaming was a process akin to the neuroses, which bedeviled his

Foundations of Psychiatric Sleep Medicine, ed. John W. Winkelman and David T. Plante. Published by Cambridge University Press.
© Cambridge University Press 2010.

patients by day. He therefore resorted to dream interpretation using the patients' free associations to their dream material to reveal and relieve the noxious unconscious force of both dreams and neurosis.

The power of this ingeniously simple but completely speculative hypothesis grew to dominate European psychiatry. Followers of Freud, including Ernest Jones, spread psychoanalysis to America where it flourished to the point that by 1950, practically every department chairman and every professor of psychiatry in the United States was a psychoanalyst. Serious critics of psychoanalysis were few and far between. Those who were critical of psychoanalytic theory were often marginalized within the psychiatric community.

The discovery of REM sleep

In 1953, Eugene Aserinsky, then a graduate student studying physiology at the University of Chicago, wired up his 9-year-old son, Armand, and other children to perform electroencephalogram (EEG) and electrooculogram (EOG) recordings in his rebellious experiments on attention carried out with the encouragement of the neurophysiologist, Ralph Gerard. As is so often the case, the monumental scientific discovery of REM sleep occurred in part by happenstance. When the child subjects became bored by Aserinsky's protocols, they fell asleep and, because they were young, evinced rapid eye movement (REM) periods shortly after sleep onset during which they dreamt. Aserinsky reported his observations to his supervisor, Nathaniel Kleitman, who suggested that they record the sleep of adults. The rest is history. All of Aserinsky and Kleitman's adult subjects showed EEG activation, REM periods, and when awakened reported long complex dreams, not at sleep onset but at 90–100 minute intervals throughout the night (Figure 1.1). Thus was modern sleep and dream science born [5].

Dream deprivation

William Dement, widely recognized as a pioneer in the field of sleep medicine, and a graduate student and psychiatrist working in Kleitman's laboratory at that time, was more interested in the dream story than his physiologist colleagues [6,7]. Dement was motivated by the conviction that he could test Freud's dream theory rigorously using the burgeoning knowledge of sleep physiology and REM sleep. By preventing subjects from entering REM with enforced awakenings, he and the neurobiologically educated psychoanalyst,

Charles Fisher, theorized they could prevent dreaming and thus cause psychological distress in their subjects [8]. Although their subjects did become psychologically distressed, they were perhaps more importantly increasingly difficult to awaken from sleep. By the fifth night of the experiment, subjects made no less than 50 attempts to enter REM (up tenfold from five such attempts on the first night). This observation indicated that REM sleep, if not dreaming, was carefully conserved, and therefore must be important.

In the years to follow, the National Institutes of Health (NIMH) funded a significant number of laboratories focused on dream research. Subjects, usually students, were awakened during sleep so as to give reports of antecedent mental activity that were then correlated with polysomnographic data. The results were inconclusive and often contradictory. Controlled experiments by Anthony Kales, another psychiatrist involved in the early development of sleep research, revealed that NREM sleep interruption was every bit as psychonoxious as the enforced REM sleep awakenings [9], a finding that did not fit with the dominant psychoanalytic paradigm of the time. By 1975, when the NIMH ceased funding of "dream lab" research, the psychiatric community had made relatively few inroads into the scientific status of Freud's dream theory.

Neurobiological progress of sleep medicine

During the same period in which dream laboratory research was flourishing, remarkable progress was being made using the (feline) animal model of sleep that William Dement had also given the field [10]. The prime mover of this initiative was Michel Jouvet, a French neurosurgeon working in Lyon, who had spent a year at the University of California at Los Angeles (UCLA) founded by Horace Magoun, the co-discoverer with Giuseppe Moruzzi of the reticular activating system [11]. Jouvet quickly localized the REM generator system to the pons [12] and suggested that the forebrain was activated, the eyes were caused to move, and spinal reflexes were inhibited [13] during REM sleep all from that central locale. With this discovery, dreaming could thus be redefined as the inevitable subjective experience of a specific physiological pattern of brain activation in sleep. As it turned out, all mammals shared this brain activation process in sleep, casting doubt, albeit

(a)

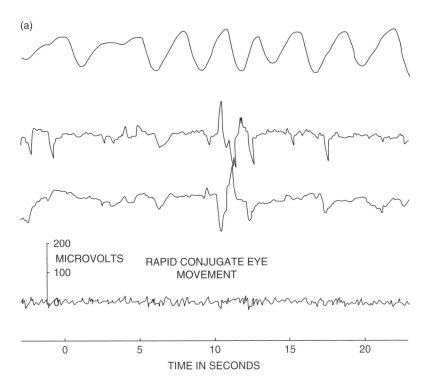

200
MICROVOLTS
100

RAPID CONJUGATE EYE
MOVEMENT

TIME IN SECONDS

Figure 1.1 Rapid eye movement sleep. The state most highly correlated with dreaming is shown at three levels of temporal detail. (a) *Polygraphic level*: a 20 s segment shows conjugate REMs as out of phase; EOG tracings (Channel (Ch) 2+3) together with respiration (Ch 1) and EEG (Ch 4). (b) *Cycle level*: the coordination of events in the six polygraphic channels shown indicates that the NREM–REM sleep cycle is an organismic whole body phenomenon. One cycle of polygraphic data lasting 100 min shows distribution in time of eye movements (Ch 1); EEG sleep stage (Ch 2); systolic blood pressure (Ch 3); respiratory irregularity (Ch 4); heart rate irregularity (Ch 5); and body movement (Ch 6). (c) *All night level*: three nights of sleep showing evolution of EEG stages with time. Note that Stages III and IV of NREM sleep occur predominantly in the first two cycles while Stage II and Stage I REM predominate in the last two cycles of the night.

(b)

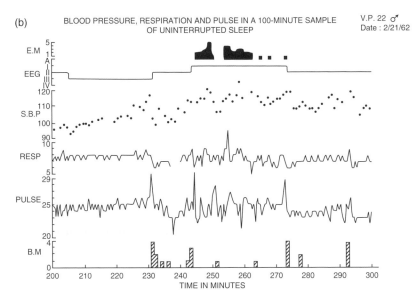

BLOOD PRESSURE, RESPIRATION AND PULSE IN A 100-MINUTE SAMPLE OF UNINTERRUPTED SLEEP

V.P. 22 ♂
Date : 2/21/62

TIME IN MINUTES

indirectly, on Freud's dream hypothesis. Under this new paradigm, REM sleep must be doing something besides serving purely as a substrate for unconsciously driven dreaming.

How was REM sleep instantiated by the pons? Jouvet's first guess, that it was enhanced cholinergic

neuromodulation, turned out to be correct [12]. But when he read Kjell Fuxe and Anica Dahlstrom's description [14] of the noradrenergic and serotonergic neuronal systems of the pontine brainstem, he was sidetracked from his original (correct) hypothesis. Jouvet then suggested that norepinephrine drove

(c)

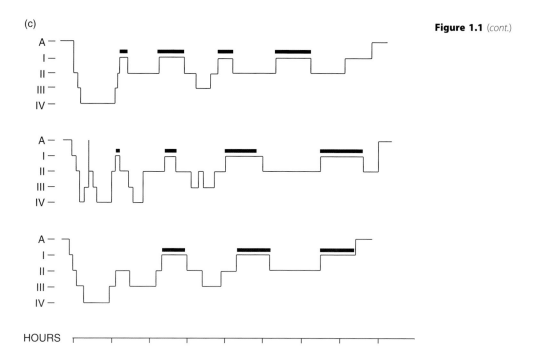

Figure 1.1 (*cont.*)

HOURS

REM sleep and that serotonin drove NREM sleep while waking was the responsibility of dopamine [15]. By 1975, it was clear from single brainstem cell recording experiments that both norepinephrine and serotonin cells enhanced waking rather than sleep. Instead of being excited in REM, the aminergic neurons needed to be *inhibited* for REM sleep to occur. Acetylcholine-containing cells, on the other hand, turned back on during REM, firing at levels as high as or higher than during waking. Subsequent experiments utilizing cholinergic microstimulation demonstrated that REM sleep could be induced by these compounds. As was later discovered, dopamine-containing cells fired throughout the sleep–wake cycle eliminating any specific role for that neuromodulator in state (i.e. wake, REM, or NREM) determination. However, this does not mean this neurotransmitter has no role in sleep or dreaming, as it has been theorized that dopamine – acting in the absence of noradrenergic and serotonergic influence – may contribute to the psychosis-like quality of dreaming.

Robert McCarley (who at the time was my student at Harvard) and I, having trained in Jouvet's laboratory in the 1960s, recorded from individual pontine neurons for almost 10 years before we realized that the brainstem had its own switching device for waking and dreaming and that dreaming had a specific neurophysiological basis. From these findings, we constructed our "reciprocal interaction model", that posited the level of activation (e.g. wake, NREM, or REM) was determined by the aforementioned interaction of pontine cholinergic neurons with aminergic systems (Figure 1.2) [16,17]. In 1977, we published our corresponding "activation-synthesis hypothesis" of the dream process in the *American Journal of Psychiatry* [18], 1 month after issuing a paper that outlined the inaccuracies of Freud's neuro-biological assumptions underlying psychoanalytic dream theory [19]. The activation-synthesis model proposed that an automatically activated forebrain synthesizes the dream by comparing information generated in specific brainstem circuits with information stored in memory. For the first time in 75 years, an alternative to Freud's theory of dreams became available with this model. The ensuing negative response from psychoanalytically oriented psychiatrists was fervent at the time, and this issue is still hotly debated, reflecting how deep the roots of Freudian psychology had grown within psychiatry.

The rise of sleep medicine

By the mid-1970s, experimental dream laboratories were failing, but modern sleep medicine was burgeoning. There was an exponential increase in pharmaceutical promotion of hypnotic sedatives and other

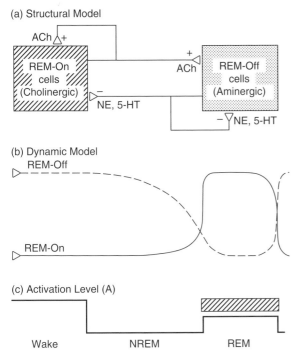

(a) Structural Model

(b) Dynamic Model

(c) Activation Level (A)

Figure 1.2 The original reciprocal interaction model of physiological mechanisms determining alterations in activation level. (a) Structural model of reciprocal interaction. REM-on cells of the pontine reticular formation are cholinoceptively excited and/or cholinergically excitatory (ACH1) at their synaptic endings. Pontine REM-off cells are noradrenergically (NE) or serotonergically (5HT) inhibitory [2] at their synapses. (b) Dynamic model. During waking, the pontine aminergic system is tonically activated and inhibits the pontine cholinergic system. During NREM sleep, aminergic inhibition gradually wanes and cholinergic excitation reciprocally waxes. At REM sleep onset, aminergic inhibition is shut off and cholinergic excitation reaches its high point. (c) Activation level. As a consequence of the interplay of the neuronal systems shown in (a) and (b), the net activation level of the brain (A) is at equally high levels in waking and REM sleep and at about half this peak level in NREM sleep. From Hobson JA. A new model of brain-mind state: activation level, input source, and mode of processing (AIM). In: Antrobus JS, Bertini M, eds. *The neuropsychology of sleep and dreaming*. Hillsdale, NJ: Lawrence Erlbaum Associates; 1992; with permission from Taylor & Francis Group LLC.

psychoactive medications. This movement was helped by the fact that mental hospitals had already been dramatically emptied by drugs like chlorpromazine, first introduced in 1955 just 2 years after the discovery of REM sleep. By 1975, there was intense competition for market share among the sedative-hypnotics. A host of designer drugs for schizophrenia and major affective disorders was also soon developed. Many of the old dream laboratories of the 1953–1975 era were thus retooled as drug-testing laboratories. This influx of pharmaceutical money

helped to maintain laboratory sleep research; however, commercial influence undoubtedly influenced some of the science it produced.

Although this was not a focus of their work, Aserinsky and Kleitman's original description of REM sleep included the recognition of concomitant changes in cardiorespiratory measures. As has been extensively demonstrated over the past 50 years, virtually every physiological system of the body undergoes a change of state over the sleep–wake cycle (see Chapter 3: Neurophysiology and neuroimaging of human sleep). Subsequent investigation has led to the recognition that such sleep-related changes may be unhealthy and in some individuals are clearly pathological. For example, respiratory commands may not be issued (central sleep apnea) and/or the commands may become blocked (obstructive sleep apnea) with deleterious effects on sleep itself and upon cardiorespiratory functions generally (see Chapter 7: Sleep-related breathing disorders).

Here again the charismatic leadership of William Dement in the development of modern sleep medicine must be recognized. In 1970, he founded the first sleep disorders clinic at Stanford University. Additionally, he has been instrumental in the growth and development of the professional and research societies that are the foundations of sleep medicine as a field. Today there are more than 1000 sleep medicine laboratories world wide and sleep-related medical problems are now increasingly recognized and treated. Very recently, the Accreditation Council for Graduate Medical Education (ACGME) has acknowledged sleep medicine as a distinct subspecialty, and begun accrediting training fellowships in clinical sleep medicine. However, despite the growth of sleep medicine as a discipline, there continues to be a dearth of education and training in sleep and its disorders, particularly among psychiatrists-in-training [20].

As an interdisciplinary medical specialty, sleep medicine has had numerous psychiatrists contribute to the field, many of whom have provided chapters for this volume. More comprehensive reviews of the history of sleep medicine are available elsewhere [21,22]. But the sleep medicine movement, as important as it is, to date, has unfortunately contributed little or nothing to the solution of the mind–body problem within psychiatry.

I would argue that the ultimate goal of psychiatry must be the pursuit of an integrative science of human consciousness. Of course, we want to understand the biological mechanisms underlying behavioral neuroscience. Why does a person – or a snail – investigate or withdraw from an object and what molecular processes underlie these behaviors? But the field has larger, more complex questions it must seek to answer. How can awareness arise from perception? How does learning become recollection? How does language arise? Although these are daunting questions, I believe that sleep and dream research will allow some of these questions ultimately to be answered.

The AIM model

As the reciprocal interaction and activation-synthesis hypotheses evolved, they metamorphosed into the AIM model based on findings in sleep and dream research [23]. Basic sleep research has identified three factors that interact to determine brain–mind state. Whether we are awake (with waking consciousness), in NREM asleep (with little or no consciousness), or in REM asleep (with dream consciousness) depends upon: (1) activation level (A) (which is high in wake and REM); (2) input–output gates (I) (which are open in wake but closed in REM); and (3) aminergic modulatory ratio (M) (which is high in wake and low in REM). Thus, the AIM (Activation, Input Source, and Modulation) model proposes that conscious states can be defined and distinguished from one another by the values of these three parameters. The three factors can be used to construct a three-dimensional AIM state space as shown in Figure 1.3. Waking, NREM, and REM occupy discreetly different domains in the state space. The wake–NREM–REM sleep cycle is seen as an elliptical trajectory in the state space with time as a fourth dimension.

The basic neurophysiology that occurs during the three AIM domains of waking, NREM, and REM sleep is shown in Figure 1.4. During REM, not only do external input–output gates close, but REM is also characterized by very strong internal stimuli generated via ponto-geniculo-occipital (PGO) waves [24,25,26,27]. These electrical impulses arise in the pons, then travel to the lateral geniculate and to the visual cortex. It is this distinctive, internally generated pseudo-sensorimotor stimulation that most directly supports the hypothesis that REM sleep dreaming is a protoconscious rather than an unconscious state. Not only is the brain activated and kept offline [28,29], but it autoactivates in such a way as to impressively simulate waking. Although inhibited, this system is

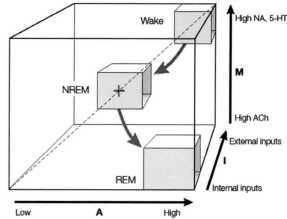

Figure 1.3 AIM model. In this figure, the fully alert, wake state is depicted in the upper right corner of the back plane of the cube. This corresponds to maximal levels of brain activation (right surface of cube), maximal external input sources with minimal internal sources (back surface), and maximal aminergic and minimal cholinergic neuromodulation (top surface). Cognitively, this corresponds to alertness with attention focused on the outside world. In the center of the cube lies deep NREM sleep, with low levels of brain activation, intermediate levels of both aminergic and cholinergic neuromodulation, and minimal levels of both external and internal input. In this state, the mind tends towards perseverative, non-progressive thinking with minimal hallucinatory activity, and this is reflected in the brevity and poverty of NREM sleep reports. As cholinergic modulation increases and aminergic modulation decreases, the modulatory function falls to its low point. The brain–mind, however, regains waking levels of activation and moves from NREM into REM sleep. AIM (here referring to the brain's location in the AIM state space) moves to the bottom front edge of the cube, with input now internally driven (front surface) and neuromodulation predominantly cholinergic (bottom surface). Note the paradox that instead of moving to the left surface of the cube – to a position diametrically opposed to waking – brain activation returns to waking level. This forces AIM to the right surface of the cube. As a result the mind is alert, but because it is demodulated and driven by powerful internal stimuli, it becomes both hallucinatory and unfocused. REM sleep's deviation from the main diagonal axis provides a visual representation of the distinctively unique phenomenology of REM sleep and shows why that state favors dreaming. Reprinted by permission from Macmillan Publishers Ltd: Nature Reviews Neuroscience (Hobson JA, Pace-Schott EF. The cognitive neuroscience of sleep: neuronal systems, consciousness and learning. 2002;3(9):679–693), copyright 2002.

also presumably used during waking to provide the brain with a model of the external world against which it compares inputs. I would hypothesize that waking provides this system with data, which it processes throughout life as dream content.

Dream consciousness

The Freudian in all of us still tends to regard dreaming as an unconscious mental activity. Even if we set aside psychoanalytic ideas about repressed infantile

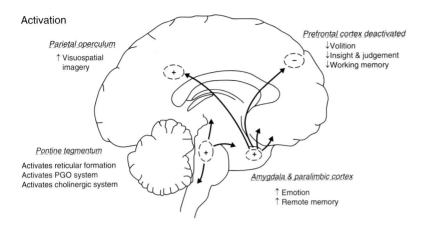

Activation

Parietal operculum

↑Visuospatial imagery

Prefrontal cortex deactivated
↓Volition
↓Insight & judgement
↓Working memory

Pontine tegmentum
Activates reticular formation
Activates PGO system
Activates cholinergic system

Amygdala & paralimbic cortex
↑ Emotion
↑ Remote memory

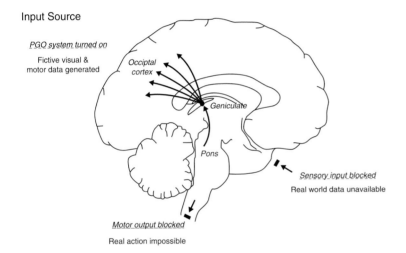

Input Source

PGO system turned on
Fictive visual & motor data generated

Occiptal cortex

Geniculate

Pons

Sensory input blocked
Real world data unavailable

Motor output blocked
Real action impossible

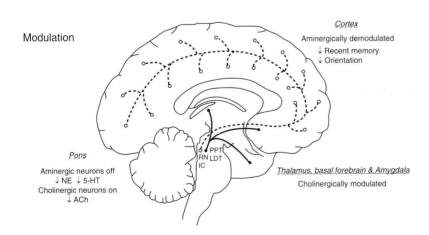

Modulation

Cortex
Aminergically demodulated
↓ Recent memory
↓ Orientation

Pons
Aminergic neurons off
↓ NE ↓ 5-HT
Cholinergic neurons on
↓ ACh

PPT
RN LDT
IC

Thalamus, basal forebrain & Amygdala
Cholinergically modulated

Figure 1.4 Physiological signs and regional brain mechanisms of REM sleep dreaming separated into the activation (A), input source (I), and modulation (M) functional components of the AIM model. Dynamic changes in A, I, and M during REM sleep dreaming are noted adjacent to each figure. Note that these are highly schematized depictions which illustrate global processes and do not attempt to comprehensively detail all the brain structures and their interactions which may be involved in REM sleep dreaming. From Hobson JA, Pace-Schott EF, Stickgold R. Dreaming and the brain: toward a cognitive neuroscience of conscious states. *Behav Brain Sci.* 2000 Dec;23(6):793–842, 2001; © Cambridge Journals, reproduced with permission.

wishes, their disguise, and their censorship, we still conceptualize dreaming as an unconscious process. Within this paradigm, dreaming, in its mysterious folds, contains insights about our secret selves discernible only through diligent study. Even if Freud was wrong about some of the details, most of psychiatry assumes he was right in this central hypothesis that dreaming is an unconscious process.

I would argue that this dogma has outlived its utility. If dreaming is not so much unconscious mental activity in a Freudian sense but is, instead, an intensely conscious experience that is not remembered, our theoretical perspective changes dramatically. Dream consciousness is vivid and distinctive, of that we can be sure, given our occasional recollection of it. Interestingly, despite the nearly 2 hours of REM sleep that occurs in a healthy adult each night, our recall of dreams comes nowhere near this amount. I argue that this discrepancy is not due to repression, but rather to the fact that the majority of dreaming (whether it occurs in REM sleep, NREM sleep, or at sleep onset) is forgotten. But if dreaming isn't disguising repressed infantile wishes, then what is it doing?

My heretical answer to this question is that dreaming is doing crucially important mental work. The mental work done by dream consciousness is far more important to waking consciousness than mere protection from unconscious infantile wishes as Freud suggested. I propose that dreaming is constantly serving consciousness in a variety of positive and progressive ways.

Aserinsky and Kleitman revisited: REM sleep and immaturity

The reason that Aserinsky stumbled onto REM sleep in the first place is because he was studying children who were bored and fell asleep and, fortunately, REM sleep occurs closer to sleep onset in the young. Not only does it occur at sleep onset but it occupies a greater proportion of a greater amount of sleep in the younger the child. The newborn human infant spends 50% of its sleep time in REM. Since infants sleep 16 hours per day, they achieve nearly 8 hours of REM sleep per day! With prematurity, these numbers increase further, until at 30 weeks of gestation, the human fetus spends 24 hours/day in a brain-activated state that is something more like REM sleep than wakefulness or NREM. Thus, I would argue that REM sleep in infancy serves brain development in the specific enhancement of cognition and consciousness.

This over-commitment to REM sleep by immature animals has not gone unnoticed. Howard Roffwarg, Joseph Muzio, and William Dement theorized in 1966 that REM favored development of the visual

system [30]. Given the REM periods themselves, the PGO waves, and the intensely visual quality of dreams, I have always liked this idea and regret that it never received its day in scientific court. But I suspect the developmental hypothesis of Roffwarg and colleagues was too modest. I would argue that it is not just vision, but consciousness itself that is the functional beneficiary of REM sleep.

Developmental considerations

Brain development proceeds, up to a point, under genetic guidance. Chemical flavors are designated and neuronal addresses are specified by the genome. When cholinergic and aminergic neurons meet in the pontine brainstem they interact automatically and spontaneously. When the cholinergic system is dominant as it is in REM, the brain is activated in one specific mode and when the aminergic system is dominant as in waking, it is activated in another specific mode. According to this theory, the aminergic system must develop later than the cholinergic system since waking consciousness follows dream consciousness by weeks or even months.

Although antecedence does not guarantee causality, this temporal sequence means that REM sleep could be a protoconscious state. What is meant by the term protoconsciousness? First, it means that a primitive sense of self could be instantiated. To paraphrase Descartes, my brain is activated, therefore I am. When my self (or ego) is activated, I move. My self is therefore an agent. This is point two. According to Rodolfo Llinás, agent-initiated movement is instantiated early in development [31]. Not only does the self-organized autoactive brain instantiate agent-initiated movement but it simulates both the sensory and emotional concomitants of that activity. These are points 3 and 4. REM sleep creates a self that acts, and feels, in a virtual world.

REM sleep and the binding problem

One of the most remarkable aspects of waking consciousness is its unity. Consciousness integrates a vast panoply of information into what seems to us to be a simple and continuous flow of awareness. Strands of data from the outside world, from our bodies, and our very complex selves are woven together into a single piece. Our subjectivity may be conflicted but it is always unified. Such an effect can only be achieved by the binding of multiple neuronal representations into an integrated whole. Rather than assuming that numerous neural pathways pump all of this information into a single place in the brain, it has been proposed that it is the synchrony of disparate brain parts that is the substrate of binding. Now we know that, in addition to synchrony, the brain utilizes modulatory chemistry to achieve the widespread harmony necessary to binding.

According to protoconsciousness theory, REM sleep serves binding automatically and spontaneously. No supervision is needed. And according to this new theory, all mammals that have REM sleep have protoconsciousness. When they wake up, they have varying degrees of what Gerald Edelman calls primary consciousness [32]. According to the complexity of their brains, they may also achieve some degree of secondary consciousness. But, as far as we know, only humans have directed thought, propositional intent, and awareness-of-awareness. This sophisticated adaptation is presumably dependent on the acquisition of symbolic language.

The interaction of dreaming and waking consciousness

Protoconsciousness develops first, even before birth. There follows, especially in humans, a prolonged period in which waking consciousness develops. It is an explicit tenet of the protoconsciousness hypothesis that dreaming and waking consciousness develop together and that each of the two states enriches the other. Furthermore, it is proposed that the two states may interact negatively in the production of psychotic states such as the organic mental syndrome, schizophrenia, and major affective disorder.

Since REM sleep brain activation precedes waking (and may occur before even birth), it follows that while it may instantiate self, self-as-agent, movement, sensation, and emotion, it could not support dreaming as we know it in adults. For adult dreaming to occur, specific content information would need to be gleaned in waking and cognitive capacity would need to evolve, as it clearly does, accounting for the fact that adult dreaming does not occur before ages 6–8 [33]. Another empirical example of this principle is the vision-free dreaming of the congenitally blind person. Vice versa, in order for a normal person to see, in either waking or dreaming consciousness, the contentless formal frame supplied by REM sleep brain activation is essential.

The emerging picture is of a two-way street: REM sleep brain activation provides the formal substrate for waking consciousness and waking consciousness provides the perceptual building blocks for dream consciousness.

Summary and conclusions

Psychiatry was born when moral and medical forces combined to separate the mentally ill from common criminals and other social undesirables. In the beginning, the medical model prevailed but no bacteria, no viruses, and no malformations were found in the brains of the vast majority of the severely mentally ill.

Frustration with the organic orientation of the field contributed to the uncritical acceptance of the psychoanalytic psychology of Sigmund Freud who based much of his speculation on the assumption that dreaming was an unconscious mental process inimical to waking consciousness. This point of view gained ascendance in the first half of the twentieth century and continues to have support within psychoanalytic circles.

The discovery of REM sleep, and its association with dreaming by Aserinsky and Kleitman in 1953, was first greeted by many in the psychiatric community as an opportunity to confirm Freud. But as the second half of the twentieth century evolved, it become more and more clear that REM sleep likely has biological significance that transcends dreaming. During this same period, the field of sleep medicine exponentially developed, with many biologically oriented psychiatrists contributing significantly to this nascent medical specialty.

Significant progress in basic sleep and dreaming research has yielded new insights previously unimaginable at the dawn of psychiatry. Now, in the twenty-first century, psychiatric sleep medicine continues to move forward with developments in sleep genetics, bioenergetics, neurophysiology, and neuropharmacology. Within modern paradigms, it seems more likely that REM sleep (and dreaming) are the handmaidens of waking consciousness, rather than the "royal road to the unconscious" as previously envisioned by Freud. I suggest that REM sleep comes to support protoconsciousness (and dreams) in a way that is specific and dynamic. It is possible that further consideration of the connection between REM sleep dreaming and waking consciousness will yield the brain–mind integration necessary to a truly scientific psychiatry. This theory is developed in more detail in a recent manuscript [34].

It is thus my deeply held belief that psychiatry might well come of scientific age through an integration of basic research of sleep, dreams, and consciousness. By this surprising means, it may be possible for psychiatry not only to contribute to, but also to profit from, a specific model of brain–mind integration that could account for both normal and abnormal mental states.

References

1. Kraeplin, E. *Dementia praecox and paraphrenia*. Translated by R. Mary Barclay. Edited by George M. Robertson. Huntington, NY: R. E. Krieger Pub. Co; 1971.

2. Bleuler E. [Dementia præcox, oder die Gruppe der Schizophrenien]. In: Aschaffenburg G, ed. *Aschaffenburg, handbuch der psychiatrie*. Leipzig: Franz Deuticke; 1911.

3. Freud S. The interpretation of dreams. In: Strachey J, ed. *The standard edition of the complete psychological works of Sigmund Freud*, Vols. 4 and 5. London: Hogarth Press; 1953.

4. Freud S. *Project for a scientific psychology*. New York: Standard Edition; 1895.

5. Aserinsky E, Kleitman N. Regularly occurring periods of ocular motility and concomitant phenomena during sleep. *Science*. 1953;**118**:361–375.

6. Dement W, Kleitman N. The relation of eye movements during sleep to dream activity: An objective method for the study of dreaming. *J Exp Psychol*. 1957;**53**:339–346.

7. Dement W, Kleitman N. Cyclic variations in EEG during sleep and their relation to eye movements, body motility, and dreaming. *Electroencephalogr Clin Neurophysiol*. 1957;**9**(4):673–690.

8. Dement W. The effect of dream deprivation. *Science*. 1960;**131**:1705–1707.

9. Kales A, Hoedemaker F, Jacobsen A, et al. Mentation during sleep: REM and NREM recall reports. *Percept Mot Skills*. 1967;**24**:556–560.

10. Dement W. The occurrence of low voltage, fast, electroencephalogram patterns during behavioral sleep in the cat. *Electroencephalogr Clin Neurophysiol*. 1958; **10**(2):291–296.

11. Moruzzi M, Magoun HW. Brainstem reticular formation and activation of the EEG. *Electroencephalogr Clin Neurophysiol*. 1949;**1**: 455–473.

12. Jouvet M. Research on the neural structures and responsible mechanisms in different phases of physiological sleep. *Arch Ital Biol*. 1962;**100**:125–206.

13. Jouvet M, Michel F. Electromyographic correlations of sleep in the chronic decorticate & mesencephalic cat. *C R Seances Soc Biol Fil*. 1959;**153**(3):422–425.

14. Dahlstrom A, Fuxe K. Evidence for the existence of monoamine-containing neurons in the central nervous system. I. Demonstration in the cell bodies of brain stem neurons. *Acta Physiologica Scandinavica*. 1964;**62**:1–55.

15. Jouvet M. Biogenic amines and the states of sleep. *Science*. 1969;**163**(862):32–41.

16. Hobson JA, McCarley RW, Wyzinski PW. Sleep cycle oscillation: reciprocal discharge by two brain stem neuronal groups. *Science*. 1975;**189**:55–58.

17. McCarley RW, Hobson JA. Neuronal excitability modulation over the sleep cycle: a structural and mathematical model. *Science*. 1975;**189**:58–60.

18. Hobson JA, McCarley RW. The brain as a dream state generator: an activation-synthesis hypothesis of the dream process. *Am J Psychiatry*. 1977;**134**(12):1335–1348.

19. McCarley RW, Hobson JA. The neurobiological origins of psychoanalytic dream theory. *Am J Psychiatry*. 1977;**134**:1211–1221.

20. Krahn LE, Hansen MR, Tinsley JA. Psychiatric residents' exposure to the field of sleep medicine: a survey of program directors. *Acad Psychiatry*. 2002;**26**(4):253–256.

21. Shepard JW Jr, Buysse DJ, Chesson AL Jr, et al. History of the development of sleep medicine in the United States. *J Clin Sleep Med*. 2005;**1**(1):61–82.

22. Dement WC. History of sleep medicine. *Sleep Med Clinics* 2008;**3**(2):147–156.

23. Hobson JA, Pace-Schott EF, Stickgold R. Dreaming and the brain: toward a cognitive neuroscience of conscious states. *Behav Brain Sci*. 2000;**23**(6):793–842.

24. Brooks DC, Bizzi E. Brain stem electrical activity during deep sleep. *Arch Ital Biol*. 1963;**101**:648–665.

25. Bowker RM, Morrison AR. The startle reflex and PGO spikes. *Brain Res*. 1976;**102**(1):185–190.

26. Lydic R, McCarley RW, Hobson JA. Serotonin neurons and sleep. II. Time course of dorsal raphé discharge, PGO waves, and behavioral states. *Arch Ital Biol*. 1987; **126**(1):1–28.

27. Nelson JP, McCarley RW, Hobson JA. REM sleep burst neurons, PGO waves, and eye movement information. *J Neurophysiol*. 1983;**50**(4):784–797.

28. Pompeiano O. The neurophysiological mechanisms of the postural and motor events during desynchronized sleep. *Res Publ Assoc Res Nerv Ment Dis*. 1967; **45**:351–423.

29. Chase MH, Morales FR. Subthreshold excitatory activity and motorneuron discharge during REM periods of active sleep. *Science*. 1983;**221**(4616):1195–1198.

30. Roffwarg HP, Muzio JN, Dement WC. Ontogenetic development of the human sleep-dream cycle. *Science*. 1966;**152**(3722):604–619.

31. Llinás R. *I of the vortex: from neurons to self*. Cambridge, MA: MIT Press; 2001.

32. Edelman GM. *Bright air, brilliant fire: on the matter of the mind*. New York: Basic Books; 1992.

33. Foulkes D. *Childrens' dreaming and the development of consciousness*. Cambridge: Harvard University Press; 1999.

34. Hobson JA. REM sleep and dreaming: towards a theory of protoconsciousness. *Nat Neurosci Rev*. 2009; **10**: 803–814.

2

Neuroanatomy and neurobiology of sleep and wakefulness

James T. McKenna, Ritchie E. Brown and Robert W. McCarley

Introduction

In recent years, loss of sleep has increasingly been recognized as a major public health issue (for review and discussion, see http://healthysleep.med.harvard.edu/ and [1,2]). Sleep disturbance due to vocational demands, such as that experienced by shift workers, physicians, nurses, and emergency responders, may contribute to decreased work performance, as well as increased accident rates. Furthermore, sleep disorders, such as obstructive sleep apnea, insomnia, narcolepsy, and restless legs syndrome, affect millions of people. In addition, many psychiatric illnesses, such as depression, anxiety, and post-traumatic stress disorder, are associated with sleep disturbance.

Investigations conducted largely in the last century revealed multiple brain systems responsible for the states of wakefulness, rapid eye movement (REM) sleep, and non-REM (NREM) sleep. Transitions between these vigilance states involve neural systems of interconnected brain regions and neurotransmitters. In recent years, knowledge of vigilance state regulation has progressed considerably due to new techniques, including pharmacological, lesioning, electrophysiological, and, most recently, molecular-level technologies. This chapter will review both the neurobiological mechanisms generating these different behavioral states, as well as the factors (homeostatic and circadian) that influence their timing.

This chapter will begin with an overview of the neural systems involved in vigilance state regulation. This will include a description of relevant brain regions/nuclei, as well as the neurotransmitters involved. We will describe the flip-flop hypothesis of sleep/wake regulation, as well as the reciprocal interaction model of REM sleep regulation. The two-process model of sleep regulation will then be explained, describing the interaction of process S (the homeostatic drive to sleep) and process C (the circadian drive to sleep). This discussion will include a description of a homeostatic sleep regulator; namely, the purine adenosine. Process C will be described, including a description of the brain nuclei and neural systems involved in circadian rhythmicity, including the suprachiasmatic and dorsomedial hypothalamic nuclei. Furthermore, we will review the proposed mechanism by which circadian rhythmicity occurs in the suprachiasmatic nucleus, involving a complex interaction of genes.

To help orient the reader to the systems important in maintaining each behavioral state, we first present an anatomical schematic of their location (Figure 2.1a), followed by figures specifically indicating the regions important in promoting wakefulness (Figure 2.1b), NREM sleep (Figure 2.1c), and REM sleep (Figure 2.1d). Figure legends for Figures 2.1b, 2.1c, and 2.1d describe the transmitter(s) important for each state. Most of the investigations reviewed in this chapter and, in turn, most of our knowledge of sleep/wakefulness regulation is derived from animal models, usually rodent, feline, or canine. Many of the nuclei to be described are anatomically interconnected, acting synergistically in vigilance state regulation. Interestingly, the majority of studies employing lesioning of wakefulness- and sleep-related nuclei have found only minor effects on the sleep–wake cycle, likely due to redundancy within the neuroanatomical circuitry involved in vigilance state regulation.

Foundations of Psychiatric Sleep Medicine, ed. John W. Winkelman and David T. Plante. Published by Cambridge University Press.
© Cambridge University Press 2010.

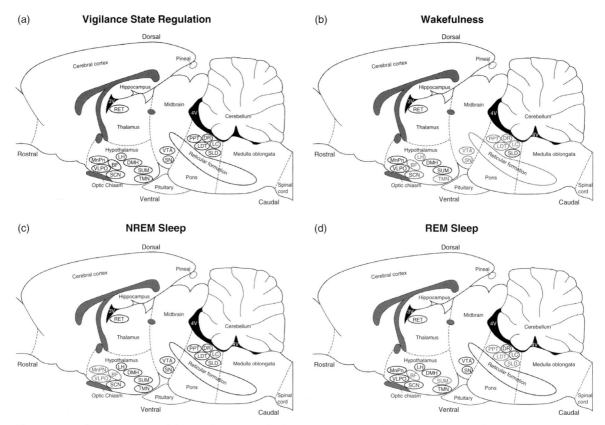

Figure 2.1 A schematic overview of the neural systems involved in vigilance state regulation. (a) Sagittal view of the rat brain (adapted from [3]) depicts nuclei and brain regions involved in vigilance state regulation (wakefulness, NREM sleep, and REM sleep) and circadian rhythmicity. In Figures 1b–d, active regions during the vigilance states are highlighted in red. (b) Nuclei that promote wakefulness, as well as regions activated during wakefulness, include: basal forebrain (BF) cholinergic, GABAergic, and putatively glutamatergic; dorsal raphe (DR) serotonergic; lateral hypothalamus (LH) orexinergic; locus coeruleus (LC) noradrenergic; pedunculopontine/laterodorsal tegmental (PPT/LDT) cholinergic; reticular formation glutamatergic; substantia nigra (SN) dopaminergic; tuberomammillary (TMN) histaminergic; and ventral tegmental area (VTA) dopaminergic nuclei. Thalamocortical and basal forebrain activity produces the EEG profile indicative of wakefulness. (c) Nuclei that promote NREM sleep include GABAergic neurons in the ventrolateral preoptic (VLPO) and median preoptic (MnPN) nuclei. Furthermore, the homeostatic sleep regulator adenosine acts to inhibit wake-promoting BF neurons. The reticular nucleus of the thalamus (RET) is responsible for NREM sleep phenomena such as sleep spindles. (d) Nuclei that promote REM sleep include the pedunculopontine/ laterodorsal tegmental nuclei (PPT/LDT), where unique "REM-on" neurons are located. The sublaterodorsal nucleus (SLD) also promotes REM sleep phenomena, including muscle atonia, by means of circuitry involving the spinal cord. The supramammillary nucleus (SUM) and medial septum of the basal forebrain (BF) are part of the circuitry responsible for theta rhythmicity in the hippocampus, which is indicative of REM sleep. Abbreviations: 3V, third ventricle; 4V, fourth ventricle; DMH, dorsomedial nucleus of the hypothalamus; SCN, suprachiasmatic nucleus. See plate section for color version.

Neural systems involved in vigilance state regulation: wakefulness

Electrical activity of the human brain was first successfully recorded by the psychiatrist Hans Berger in the late 1920s [4]. He noted that the profile of "electroencephalograms" changed across the vigilance states. In the 1930s, investigations further described the electroencephalogram (EEG) profile of the sleeping brain [5,6]. Wakefulness is characterized by a cortical EEG profile of low-voltage, fast/high-frequency field potentials of the alpha (8–12 Hz), beta (12–20 Hz), high beta (20–30 Hz), and gamma (>30 Hz, usually about 40 Hz) spectral range. However, theta (4–8 Hz) frequency activity is often also recorded in association with movement, attentional tasks, and mnemonic processing. Furthermore, wakefulness is usually accompanied with relatively high muscle tone and movement, evident in EMG (electromyogram) and EOG (electrooculogram) recordings. In contrast, NREM sleep exhibits higher voltage/ lower frequency field oscillations, accompanied by little movement. During REM sleep, the cortical EEG profile returns to low-voltage/high-frequency activity, but is accompanied by an overall lack of movement and postural tone. A more detailed review of the EEG/EMG profile of NREM and REM sleep is provided later in this chapter.

Baron Constantin Von Economo studied the worldwide flu epidemic in the late 1920s, and observed that in patients who developed *encephalitis lethargica*, a neuropsychiatric disorder characterized by either severe insomnia or hypersomnia, the anterior hypothalamus was damaged in the post-mortem tissue of patients that had suffered from insomnia; whereas damage posterior to the hypothalamus at the junction of the forebrain and brainstem was identified in patients that exhibited excessive sleepiness [7]. Therefore, he concluded that the brain's sleep-inducing regions were located in the anterior hypothalamus, and wakefulness-promoting regions were located in the posterior hypothalamus. As described below in the review of NREM sleep mechanisms of this chapter, Von Economo's hypotheses were largely correct.

In the 1930s, Frederick Bremer performed seminal studies of EEG activity in the cat [8,9]. In one preparation, termed *encephale isolé*, a cut was made in the lower part of the medulla. In the other preparation, termed *cerveau isolé*, a cut was made at the junction of the midbrain and the brainstem. Interestingly, the *encephale isolé* preparation allowed a continual presence of EEG activity reflecting the fluctuation between wake and sleep activity. In the second *cerveau isolé* preparation, though, the cat EEG profile remained in a constant sleep-like state. Therefore, it was concluded that sleep involved a deafferentation of the cerebral cortex.

Following the seminal work of Bremer, Moruzzi and Magoun reported that electrical stimulation of the brainstem reticular formation (RF) produced a cortical EEG profile indicative of wakefulness [10]. These findings lead to the concept of the reticular activating system (RAS), comprised of the reticular formation and its connections, which generate wakefulness (for review, see [11]). Subsequent investigations have revealed that the RAS is composed of a dorsal and ventral arousal pathway. The dorsal arousal pathway is composed of select nuclei in the brainstem, particularly the pontine oralis and mesencephalic RF, that project to midline thalamic nuclei, which subsequently have widespread projections throughout the neocortex. The ventral arousal pathway, initially identified by Von Economo, includes projections from the RF to the basal forebrain and posterior hypothalamic regions, which then influence cortical EEG activation by means of projections to the neocortex that bypass the thalamus [11,12,13]. Initial projections of both the dorsal and ventral branches of the ascending arousal systems are largely glutamatergic, as are the related thalamic and a portion of the basal forebrain projections to the cortex. Additionally, the ventral arousal pathway involves a number of neurotransmitter systems besides glutamate, including acetylcholine, norepinephrine, serotonin, histamine, and orexin (also known as hypocretin), that are involved in the generation and maintenance of wakefulness.

Acetylcholine

Acetylcholine not only plays a critical role in parasympathetic and neuromuscular junctions [14], but also in the control of vigilance states. Two brain regions rich in cholinergic neurons are of particular importance in both the dorsal and ventral branches of the RAS. The first region is the basal forebrain (BF, Figure 2.1), including the medial septum/vertical limb of the diagonal band of Broca, the horizontal limb of the diagonal band, magnocellular preoptic nucleus, substantia innominata, and nucleus basalis. A second region of interest is located in the midbrain tegmentum, distributed across the laterodorsal tegmental (LDT) and pedunculopontine tegmental (PPT) nuclei (see Figure 2.1).

Neuroanatomical studies have defined the BF, including cholinergic neurons, as a principal relay for ascending activation of neocortical regions in the ventral arousal pathway. Double-labeling experiments (employing immunohistochemistry techniques to determine the cholinergic phenotypes of BF neurons, in combination with retrograde tract tracing techniques) have demonstrated BF cholinergic projections to widespread cortical regions [15,16]. This technique has also been used to describe the more specific projections of the medial septum/vertical limb of the diagonal band of Broca to the hippocampus, including both GABAergic and cholinergic input (for review, see [17,18]). These septo-hippocampal projections are part of the brain circuitry involved in the generation of the EEG theta wave, recorded in the hippocampus during REM sleep, as well as during movement and specific mnemonic/cognitive tasks in waking.

Immunohistochemical detection of the protein c-Fos may be employed to indicate neuronal activation, where c-Fos immunohistochemical staining following sacrifice of the animal reflects neuronal subpopulation activation within the preceding hour [19,20]. These studies described a subpopulation of BF cholinergic neurons that express the c-Fos protein during sleep deprivation [21,22,23], in contrast to little co-localization following sleep deprivation recovery (when sleep rebound occurred) or natural spontaneous sleep. Overall, c-Fos protein expression in the cholinergic neurons of BF increased as the percentage of time awake in the hour prior to sacrifice increased. This observation is consistent with a role for BF cholinergic neurons in promoting cortical activation. Although the documentation of c-Fos and other immediate early gene protein expression is useful, it is not necessarily a faithful representation of neuronal discharge. For example, spinal alpha motor neurons do not express c-Fos with discharges, and c-Fos may reflect calcium influx even without discharge. It is thus important to realize c-Fos evidence is provisional and needs to be confirmed by electrophysiological recordings, as is discussed in a recent review [24].

Electrophysiological and pharmacological studies confirm the particular role of acetylcholine in cortical EEG activation [11,25]. Single unit recordings revealed that neurons in the BF, LDT, and PPT regions were more active during wakefulness, when compared to NREM sleep [25,26,27]. Subsequent investigations described BF neurons, determined to be cholinergic by means of *post hoc* juxtacellular labeling, which increased firing during cortical activation [28,29]. These cholinergic neurons discharged in rhythmic bursts in association with wakefulness-related cortical EEG theta and gamma wave activity [30]. Also, inactivation of BF by lesioning of cell bodies, sparing fibers of passage, decreases wakefulness [11]. Although acetylcholine is a crucial neurotransmitter in the arousal mechanism, it is also important to recognize that BF GABAergic and glutamatergic neurons also play a role in cortical activation [31,32,33].

Unlike other wakefulness-related neurotransmitter systems that are described in this chapter that are typically decreased in both NREM and REM sleep, the highest levels of acetylcholine in the cortex and thalamus occur during both wakefulness and REM

sleep, implicating acetylcholine as an important neurotransmitter in REM sleep regulation [34]. BF projections provide the cholinergic innervation of the neocortex, while LDT/PPT projections provide cholinergic innervation of thalamic regions involved in the dorsal arousal pathway. Electrophysiological studies demonstrated increased neuronal firing in BF and LDT/PPT during wakefulness and REM sleep [26,27,29]. The role of acetylcholine in REM sleep control will be further discussed in the following sections.

Serotonin

Several midbrain/brainstem regions rich in serotonin (5-HT), i.e. the dorsal, median, magnus, obscurus, and pallidus raphe nuclei [35,36], are involved in vigilance state regulation. Serotonin plays a complex role in vigilance state regulation, due to its actions in different brain regions, as well as the complexity of the multiple serotonergic auto- and heteroreceptors distributed throughout the arousal circuitry. Serotonergic neurons send projections to many areas involved in vigilance state regulation. These neurons are most active during wakefulness, have considerably decreased firing during NREM sleep, and cease activity during REM sleep [37,38]. Correspondingly, 5-HT levels in various brain regions, including the neocortex, significantly rise during wakefulness, and decrease considerably during NREM and REM sleep [39,40].

Recent neurochemical and electrophysiological investigations conclude that serotonin promotes wakefulness and inhibits REM sleep, complementing the action of noradrenergic and histaminergic systems. This contrasts with early studies which suggested a sleep-promoting role for serotonin, based mainly on experiments which showed that depletion of serotonin by means of *p*-chlorophenylalanine (PCPA) led to insomnia [41,42]. Amounts of REM sleep increased following specific serotonergic inhibition by means of injection of 8-OH-DPAT into the dorsal raphe nucleus (acting on the 5-HT_{1A} inhibitory autoreceptor) [43,44]. Furthermore, infusion of 8-OH-DPAT in the median raphe nucleus promoted hippocampal theta activity [45,46].

Recent studies in mice have reinforced the hypothesis that serotonin is involved in both depression and sleep. In the serotonin transporter knockout mouse, extracellular serotonin levels were significantly elevated, REM sleep was enhanced, and these animals exhibited depression-like behavior [47,48,49,50]. The seemingly paradoxical increase in REM sleep in these knock-out mice is likely due to compensatory developmental adaptations in these animals, such as downregulation of the 5-HT$_{1A}$ receptor (which normally inhibits REM sleep) on cholinergic neurons in response to the enhanced serotonergic tone. Blockade of the 5-HT$_{1A}$ receptor early in development reversed such phenomena in the knock-out mouse [51]. Furthermore, neonatal treatment of normal (non-knock-out) female mice with the selective serotonin reuptake inhibitor, escitalopram, induced depression- and anxiety-like behavior, as well as an increase in REM sleep [52].

Noradrenaline (NA)

The locus coeruleus, located bilaterally in the dorsolateral pons, contains a large group of noradrenergic neurons. Similar to serotonergic neurons, noradrenergic neurons of LC project to widespread areas of the neuraxis, and are most active during wakefulness, minimally active during NREM sleep, and cease activity during REM sleep [53,54,55]. Non-specific lesions of the LC lead to a minimal decrease in wakefulness behavior and attenuation of the cortical EEG indicative of wakefulness [56]. This may be due to the redundancy of systems involved in vigilance state regulation, for the many wakefulness-related neurotransmitter systems described here act similarly on the brain nuclei comprising the dorsal and ventral arousal pathways, as well as in the cortex. Emotional states that involve an increase of NA activity (e.g. stress) may lead to overexcitation of arousal regions, causing vigilance state dysregulation, such as that seen in insomnia [57].

Interestingly, the actions of NA may be either excitatory or inhibitory, depending on the type of adrenoreceptor on the efferent neurons of interest. Overall, it appears that NA projections to nuclei of arousal systems in the brainstem, BF, and spinal cord are excitatory, acting on alpha 1 receptors [58,59]. In contrast, noradrenergic projections to sleep-related neurons, such as preoptic region neurons (to be reviewed later), as well as noradrenaline neurons themselves, and LDT/PPT neurons, are inhibitory, acting on alpha 2 receptors [60,61]. In particular, noradrenergic LC neurons may be involved in maintaining muscle tone during wakefulness (to be reviewed later).

Dopamine

It is unclear what role, if any, dopamine (DA) plays in vigilance state regulation. Substantia nigra and midbrain dopaminergic neurons project to wakefulness-related brain regions, including BF and prefrontal cortex [62,63]. These neurons fire in bursts, correlated to arousal and reward [64]. Single-unit recordings in the substantia nigra and ventral tegmental area, though, were not able to determine firing rate fluctuation between wakefulness versus sleep states [65]. Recently, another group of dopaminergic neurons in the ventral periaqueductal gray (vlPAG) was described, where c-Fos protein expression correlated most strongly with wakefulness [66]. These neurons were located near the dorsal raphe nucleus, interspersed with serotonergic wakefulness-active cells, and projected to many of the wakefulness-related nuclei. Further investigations, including electrophysiological profiling of these neurons, will allow conclusive evidence of a role these neurons may play in vigilance state regulation. Interestingly, drugs that block the reuptake of DA and NA and thus enhance dopaminergic and noradrenergic release, such as cocaine and amphetamine, are usually associated with stimulatory effects. Additionally, DA-stimulating compounds are used to treat disorders of central hypersomnolence such as narcolepsy (see Chapter 9: Hypersomnias of central origin) [67,68].

Histamine

Older generation antihistamines, known to cross the blood/brain barrier, have sedating effects, acting as antagonists largely on the histamine 1 (H1) receptor of wakefulness-related nuclei [69]. Histaminergic neurons are located in the tuberomammillary nucleus of the posterior hypothalamus (TMN), and project to a number of the arousal-related brain nuclei, as well as directly to the cortex [70,71]. The discharge profile of these neurons matches that of noradrenergic and serotonergic neurons, where most action potential firing occurs during wakefulness, considerably less firing is observed during NREM sleep, and firing ceases during REM sleep [72,73,74]. Histamine release in the posterior hypothalamus is highest during wake, lower during NREM sleep, and minimal during REM sleep [75], matching the discharge profile.

Non-specific lesioning of the TMN region, as well as histaminergic-specific lesions and chemical manipulations, support the suggestion that this region may contain neurons that promote wakefulness [73,76].

An investigation by Siegel and colleagues recently revealed a unique role of histaminergic neurons in the maintenance of wakefulness [74]. Cataplexy is a sudden loss of muscle tone in waking with preservation of conscious awareness, and is a symptom of the sleep disorder narcolepsy. During cataplectic attacks in the dog, NA neurons ceased firing, serotonergic neurons reduced firing, but histaminergic neurons remained active. Thus, while NA and serotonergic neurons particularly appear to maintain muscle tone during wakefulness, histamine neurons may help to maintain cortical activity indicative of wakefulness. Most recently, reduced histamine levels have also been reported in the cerebrospinal fluid of narcoleptic patients [77,78].

Orexin (hypocretin)

Neurons containing the neuropeptide orexin (also called hypocretin) are located largely in the perifornical region (near the fornix) of the lateral hypothalamus. Recent investigations reveal a unique role of orexin neurons in vigilance state regulation, as well as in the sleep disorder narcolepsy, by means of their extensive input to a number of sleep/wake-related nuclei [79,80].

Narcolepsy is characterized by symptoms including excessive daytime sleepiness (hypersomnolence), hypnagogic hallucinations, cataplexy, sleep-onset REM periods, and sleep paralysis (see Chapter 9: Hypersomnias of central origin). In 1999, two seminal investigations suggested that orexin plays a role in this disease. A deficit of the orexin type II receptor was discovered in a strain of dogs that exhibit narcolepsy [81]. In another study, orexin knock-out mice (lacking the prepro-orexin gene, the precursor for the orexin protein) exhibited decreased wakefulness and behavioral arrest during transitions from wakefulness to sleep, similar to the narcoleptic symptoms of sleep-onset REM episodes and cataplexy [82]. Behavioral arrest was described as a sudden cessation of motor activity, including a change in posture, which then abruptly ended with resumption of motor activity. Follow-up orexin-specific lesioning and knock-down studies described an increase in the number of transitions between vigilance states, and abnormal expression of REM-related characteristics during wakefulness, similar to the symptomology of narcolepsy [83,84,85,86]. An examination of post-mortem tissue of narcoleptic humans revealed an almost total

absence of orexin neurons [87,88]. Furthermore, low cerebrospinal fluid orexin levels occur in many narcoleptic patients, and prominently in cases with cataplexy [89,90]. Therefore, orexin plays a central role in the maintenance of wakefulness, and abnormalities may lead to sleep-related pathology such as narcolepsy. Of note, because there are no marketed medications that directly affect orexigenic neurotransmission, amphetamine-like stimulants and DA reuptake inhibitors have been prescribed to treat excessive sleepiness in narcolepsy, but appear to have little effect on cataplexy, for which compounds that inhibit adrenergic and serotonergic reuptake are effective [68].

Direct application of wake-promoting agents into the LH increases orexinergic neuronal activity [91]. Similar to the majority of wakefulness-related nuclei, orexinergic cell firing largely occurs during wakefulness, decreases considerably during NREM sleep, and ceases during REM sleep, except for some activity during REM-related muscle twitches [92]. Microdialysis sampling in the lateral hypothalamus found highest orexin levels during wakefulness [93], and following examination of c-Fos protein expression it was concluded that orexinergic neurons were wakefulness-active [94]. The unique role orexin may play in vigilance state regulation has been conceptualized in a "flip-flop" model of wakefulness/sleep transitions, in which orexin serves to stabilize transitions between sleep and wakefulness (see below).

Neural systems involved in vigilance state regulation: NREM sleep

NREM sleep may be classified into four stages in humans according to criteria developed by Rechtschaffen and Kales (R&K Criteria), or three stages (N1, N2, N3) according to recent criteria of the American Academy of Sleep Medicine (AASM). Stage 1 NREM sleep (N1) activity usually exhibits a mixture of theta (4–8 Hz) and alpha (8–12 Hz) cortical EEG activity. During stage 2 NREM sleep (N2), sleep spindles and K-complexes become evident. Sleep spindles, usually of the frequency of 12–16 Hz and lasting 0.5 to 1.5 seconds, are generated from the interplay between thalamic and cortical regions, and are present throughout the deeper stages (2–4) of sleep (for review, see [11]). K-complexes are brief, high-voltage ($<100 \,\mu V$) spikes that last approximately 0.5 seconds, and are unique to stage 2 sleep. Stages 3 and 4 (together form N3) are considered "deeper" NREM sleep, and are characterized by large/high-amplitude, low-frequency delta range (1–4 Hz) activity; hence, it is also termed slow-wave sleep (SWS). NREM sleep states recorded in animals usually are not subdivided into the stages employed in human sleep, although delta (deep) sleep is often differentiated from light sleep. Furthermore, neocortical slow oscillations (0.5–1 Hz) are evident throughout NREM sleep, and play a role in facilitation of thalamic and intracortical synchronization (for review, see [11]). This slow oscillation may further act to synchronize NREM delta activity with sleep spindles. NREM sleep is characterized by low muscle tone and moderate/lack of movement, evident in EMG and EOG recording.

Sleep spindles during NREM sleep

It has been proposed that spindle activity is important for the disconnection of the cerebral cortex from the external environment during sleep. The bilateral reticular nucleus of the thalamus (RET) is the pacemaker of spindle oscillations, which are generated by means of RET GABAergic inhibitory projections to thalamocortical neurons that are responsible for cortical EEG activation [95,96]. Spindle oscillations may be readily recorded in both thalamic and cortical regions during stages 2–4 of NREM sleep, and lesioning of the reticular nucleus-rostral thalamic nuclei pathway attenuates spindle activity [97].

Cholinergic projections from the brainstem LDT/PPT excite thalamocortical relay neurons, and directly inhibit RET. These actions desynchronize the thalamic reticular network, and lead to arousal [11]. Particularly, stimulation of PPT prevents spindle activity in RET [98]. Basal forebrain projections may play a role in spindle blockage, by means of GABA-ergic and cholinergic projections to the rostral sub-regions of the RET [99], and chemical lesions of the BF have been shown to produce increased spindle activity [100].

K-complexes during NREM sleep

Animal studies demonstrate that the K-complex, most often observed in human sleep during stage 2 NREM sleep, represents a combination of the neocortical slow oscillations and sleep spindles. A cycle of the slow oscillation is followed by a brief spindle sequence in thalamocortical neurons, which is transferred to the cortical EEG, and is seen as a surface-negative (upward) EEG transient, corresponding to the excitation in deeply lying neocortical neurons, followed by a surface-positive (downward) component and a short sequence of spindle waves. For a more detailed review of K-complexes during NREM sleep, the reader is referred to [11].

Delta frequency (1–4 Hz) EEG activity during NREM sleep

The cellular basis of delta waves (0.5–4 Hz) originating in thalamocortical neurons is that a hyperpolarized membrane potential in cortically projecting thalamic neurons permits the occurrence of delta waves in thalamocortical circuits. In both the thalamus and cortex, a phasic input to the hyperpolarized membrane causes a calcium-mediated depolarization (low threshold spike, LTS) on which a burst of sodium-mediated spikes occur (low threshold burst). The slow time course of delta waves is determined by the time course of the LTS and the subsequent hyperpolarization to re-enable another LTS. Any factors persistently depolarizing the membrane in either thalamic or cortical neurons will block delta waves through inactivation of the calcium channels mediating the LTS, and these are the wake–active systems illustrated in Fig. 2.1b. Cholinergic input from BF to the cortex, and from LDT/PPT to the thalamus, is thought to be especially important in arresting delta waves. Also, brainstem noradrenergic and serotonergic projections may disrupt delta activity in waking, although they are inactive during REM sleep. Thus, delta waves during sleep may be seen to represent thalamocortical oscillations occurring in the absence of activating inputs. For a more detailed review of delta frequency EEG activity during NREM sleep, the reader is referred to [11].

Neocortical slow (~0.5 Hz) EEG activity/oscillation during NREM sleep

The neocortical slow oscillation plays a role in grouping delta and fast rhythms (gamma and fast beta). This slow oscillation (~0.5 Hz) was first described by Steriade and collaborators in anaesthetized animals (for review, see [11]), and has been confirmed in both naturally sleeping animals and in the human EEG and magnetoencephalogram (MEG), which measures the magnetic field produced by electrical brain activity. The cortical nature of the slow oscillation was demonstrated by its persistence after disconnecting input to the cortex, and is found in cortical neurons of all layers. The slow oscillation consists of prolonged depolarizations, associated with brisk firing (~8–40 Hz, "up states", lasting 0.3–0.6 s), and prolonged hyperpolarizations during which neurons are silent ("down states"). The depolarizing phase consists of excitatory synaptic input (N-methyl-D-aspartic acid (NMDA) and non-NMDA mediated) and a voltage-dependent persistent sodium current, as well as fast inhibitory input (beta/gamma band) reflecting the action of synaptically coupled GABAergic local-circuit cortical cells. The hyperpolarizing phase is thought to result from the removal of excitatory input (disfacilitation). Although the literature consistently refers to it as an oscillation, its periodic occurrence has been difficult to demonstrate definitively, unlike, for example, sleep spindles.

GABAergic preoptic nuclei

Gamma-aminobutyric acid (GABA) is the most prominent inhibitory neurotransmitter in the central nervous system. A variety of anesthetics and hypnotics act on GABA receptors. For example, benzodiazepines depress wakefulness/arousal circuitry by means of modulation of the GABA-A receptor. Although GABA is an important neurotransmitter for sleep induction, some groups of GABA neurons may be involved in wakefulness as well as REM sleep control (see below).

Early evidence from studies employing lesioning and electrophysiological recordings suggested that a proportion of neurons in the basal forebrain and neighboring preoptic regions act to promote sleep [12,101]. Recordings of preoptic neuronal activity demonstrated increased firing of many neurons in these areas during sleep, compared to activity during wakefulness. Juxtacellular labeling further defined these particular neurons as GABAergic[29]. c-Fos protein expression studies described the location of these sleep-active populations as being largely in the preoptic nuclei, and double-labeling of these neurons with antibody for the GABA-synthesizing enzyme glutamic acid decarboxylase (GAD) led to the conclusion that the majority of sleep-active neurons were GABAergic, located in the median preoptic nucleus and the bilateral ventrolateral preoptic nuclei [102,103].

The ventrolateral preoptic nucleus (VLPO) receives input from a variety of different nuclei of the arousal circuitry, including serotonergic and noradrenergic input [104]. VLPO projections to a variety of the wakefulness-related nuclei use the neurotransmitters galanin and GABA [105]. The core of VLPO contains neurons that largely project to TMN, while the extended cluster surrounding region is more connected to other arousal-related regions, such as LC and the raphe nuclei [105]. Specific lesions located in the central cluster of VLPO led largely to decreases of NREM sleep, but lesions of the surrounding extended region of VLPO produced largely decreases of REM sleep [106].

A subset of GABAergic neurons in the median preoptic nuclei (MnPN) are also active during NREM sleep, determined by electrophysiological studies as well as c-Fos protein expression investigations (for review, see [101]). Comparisons of MnPN versus VLPO activity demonstrated that MnPN cells fired immediately preceding sleep states, and continued to fire during sleep [107]. In contrast, VLPO cell firing occurred once NREM sleep began. Therefore, it was concluded that MnPN neurons may be more involved in NREM sleep initiation and maintenance, while VLPO neurons are more involved solely in NREM sleep maintenance.

Wakefulness–sleep transitions: the flip-flop switch (Figure 2.2)

As described above, the VLPO is reciprocally connected with a number of the arousal-related nuclei. It was therefore proposed that mutual inhibition would occur between the VLPO and arousal-related nuclei [108]. For example, in vitro investigations showed that VLPO neurons are inhibited by 5-HT and NA [109]. Arousal systems therefore act to inhibit VLPO sleep-promoting activity and, as discussed above, VLPO inhibits wakefulness-promoting systems. Thus, these arousal and sleep-related nuclei are mutually inhibitory. This reciprocal relationship is reminiscent of a "flip flop" switch, as described in electrical engineering [110,111]. As depicted in Figure 2.2, distinct transitions occur between states, and intermediary states do not normally occur in such a system. Since TMN neurons project to VLPO [104], it was assumed that histaminergic input would inhibit VLPO activity. In vitro, histamine had no post-synaptic effect on VLPO activity [112].

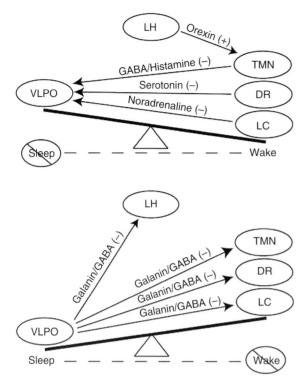

Figure 2.2 Graphic depiction of the flip-flop switch model of wakefulness and sleep systems. GABAergic/galaninergic ventrolateral preoptic (VLPO) neurons, active during sleep, are connected to wakefulness-promoting brain nuclei, including GABAergic/histaminergic neurons of the tuberomammillary nucleus (TMN), serotonergic neurons of the dorsal raphe nucleus (DR), and noradrenergic neurons of the locus coeruleus (LC). Mutual inhibition between these sleep-related and arousal-related neurons allows distinct transitions between states (Wake and Sleep). Orexinergic input from the lateral hypothalamus (LH) to the wakefulness-related nuclei stabilizes the wakefulness state, and during sleep, VLPO inhibits orexinergic activity, as well as the other arousal mechanisms.

However, other indirect inhibitory TMN mechanisms are possible, including presynaptic effects of histamine on inputs to VLPO. Also, TMN neurons contain GAD65, a synthesizing enzyme for GABA, which may allow inhibition of VLPO neurons during wake. It was hypothesized that orexin plays a crucial role in stabilizing the waking state of the switch, due to its widespread projections to the arousal nuclei [110]. Therefore, abnormalities in orexin systems, such as that seen in narcolepsy, would result in more frequent and abnormal state transitions. Consistent with this model, orexin knock-out mice exhibited increased transitions between wakefulness and sleep states [85]. An incompletely answered question in this model is how the system exits states of wakefulness and sleep; a switch remains flipped or flopped unless a third agent

causes a transition. The mechanism of this transition, the agent flipping the switch, is not clearly described, as reflected in the figure.

Neural systems involved in vigilance state regulation: REM sleep

Aserinsky and Kleitman in the 1950s first documented the rapid eye movements indicative of REM sleep in humans, and coined the term "REM sleep" [113,114]. REM sleep mechanisms involve brain regions and systems that differ from those involved with NREM sleep induction and maintenance. Jouvet and colleagues, employing transections, determined that regions of the brain rostral to the midbrain and caudal to the medulla were not necessary for the brainstem activity seen during REM sleep [115,116]. Lesion and transection studies in cats of the dorsolateral pons abolished the REM state. As described previously, this area includes the wakefulness-active noradrenergic, serotonergic and wakefulness/REM-active cholinergic neurons [117,118].

REM sleep is characterized by a return from the high-amplitude, slow-frequency cortical EEG profile evident during deep NREM sleep to fast-frequency, low-voltage EEG activity, such as that seen during wakefulness. Hence, REM sleep is also referred to as "paradoxical sleep." In contrast to wakefulness, EMG recordings during REM sleep exhibit a lack of postural muscle activity. In addition, EOG recordings reveal the characteristic rapid eye movements of REM sleep. REM sleep exhibits further phenomena, including pontine-geniculo-occipital (PGO) waves, and theta rhythmicity evident in the hippocampal EEG.

Pontine-geniculo-occipital (PGO) waves preceding and during REM sleep

One of the important advantages of animal work is the ability to record intracranial EEG and neuronal activity. Thus, investigators are able to detect a transitional state that occurs just before the onset of REM sleep, often termed REM-T. The sleep researcher monitoring pontine reticular neuronal activity easily detects the impending onset of REM by the flurry of activity on the oscilloscope or an audio monitor – all of this stigmatic subcortical activity occurring before the change of externally recorded polysomnographic signs of REM. As depicted in Figure 2.3, REM-T is

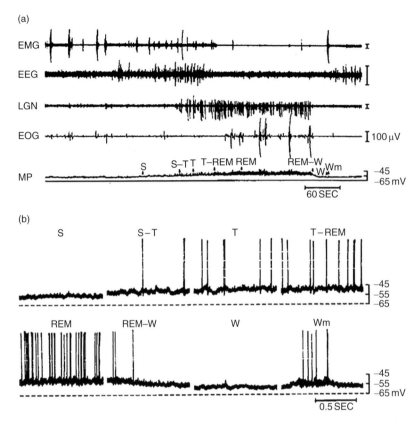

Figure 2.3 Changes in the membrane potential (MP) of a pontine tegmental neuron over the sleep–wake cycle in the cat. These EEG and neuronal recordings illustrate the paucity of reticular activity during NREM sleep and the frenzy of activity during REM sleep. As well, the premonitory transition period of the approach of REM sleep is not visible in the cortical EEG. The first trace of the top panel (a) is EMG from the deep nuchal muscles. The second trace is EEG from the frontal cortex. The third trace is LGN activity, showing PGO waves, which consist of high-amplitude pre-REM waves (REM-T), irregular, high-frequency waves during REM sleep, and rather high-amplitude waves near the end of REM sleep. The fourth trace is EOG from the lateral rectus extraocular muscles. The fifth trace is the ink writer membrane potential record of the pontine tegmental neuron, in which the many single spike-like deflections on the trace are prominent EPSPs, or compounds of EPSPs and actual action potentials (the inkwriter sensitivity is not high enough to trace individual action potentials in the MP trace). In the bottom panel (b), oscilloscope photographs detail changes in the frequency of action potentials together with the MP level. The MP records in the bottom panel are eight photographs of the oscilloscope display of the tape-recorded MP. The labels indicate the corresponding segment on the inkwriter MP trace (arrows). Adapted from [121].

marked by the onset of ponto-geniculo-occipital (PGO) EEG waves, which are characteristic field potentials in the pontine tegmentum (P), lateral geniculate nucleus (G), and the occipital cortex (O). These potentials first arise in the pons and propagate via the lateral geniculate nucleus to the occipital cortex, with PGO activity continuing in REM proper. The source of the pontine initiator of these PGO waves was located in the dorsolateral pons, neighboring the brachium conjunctivum and overlapping the SubC/SLD region important for muscle atonia [119,120,121]. These waves occur immediately preceding REM sleep, and continue to occur during the REM sleep state [11,116,121]. Using positron emission tomography (PET), Maquet and colleagues found that in humans, the right geniculate body and occipital cortex were more active during REM sleep when compared to the other vigilance states [122], supporting the possibility that PGO waves may be present in humans during REM sleep. Recent work has reported PGO-like field potentials in humans [123].

Hippocampal theta (4–8 Hz) rhythmicity during REM sleep

The hippocampal theta rhythm is a sinusoidal wave of neuronal field activity in the frequency range of 4–8 Hz. Theta rhythmicity is evident throughout the REM state in all mammals, and is also present during certain specific wakefulness behaviors/conditions, including attentional processing, spatial navigation, and voluntary movement [124,125]. The origin of hippocampal theta rhythm generation is thought to be brainstem sites within the reticular formation, particularly the rostral pontis oralis, nucleus giganto-cellularis, and pontis caudalis. Such nuclei fire tonic-ally during states when hippocampal theta occurs. These RF nuclei project to the supramammillary nucleus, and here the tonic glutamatergic input from RF is transformed into rhythmic firing. These nuclei then initiate and modulate hippocampal activity, either directly by means of projections to the hippo-campus, or indirectly through the medial septum/diagonal band, which in turn projects by means of GABAergic and cholinergic projections to hippocampal regions.

Pontine cholinergic activation during REM sleep

Pharmacological experiments have indicated a particular role of cholinergic transmission in both wakefulness and REM sleep promotion. The cholinergic neurons of the midbrain tegmentum, particularly of LDT/PPT, are crucial for control of both wakefulness and REM sleep. Non-specific lesioning of this region, by means of intracerebral kainic acid injections, attenuates REM sleep, and the amount of cholinergic cell loss correlates with the REM sleep loss [126]. Of particular interest, some neurons of LDT/PPT discharge selectively during wakefulness and/or REM sleep [26,27]. The LDT/PPT neurons that fire preferentially during REM sleep are often termed "REM-on" neurons. A separate subpopulation of LDT/PPT cholinergic neurons is active during both wakefulness and REM sleep and is referred to as "wake/REM-on" neurons. Systemic administration of the acetylcholine-esterase (AChE) inhibitor physo-stigmine during NREM sleep induces REM sleep [127]. Direct injections of the cholinergic agonist carbachol, muscarinic agonists, or AChE inhibitors (physostigmine or neostigmine) into the RF, particu-larly pontine dorsolateral regions, induce a REM-like state (for review, see [11]).

Noradrenergic and serotonergic inhibition of REM-active neurons

Noradrenergic and serotonergic neurons have been described as "wake-on/REM-off." These neurons decrease activity as REM sleep approaches, and are largely silent during REM sleep. LC noradrenergic and raphe serotonergic neurons counteract the "REM-on" neuronal activity of LDT/PPT neurons, by means of a substantial projection to LDT/PPT that acts on inhibitory alpha 2 adrenergic and 5-HT$_{1A}$ receptors, respectively (for review, see [25]). As depicted in Figure 2.4, Thakkar and colleagues dem-onstrated that "REM-on" neurons of LDT/PPT, but not "wake/REM-on" neurons, were inhibited by 8-OH-DPAT, a selective 5-HT$_{1A}$ agonist [128]. Sero-tonergic "REM-off" neurons act on LDT/PPT neurons, thus accounting for their REM-selective dis-charge (with the same effect postulated for LC nor-adrenergic neurons). Therefore, during REM sleep, as serotonergic raphe and noradrenergic LC neurons cease activity, LDT/PPT neurons are disinhibited.

Pontine sublaterodorsal nucleus activation during REM sleep

Excitatory cholinergic projections from LDT/PPT to regions of the pontine RF may be responsible for some of the characteristic phenomena of REM sleep. One pontine RF region important for muscle atonia, just ventral to LC, was later defined as the perilocus coeruleus alpha in the cat (also termed the subcoer-uleus (SubC) or sublaterodorsal nucleus (SLD) in the rodent). Seminal investigations by Jouvet and col-leagues revealed that lesions of the perilocus coeruleus alpha in the cat produced suppression of muscle ato-nia during REM sleep [129]. Larger lesions of this area, including neighboring pontine regions con-nected to the superior colliculus and amygdala, caused "oneiric" (i.e. dream-like) behavior during REM sleep, including locomotion, attack behavior, and head movement [130]. Recent models of REM sleep suggest that these muscle atonia-on neurons are kept silent during wakefulness by means of GABAergic inputs from neighboring RF regions.

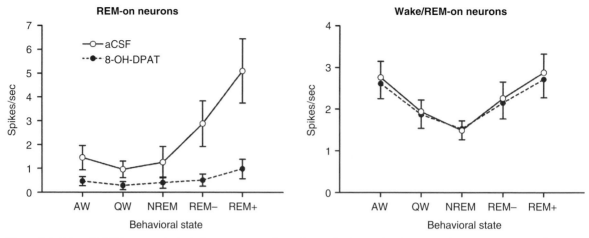

Figure 2.4 Select LDT/PPT, presumptively cholinergic, neurons fire preferentially during REM sleep, termed "REM-on" neurons. Left panel: "REM-on" unit firing of LDT/PPT neurons was suppressed, comparing discharge during aCSF control perfusion (open circles) to activity following 8-OH-DPAT perfusion directly into LDT/PPT (filled circles). Right panel: "Wake/REM-on" neurons were not affected by 8-OH-DPAT perfusion. Abbreviations: AW, active wake; QW, quiet wake; REM, REM sleep. Data expressed as mean ±SEM. Adapted from [128].

These GABAergic neurons may be inhibited by cholinergic input during REM sleep [131,132,133].

Magoun and Rhines discovered a zone in the ventral medulla important for the muscle atonia seen during REM sleep [134]. SubC sends descending projections to glycinergic neurons in this area that, in turn, project to spinal cord motor neurons responsible for postural muscle tone [135]. Recent investigations, employing neuroanatomical and c-Fos expression techniques, suggest that there may also be a glutamatergic direct projection from the SubC region to spinal cord interneurons, bypassing the medial medulla region [66], which in turn inhibit the motor neurons of the spinal cord via spinal glycinergic and GABAergic neurons.

The reciprocal interaction model

McCarley and Hobson proposed the reciprocal interaction model to explain the transitions into and out of REM sleep states, described by the Lotka–Volterra equations, derived from population models of predator/prey interaction [136]. The limit cycle model, an update of the reciprocal interaction model, incorporated circadian and local GABAergic influences on REM sleep regulation [118,137].

As reviewed in Figure 2.5, select cholinergic neurons of LDT/PPT increase firing prior to and during REM sleep. These cholinergic neurons specifically direct the firing of reticular formation neurons

(SubC, parabrachial nucleus, and PnO), whose glutamatergic output is responsible for the activation of the various components of REM sleep described above, including muscle atonia, PGO wave generation, and hippocampal theta activity. LDT/PPT neurons also project to GABAergic interneurons of RF. Therefore, inhibition of these GABAergic RF neurons, which inhibit REM-on RF neurons, provides positive feedback, where glutamatergic RF neurons are disinhibited as REM sleep begins. Cholinergic projections to both DR and LC have been described, although *in vitro* evidence only supports a direct excitatory role of acetylcholine on LC neurons [138]. The original model suggested that there was a very slow modulation of LC firing by LDT/PPT due to a slowly acting intracellular cascade leading to significant excitation. However it now seems much more likely that removal of a GABAergic input to LC/DR is important. We now postulate that, during REM sleep, GABAergic neurons, excited by LDT/PPT cholinergic output, inhibit these serotonergic and noradrenergic REM-off neurons (evidence reviewed in [132]). In contrast, raphe serotonergic and locus coeruleus noradrenergic neurons act as REM-off neurons, inhibiting the REM-on neurons of LDT/PPT during waking and NREM sleep. During wakefulness and NREM sleep, serotonergic and noradrenergic levels build up, activating autoreceptors that inhibit these systems, allowing REM state expression.

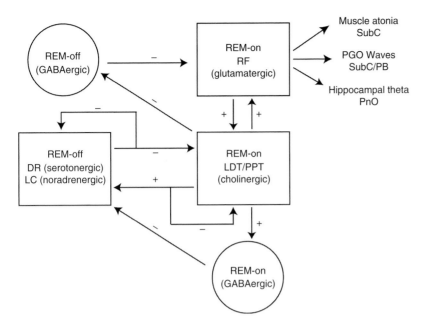

Figure 2.5 Graphic depiction of the modified reciprocal interaction model of REM sleep control, originally proposed by McCarley and Hobson [136]. REM-off neurons inhibit the REM-on neurons during waking and NREM sleep. During NREM sleep, REM-off cell firing significantly decreases as a result of self-inhibition of the REM-off neurons; this results in disinhibition of REM-on neurons, and REM sleep then occurs. As REM sleep progresses, REM-on cells begin to excite the REM-off cells, which become gradually more active and eventually terminate REM sleep. Cholinergic (REM-on) LDT/PPT output excites local GABAergic interneurons that in turn inhibit REM-off neurons. Also, this cholinergic output acts to inhibit local GABAergic REM-off interneurons, which in turn inhibit the glutamatergic REM-on reticular formation neurons.

The two-process model of sleep regulation

Process S: the homeostatic drive to sleep

As proposed by Borbély and colleagues, both a homeostatic drive (termed process S) and a circadian drive (termed process C) play a role in regulating sleep [139]. Process S is an increase in the propensity to sleep proportional to the time spent awake. That is, as time awake is extended, the drive to sleep increases. During slow-wave sleep, spectral activity in the delta range (1–4 Hz) is predominant. It was proposed that this delta activity, particularly during NREM sleep, is an electrophysiological correlate of the homeostatic sleep drive. Following short-term sleep deprivation, an elevation of NREM delta activity, compared to control times of day, is noted in numerous studies. However, recent investigations have suggested that, following multiple days of sleep restriction, NREM delta power does not directly reflect sleep loss [140,141].

We will review here the best characterized homeostatic sleep regulators. Such "homeostatic sleep factors" may be defined by two main criteria: (1) exogenous application of the substance should induce sleep; and (2) endogenous levels of the substance should correlate with time spent awake (process S).

Sleep may serve the purpose of replenishment of energy stores/restoration of the brain [142,143].

Various somnogens have been described, and it has been proposed that the endogenous neuromodulator adenosine may be a homeostatic sleep factor [144,145,146]. Adenosine plays a central role in cellular metabolism, as a product of adenosine triphosphate (ATP) use/degradation. Its potent inhibition of wakefulness-active neurons in BF has led to the proposal that adenosine may be a homeostatic cellular regulator of energy in the brain.

An early study showed that subcutaneous injection of adenosine in the guinea pig resulted in sleep-like behavior, although it is unlikely that this was a reaction to adenosine receptor activation in the brain [147]. More recent pharmacological studies have described the sleep-inducing effects of adenosine, when exogenous adenosine or adenosine agonists were systemically or intracerebrally administered [144,145]. Conversely, antagonism of the adenosine receptor, by substances such as coffee (caffeine) and tea (theophylline), increases alertness.

Adenosine accumulates specifically in the basal forebrain and cortex of the rat and cat as wakefulness is extended by means of sleep deprivation or disruption [21,148,149,150,151,152]. Inhibition of wakefulness-active, cortically projecting neurons in these regions (including those of cholinergic phenotype) by adenosine could contribute to the homeostatic sleep drive [25,144,145]. A diurnal rhythm of adenosine in the rat has been reported, where levels increased as the dark (active) period progressed, and decreased during the light (inactive) period [150,151,153]. Of particular interest, a recent study in epileptic patients included microdialysis sampling of the cortex, hippocampus, and amygdala, where a diurnal oscillation of adenosine levels was found [154].

The subarachnoid space ventral to the BF may be another region where adenosinergic mechanisms promote sleep. When prostaglandin (PGD) 2, another proposed somnogen, was injected into the subarachnoid space ventral to VLPO, the amounts of NREM sleep increased significantly [155]. Activation of prostaglandin receptors in the leptomeninges of the subarachnoid space also led to adenosine release [156]. The A2A receptors of the meninges ventral to VLPO may be activated, which in turn disinhibit VLPO GABAergic/galaninergic sleep-active neurons [109]. In addition, c-Fos protein expression was increased in neurons of the neighboring VLPO region following PGD2 injections [157]. A1 receptor activation in these regions may also lead to disinhibition of VLPO neurons [158]. However, adenosine levels in these preoptic regions did not rise during sleep deprivation in the cat [149]. Therefore, it remains to be determined what specific role extracellular adenosine plays in this region, and if adenosine in this region truly acts as a "homeostatic sleep factor," meeting the above defined criteria.

Recent investigations have proposed a link between nitric oxide (NO) production and the increase of BF adenosine levels during sleep deprivation (for review, see [159]). Administration of inhibitors of NO synthase (the NO-synthesizing enzyme) decreased amounts of sleep. Administration of NO or NO donors increased adenosine levels in both *in vitro* hippocampal and forebrain investigations [160,161], and NO donor infusion (diethylamine-NONOate) into the basal forebrain mimicked sleep deprivation effects, including an increased amount of NREM sleep and extracellular adenosine levels [162]. Therefore, the local release of NO in BF during sleep deprivation may lead to an increase of the homeostatic sleep drive, as well as a rise in extracellular adenosine levels.

Process C: the circadian drive to sleep

As previously mentioned, sleep/wakefulness cycling is influenced by two different processes: a homeostatic drive (termed process S) and the circadian drive

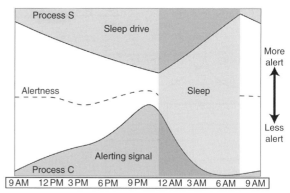

Figure 2.6 The two-process model of sleep regulation, as originally proposed by Borbély and colleagues [139], described the interaction of both homeostatic and circadian processes. In this updated representation of the model [164], the sleep drive due to process S (homeostatic process), represented in the upper portion, increases as the day progresses, and declines during sleep. The alerting signal due to process C (circadian process), represented in the bottom portion, increases during the day, and declines during sleep. The propensity for alertness (dashed line) is the result of the interaction of these two processes. During the late afternoon, alertness declines due to a dip in the circadian rhythm [163]. During sleep, both the homeostatic sleep drive and the circadian drive for alertness decline.

(termed process C), described as the two-process model of sleep regulation (Figure 2.6) [139]. Circadian rhythms are cyclical rhythms of behavior or physiological processes, exhibiting a periodicity of approximately 24 hours. These rhythms are controlled by both external cues (zeitgebers; German for "timegiver"), which synchronize and/or reset this rhythm, and by internal oscillators. The circadian rhythm of an animal may be reset by the introduction of a zeitgeber, such as light, at an unusual time of day. Morning light is the primary zeitgeber in humans. A biphasic pattern of alertness/sleepiness has been described, for sleep propensity reaches its highest levels during the predicted time of 11 p.m.–7 a.m., as well as a brief time during the afternoon between 2 and 6 p.m. [163]. It is theorized that the interaction between homeostatic sleep propensity and the circadian drive for alertness allows for this relatively circumscribed pattern of diurnal wakefulness and nocturnal sleep in humans (Figure 2.6) [164].

The suprachiasmatic nucleus (SCN) is located in the hypothalamus, dorsal to the optic chiasm, and serves as the primary biological clock of mammals (for review, see [165]). Lesions of the SCN disrupt vigilance state regulation, behavior, and physiological processes such as hormonal secretion. Interestingly, these lesions of the SCN drastically alter the periodicity of wakefulness and sleep bouts, but the overall amount of sleep over the 24-hour period remains constant. Studies of neuronal activation in the rodent, indicated by c-Fos protein expression, conclude that neurons of SCN are active during the light (inactive) period, and silent during the dark (active) period [166].

The molecular mechanisms of circadian rhythmicity are highly conserved evolutionarily. The mechanism by which rhythmicity occurs in SCN neurons of mammals involves two autoregulatory loops. The primary core loop includes the cryptochrome gene products CRY1 and CRY2, the period gene products PER1 and PER2, as well as the transcription factors CLOCK and BMAL1 (also known as MOP3, ARNTL, and CYCLE) [167,168]. Although the complexity of this oscillation continues to be a line of scientific inquiry, the basic feedback loop is described below and depicted in Figure 2.7. CLOCK and BMAL1 proteins heterodimerize and bind to E-box enhancer sequences, thereby providing a constitutive drive to induce the expression of multiple genes, including the Per and Cry family genes. A negative feedback loop is formed by the proteins PER and CRY in the cytoplasm, which form heterodimers and translocate back into the nucleus to inhibit the transcription initiated by CLOCK/BMAL1. At the beginning of the subjective day (circadian time hour 0), which for humans corresponds to the light period, the level of PER/CRY is low. The CLOCK/BMAL heterodimer promotes the transcription and the synthesis of gene products CRY1 and 2, and PER1 and 2, leading to increased levels as the subjective day progresses. The resulting CRY/PER protein complex is phosphorylated by casein kinase 1 and glycogen synthase kinase-3 in the cytoplasm. Heterodimerization and phosphorylation is an important determinant of the 24-hour duration of the circadian cycle. The resulting phosphorylated heterodimer is translocated back into the nucleus, where it provides negative feedback by inhibiting CLOCK/BMAL1 transcription. As depicted in Figure 2.7b, by circadian time hour 12, CRY/PER proteins have reached the zenith of expression, inhibiting CLOCK/BMAL transcription. Levels of CRY/PER proteins in the nucleus then begin to attenuate, degraded by means of mechanisms such as proteolysis. Feedback inhibition of CLOCK/BMAL1 at hours 12–24 then attenuates CRY and PER levels. As time approaches hour 24, CLOCK/BMAL1-induced transcription is disinhibited, completing the cycle. This

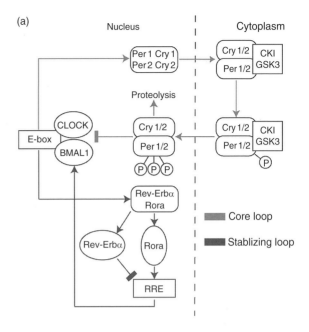

(a)

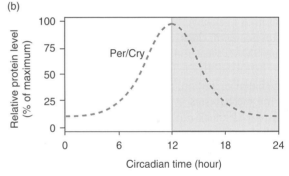

(b)

Figure 2.7 Schematic representation of the interaction of mammalian clock genes contributing to cellular circadian oscillations, adapted from [170]. (a) As described in the core feedback loop (depicted in red), a heterodimeric transcription factor, including CLOCK and BMAL1, by acting on the E-box DNA control element, initiates the expression of the negative regulators PER1 and PER2 (period proteins), as well as CRY1 and CRY 2 (cryptochromes). PER and CRY accumulate as the day progresses, multimerize in the cytoplasm, and are phosphorylated by the enzymes casein kinase I (CKI) and glycogen synthase kinase-3 (GSK3). The PER/CRY complex is then translocated to the nucleus, and represses CLOCK/BMAL1 expression. PER and CRY proteins are then degraded at the end of the circadian cycle (CKI dependent), disinhibiting CLOCK and BMAL1 transcription. As described in the stabilizing feedback loop (depicted in blue), BMAL1 transcription can activate the orphan nuclear receptors Rora and Rev-Erbα, which suppress and activate BMAL1 expression respectively through the intermediary ROR-response element (RRE). (b) Graphic depiction of Per/Cry protein levels in the suprachiasmatic nucleus across the 24-hour day, adapted from [168]. Circadian time 0 is the beginning of the subjective day/light period for humans. Abbreviations: P, phosphate. See plate section for color version.

feedback loop takes approximately 24 hours to complete, and is therefore responsible for the cycling of the circadian clock [169].

In addition to this primary core loop, a stabilizing feedback loop helps maintain 24-hour periodicity; this involves the orphan nuclear receptors Rev-Erbα and the retinoid-related orphan receptor alpha (Rora), which suppress and activate BMAL1 expression respectively [169–171]. The CLOCK/BMAL1 heterodimer interacts with the E-box response element of the promoter region of the Rev-Erbα and Rora genes. Rev-Erbα and Rora compete to bind to the retinoid-related orphan receptor response elements (RRE) in the BMAL1 promoter region. In this manner the circadian oscillation of BMAL is regulated by these orphan nuclear receptors [170,171].

Investigations have begun to describe how these genetic transcriptional/translation interactions may regulate circadian-related events including SCN neuronal activity [167,168]. Clock controlled genes (CCGs), such as vasopressin prepropressophysin and albumin D-element binding protein, are promoted by expression of clock-related genes, such as CLOCK and BMAL. Electrical activity of the SCN is enhanced by increased expression of CCGs through receptor-mediated excitation, as well as autocrine and paracrine mechanisms. A number of investigations have employed knock-out technology to breed mice that possess abnormal expression of a variety of these circadian-related genes. For example, a mouse model knock-out of the CLOCK gene lengthened the circadian rhythm by 4 hours. These animals, when deprived of zeitgeber cues (free-running) did not exhibit circadian rhythmicity in a number of physiological processes [172]. Interestingly, some studies have suggested mutations in various clock-related genes may contribute to human circadian rhythm sleep disorders (CRSDs) such as advanced and delayed sleep phase disorder (for review, see [173]).

Visual input reaches the SCN by means of the retinohypothalamic pathway, which is largely glutamatergic. Freedman and colleagues did not observe altered circadian rhythms with targeted gene knock-out of either the rods or cones in the mouse [174]. Removal of the eyes, though, did affect rhythmicity, and it was later determined that melanopsin, unique to the ganglion cells of the retina, was a photosensitive molecule responsible for changes in excitability of ganglion cells in the retina [175]. Furthermore, anatomical studies have revealed a monosynaptic connection between melanopsin-positive cells and the SCN, suggesting melanopsin is the "circadian photoreceptor" [176,177].

Besides circadian rhythms that occur over an approximate 24-hour period, biological rhythms with other periodicities occur and are often related to interactions with the circadian system and changing external time cues. Seasonal rhythms are regulated by melatonin secretion by means of a well-investigated anatomical circuit involving the SCN, paraventricular nucleus of the hypothalamus, and preganglionic neurons in the sympathetic nervous system [178]. Postganglionic cells in turn project directly to the pineal gland, which is responsible for the secretion of melatonin. Because the amount of light (day) and dark (night) hours fluctuates across seasons, this may be the mechanism by which a seasonal clock occurs. Although the effectiveness of melatonin for jet lag is disputed, some people take melatonin to "reset" their biological clock, for travel across time zones [179]. Melatonin is administered at the beginning of what would be the "new" night period, for melatonin levels are highest at the beginning of the night.

Recent reports have proposed that another internal clock may exist, which is entrainable based on food availability. Food availability, only in the animal's inactive period, can shift rhythms, superseding the photic zeitgeber cues. Such a shift in this rhythm may be an adaptive response for survival of the organism. The dorsomedial nucleus of the hypothalamus (DMH) may correspond to this food-entrainable oscillator. Lesions of DMH block the food-entrainability of the vigilance states [180]. Interestingly, in a mouse with knock-out of the BMAL clock gene, viral vector injection of BMAL in the SCN restored light entrainment of the circadian rhythm [181]. When the BMAL viral vector was injected into DMH, animals were able to entrain to food, but not light. Therefore, it was concluded that a food-entrainable clock is located in this region, although this is presently controversial [182]. As one may predict, interplay between vigilance state and circadian drive circuitry is due to interconnections between the two systems, however the nature of these connections is not fully understood at present. It is notable that the DMH projects directly to the VLPO, as well as to the lateral hypothalamus, rich in wakefulness-active orexinergic neurons. Therefore, DMH may be a key player in the timing of circadian rhythmicity with the homeostatic drive. Future investigations in this exciting avenue of sleep research may further elucidate the interaction of the SCN with vigilance state regulation systems.

Conclusion

The field of sleep medicine has seen a recent investigational surge, due to the development of novel experimental techniques, as well as an increased public awareness of sleep disorders and their implications. Only within the last century have investigations attempted to explain the neural mechanisms responsible for vigilance state regulation. This chapter provides a review of both the neurobiological mechanisms generating wakefulness, NREM sleep, and REM sleep, as well as the major homeostatic and circadian factors that influence the timing of these states. All human life, and indeed the life of most animals, is shaped by periods of wakefulness and sleep, and thus knowledge of the underlying mechanisms is of great biological, social, and medical significance. By furthering understanding of the neural circuitry involved in vigilance state regulation, pharmacological and behavioral treatments may then be developed to reverse the symptomology of a number of sleep-related disorders.

References

1. Committee on Sleep Medicine and Research, Board on Health Sciences Policy, Institute of Medicine of the National Academies. *Sleep disorders and sleep deprivation: an unmet public health problem*. Colten HR, Altevogt BM, eds. Washington, DC: National Academies Press; 2006.

2. Mitler ME, Dement WC, Dinges DF. Sleep medicine, public policy, and public health. In Kryger MH, Roth T, Dement WC, eds. *Principles and practice of sleep medicine*, 3rd ed. Philadelphia, PA: WB Saunders; 2000:580–588.

3. Paxinos G, Watson C. *The rat brain in stereotaxic coordinates*, 3rd ed. San Diego, CA: Academic Press Limited; 1997.

4. Berger H. [Ueber das Elektronkelogramm des Menchen]. *J Psychol Neurol*. 1930;**40**:160–179.

5. Davis H, Davis PA, Loomis AL, Harvey EN, Hobart G. Changes in human brain potentials during the onset of sleep. *Science*. 1937;**86**(2237):448–450.

6. Loomis AL, Harvey EN, Hobart G. Potential rhythms of the cerebral cortex during sleep. *Science*. 1935;**81**(2111):597–598.

7. Von Economo C. [Die Pathologie des Schlafes]. In: Von Bethe A, Von Bergmann A, Embden G, Ellinger A, eds. *Handbuch des normalen und pathologischen physiologie*. Berlin: Springer; 1926:591–610.

8. Bremer F. [Cerveau isole et physiologie du sommeil]. *C R Soc Biol*. 1935;**118**:1235–1241.

9. Bremer F. [Cerveau. Nouvelles recherches sur le mechanisme dur sommeil]. *C R Soc Biol*. 1936;**122**:460–464.

10. Moruzzi G, Magoun HW. Brain stem reticular formation and activation of the EEG. *Electroencephalogr Clin Neurophysiol*. 1949;**1**(4):455–473.

11. Steriade M, McCarley RW. *Brain control of wakefulness and sleep*, 2nd ed. New York, NY: Kluwer Academic/Plenum Publishers; 2005.

12. Jones BE. From waking to sleeping: neuronal and chemical substrates. *Trends Pharmacol Sci*. 2005;**26**(11):578–586.

13. Jones BE. Modulation of cortical activation and behavioral arousal by cholinergic and orexinergic systems. *Ann N Y Acad Sci*. 2008;**1129**:26–34.

14. Dale, H. Pharmacology and nerve endings. *Proc R Soc Med*. 1935;**28**:319–332.

15. Gritti I, Mainville L, Mancia M, Jones BE. GABAergic and other noncholinergic basal forebrain neurons, together with cholinergic neurons, project to the mesocortex and isocortex in the rat. *J Comp Neurol*. 1997;**383**(2):163–177.

16. Henry P, Jones BE. Projections from basal forebrain to prefrontal cortex comprise cholinergic, GABAergic and glutamatergic inputs to pyramidal cells or interneurons. *Eur J Neurosci*. 2008;**27**(3):654–670.

17. Smythe JW, Colom LV, Bland BH. The extrinsic modulation of hippocampal theta depends on the coactivation of cholinergic and GABA-ergic medial septal inputs. *Neurosci Biobehav Rev*. 1992;**16**(3):289–308.

18. Vertes RP, Kocsis B. Brainstem-diencephalo-septohippocampal systems controlling the theta rhythm of the hippocampus. *Neuroscience*. 1997;**81**(4):893–926.

19. Morgan JI, Curran T. Stimulus-transcription coupling in the nervous system: involvement of the inducible proto-oncogenes fos and jun. *Annu Rev Neurosci*. 1991;**14**:421–451.

20. Kovács KJ. c-Fos as a transcription factor: a stressful (re)view from a functional map. *Neurochem Int*. 1998;**33**(4):287–297.

21. Basheer R, Porkka-Heiskanen T, Stenberg D, McCarley RW. Adenosine and behavioral state control: adenosine increases c-Fos protein and AP1 binding in

basal forebrain of rats. *Brain Res Mol Brain Res.* 1999;**73**(1–2):1–10.

22. Greco MA, Lu J, Wagner D, Shiromani PJ. c-Fos expression in the cholinergic basal forebrain after enforced wakefulness and recovery sleep. *Neuroreport.* 2000;**11**(3):437–440.

23. Modirrousta M, Mainville L, Jones BE. Gabaergic neurons with alpha2-adrenergic receptors in basal forebrain and preoptic area express c-Fos during sleep. *Neuroscience.* 2004;**129**(3):803–810.

24. Kovács KJ. Measurement of immediate-early gene activation- c-fos and beyond. *J Neuroendocrinol.* 2008;**20**(6):665–672.

25. McCarley RW. Neurobiology of REM and NREM sleep. *Sleep Med.* 2007;**8**(4):302–330.

26. El Mansari M, Sakai K, Jouvet M. Unitary characteristics of presumptive cholinergic tegmental neurons during the sleep-waking cycle in freely moving cats. *Exp Brain Res.* 1989;**76**(3):519–529.

27. Steriade M, Paré D, Datta S, Oakson G, Curró Dossi R. Different cellular types in mesopontine cholinergic nuclei related to ponto-geniculo-occipital waves. *J Neurosci.* 1990;**10**(8):2560–2579.

28. Manns ID, Alonso A, Jones BE. Discharge properties of juxtacellularly labeled and immunohistochemically identified cholinergic basal forebrain neurons recorded in association with the electroencephalogram in anesthetized rats. *J Neurosci.* 2000;**20**(4):1505–1518.

29. Manns ID, Alonso A, Jones BE. Rhythmically discharging basal forebrain units comprise cholinergic, GABAergic, and putative glutamatergic cells. *J Neurophysiol.* 2003;**89**(2):1057–1066.

30. Lee MG, Hassani OK, Alonso A, Jones BE. Cholinergic basal forebrain neurons burst with theta during waking and paradoxical sleep. *J Neurosci.* 2005;**25**(17): 4365–4369.

31. Blanco-Centurion C, Xu M, Murillo-Rodriguez E, et al. Adenosine and sleep homeostasis in the basal forebrain. *J Neurosci.* 2006;**26**(31):8092–8100.

32. Kaur S, Junek A, Black MA, Semba K. Effects of ibotenate and 192IgG-saporin lesions of the nucleus basalis magnocellularis/substantia innominata on spontaneous sleep and wake states and on recovery sleep after sleep deprivation in rats. *J Neurosci.* 2008;**28**(2):491–504.

33. Kalinchuk AV, McCarley RW, Stenberg D, Porkka-Heiskanen T, Basheer R. The role of cholinergic basal forebrain neurons in adenosine-mediated homeostatic control of sleep: lessons from 192 IgG-saporin lesions. *Neuroscience.* 2008; **157**(1):238–253.

34. Steriade M. Acetylcholine systems and rhythmic activities during the waking-sleep cycle. *Prog Brain Res.* 2004;**145**:179–196.

35. Dahlström A, Fuxe K. Localization of monoamines in the lower brain stem. *Experientia.* 1964;**20**(7): 398–399.

36. Jacobs BL, Azmitia EC. Structure and function of the brain serotonin system. *Physiol Rev.* 1992;**72**(1): 165–229.

37. McGinty DJ, Harper RM. Dorsal raphe neurons: depression of firing during sleep in cats. *Brain Res.* 1976;**101**(3):569–575.

38. Trulson ME, Jacobs BL. Raphe unit activity in freely moving cats: correlation with level of behavioral arousal. *Brain Res.* 1979;**163**(1):135–150.

39. Wilkinson LO, Auerbach SB, Jacobs BL. Extracellular serotonin levels change with behavioral state but not with pyrogen-induced hyperthermia. *J Neurosci.* 1991;**11**(9):2732–2741.

40. Portas CM, McCarley RW. Behavioral state-related changes of extracellular serotonin concentration in the dorsal raphe nucleus: a microdialysis study in the freely moving cat. *Brain Res.* 1994;**648**(2):306–312.

41. Mouret J, Froment JL, Bobillier P, Jouvet M. Neuropharmacologic and biochemical study of insomnia induced by P.chlorophenylalanine. *J Physiol (Paris).* 1967;**59**(4 Suppl):463–464.

42. Jouvet M. Sleep and serotonin: an unfinished story. *Neuropsychopharmacology.* 1999;**21**(2 Suppl):24S–27S.

43. Monti JM, Jantos H. Dose-dependent effects of the 5-HT1A receptor agonist 8-OH-DPAT on sleep and wakefulness in the rat. *J Sleep Res.* 1992;**1**(3):169–175.

44. Portas CM, Thakkar M, Rainnie D, McCarley RW. Microdialysis perfusion of 8-hydroxy-2-(di-n-propylamino)tetralin (8-OH-DPAT) in the dorsal raphe nucleus decreases serotonin release and increases rapid eye movement sleep in the freely moving cat. *J Neurosci.* 1996;**16**(8):2820–2828.

45. Vertes RP, Kinney GG, Kocsis B, Fortin WJ. Pharmacological suppression of the median raphe nucleus with serotonin1A agonists, 8-OH-DPAT and buspirone, produces hippocampal theta rhythm in the rat. *Neuroscience.* 1994;**60**(2):441–451.

46. Kinney GG, Kocsis B, Vertes RP. Medial septal unit firing characteristics following injections of 8-OH-DPAT into the median raphe nucleus. *Brain Res.* 1996;**708**(1–2):116–122.

47. Fabre V, Beaufour C, Evrard A, et al. Altered expression and functions of serotonin 5-HT1A and 5-HT1B receptors in knock-out mice lacking the 5-HT transporter. *Eur J Neurosci.* 2000;**12**(7): 2299–2310.

48. Li Q, Wichems C, Heils A, Lesch KP, Murphy DL. Reduction in the density and expression, but not G-protein coupling, of serotonin receptors (5-HT1A) in 5-HT transporter knock-out mice: gender and brain region differences. *J Neurosci*. 2000;**20**(21):7888–7895.

49. Holmes A, Murphy DL, Crawley JN. Abnormal behavioral phenotypes of serotonin transporter knockout mice: parallels with human anxiety and depression. *Biol Psychiatry*. 2003;**54**(10):953–959.

50. Wisor JP, Wurts SW, Hall FS, et al. Altered rapid eye movement sleep timing in serotonin transporter knockout mice. *Neuroreport*. 2003;**14**(2):233–238.

51. Alexandre C, Popa D, Fabre V, et al. Early life blockade of 5-hydroxytryptamine 1A receptors normalizes sleep and depression-like behavior in adult knock-out mice lacking the serotonin transporter. *J Neurosci*. 2006;**26**(20):5554–5564.

52. Popa D, Léna C, Alexandre C, Adrien J. Lasting syndrome of depression produced by reduction in serotonin uptake during postnatal development: evidence from sleep, stress, and behavior. *J Neurosci*. 2008;**28**(14):3546–3554.

53. Hobson JA, McCarley RW, Wyzinski PW. Sleep cycle oscillation: reciprocal discharge by two brainstem neuronal groups. *Science*. 1975;**189**(4196):55–58.

54. Aston-Jones G, Bloom FE. Activity of norepinephrine-containing locus coeruleus neurons in behaving rats anticipates fluctuations in the sleep-waking cycle. *J Neurosci*. 1981;**1**(8):876–886.

55. Rasmussen K, Morilak DA, Jacobs BL. Single unit activity of locus coeruleus neurons in the freely moving cat. I. During naturalistic behaviors and in response to simple and complex stimuli. *Brain Res*. 1986;**371**(2): 324–334.

56. Jones BE. Paradoxical sleep and its chemical/structural substrates in the brain. *Neuroscience*. 1991;**40**(3): 637–656.

57. Saper CB, Cano G, Scammell TE. Homeostatic, circadian, and emotional regulation of sleep. *J Comp Neurol*. 2005;**493**(1):92–98.

58. Vandermaelen CP, Aghajanian GK. Electrophysiological and pharmacological characterization of serotonergic dorsal raphe neurons recorded extracellularly and intracellularly in rat brain slices. *Brain Res*. 1983; **289**(1–2):109–119.

59. Brown RE, Sergeeva OA, Eriksson KS, Haas HL. Convergent excitation of dorsal raphe serotonin neurons by multiple arousal systems (orexin/hypocretin, histamine and noradrenaline). *J Neurosci*. 2002;**22**(20):8850–8859.

60. Aghajanian GK, Vandermaelen CP. Alpha 2-adrenoceptor-mediated hyperpolarization of locus coeruleus neurons: intracellular studies in vivo. *Science*. 1982;**215**(4538):1394–1396.

61. Williams JA, Reiner PB. Noradrenaline hyperpolarizes identified rat mesopontine cholinergic neurons in vitro. *J Neurosci*. 1993;**13**(9):3878–3883.

62. Swanson LW. The projections of the ventral tegmental area and adjacent regions: a combined fluorescent retrograde tracer and immunofluorescence study in the rat. *Brain Res Bull*. 1982;**9**(1–6):321–353.

63. Gaykema RP, Zaborszky L. Direct catecholaminergic-cholinergic interactions in the basal forebrain. II. Substantia nigra-ventral tegmental area projections to cholinergic neurons. *J Comp Neurol*. 1996;**374**(4): 555–577.

64. Horvitz JC. Mesolimbocortical and nigrostriatal dopamine responses to salient non-reward events. *Neuroscience*. 2000;**96**(4):651–656.

65. Miller JD, Farber J, Gatz P, Roffwarg H, German DC. Activity of mesencephalic dopamine and non-dopamine neurons across stages of sleep and walking in the rat. *Brain Res*. 1983;**273**(1): 133–141.

66. Lu J, Jhou TC, Saper CB. Identification of wake-active dopaminergic neurons in the ventral periaqueductal gray matter. *J Neurosci*. 2006;**26**(1):193–202.

67. Nishino S, Mignot E. Pharmacological aspects of human and canine narcolepsy. *Prog Neurobiol*. 1997;**52**(1):27–78.

68. Mignot E, Nishino S. Emerging therapies in narcolepsy-cataplexy. *Sleep*. 2005;**28**(6):754–763.

69. Brown RE, Stevens DR, Haas HL. The physiology of brain histamine. *Prog Neurobiol*. 2001;**63**(6):637–672.

70. Watanabe T, Taguchi Y, Shiosaka S, et al. Distribution of the histaminergic neuron system in the central nervous system of rats: a fluorescent immunohistochemical analysis with histidine decarboxylase as a marker. *Brain Res*. 1984;**295**(1): 13–25.

71. Panula P, Yang HY, Costa E. Histamine-containing neurons in the rat hypothalamus. *Proc Natl Acad Sci U S A*. 1984;**81**(8):2572–2576.

72. Vanni-Mercier G, Sakai K, Jouvet M. [Specific neurons for wakefulness in the posterior hypothalamus in the cat]. *C R Acad Sci III*. 1984;**298**(7):195–200.

73. Monti JM. Involvement of histamine in the control of the waking state. *Life Sci*. 1993;**53**(17):1331–1338.

74. John J, Wu MF, Boehmer LN, Siegel JM. Cataplexy-active neurons in the hypothalamus: implications for the role of histamine in sleep and waking behavior. *Neuron*. 2004;**42**(4):619–634.

75. Strecker RE, Nalwalk J, Dauphin LJ, et al. Extracellular histamine levels in the feline preoptic/anterior hypothalamic area during natural sleep-wakefulness and prolonged wakefulness: an in vivo microdialysis study. *Neuroscience.* 2002;**113**(3):663–670.

76. Lin JS, Sakai K, Jouvet M. Evidence for histaminergic arousal mechanisms in the hypothalamus of cat. *Neuropharmacology.* 1988;**27**(2):111–122.

77. Kanbayashi T, Kodama T, Kondo H, et al. CSF histamine contents in narcolepsy, idiopathic hypersomnia and obstructive sleep apnea syndrome. *Sleep* 2009;**32**(2):181–187.

78. Nishino S, Sakurai E, Nevsimalova S, et al. Decreased CSF histamine in narcolepsy with and without low CSF hypocretin-1 in comparison to healthy controls. *Sleep* 2009;**32**(2):175–180.

79. Peyron C, Tighe DK, van den Pol AN, et al. Neurons containing hypocretin (orexin) project to multiple neuronal systems. *J Neurosci.* 1998;**18**(23): 9996–10015.

80. de Lecea L, Kilduff TS, Peyron C, et al. The hypocretins: hypothalamus-specific peptides with neuroexcitatory activity. *Proc Natl Acad Sci U S A.* 1998;**95**(1):322–327.

81. Lin L, Faraco J, Li R, et al. The sleep disorder canine narcolepsy is caused by a mutation in the hypocretin (orexin) receptor 2 gene. *Cell.* 1999;**98**(3):365–376.

82. Chemelli RM, Willie JT, Sinton CM, et al. Narcolepsy in orexin knockout mice: molecular genetics of sleep regulation. *Cell.* 1999;**98**(4):437–451.

83. Gerashchenko D, Kohls MD, Greco M, et al. Hypocretin-2-saporin lesions of the lateral hypothalamus produce narcoleptic-like sleep behavior in the rat. *J Neurosci.* 2001;**21**(18):7273–7283.

84. Gerashchenko D, Blanco-Centurion C, Greco MA, Shiromani PJ. Effects of lateral hypothalamic lesion with the neurotoxin hypocretin-2-saporin on sleep in Long-Evans rats. *Neuroscience.* 2003;**116**(1):223–235.

85. Mochizuki T, Crocker A, McCormack S, et al. Behavioral state instability in orexin knock-out mice. *J Neurosci.* 2004;**24**(28):6291–6300.

86. Chen L, Thakkar MM, Winston S, et al. REM sleep changes in rats induced by siRNA-mediated orexin knockdown. *Eur J Neurosci.* 2006;**24**(7): 2039–2048.

87. Peyron C, Faraco J, Rogers W, et al. A mutation in a case of early onset narcolepsy and a generalized absence of hypocretin peptides in human narcoleptic brains. *Nat Med.* 2000;**6**(9):991–997.

88. Thannickal TC, Moore RY, Nienhuis R, et al. Reduced number of hypocretin neurons in human narcolepsy. *Neuron.* 2000;**27**(3):469–474.

89. Nishino S, Ripley B, Overeem S, Lammers GJ, Mignot E. Hypocretin (orexin) deficiency in human narcolepsy. *Lancet.* 2000;**355**(9197):39–40.

90. Mignot EM, Lammers GJ, Ripley B, et al. The role of cerebrospinal fluid hypocretin measurement in the diagnosis of narcolepsy and other hypersomnias. *Arch Neurol.* 2002;**59**(10):1553–1562.

91. Brown RE. Involvement of hypocretins/orexins in sleep disorders and narcolepsy. *Drug News Perspect.* 2003;**16**(2):75–79.

92. Mileykovskiy BY, Kiyashchenko LI, Siegel JM. Behavioral correlates of activity in identified hypocretin/orexin neurons. *Neuron.* 2005;**46**(5): 787–798.

93. Kiyashchenko LI, Mileykovskiy BY, Maidment N, et al. Release of hypocretin (orexin) during waking and sleep states. *J Neurosci.* 2002;**22**(13): 5282–5286.

94. Estabrooke IV, McCarthy MT, Ko E, et al. Fos expression in orexin neurons varies with behavioral state. *J Neurosci.* 2001;**21**(5):1656–1662.

95. Morison RS, Bassett DL. Electrical activity of the thalamus and basal ganglia in decorticate cats. *J Neurophysiol.* 1945;**8**(5):309–314.

96. Steriade M, Deschenes M. The thalamus as a neuronal oscillator. *Brain Res.* 1984;**320**(1):1–63.

97. Steriade M, Domich L, Oakson G, Deschênes M. The deafferented reticular thalamic nucleus generates spindle rhythmicity. *J Neurophysiol.* 1987;**57**(1): 260–273.

98. Hu B, Steriade M, Deschênes M. The effects of brainstem peribrachial stimulation on perigeniculate neurons: the blockage of spindle waves. *Neuroscience.* 1989;**31**(1):1–12.

99. Guillery RW, Harting JK. Structure and connections of the thalamic reticular nucleus: Advancing views over half a century. *J Comp Neurol.* 2003;**463**(4): 360–371.

100. Buzsaki G, Bickford RG, Ponomareff G, et al. Nucleus basalis and thalamic control of neocortical activity in the freely moving rat. *J Neurosci.* 1988; **8**(11):4007–4026.

101. Szymusiak R, McGinty D. Hypothalamic regulation of sleep and arousal. *Ann N Y Acad Sci.* 2008;**1129**:275–286.

102. Sherin JE, Shiromani PJ, McCarley RW, Saper CB. Activation of ventrolateral preoptic neurons during sleep. *Science.* 1996;**271**(5246):216–219.

103. Gong H, McGinty D, Guzman-Marin R, et al. Activation of c-fos in GABAergic neurones in the preoptic area during sleep and in response to sleep deprivation. *J Physiol.* 2004;**556**(3):935–946.

104. Chou TC, Bjorkum AA, Gaus SE, et al. Afferents to the ventrolateral preoptic nucleus. *J Neurosci.* 2002;**22**(3):977–990.

105. Sherin JE, Elmquist JK, Torrealba F, Saper CB. Innervation of histaminergic tuberomammillary neurons by GABAergic and galaninergic neurons in the ventrolateral preoptic nucleus of the rat. *J Neurosci.* 1998;**18**(12):4705–4721.

106. Lu J, Bjorkum AA, Xu M, et al. Selective activation of the extended ventrolateral preoptic nucleus during rapid eye movement sleep. *J Neurosci.* 2002; **22**(11):4568–4576.

107. Suntsova N, Szymusiak R, Alam MN, Guzman-Marin R, McGinty D. Sleep-waking discharge patterns of median preoptic nucleus neurons in rats. *J Physiol.* 2002; **543**(2):665–677.

108. McGinty D, Szymusiak R. The sleep-wake switch: A neuronal alarm clock. *Nat Med.* 2000; **6**(5):510–511.

109. Gallopin T, Luppi PH, Cauli B, et al. The endogenous somnogen adenosine excites a subset of sleep-promoting neurons via A2A receptors in the ventrolateral preoptic nucleus. *Neuroscience.* 2005; **134**(4):1377–1390.

110. Saper CB, Chou TC, Scammell TE. The sleep switch: hypothalamic control of sleep and wakefulness. *Trends Neurosci.* 2001;**24**(12):726–731.

111. Lu J, Sherman D, Devor M, Saper CB. A putative flip-flop switch for control of REM sleep. *Nature.* 2006; **441**(7093):589–594.

112. Gallopin T, Fort P, Eggermann E, et al. Identification of sleep-promoting neurons in vitro. *Nature.* 2000;**404** (6781):992–995.

113. Aserinsky E, Kleitman N. Regularly occurring periods of eye motility, and concomitant phenomena, during sleep. *Science.* 1953;**118**(3062):273–274.

114. Dement WC. Knocking on Kleitman's door: the view from 50 years later. *Sleep Med Rev.* 2003;**7**(4): 289–292.

115. Jouvet M. Paradoxical sleep – a study of its nature and mechanisms. *Prog Brain Res.* 1965;**18**:20–62.

116. Jouvet M. Paradoxical sleep mechanisms. *Sleep.* 1994;**17**(8 Suppl):S77–S83.

117. Jones BE. The role of noradrenergic locus coeruleus neurons and neighboring cholinergic neurons of the pontomesencephalic tegmentum in sleep-wake states. *Prog Brain Res.* 1991;**88**:533–543.

118. McCarley RW. Mechanisms and models of REM sleep control. *Arch Ital Biol.* 2004;**142**(4):429–467.

119. Sakai K, Petitjean F, Jouvet M. Effects of ponto-mesencephalic lesions and electrical stimulation upon PGO waves and EMPs in unanesthetized cats. *Electroencephalogr Clin Neurophysiol.* 1976; **41**(1):49–63.

120. McCarley RW, Nelson JP, Hobson JA. Ponto-geniculo-occipital (PGO) burst neurons: correlative evidence for neuronal generators of PGO waves. *Science.* 1978;**201**(4352):269–272.

121. Ito K, Yanagihara M, Imon H, Dauphin L, McCarley RW. Intracellular recordings of pontine medial gigantocellular tegmental field neurons in the naturally sleeping cat: behavioral state-related activity and soma size difference in order of recruitment. *Neuroscience.* 2002;**114**(1):23–37.

122. Peigneux P, Laureys S, Fuchs S, et al. Generation of rapid eye movements during paradoxical sleep in humans. *Neuroimage.* 2001;**14**(3):701–708.

123. Lim AS, Lozano AM, Moro E, et al. Characterization of REM-sleep associated ponto-geniculo-occipital waves in the human pons. *Sleep.* 2007;**30**(7):823–827.

124. Bland BH. The power of theta: providing insights into the role of the hippocampal formation in sensorimotor integration. *Hippocampus.* 2004; **14**(5):537–538.

125. Vertes RP, Hoover WB, Viana Di Prisco G. Theta rhythm of the hippocampus: subcortical control and functional significance. *Behav Cogn Neurosci Rev.* 2004;**3**(3):173–200.

126. Webster HH, Jones BE. Neurotoxic lesions of the dorsolateral pontomesencephalic tegmentum-cholinergic cell area in the cat. II. Effects upon sleep-waking states. *Brain Res.* 1988;**458**(2):285–302.

127. Sitaram N, Wyatt RJ, Dawson S, Gillin JC. REM sleep induction by physostigmine infusion during sleep. *Science.* 1976;**191**(4233):1281–1283.

128. Thakkar MM, Strecker RE, McCarley RW. Behavioral state control through differential serotonergic inhibition in the mesopontine cholinergic nuclei: a simultaneous unit recording and microdialysis study. *J Neurosci.* 1998;**18**(14):5490–5497.

129. Sastre JP, Jouvet M. Oneiric behavior in cats. *Physiol Behav.* 1979;**22**(5):979–989.

130. Hendricks JC, Morrison AR, Mann GL. Different behaviors during paradoxical sleep without atonia depend on pontine lesion site. *Brain Res.* 1982;**239**(1): 81–105.

131. Xi MC, Morales FR, Chase MH. Interactions between GABAergic and cholinergic processes in the nucleus pontis oralis: neuronal mechanisms controlling active (rapid eye movement) sleep and wakefulness. *J Neurosci.* 2004;**24**(47):10670–10678.

132. Luppi PH, Gervasoni D, Verret L, et al. Paradoxical (REM) sleep genesis: the switch from

aminergic-cholinergic to a GABAergic-glutamatergic hypothesis. *J Physiol Paris.* 2006;**100**(5–6):271–283.

133. Brown RE, McKenna JT, Winston S, et al. Characterization of GABAergic neurons in rapid-eye-movement sleep controlling regions of the brainstem reticular formation in GAD67-green fluorescent protein knock-in mice. *Eur J Neurosci.* 2008;**27**(2): 352–363.

134. Magoun HW, Rhines R. An inhibitory mechanism in the bulbar reticular formation. *J Neurophysiol.* 1946;**9**:165–171.

135. Chase MH, Morales FR. The atonia and myoclonia of active (REM) sleep. *Annu Rev Psychol.* 1990;**41**:557–584.

136. McCarley RW, Hobson JA. Neuronal excitability modulation over the sleep cycle: a structural and mathematical model. *Science.* 1975;**189**(4196): 58–60.

137. McCarley RW, Massaquoi SG. A limit cycle mathematical model of the REM sleep oscillator system. *Am J Physiol.* 1986;**251**(6 Pt 2):R1011–R1029.

138. Li X, Rainnie DG, McCarley RW, Greene RW. Presynaptic nicotinic receptors facilitate monoaminergic transmission. *J Neurosci.* 1998;**18**(5): 1904–1912.

139. Borbély AA, Achermann P. Sleep homeostasis and models of sleep regulation. *J Biol Rhythms.* 1999;**14**(6): 557–568.

140. Van Dongen HP, Maislin G, Mullington JM, Dinges DF. The cumulative cost of additional wakefulness: dose-response effects on neurobehavioral functions and sleep physiology from chronic sleep restriction and total sleep deprivation. *Sleep.* 2003;**26**(2): 117–126.

141. Kim Y, Laposky AD, Bergmann BM, Turek FW. Repeated sleep restriction in rats leads to homeostatic and allostatic responses during recovery sleep. *Proc Natl Acad Sci U S A.* 2007;**104**(25):10697–10702.

142. Benington JH, Heller HC. Restoration of brain energy metabolism as the function of sleep. *Prog Neurobiol.* 1995;**45**(4):347–360.

143. Scharf MT, Naidoo N, Zimmerman JE, Pack AI. The energy hypothesis of sleep revisited. *Prog Neurobiol.* 2008;**86**(3):264–280.

144. Strecker RE, Morairty S, Thakkar MM, et al. Adenosinergic modulation of basal forebrain and preoptic/anterior hypothalamic neuronal activity in the control of behavioral state. *Behav Brain Res.* 2000;**115**(2):183–204.

145. Basheer R, Strecker RE, Thakkar MM, McCarley RW. Adenosine and sleep-wake regulation. *Prog Neurobiol.* 2004;**73**(6):379–396.

146. Radulovacki M. Adenosine sleep theory: how I postulated it. *Neurol Res.* 2005;**27**(2):137–138.

147. Drury AN, Szent-Györgyi A. The physiological activity of adenine compounds with especial reference to their action upon the mammalian heart. *J Physiol.* 1929;**68**(3):213–237.

148. Porkka-Heiskanen T, Strecker RE, Thakkar M, et al. Adenosine: a mediator of the sleep-inducing effects of prolonged wakefulness. *Science.* 1997; **276**(5316):1265–1268.

149. Porkka-Heiskanen T, Strecker RE, McCarley RW. Brain site-specificity of extracellular adenosine concentration changes during sleep deprivation and spontaneous sleep: an in vivo microdialysis study. *Neuroscience.* 2000;**99**(3):507–517.

150. McKenna JT, Dauphin LJ, Mulkern KJ, et al. Nocturnal elevation of extracellular adenosine in the rat basal forebrain. *Sleep Research Online.* 2003;**5**: 155–160.

151. Murillo-Rodriguez E, Blanco-Centurion C, Gerashchenko D, Salin-Pascual RJ, Shiromani PJ. The diurnal rhythm of adenosine levels in the basal forebrain of young and old rats. *Neuroscience.* 2004;**123**(2):361–370.

152. McKenna JT, Tartar JL, Ward CP, et al. Sleep fragmentation elevates behavioral, electrographic and neurochemical measures of sleepiness. *Neuroscience.* 2007;**146**(4):1462–1473.

153. Chagoya de Sánchez V, Hernández Múñoz R, Suárez J, Vidrio S, Yáñez L, Díaz Múñoz M. Day-night variations of adenosine and its metabolizing enzymes in the brain cortex of the rat – possible physiological significance for the energetic homeostasis and the sleep-wake cycle. *Brain Res.* 1993;**612**(1–2): 115–121.

154. Zeitzer JM, Morales-Villagran A, Maidment NT, et al. Extracellular adenosine in the human brain during sleep and sleep deprivation: an in vivo microdialysis study. *Sleep.* 2006;**29**(4):455–461.

155. Satoh S, Matsumura H, Suzuki F, Hayaishi O. Promotion of sleep mediated by the A2a-adenosine receptor and possible involvement of this receptor in the sleep induced by prostaglandin D2 in rats. *Proc Natl Acad Sci U S A.* 1996;**93**(12): 5980–5984.

156. Hayaishi O. Molecular mechanisms of sleep-wake regulation: a role of prostaglandin D2. *Philos Trans R Soc Lond B Biol Sci.* 2000;**355**(1394):275–280.

157. Scammell TE, Gerashchenko DY, Mochizuki T, et al. An adenosine A2a agonist increases sleep and induces Fos in ventrolateral preoptic neurons. *Neuroscience.* 2001;**107**(4):653–663.

158. Morairty S, Rainnie D, McCarley R, Greene R. Disinhibition of ventrolateral preoptic area sleep-active neurons by adenosine: a new mechanism for sleep promotion. *Neuroscience*. 2004;**123**(2):451–457.

159. Gautier-Sauvigné S, Colas D, Parmantier P, et al. Nitric oxide and sleep. *Sleep Med Rev*. 2005;**9**(2):101–113.

160. Fallahi N, Broad RM, Jin S, Fredholm BB. Release of adenosine from rat hippocampal slices by nitric oxide donors. *J Neurochem*. 1996;**67**(1):186–193.

161. Rosenberg PA, Li Y, Le M, Zhang Y. Nitric oxide-stimulated increase in extracellular adenosine accumulation in rat forebrain neurons in culture is associated with ATP hydrolysis and inhibition of adenosine kinase activity. *J Neurosci*. 2000;**20**(16):6294–6301.

162. Kalinchuk AV, Lu Y, Stenberg D, Rosenberg PA, Porkka-Heiskanen T. Nitric oxide production in the basal forebrain is required for recovery sleep. *J Neurochem*. 2006;**99**(2):483–498.

163. Richardson GS, Carskadon MA, Orav EJ, Dement WC. Circadian variation of sleep tendency in elderly and young adult subjects. *Sleep*. 1982;**5**(Suppl 2):S82–S94.

164. Dijk DJ, Edgar DM. Circadian and homeostatic control of wakefulness and sleep. In: Turek FW, Zee PC, eds. *Regulation of sleep and circadian rhythms*. New York: Marcel Dekker Inc.; 1999:111–147.

165. Harrington ME, Mistlberger RE. Anatomy and physiology of the mammalian circadian system. In: Kryger MH, Roth T, Dement WC, eds. *Principles and practice of sleep medicine*, 3rd ed. Philadelphia, PA: WB Saunders; 2000:334–345.

166. Morin LP. The circadian visual system. *Brain Res Brain Res Rev*. 1994;**19**(1):102–127.

167. King DP, Takahashi JS. Molecular genetics of circadian rhythms in mammals. *Annu Rev Neurosci*. 2000;**23**:713–742.

168. Reppert SM, Weaver DR. Molecular analysis of mammalian circadian rhythms. *Annu Rev Physiol*. 2001;**63**:647–676.

169. Ko CH, Takahashi JS. Molecular components of the mammalian circadian clock. *Hum Mol Genet*. 2006;**15**(2):R271–R277.

170. Gallego M, Virshup DM. Post-translational modifications regulate the ticking of the circadian clock. *Nat Rev Mol Cell Biol*. 2007;**8**(2):139–148.

171. Jetten AM. Retinoid-related orphan receptors (RORs): critical roles in development, immunity, circadian rhythm, and cellular metabolism. *Nucl Recept Signal*. 2009;**7**:1–32.

172. Challet E, Takahashi JS, Turek FW. Nonphotic phase-shifting in clock mutant mice. *Brain Res*. 2000;**859**(2): 398–403.

173. Sack RL, Auckley D, Auger RR, et al. Circadian rhythm sleep disorders: part II, advanced sleep phase disorder, delayed sleep phase disorder, free-running disorder, and irregular sleep-wake rhythm. An American Academy of Sleep Medicine review. *Sleep*. 2007;**30**(11):1484–1501.

174. Freedman MS, Lucas RJ, Soni B, et al. Regulation of mammalian circadian behavior by non-rod, non-cone, ocular photoreceptors. *Science*. 1999;**284**(5413): 502–504.

175. Provencio I, Rodriguez IR, Jiang G, et al. A novel human opsin in the inner retina. *J Neurosci*. 2000; **20**(2):600–605.

176. Berson DM, Dunn FA, Takao M. Phototransduction by retinal ganglion cells that set the circadian clock. *Science*. 2002;**295**(5557):1070–1073.

177. Hattar S, Liao HW, Takao M, Berson DM, Yau KW. Melanopsin-containing retinal ganglion cells: architecture, projections, and intrinsic photosensitivity. *Science*. 2002;**295**(5557): 1065–1070.

178. Buijs RM, Scheer FA, Kreier F, et al. Organization of circadian functions: interaction with the body. *Prog Brain Res*. 2006;**153**:341–360.

179. Deacon S, Arendt J. Adapting to phase shifts, II. Effects of melatonin and conflicting light treatment. *Physiol Behav*. 1996;**59**(4–5):675–682.

180. Gooley JJ, Schomer A, Saper CB. The dorsomedial hypothalamic nucleus is critical for the expression of food-entrainable circadian rhythms. *Nat Neurosci*. 2006;**9**(3):398–407.

181. Fuller PM, Lu J, Saper CB. Differential rescue of light- and food-entrainable circadian rhythms. *Science*. 2008;**320**(5879):1074–1077.

182. Mistlberger RE, Yamazaki S, Pendergast JS, et al. Comment on "Differential rescue of light- and food-entrainable circadian rhythms." *Science*. 2008; **322**(5902):675.

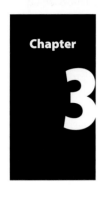

Chapter 3

Neurophysiology and neuroimaging of human sleep

Fabio Ferrarelli and Ruth M. Benca

Sleep is a behavior universally present in the animal kingdom, occurring in a range of species from drosophila to human beings [1]. Sleep occupies about one-third of the human life-span [2] and, although its functions are still not understood, regular sleep is essential for survival. Aspects of normal and abnormal human sleep can be characterized by employing electrophysiological tools including electroencephalogram (EEG), electromyogram (EMG), and electrooculogram (EOG). Sleep can be subdivided into two types: rapid eye movement (REM) and non-rapid eye movement (NREM), with specific behavioral and neurophysiological correlates [3,4]. Over the last four decades numerous studies have revealed the organization of REM and NREM sleep in healthy subjects and patients with a broad range of neuropsychiatric disorders [5,6,7]. Additionally, the development of neuroimaging techniques has allowed sleep researchers to explore the neurobiological systems and mechanisms underlying sleep organization [8], as well as the consequences of sleep disruption on cognitive functions [9].

This chapter reviews the characteristics of human sleep, with particular emphasis on REM/NREM sleep stages and their physiological correlates, and describes the electrophysiological assessment of normal sleep and sleep disorders with polysomnography (PSG), as well as the standardized clinical tests utilized to establish the daytime consequences of sleep disorders: the multiple sleep latency test (MSLT) and the maintenance of wakefulness test (MWT). The organization of sleep (sleep architecture) in young healthy adults, and the effects of age, psychiatric disorders, and psychoactive medications on sleep architecture are discussed. Finally, several neuroimaging techniques are described, including functional magnetic resonance imaging (f-MRI), positron emission tomography (PET), and high-density

(hd)-EEG, which are increasingly utilized in sleep research to investigate the neural correlates of normal sleep and the effects of sleep deprivation on cognitive functions.

Characteristics of human sleep
Definition of sleep

Sleep is defined by a combination of behavioral and physiological characteristics. Behaviorally, sleeping humans tend to lie still in stereotypical postures. This condition, which is characterized by a markedly reduced awareness of the outside world, is different, however, from other unconscious states like coma or anesthesia because of its prompt reversibility [10]. Using electrophysiological criteria, human sleep can be divided into two types, REM and NREM sleep. During REM sleep, bursts of eye movement activity frequently occur. REM sleep is also called *paradoxical sleep* because of EEG activity similar to that observed during wakefulness. On the other hand, during NREM sleep, which is also described as *orthodox sleep*, the EEG shows low-frequency activity.

Sleep stages

Human sleep occurs in several cycles of NREM–REM sleep across the night, each approximately 90 to 110 minutes long, which can be further classified into different sleep stages [11]. Sleep stages are identified based on three electrophysiological parameters: EEG, EOG, and EMG activity, the latter usually recorded from neck or chin muscles. For clinical and research purposes, sleep is usually scored in 30 second epochs. The criteria of sleep stage scoring, established by Rechtschaffen and Kales (R&K) [12], have been

Foundations of Psychiatric Sleep Medicine, ed. John W. Winkelman and David T. Plante. Published by Cambridge University Press.

Table 3.1 Stages of sleep: electrophysiological criteria

	EEG	EOG	EMG
Wakefulness Stage W	Low-amplitude, mixed frequency; alpha rhythm (8–12 Hz) with eye closure, attenuating with eye opening	Eye movements and eye blinks (0.5–2 Hz)	High tonic activity in skeletal muscles
NREM sleep Stage N1	Low-amplitude, mixed frequency; theta rhythm (4–7 Hz), with Vertex sharp waves (V waves, $\leq$0.5 seconds)	Slow eye movements (SEM)	Slight decrease in tonic muscle activity
NREM sleep Stage N2	Low-voltage background activity with sleep spindles (11–16 Hz bursts) and K-complexes (biphasic waves lasting $\geq$0.5 seconds)	No eye movements	Further decrease in tonic muscle activity
NREM sleep Stage N3	High-amplitude ($\geq$75 μV), slow ($\leq$2 Hz) waves lasting $\geq$20% of the epoch	No eye movements	Low tonic activity
REM sleep	Low-voltage, saw-tooth waves (2–6 Hz), predominant theta activity	Rapid eye movements (REM)	Muscle atonia with phasic twitches

recently modified by the American Academy of Sleep Medicine (AASM) [13]. In this chapter, the AASM scoring criteria are used.

During wakefulness, the EEG is characterized by low-amplitude, fast-frequency activity (>8 Hz) while the EMG shows a high-voltage, tonic activity combined with phasic increases related to voluntary movements. Also, eye blinks or eye movements are detected by the EOG when the subject is resting with the eyes open or is engaged in a specific task. When eyes are closed in preparation for sleep, EEG alpha activity (8 to 12 Hz) increases and becomes the fundamental rhythm, especially in the occipital cortex.

NREM sleep, which usually initiates each sleep cycle, can be further divided into three stages: N1, N2, and N3 (Table 3.1 and Figure 3.1). During stage N1 (stage 1 according to R&K) the alpha rhythm wanes, while the EEG is characterized by activity in the theta range (4–7 Hz) combined with sporadic high-voltage sharp waves over the central region. Slow, rolling eye movements and a generalized reduction in muscle tone are also present. Subjectively, stage N1 is accompanied by a decreased awareness of environmental stimuli and dream-like mentation. Some individuals report having hypnagogic hallucinations at sleep onset, which can range from vague and brief to vivid perceptual experiences. Sudden muscle

twitches can also occur at the transition into sleep. These hypnic jerks, also known as positive myoclonus, are sporadic, generally benign, and are more common after sleep deprivation. Brief episodes of Stage N1, usually lasting a few seconds, tend to occur during the daytime in sleepy subjects, either due to sleep disorders or sleep deprivation, and can have dire consequences in situations that require a constant high level of awareness, such as driving.

Stage N2 (stage 2 sleep according to R&K) usually follows stage N1, and is characterized by two EEG elements: (1) sleep spindles (waxing and waning oscillations at 11–16 Hz, lasting 0.5–2 seconds); and (2) K-complexes (high-voltage, biphasic waves 0.5–1.0 seconds long with an initial, sharp, upward component followed by a slower downward peak). The transition from stage N2 to N3 is heralded by the occurrence, in the EEG, of slow waves: low-frequency (0.5–2 Hz) oscillations with a peak-to-peak amplitude $\geq$75 μV. Indeed, when sleep epochs display at least 20% slow waves they are scored as stage N3. N3 is also described as slow-wave sleep (SWS), or deep sleep, because of the increased arousal threshold from N1 to N3. SWS was previously subdivided according to R&K criteria, based on the amount of slow waves in the sleep epoch, into NREM stage 3 (20–50% slow waves) and stage 4 (>50% slow waves). However, the biological relevance of this distinction has never been

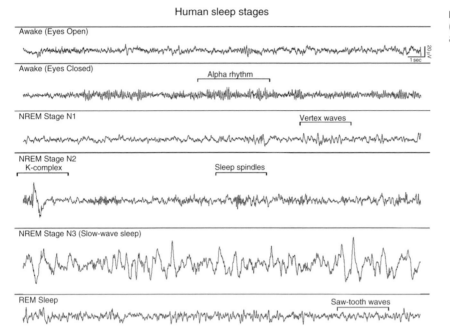

Human sleep stages

Figure 3.1 Electroencephalogram (EEG) patterns for wakefulness and stages of sleep.

established; thus, the AASM has recently combined these sleep stages into N3. Eye movements are usually absent during both N2 and N3, and EMG activity progressively decreases from N1 to N3.

REM sleep, or stage R, usually follows a NREM sleep episode and consists of tonic (persistent) and phasic (episodic) components. REM tonic activity is characterized by low-voltage, mixed frequency EEG patterns with a predominance of theta rhythm and a marked decrease of skeletal muscle tone (atonia), except for the extraocular muscles and the diaphragm. One of these tonic EEG patterns, called saw-tooth waves because of their notched morphology, is rather common particularly before the onset of eye movements. The phasic components of REM sleep consist of irregular bursts of rapid eye movements, which occur more often and for longer periods of time in later REM episodes, along with (mostly distal) muscle twitches.

Physiological changes occurring in sleep stages

Several physiological parameters, including some pertaining to the autonomic and endocrine systems, undergo significant changes during sleep. A brief review of these changes is helpful for understanding sleep abnormalities in medical and psychiatric disorders.

Autonomic nervous system (ANS)

During NREM and tonic REM sleep the sympathetic activity ("fight or flight") of the ANS decreases [14], whereas the parasympathetic activity ("rest and repose") progressively increases until it peaks in deep sleep (SWS) [15], where blood pressure and heart and respiratory rates reach their lowest values [16]. Notably, increased sympathetic activation observed in individuals affected by sleep apnea, a condition characterized by chronic SWS deficits, may theoretically increase their risk of developing diabetes [17]. Abnormal peaks of sympathetic activity have also been reported during phasic REM in patients affected by melancholic depression, although their relationship with this psychiatric disorder is not clear [18].

Cardiovascular system

Blood pressure and cardiac output are markedly reduced during NREM sleep relative to wakefulness. During REM sleep these cardiovascular parameters reach their peak values during sleep, although mean values are generally lower than during waking [16]. Episodes of arrhythmia are also more common during REM sleep, which could partially explain the higher incidence of cardiovascular events early in the morning, when REM episodes are longer [19]. It could also contribute to the higher cardiovascular mortality seen in patients with major depression, who show increased REM sleep period duration and greater phasic REM activity relative to healthy subjects, although this is theoretical [20].

Respiratory system

During sleep, air exchange decreases because of the loss of waking-related respiratory drive and a reduction in respiratory rate and minute ventilation. At the same time, the resistance in the upper airways increases as a result of muscle relaxation [21]. Reduced sensitivity of central chemoreceptors to higher levels of CO_2 or to lower levels of O_2 is also observed, especially during REM sleep [22]. These changes, usually present in normal sleep, contribute to sleep disorders such as sleep apnea [23].

Thermoregulation

During NREM sleep, homeostatic thermoregulation is preserved and is characterized, particularly in SWS, by a reduction in body temperature that follows a decrease in the hypothalamic temperature set point [24]. Conversely, during REM sleep the ability to regulate body temperature through sweating and shivering is markedly reduced [25]. Intriguingly, hypothermia and other abnormalities in thermoregulation are reported in psychiatric disorders, such as anorexia nervosa [26], which are also characterized by sleep abnormalities (i.e. SWS deficits) [27].

Neuroendocrine system

Several hormones are released during sleep. *Growth hormone (GH)* secretion occurs early in the night, and peaks during SWS [28], while *prolactin* is usually released in the middle of the night [29]. Both of these hormones have feedback effects on sleep: GH on SWS [30], prolactin on REM [31]. *Adrenocorticotropic hormone (ACTH)* and *cortisol*, two hormones of the *hypothalamic-pituitary-adrenal* (HPA) *axis*, are downregulated at sleep onset but increase and peak toward the end of sleep, when they likely contribute to morning arousal [32]. In contrast, the secretion of *thyroid-stimulating hormone (TSH)* is maximal in the evening before sleep onset, inhibited by sleep, and enhanced by sleep deprivation [33]. *Melatonin*, whose secretion by the pineal gland is permitted only at night by the circadian system, is also inhibited by light and promoted by darkness, thus providing information to the brain regarding seasonal day length. Melatonin is often used as a sleep-promoting agent,

due to its ability to induce drowsiness and lower body temperature [34]. Altogether, while hormones such as prolactin and GH show a significant sleep-dependent secretion, melatonin and cortisol levels are circadian-regulated and thus are relatively unaffected by sleep [35].

Chronic sleep disruption or sleep deprivation can have dramatic effects on the endocrine system. For example, the secretion of GH and prolactin is markedly decreased in sleep apnea patients [36]. Furthermore, there is increasing evidence that sleep loss is associated with decreased insulin sensitivity, which eventually could result in elevated risk for diabetes [37]. In addition, severe sleep restriction may result in a reduction of satiety hormones (e.g. *leptin*) as well as an increase in hunger-promoting hormones (e.g. *ghrelin*), which could lead to higher body mass index and obesity [38].

Reproductive system

During REM sleep, men commonly experience nocturnal penile tumescence (NPT) [39]. The occurrence of NPT, which is unrelated to the sexual content of dreaming and persists into old age, can be used to establish whether cases of impotence are biological or psychogenic in origin. However, testing for NPT is no longer commonly performed due to newer pharmacological methods of evaluating impotence [40]. In women, during REM sleep, a phasic increase in vaginal blood flow as well as clitoral engorgement and erection occur, phenomena which are also unrelated to the sexual content of dreaming activity [41].

Electrophysiological tools to monitor sleep

Monitoring normal human sleep

EEG, since it was first utilized by Hans Berger in 1929 to describe brain rhythms (alpha, beta) generated during waking [42], has been extensively employed to investigate sleep activity. In combination with EMG (which assesses muscle activity) and EOG (which measures eye movement), EEG has played a critical role in characterizing the different stages of NREM as well as REM sleep.

EEG is recorded from electrodes placed on different scalp locations according to the 10–20 system [43]. This is a standardized electrode placement method developed to ensure high within- and across-subject reproducibility. Electrodes localized in different scalp regions (frontal, central, and occipital) can best identify specific EEG patterns of waking

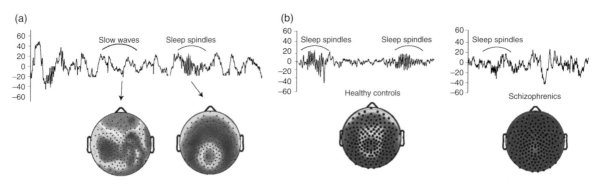

Figure 3.2 (a) NREM sleep EEG traces and topographies of slow waves and sleep spindles in a healthy control. (b) Topographic analysis of sleep spindles revealed that schizophrenics had reduced spindle activity localized in a centroparietal area (adapted from [1]). See plate section for color version.

and sleep. For example, a frontal electrode can optimally record K-complexes (NREM stage N2) and slow waves (NREM stage N3), whereas a central electrode is ideally located to detect sleep spindles (NREM stage N2). Conversely, an occipital electrode can best record alpha rhythm, EEG oscillations at 8–12 Hz occurring during resting wakefulness with the eyes closed. The current availability of high-density (≥ 60 channels) EEG (hd-EEG) systems has made it possible to describe a highly detailed topography of characteristic waking as well as sleep rhythms, such as slow waves and sleep spindles (Figure 3.2a). A recent study has also shown the potential of hd-EEG in identifying local deficits in sleep rhythms in patients with schizophrenia (Figure 3.2b) [44].

EOG electrodes are placed in pairs (above and below the eye or to the left and right of it) in order to track vertical and horizontal eye movements. EOG electrodes can detect the slow, rolling eye movement associated with NREM sleep stage N1 as well as the rapid eye movements that occur during REM sleep. EMG recordings are performed to monitor changes in tonic and phasic muscle activity during sleep. For example, EMG activity is markedly decreased during REM sleep, when skeletal muscles are virtually paralyzed (atonia). EMG is usually recorded from chin electrodes over the submentalis muscle. Additional electrodes can be placed over the anterior tibialis and intercostal muscles to monitor leg movements and respiratory efforts, respectively.

Monitoring abnormal sleep: polysomnography

Polysomnography (PSG) is an overnight procedure that involves continuous recording of several physiological variables for the characterization of sleep for the diagnosis of sleep disorders or for clinical research [45]. In addition to EEG, EOG, and EMG activity, the variables monitored during clinical PSG include: (a) limb movements via EMG electrodes on arms and/or legs; (b) electrocardiogram (ECG) using chest leads; (c) respiratory effort with thoracic and abdominal piezoelectric belts or respiratory inductive plethysmography (RIP) belts; (d) airflow at nose/mouth via heat-sensitive devices called thermistors and/or nasal pressure transducers; and (e) oxygen saturation via pulse oximetry. PSG is commonly indicated for: (1) the diagnosis of sleep-related breathing disorders (SRBDs); (2) titrating positive airway pressure (PAP) in patients with SRBDs; (3) cases of suspected narcolepsy; and (4) monitoring sleep behaviors (parasomnias) that are potentially harmful or are particularly unusual for age of onset, duration, and frequency of occurrence [46]. PSG is also employed in patients with neuromuscular disorders reporting sleep complaints, in patients with parasomnias unresponsive to therapy, and in order to support diagnoses of seizure-related paroxysmal arousals or periodic limb movement disorder [46]. Conversely, PSG is usually not indicated in cases of insomnia, circadian rhythm disorders, typical, uncomplicated parasomnias, or to confirm sleep abnormalities (i.e. insomnia) in subjects affected by psychiatric disorders, such as depression or schizophrenia [46].

Clinical tests to establish daytime sleepiness

Daytime sleepiness is characterized by difficulties in maintaining wakefulness while performing daytime activities. It is a chronic problem for about 5% of the general population, and it is the most common sleep-related complaint reported by patients seen in sleep disorder centers [47]. Sleepiness can be caused by sleep deprivation, sleep fragmentating disorders (e.g. sleep apnea) [48], disorders of central hypersomnolence (e.g. narcolepsy), or certain types of medications [49]. Decreased productivity, problems in interpersonal relationships, and increased risk for motor vehicle accidents are some of the most common consequences of excessive sleepiness [50].

Daytime sleepiness can be measured with subjective questionnaires, such as the Stanford sleepiness scale (SSS) [51] and the Epworth sleepiness scale (ESS) [52], or by using objective electrophysiological tests. The SSS ratings reflect the subject's self-reported level of sleepiness at the time of report, while the ESS scores indicate the subject's self-evaluated propensity to fall asleep under various circumstances. Both questionnaires, although inexpensive and easy to administer, can be confounded by factors such as the individuals' ability to assess their own level of vigilance or their motivation to seek medical treatment. Also, subjective scales may not measure the same parameter across subjects (e.g. fatigue vs. sleepiness) [53]. Objective tests of sleepiness are more time-consuming, but more accurate. Among them, the two most commonly employed to assess daytime sleepiness are the MSLT [54] and the MWT [55].

The MSLT measures the ability to fall asleep under standardized conditions across the day, and consists of four or five nap opportunities repeated 2 hours apart. At the beginning of each test, the individual lies in a quiet, darkened room and tries to fall asleep. Sleep latency, measured from lights out to the first epoch of any stage of sleep, is recorded and the test is terminated if sleep does not occur within 20 minutes. When the MSLT is used for clinical purposes, patients are allowed to sleep for 15 minutes after falling asleep to establish whether they go into REM sleep during the nap. In combination with other symptoms, two or more naps with REM sleep are highly suggestive of narcolepsy. In general, sleep latency values ≤5 minutes indicate severe, excessive sleepiness, and the majority of patients with narcolepsy or idiopathic hypersomnias have an average sleep latency ≤8 minutes, whereas values ≥15 minutes are considered normal [56]. Notably, while this test is extremely helpful in identifying subjects with narcolepsy, there is evidence that patients with psychiatric disorders who complain of excessive daytime sleepiness (EDS) often have relatively normal sleep latencies on MSLT [57].

The MWT measures the ability to stay awake while sitting in a quiet and dimly lit room for a period of time ranging from 20 to 40 minutes. As in the MSLT, four or five trials are performed about 2 hours apart. The 40-minute protocol is used to prevent ceiling effects, and a mean sleep latency >35 minutes is considered normal [55]. Although both tests measure sleep-onset latency, the MSLT reflects the tendency to fall asleep (sleepiness), while the MWT indicates the ability to stay awake in spite of sleep pressure levels (alertness). Results of these tests are used to help diagnose sleep disorders [58], evaluate their treatment [59], and to support recommendations to patients regarding daily activities that require an adequate level of vigilance, such as driving [60]. It is therefore critical to interpret the findings of these tests in light of the individual's prior sleep history. For example, short sleep latency values at the MSLT are irrelevant in cases where the patient is sleep-deprived [61]. Conversely, a careful assessment of the patient's sleep habits in the week preceding the tests as well as monitoring of the patient's sleep during an adaptation night in the sleep laboratory can maximize the clinical significance of these tests [62]. In some cases, patients may be asked to wear a device on their wrist that detects and records motion, a correlate of wakefulness, for several weeks before the laboratory test. This procedure (actigraphy) is sometimes also utilized to collect a longitudinal objective measure of sleep in subjects complaining of chronic insomnia [63]. Also, urine toxicology screening may be performed on the day of MSLT/MWT testing to document that the subject is not using stimulants to stay awake or illicit substances that can cause daytime sedation.

Organization of sleep
Sleep architecture

Sleep architecture refers to the organization of sleep across the recording period. Sleep recording is divided into 30-second epochs across the night, and each epoch is classified into a stage based on the predominant pattern (>50% of the epoch). Sleep stage scoring is a standardized procedure established about 40 years ago [12] and is still routinely employed, with some recent modifications [13], in clinical and research settings. Sleep scoring provides several measures of sleep quality and quantity. For example, sleep scoring quantifies the amount of time spent in each sleep stage. In a healthy young adult, NREM stage N1

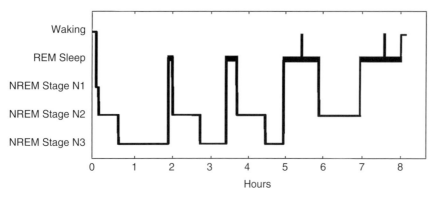

Figure 3.3 Hypnogram of a night of sleep in a healthy subject.

Table 3.2 Sleep architecture variables

Sleep architecture parameters	Definition
Total sleep time (minutes)	The amount of sleep time during the recording
Sleep onset latency (minutes)	The time from lights out to the onset of any sleep stage
Sleep efficiency (%)	The ratio of total sleep time to time in bed
Wake after sleep onset (minutes)	The amount of wake during the recording following the first sleep epoch

occupies about 5% of the total sleep time, stage N2 50–60%, and stage N3 20–25%, while REM sleep (stage R) accounts for the remaining 20–25%. Periods of NREM and REM alternate in a relatively predictable temporal pattern (approximately 90–120-minute intervals) through the course of the night, with the first REM period usually occurring about 70–100 minutes after sleep onset. SWS (stage N3) time peaks during the first sleep cycle, and markedly declines across the night. Conversely, as the night progresses, REM sleep episodes increase in length and are characterized by more intense dreaming as experienced subjectively [11] (Fig. 3.3). A number of sleep architecture parameters are typically calculated in clinical studies and research settings. These parameters are listed in Table 3.2.

Sleep architecture is fairly consistent in healthy adults, but changes significantly across the life-span [64], in psychiatric patients [65], or in subjects taking psychotropic medications [66].

Sleep changes across the life-cycle

The sleep–wake cycle begins in the second trimester of fetal life, and in the last trimester prior to birth and the first months of life sleep can be differentiated into active and quiet sleep, which are the precursors of REM and NREM sleep, respectively. Quiet (NREM) sleep is characterized by: even respiration; discontinuous EEG with bursts of high-amplitude delta frequency oscillations lasting 2–4 seconds; low-voltage, inter-burst activity in the theta range; and an absence of body or eye movements. Conversely, active (REM) sleep shows uneven respiration, continuous EEG activity, and atonia with frequent myoclonic jerks as well as rapid eye movements [67]. Newborns spend 16 to 18 hours per day sleeping; REM sleep represents about half of total sleep time, and tends to initiate each sleep episode [68]. After the first 3 months of life, infants start developing more adult-like sleep characteristics: (a) time spent in REM sleep decreases progressively; (b) sleep is initiated through NREM sleep at the beginning of each sleep cycle; (c) NREM stages differentiate; and (d) sleep spindles and slow waves emerge in the NREM sleep EEG [69].

Childhood is characterized by a reduction of REM sleep (from 50% to 20–25%), while SWS, which represents the deepest stage of NREM sleep, markedly increases and is accompanied by a higher arousal threshold [68]. This explains why children are difficult to awaken, especially at the beginning of the sleep period, and are prone to experience SWS-related sleep disorders, such as night terrors and somnambulism [70].

During adolescence, SWS decreases considerably, likely as a result of a neuronal regulatory process called synaptic pruning [71]. Synaptic pruning eliminates weak neuronal connections, making the brain more efficient and organized. Intriguingly, because of its critical role in shaping brain connectivity, it has been suggested that synaptic pruning abnormalities underlie the increased incidence of schizophrenia in adolescent/young adult individuals [72]. Adolescents also show a reduction in total sleep time, and a tendency of "eveningness" over "morningness," probably related to a shift in the intrinsic period of the circadian clock [73]. Healthy adults sleep about 8 hours per night, and their sleep period is usually divided into four NREM–REM sleep cycles. The amount of SWS progressively decreases across the adult life, while the duration of REM sleep is virtually unchanged.

In older individuals the presence of medical ailments as well as primary sleep disorders (e.g. sleep apnea) makes it more difficult to identify sleep changes related to "normal" aging. Elderly subjects show difficulty initiating and maintaining sleep, experience early awakenings, tend to nap during the daytime, and get sleepy earlier in the evening [64]. Altogether, ability to maintain consolidated sleep decreases with age, although it is unclear whether sleep need does. From early adulthood into late life SWS declines progressively from 20% to 3.5%, whereas REM sleep is only slightly reduced. However, older individuals with disorders of the central nervous system, including Alzheimer's disease and other dementias, show a significant decrease in REM sleep as well as fragmentation of the sleep–waking cycle [74].

Sleep architecture abnormalities in psychiatry

Sleep disturbances are often associated with psychiatric illnesses. Psychiatric patients often report sleep complaints, and sleep symptoms are part of the primary diagnostic criteria for several psychiatric disorders [65]. In an attempt to characterize the nature of this relationship better, numerous studies over the past 50 years have investigated the sleep EEG patterns of different psychiatric populations, and have consistently reported sleep architecture abnormalities in psychiatric patients [75] (Table 3.3).

The majority of sleep EEG studies have focused on patients with *major depressive disorders*, and have found three main abnormalities [76]: (1) reduced sleep continuity; (2) SWS deficits; and (3) REM sleep abnormalities. Reduced sleep continuity manifests in subjects with depression as longer sleep latency, increased waking periods after sleep onset, frequent early morning awakenings, decreased sleep efficiency, and less total sleep time compared to age-matched healthy controls. Depressed patients exhibit a reduction in total minutes of SWS [77] that is particularly evident during the first sleep cycle, when SWS activity in healthy subjects peaks. REM sleep abnormalities are present in patients with depression, who show reduced REM sleep latency, a longer first REM sleep episode, enhanced phasic REM activity, and increased total minutes of REM sleep [65,76]. Intriguingly, similar sleep architecture disturbances have been found in *bipolar patients*, during both manic and depressive episodes [78].

Anxiety disorders are the most common psychiatric illnesses and show a strong correlation with several sleep complaints, including insomnia [79]. The most consistent sleep abnormality found in *patients with anxiety disorders* is reduced sleep continuity, which manifests itself as increased sleep latency, and decreased sleep efficiency and total amount of sleep (see Table 3.3). Some studies focusing on subgroups of anxiety disorder patients have also reported REM sleep disturbances, including increased REM density (post-traumatic stress disorders) [80] and reduced REM sleep latency (obsessive-compulsive disorders) [81].

The study of sleep architecture in *schizophrenia patients* has a long history. Starting from the observation that dreaming and psychosis share common features, an early hypothesis suggested that schizophrenia was determined by a dysregulation of REM sleep [82]. Although this hypothesis has been discounted by subsequent studies, several REM abnormalities, including reduced REM latency [83], as well as a decrease in SWS time, have been found in patients with schizophrenia [84]. However, sleep disturbances other than reduced sleep continuity have shown high variability across studies [85].

Sleep patterns have been less extensively explored in other psychiatric disorders. Some studies have investigated the sleep EEG of *eating disorder patients*, who may report sleep disturbances including abnormal nocturnal eating behaviors. The main findings of these studies were sleep continuity decrements, reduced REM sleep latency, and excessive numbers of arousals from NREM sleep [86]. *Patients with substance abuse disorders* also frequently complain of sleep difficulties [87]. Most studies have been conducted in alcoholic patients, who have shown reduced sleep continuity, SWS (stage N3) deficits, decreased REM sleep latency, and increased REM percentage of total sleep time even after prolonged periods of sobriety [88].

Table 3.3 Sleep abnormalities in psychiatric disorders

Psychiatric diagnosis	Subjective complaints	Polysomnographic findings
Major depressive disorder	Difficulty falling asleep (initial insomnia), increased awakening at night/restless sleep (middle insomnia), and early morning awakening (terminal insomnia)	↓ Sleep continuity[1] (↑ SL[2], ↓ TST[3], ↓ SE[4]) ↓ SWS (stage N3) ↓ SWS % of TST ↓ REML[5] ↑ REMD[6] ↑ REM % of TST
Bipolar disorder	Decreased need for sleep in manic phase, increased sleep in depressed phase. Sleep deprivation associated with elevation in mood	Similar to major depressive disorder
Panic disorder (PD)	Nocturnal panic attacks: in 40–70% of PD patients, same symptoms of daytime episodes	Normal or ↓ sleep continuity[1]
Generalized anxiety disorder	Sleep-onset delay and sleep-maintenance insomnia	↓ Sleep continuity[1]
Post-traumatic stress disorder	Trauma-related dreams. Hyperarousability (insomnia)	↑ REMD[6] ↓ SWS (stage N3)
Obsessive-compulsive disorder	Initial insomnia caused by obsessions or compulsions	Normal or ↓ sleep continuity[1] Normal or ↓ REML[5]
Eating disorders	Insomnia (anorexia nervosa). Sleep-related eating (bulimia nervosa)	↓ Sleep continuity[1] Normal or ↓ REML[5]
Alcohol abuse	Insomnia. Light, fragmented sleep. Vivid dreaming (delirium)	↓ Sleep continuity[1] ↓ SWS (stage N3) ↑ REM % of TST
Schizophrenia	Severe early insomnia. Inversion of wake–sleep cycle. Polyphasic sleep pattern	↓ Sleep continuity[1] Normal or ↓ SWS (stage N3) Normal or ↓ REML[5], ↑ REMD[6]

Notes: [1] Sleep continuity: measures the ability to fall asleep (SL[2]) and remain asleep (TST[3], SE[4]).
[2] Sleep latency: the amount of time from "lights out" to the onset of sleep.
[3] Total sleep time: the amount of actual sleep time in a sleep period.
[4] Sleep efficiency: measured as the ratio between TST and time in bed.
[5] REM latency: the amount of time from sleep onset to the first REM epoch.
[6] REM density: the ratio of rapid eye movement activity to total REM sleep time.

Effects of medications on sleep architecture

Several medications that reach the central nervous system and affect brain function (i.e. psychoactive drugs) can alter sleep activity (Table 3.4). For example, *first-generation antiepileptic drugs* (AEDs) increase somnolence and may affect sleep architecture by increasing NREM stage N1 (phenytoin) or decreasing REM sleep (phenytoin, carbamazepine) [89]. *Newer AEDs* are relatively less sedating and have variable effects on sleep architecture, which may reflect heterogeneity in their mechanisms of action [90].

On the other hand, many *antidepressant agents* suppress REM sleep, resulting in dramatic reduction of REM sleep and prolongation of REM sleep latency. Monoamine oxidase inhibitors (MAOIs) show the strongest REM suppression effect [91], while tricyclic antidepressants (TCAs), selective-serotonin and serotonin-norepinephrine reuptake inhibitors (SSRIs and SNRIs) may cause a more moderate reduction in REM sleep, often associated with increased eye movement (REM density) during the REM episode [92]. Preclinical studies indicate that the mechanism of REM suppression is related to increased levels of serotonin and it is most likely mediated via post-synaptic 5-HT$_{1A}$ receptors [93]. In humans, selective serotonergic (5-HT$_{1A}$) agonists

Table 3.4 Effects of common psychoactive medications on sleep

Type of medication	Subtype	Sleep effects
Antiepileptic drugs (AEDs)	Older AEDs Carbamazepine Phenytoin Valproic acid	↑ Daytime somnolence ↓ REM sleep* ↓ SL[1], ↑ NREM Stage N1, ↓ REM sleep ↑ NREM Stage N1
	Newer AEDs Gabapentin Lamotrigine Tiagabine	No common effect on sleep ↓ Stage N1, ↑ SWS (Stage N3), ↑ REM sleep ↓ SWS, ↑ REM sleep ↑ SE[2], ↑ SWS
Antidepressant drugs	Tricyclic antidepressants Amitryptiline, nortryptiline, doxepin, clomipramine	↑ Sedation ↑ NREM Stage N2 ↓ REM sleep
	Monoamine oxidase inhibitors Phenelzine, tranylcypromine	↑ SL[1], ↓ TST[3], insomnia ↓ REM sleep
	Serotonin reuptake inhibitors	↑ SL[1], ↓ TST[3], insomnia ↓ REM sleep ↑ Eye movements in NREM
	Serotonin-norepinephrine reuptake inhibitors Venlafaxine, duloxetine	↑ SL[1], ↓ TST[3], insomnia ↓ REM sleep ↑ Eye movements in NREM
	Other antidepressants Trazodone Bupropion Mirtazipine	No common effect on sleep Sedation Insomnia/activation Sedation, ↓ REM sleep
Sedative/hypnotic drugs	Benzodiazepine receptor agonists Flurazepam, temazepam Lorazepam Triazolam Zolpidem	↑ Daytime somnolence ↑ NREM stage N2, ↓ SWS, ↓ REM sleep
Lithium		↑ Daytime somnolence ↑ TST[3] ↓ NREM stage N1 ↑ SWS ↓ REM sleep ↑ REM latency
Antipsychotic drugs	First-generation antipsychotics Chlorpromazine Haloperidol	↑ Daytime somnolence, ↑ TST[3] ↑ SE[2], ↑ REM latency
	Second-generation antipsychotics Clozapine Olanzapine Quetiapine Risperidone Ziprasidone	No common effect on sleep ↑ TST[3], ↑ SE[2], ↑ REM density ↓ SL[1], ↑ TST[3], ↑ SE[2], ↓ Stage N1, ↑ SWS ↓ SL[1], ↑ TST[3], ↑ SE[2] ↓ REM sleep ↑ TST[3], ↑ SE[2], ↑ REM latency
Nicotine		↓ TST[3] ↑ SL[1] ↓ REM sleep
Opioid drugs	Morphine, heroin, codeine	↑ Daytime somnolence ↓ TST[3], ↓ SC[4]

Table 3.4 (cont.)

Type of medication	Subtype	Sleep effects
Stimulant drugs	Amphetamines D-amphetamine, methamphetamine	↓ Daytime somnolence ↑ SL[1], ↓ TST[3] ↑ REM latency, ↓ REM sleep
	Xanthines Caffeine, theophylline	↓ Daytime somnolence ↑SL[1], ↓ TST[3], ↑ NREM stage N1
	Cocaine	↓ Daytime somnolence ↓ TST[3]
	Methylphenidate	↓ Daytime somnolence ↓ TST[3], ↓ SC[4] ↑ NREM stage N1, ↓ NREM Stage N2 ↑ REM latency, ↓ REM sleep

Notes: Bold items refer to classes of medications and to their class-specific sleep effects; non-bold items to specific agents within a class and to their agent-specific sleep effects.
*With short-term use only.
[1] SL: sleep latency.
[2] SE: sleep efficiency.
[3] TST: total sleep time.
[4] SC: sleep continuity.

strongly suppress REM [94]. Additionally, antidepressants that bind to serotonergic reuptake proteins (SSRIs and SNRIs) cause an increase in sleep latency and a reduced total sleep time, often accompanied by subjective complaints of insomnia, likely related to their activating effects on the brain [66]. The molecular mechanism underlying the differential effects of antidepressants on sleep continuity is still unclear. Different antagonism of H1 histaminergic or cholinergic receptors, or alterations in GABAergic activity have been proposed as possible explanations [95,96].

Hypnotic drugs, which are usually utilized to treat insomnia, improve several sleep continuity parameters (e.g. they decrease sleep latency, increase total sleep time). *Benzodiazepines* and *benzodiazepine receptor agonists* (*BzRAs*) are widely prescribed hypnotic agents, and generally have replaced *barbiturates* because of fewer side-effects [97]. In addition to improving sleep continuity, benzodiazepines and BzRAs increase NREM stage N2, whereas they dramatically reduce SWS (NREM stage N3) and REM sleep [98]. Benzodiazepines bind with various levels of affinity to GABA-A receptors, causing an increased flow of chloride ions into the neuron. As a result, the neuron is hyperpolarized, and its activity is reduced. BzRAs generally represent an improvement over benzodiazepines as a result of enhanced binding selectivity and pharmacokinetic

profiles. Another, newly discovered group of hypnotic drugs are the selective extrasynaptic GABA-A receptor agonists (SEGAs). Intriguingly, recent studies have shown that SEGAs, which target the synaptic junctions of thalamic and cortical neurons, can help regulate some sleep parameters, including sleep onset and maintenance [99].

Antipsychotic medications can facilitate sleep by: (1) attenuating psychotic symptoms, such as hallucinations and delusions; (2) reducing psychomotor agitation; and (3) increasing sedation through antagonistic effects on histaminergic, cholinergic, adrenergic, and dopaminergic receptors. The effects of these drugs on sleep architecture include reduced sleep latency and improved sleep continuity [100], with an increase in SWS reported with some agents [101] but not all [102]. In general antipsychotics (APs) improve sleep efficiency and have a strong sedative effect [103]. The lower sedation rates reported with some APs, including haloperidol and aripiprazole, are likely related to a stronger affinity for serotonin $5\text{-}HT_{2B}$ receptors, combined with a weaker affinity for dopaminergic D2 receptors.

Opioids have several clinical applications but are also drugs of abuse. Although the analgesic properties of these drugs permit sleep in patients with chronic pain or restless legs syndrome, repeated use of *morphine* or *heroin* may cause sleep disturbances such as reduction in total sleep and sleep continuity [7]. Similar effects on sleep are caused by *stimulants*, which include *caffeine, amphetamine,* or related compounds (i.e. *methylphenidate, cocaine*). Stimulants also increase wakefulness, prolong sleep latency, and decrease total sleep time, SWS (NREM stage N3), and REM sleep [104–106]. For a more detailed review of the effects of drugs of abuse/dependence on sleep, please refer to Chapter 19: Sleep in substance use disorders.

Applications of neuroimaging techniques in sleep medicine

Over the last two decades, several neuroimaging techniques, including positron emission tomography (PET), anatomical and functional magnetic resonance imaging (MRI and fMRI), magnetic resonance spectroscopy (MRS), single photon emission computed tomography (SPECT), and high-density electroencephalography (hd-EEG), have been increasingly utilized in research and clinical settings (Table 3.5). For example, neuroimaging techniques have been employed in a range of experimental conditions to further our understanding of normal brain activity during wakefulness. Additionally, given their ability to provide valuable information on brain activity changes in different states of vigilance (e.g. sleep–wake cycle) [8] as well as in various pathological conditions (e.g. psychiatric and sleep disorders) [107,108], these techniques have been used in sleep research to better characterize fundamental aspects of normal sleep and of sleep disruption. Some of these aspects include: (a) the functional neuroanatomy of sleep stages; (b) the relationship between waking neuronal plastic changes (e.g. learning tasks, sensory deprivation) and sleep; and (c) the effects of sleep deprivation on waking brain activities, especially on the neuronal circuits underlying key cognitive functions (e.g. memory, attention). The most relevant neuroimaging findings related to each of these aspects are reviewed below.

Functional neuroanatomy of sleep stages

Whereas traditional EEG recordings have revealed brain activity patterns characteristic of the sleep–wake cycle, neuroimaging studies employing PET and fMRI have significantly contributed to characterize the functional neuroanatomy underlying these EEG patterns. Specifically, these studies have shown that both global and local brain activity changes occur in sleep compared to waking and that different patterns of activity are present in REM and NREM sleep.

NREM sleep is characterized by a global reduction in brain metabolism and cerebral blood flow relative to waking, as well as a decrease in regional cerebral blood flow (rCBF) in several subcortical (dorsal pons, cerebellum, midbrain, basal ganglia, basal forebrain, thalamus) [109,111] and cortical regions (anterior cingulate, inferior parietal, dorsolateral prefrontal cortex) [110,112–114] (Figure 3.4). A recent meta-analysis of PET data has shown an inverse correlation between slow waves and the rCBF of all of these brain structures, with the exception of the thalamus [115]. Notably, these findings are consistent with evidence from electrophysiological studies showing that disruption of thalamocortical connections leaves the slow oscillation intact, whereas damaging corticocortical connections disrupts the synchronization of the slow oscillation [116,117].

Neuroimaging studies have also revealed that decreases in cortical rCBF during NREM sleep mainly occur in associative areas (dorsolateral prefrontal, orbitofrontal, and parietal cortices) and the precuneus [109,111,112], while primary cortices are the least affected [109] (Figure 3.4). The marked decrease of rCBF in the associative areas likely reflects the high level of activity of these areas during wakefulness, while the rCBF reduction in the precuneus possibly indicates the loss of wakefulness-promoting mechanisms, as suggested by the deactivation observed in the precuneus during states of decreased consciousness (vegetative state, anesthesia) [118].

A pivotal contribution to understanding the functional neuroanatomy of NREM sleep EEG rhythms, such as slow waves and sleep spindles, is expected from a newly introduced neuroimaging technique, EEG/fMRI. By recording EEG with simultaneous fMRI, this technique provides a unique opportunity to combine high spatial (fMRI) and temporal (EEG) resolution. For example, a recent EEG/fMRI study found that the thalamus, in combination with limbic areas and superior temporal gyri, was significantly activated during sleep in healthy subjects when sleep spindles occurred [119]. While several electrophysiological studies in animals had previously revealed that thalamic nuclei are critically involved in generating

Table 3.5 Neuroimaging techniques commonly utilized in sleep

Neuroimaging technique	Parameters measured	Clinical and research use	Advantages	Limitations
Magnetic resonance imaging (MRI)	Voxel-based morphometry (VBM)[1]	Examine gray/white matter changes related to aging, neurodegenerative, or other chronic diseases (dementia, schizophrenia) which affect brain tissues	High spatial resolution, automatic procedure faster than traditional morphometric analyses (ROI)[2]	Expensive, provide no functional data
Magnetic resonance spectroscopy (MRS)	Metabolite levels	Measure metabolite levels in tumors or other disorders (OSAS[3]) where metabolite deficits (i.e. choline) can occur	Combine anatomical and functional data, confirm involvement of certain metabolites in specific brain disorders	Expensive, lower spatial resolution than MRI
Functional magnetic resonance imaging (fMRI)	Blood-oxygen-level-dependent (BOLD[4]) signal	Assess BOLD (O_2 supply) changes in brain regions involved in cognitive tasks or affected by acute and chronic brain disorders	High spatial resolution, safe, non-invasive, allows repetitive measures within a session and over time	Low temporal resolution (~4 sec), indirect measure of neural activity
Single photon emission computed tomography (SPECT)	Regional cerebral blood flow (or rCBF[5], with ^{99m}Tc-HMPAO[6])	Diagnosis of dementia, rCBF changes in other chronic brain disorders	Inexpensive relative to other imaging tools, good spatial resolution	Poor temporal resolution (1 min), radiation exposure
Positron emission tomography (PET)	rCBF[5] (with ^{18}[F] DG, H_2^{15}O)[7] receptor binding (radioligands)[8]	Differentiate Alzheimer from other types of dementia, assess receptor deficits in psychiatric disorders	Less expensive than fMRI, good spatial resolution, imaging of neuroreceptors' activity	Low temporal resolution (40 sec), radiation exposure
High-density (hd)-EEG	EEG patterns during waking as well as sleep	Differentiate delirium from catatonia, identify seizures as well as other waking and sleep rhythm abnormalities	Exquisite temporal and good spatial resolution (relative to standard EEG), safe, inexpensive	Limited ability to localize cortical sources of activity and gather data from deep regions

Notes: [1] Identifies gray and white matters in all brain regions from high-resolution MRI scans.
[2] ROI: region of interests manually drawn on MRI scannings.
[3] OSAS: obstructive sleep apnea syndrome.
[4] BOLD: Measures the level of blood oxygenated hemoglobin, which increases with higher neural activity.
[5] rCBF: the blood supplied to the different brain regions in a given time.
[6] Technetium-hexamethylpropylene amine oxime = radiotracer which accumulates in brain regions proportional to blood flow.
[7] (^{18}Fluorodeoxyglucose, H_2^{15}O) = radiotracers which measure CBF to brain regions.
[8] These agents permit visualization of neuroreceptors in a plurality of neuropsychiatric illnesses.

sleep spindles [120], this study was the first to establish a similar role for the thalamus in humans. This study also characterized the brain areas that were specifically activated during slow (11–13 Hz) and fast (13–15 Hz) spindles, the superior frontal gyrus and the sensorimotor/hippocampal regions respectively, thus suggesting that these two spindle types might have different functional roles during NREM sleep [119].

In comparison to NREM sleep, REM sleep is characterized by an increase in neuronal activity, brain metabolism, and rCBF in the pons, midbrain,

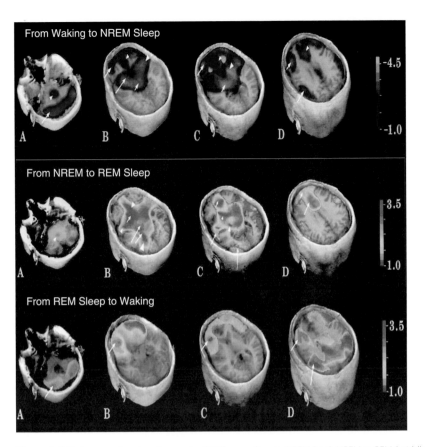

Figure 3.4 Brain maps showing changes in rCBF from waking to NREM (top), NREM to REM (middle), and REM to waking (bottom), measured with H$_2$^{15}O PET. *Top panel*: brain regions with decreased rCBF during NREM sleep compared with presleep wakefulness. The reduction is expressed in Z scores, ranging from −1 (light purple) to −4.5 (deep purple). Significant rCBF reductions were observed in the pons (A, arrowhead), midbrain (B, short arrow), basal ganglia (B, long arrow; C, medium arrowhead), thalamus (C, short arrow), caudal orbital cortex (B, small arrowhead), and cerebellum (A, arrow). Similar rCBF decreases were found in the anterior insula (B, medium arrowhead), anterior cingulate (C and D, small arrowheads), as well as in the orbital (B, medium arrow), dorsolateral prefrontal (C, medium arrow; D, small arrow), and inferior parietal lobes (D, medium arrow). *Middle panel*: brain regions with increased rCBF during REM sleep compared with NREM sleep. Z-scores values range from 1 (green) to 3.5 (red). Significant increases in rCBF during REM sleep were observed in the pons (A, arrowhead), midbrain (B, long arrow), basal ganglia (B, short arrow; C, small arrowhead), thalamus (C, medium arrowhead), and caudal orbital cortex (B, medium arrowhead). Increases were also found in anterior insula (B, small arrowhead), anterior cingulate (C, small arrow; D, medium arrow), mesial temporal (parahippocampal) (B, medium arrow), fusiform–inferotemporal (B, large arrowhead), lateral occipital (C, long arrow), auditory association (C, medium arrow), and medial prefrontal cortices (D, small arrow). *Bottom panel*: brain regions with rCBF increase during post-sleep wakefulness compared to REM sleep. Z-scores values are from 1 (green) to 3.5 (red). Significant increases in rCBF occurred in the orbital (B, small arrow), dorsolateral prefrontal (C and D, small arrows), and inferior parietal lobes (D, medium arrow), as well as in the cerebellar hemispheres (A, small arrow). Reproduced, with permission, from [2]. See plate section for color version.

basal ganglia, thalamus [109], amygdala, anterior cingulate, and temporal and orbito-medial prefrontal cortices [121] (Figure 3.4). Activation of the pons, the midbrain, and the thalamus during REM is consistent with electrophysiological evidence showing that REM activity is initiated by pontine cholinergic nuclei [122,123], which then induce widespread cortical activation through a dorsal (thalamic) and a ventral (midbrain) pathway [124,125]. Furthermore, electrophysiological studies in animals have shown an

involvement of neurons of the amygdala in generating ponto-geniculo-occipital (PGO) waves, key components of phasic REM sleep underlying rapid eye movements [126,127]. In humans, dreaming activity occurring during REM sleep is associated with an increased activation in the temporal cortex, in a region anatomically connected to the visual areas [113], as well as in the cingulate [113,128] and orbito-medial prefrontal cortices, both part of the limbic system. This pattern of activation may account for the visually vivid, emotionally laden conscious experience occurring during dreams [121].

Neuroimaging studies also demonstrate that several areas are significantly deactivated during REM sleep when compared to wakefulness, including the precuneus, the posterior cingulate, and the dorsolateral prefrontal and the inferior parietal cortices [109,129,130] (Figure 3.4). Specifically, PET data reveal that, in these brain regions, a decrease in rCBF occurs at the onset of NREM sleep, and remains constant during REM episodes. Deactivation of prefrontal areas during REM sleep has been confirmed by fMRI studies [131,132], and suggests that during REM sleep the brain is generally active with the exception of higher-order associative cortical areas. Intriguingly, these areas are involved in coherently integrating multimodal neural information and in planning behavioral output based on this information. Thus, a reduction in the activity of these areas during REM would explain the sense of "passivity" and "incongruity" that is often subjectively experienced while dreaming [133].

Neuroplasticity and sleep

Neuroimaging studies have begun to reveal the relationship between waking activities such as learning and memory, which induce brain plasticity, and sleep. For example, recent PET studies found that several brain areas, including sensorimotor, premotor, and anterior cingulate cortices, which were activated during a serial reaction time task, had higher rCBF and showed a stronger functional connectivity during REM sleep in previously trained, relative to untrained, subjects [134,135]. Furthermore, two fMRI studies that employed either motor-sequence memory [136] or visual texture discrimination [137] tasks reported that the brain areas involved in learning these tasks showed higher activity 12 hours after a training session in subjects who were allowed to sleep relative to the subjects who were kept awake. These findings suggest that neuronal plasticity occurring during waking has an effect on subsequent sleep and that sleep might have a role in modulating these plastic changes.

In this regard, the most direct evidence of the relationship between waking plastic changes and sleep regulation comes from several recent EEG studies [138–140]. By employing a 256-channel high-density EEG system, these studies have shown that changes in sleep activity, and particularly in local slow-wave activity (SWA) during NREM sleep, are highly sensitive markers of plastic changes in the cortex. For example, it was found that a brief (~1 hour), simple motor learning task induced an increase in the SWA of the involved parietal cortex [140] (Figure 3.5a); conversely, immobilization of the non-dominant (left) arm led to a decrease in SWA at the corresponding cortical region [139] (Figure 3.5b). Local increases in SWA were also found in healthy subjects following high-frequency (5 Hz) repetitive transcranial magnetic stimulation (rTMS), a paradigm known to induce potentiation [138] (Figure 3.5c), while in stroke patients with expressive (Broca's area) aphasia a 4-hour program of speech therapy produced focal increases in SWA in the perilesional area (Figure 3.5d). Additional findings from other EEG studies, showing local increases in SWA or sleep spindle activity that were significantly correlated with performance improvement in various learning and memory tasks, support the notion that sleep-specific rhythms contribute to neuroplasticity [141,142].

Effects of sleep deprivation

Sleep deprivation (SD) is a fairly common event that can be experienced sporadically (e.g. following traumatic events or periods of high stress) or chronically (e.g. living in a noisy environment or working under an irregular schedule) [8]. SD is also a leading cause of serious accidents, for instance at work or while driving, which can result in injuries or death [50,143]. While it is established that SD results in impaired cognitive functions, the effects of SD on waking brain activity are still largely unknown. However, several recent neuroimaging studies have begun addressing this issue. Specifically, these studies have investigated with imaging scans the cognitive functions of sleep-deprived healthy subjects, in order to identify the neuroanatomical correlates of both impaired cognitive performance and of possible compensatory mechanisms. The cognitive domains most characterized include working memory [144–150] and attention [151–153]. Other cognitive aspects, including inhibitory control [154] and emotional processing [155], have also been explored.

Working memory (WM) requires temporarily storing and manipulating information in specific brain areas. Neuroimaging studies have consistently shown an involvement of dorsolateral prefrontal [156] and parietal cortices [157] during WM tasks. However, the

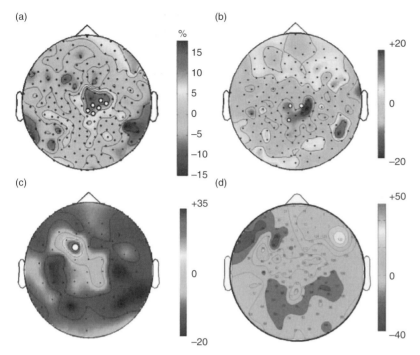

Figure 3.5 Cortical plasticity is reflected by local changes in SWA. In each panel regions with SWA increase are in red, while in blue are regions with SWA decrease. White circles indicate electrodes with significant SWA activity change. (a) Increased SWA after a rotation learning task. Six electrodes with significant differences from baseline located in the right sensorimotor area were found [3]. (b) Decreased SWA following left arm immobilization for one day was found in three electrodes in the right sensorimotor cortex [4]. (c) Increased SWA following rTMS of the left premotor cortex [5]. (d) Increased SWA at the right inferior frontal gyrus, symmetrical to Broca's area, in a stroke patient with expressive aphasia following 4 hours of speech therapy. See plate section for color version.

effects of SD on these cortical areas vary across studies as a result of multiple factors, including type of task, task difficulty, or interindividual variability. For example, it has been shown that, after SD, activation of the frontal and parietal cortices increases in experiments involving verbal learning [158,159], while it decreases in experiments involving serial subtraction [152,160]. Furthermore, a recent fMRI study reported that increasing the complexity of a verbal WM task elicited greater activation in prefrontal cortex after 24 hours of SD than after sleep, possibly reflecting a "compensatory" mechanism [161]. Additionally, two fMRI studies found that task-related activation of frontal and parietal areas before SD predicted the individual's reduction in task performance after SD (the lower the BOLD activation pre-SD, the worse the performance post-SD) [146,148], while another fMRI study found that 19 healthy subjects showed a decrease in task-related BOLD activation of parietal cortex after SD, which was correlated with their decline in task performance [144].

The effects of SD on attentional tasks and their neural correlates have been investigated in both PET and fMRI studies. The most consistently reported findings include an increase in the activation of sensory (and particularly visual) cortical areas and a reduced activation of the prefrontal cortex.

Specifically, an early [18] FDG PET study found that, after 32 hours of SD, the performance in an attentional task (detection of degraded visual targets) was significantly reduced from baseline while glucose metabolism (CMRGlu) was decreased in frontotemporal areas and increased in the visual cortex [153]. By employing different durations of SD (24, 48, and 72 hours) and a different visual attentional task (serial subtraction), another PET study reported a progressive increase of CMRGlu in visual areas from 24 to 72 hours of SD. The authors also reported a decrease in prefrontal cortex CMRGlu, which was larger after 48 or 72 hours of SD than after 24 hours of SD [152]. A similar, marked reduction in prefrontal activity following SD was found using the same visual attentional task in healthy subjects before and after 35 hours of SD [160]. However, other fMRI studies employing different attentional tasks (i.e. divided attention tasks [162] and psychomotor vigilance tests [151]) have shown an increase in prefrontal and parietal BOLD activity following SD, which has been explained as adaptive responses of the brain. Consistent with this interpretation, in these studies the cognitive performances were only slightly affected by SD. In sum, these neuroimaging findings suggest that prefrontal deactivation underlies SD-related attentional impairments, and that some of these deficits can be compensated for by enhanced activity in prefrontal, parietal, and visual cortical areas.

The ability to inhibit inappropriate responses (inhibitory efficiency) is reduced by sleep loss. The effect of SD on inhibitory efficiency varies across individuals [9]. In a recent fMRI study employing a go/no-go inhibitory task, the task-related activation of the anterior insula and ventral and anterior prefrontal cortices decreased in all participants after 24 hours of SD [154]. However, individuals who showed a lower no-go-related activation of the right inferior frontal region before SD performed better following SD (higher inhibitory efficiency). The authors suggested that these subjects were able to enhance the level of engagement of this region after SD, whereas the poor performers had already reached a "maximal" activation of this region before SD [154].

Sleep deprivation can also influence different aspects of emotion regulation, including the processing of emotionally salient stimuli and the modulation of emotional responses. A recent fMRI study has begun to reveal the neural effects of SD on emotional processing. Specifically, in this study it was found that amygdala activation to emotionally charged (aversive) pictures as well as its connectivity with the limbic system increased after SD, while the amygdala-medio-prefrontal (MPFC) connectivity was decreased relative to the normal sleep condition [155]. The combination of enhanced limbic-subcortical responses and reduced MPFC activation to aversive stimuli suggests a failure of top-down, prefrontal regulation of emotions after SD.

Conclusion

In this chapter we briefly reviewed the neurophysiology of normal human sleep, including the electrophysiological and neuroendocrine characteristics of the REM/NREM sleep stages, and described the electrophysiological assessment of sleep disorders with polysomnography (PSG). We also discussed the organization of sleep (sleep architecture) in young healthy adults, and reported the effects of age, psychiatric disorders, and psychoactive medications on sleep architecture. Finally, we presented several neuroimaging techniques, including fMRI, PET, and hd-EEG, which have been increasingly utilized in sleep research to explore the neuroanatomy of normal sleep and the effects of sleep deprivation on cognitive functions.

The science of sleep has progressed tremendously in the last 50 years, from the early description of NREM/REM sleep stages, through the investigation of sleep architecture in healthy subjects as well as in neuropsychiatric patients with various sleep disorders, and now to the study of the neural correlates of sleep activity with state-of-the-art neuroimaging techniques. In particular, the exquisite spatial and temporal resolution provided by neuroimaging tools such as fMRI and hd-EEG has recently enabled us to explore sleep activity in greater detail and to begin to address some of the fundamental questions regarding the function of sleep.

For example, what is the exact relationship between sleep and fundamental waking activities, such as memory and learning? Are local changes in sleep activity (occurring in the same area where waking plastic changes have taken place) more relevant to the function of sleep than the overall global activity? Are specific brain areas more in need of sleep, and therefore more sensitive to the effects of sleep deprivation? Are some sleep-specific rhythms (e.g. sleep slow waves, sleep spindles) more involved in implementing these waking-related plastic changes in the healthy brain? And are deficits in some of these sleep EEG rhythms relevant to the neurobiology of psychiatric disorders?

In general, the study of spontaneous neural activity during sleep offers some important advantages for investigating brain function in psychiatric patients. Sleep recordings minimize possible confounding factors related to waking activities, including changes in the level of attention, decreased motivation, or cognitive capacity, and the presence of active symptoms. Intriguingly, in a recent study employing hd-EEG during sleep it was found that sleep spindles were markedly reduced in schizophrenic patients compared to healthy subjects as well as psychiatric controls, and that these spindle activity deficits provided a 90% separation between schizophrenics and subjects from the other two groups [44]. These findings, whose relevance will be established by future studies on larger populations of psychiatric patients and healthy subjects, show the importance of sleep research in psychiatry, and underscore how imaging techniques applied to the sleeping brain may contribute not only to diagnoses but also, ultimately, to a better understanding of the neurobiology of neuropsychiatric disorders.

References

1. Greenspan RJ, Tononi G, Cirelli C, Shaw PJ. Sleep and the fruit fly. *Trends Neurosci.* 2001;**24**(3):142–145.

2. Banks S, Dinges DF. Behavioral and physiological consequences of sleep restriction. *J Clin Sleep Med.* 2007;**3**(5):519–528.

3. Aserinsky E. The discovery of REM sleep. *J Hist Neurosci.* 1996;**5**(3):213–227.

4. Kryger MH, Roth T, Dement WC. *Principles and practices of sleep medicine*, 3rd ed. Philadelphia: WB Saunders Co.; 2000.

5. Benca RM, Obermeyer WH, Thisted RA, Gillin JC. Meta-analysis of sleep changes in psychiatric disorders. *Sleep Res.* 1991;**20**:169.

6. Markov D, Goldman M. Normal sleep and circadian rhythms: neurobiologic mechanisms underlying sleep and wakefulness. *Psychiatr Clin North Am.* 2006; **29**(4):841–853; abstract vii.

7. Wang D, Teichtahl H. Opioids, sleep architecture and sleep-disordered breathing. *Sleep Med Rev.* 2007;**11** (1):35–46.

8. Dang-Vu TT, Desseilles M, Petit D,et al. Neuroimaging in sleep medicine. *Sleep Med.* 2007; **8**(4):349–372.

9. Chee MW, Chuah LY. Functional neuroimaging insights into how sleep and sleep deprivation affect memory and cognition. *Curr Opin Neurol.* 2008; **21**(4):417–423.

10. Boveroux P, Bonhomme V, Boly M, et al. Brain function in physiologically, pharmacologically, and pathologically altered states of consciousness. *Int Anesthesiol Clin.* 2008;**46**(3):131–146.

11. Hirshkowitz M. Normal human sleep: an overview. *Med Clin North Am.* 2004;**88**(3):551–565, vii.

12. Rechtschaffen A, Kales A. *A manual of standardized terminology, techniques, and scoring system for sleep stages of human subjects.* UCLA, Los Angeles: Brain Information Service/Brain Research Institute; 1968.

13. Silber MH, Ancoli-Israel S, Bonnet MH, et al. The visual scoring of sleep in adults. *J Clin Sleep Med.* 2007;**3**(2):121–131.

14. Trinder J, Kleiman J, Carrington M, et al. Autonomic activity during human sleep as a function of time and sleep stage. *J Sleep Res.* 2001;**10**(4):253–264.

15. Brandenberger G, Ehrhart J, Piquard F, Simon C. Inverse coupling between ultradian oscillations in delta wave activity and heart rate variability during sleep. *Clin Neurophysiol.* 2001;**112**(6):992–996.

16. Murali NS, Svatikova A, Somers VK. Cardiovascular physiology and sleep. *Front Biosci.* 2003;**8**:s636–652.

17. Tasali E, Leproult R, Ehrmann DA, Van Cauter E. Slow-wave sleep and the risk of type 2 diabetes in humans. *Proc Natl Acad Sci U S A.* 2008; **105**(3):1044–1049.

18. Vgontzas AN, Bixler EO, Papanicolaou DA, et al. Rapid eye movement sleep correlates with the overall activities of the hypothalamic-pituitary-adrenal axis and sympathetic system in healthy humans. *J Clin Endocrinol Metab.* 1997;**82**(10): 3278–3280.

19. Verrier RL, Muller JE, Hobson JA. Sleep, dreams, and sudden death: the case for sleep as an autonomic stress test for the heart. *Cardiovasc Res.* 1996; **31**(2):181–211.

20. Bankier B, Littman AB. Psychiatric disorders and coronary heart disease in women – a still neglected topic: review of the literature from 1971 to 2000. *Psychother Psychosom.* 2002;**71**(3): 133–140.

21. Penzel T, Wessel N, Riedl M, et al. Cardiovascular and respiratory dynamics during normal and pathological sleep. *Chaos.* 2007;**17**(1):015116.

22. Nattie E. CO2, brainstem chemoreceptors and breathing. *Prog Neurobiol.* 1999;**59**(4):299–331.

23. Owens RL, Eckert DJ, Yeh SY, Malhotra A. Upper airway function in the pathogenesis of obstructive sleep apnea: a review of the current literature. *Curr Opin Pulm Med.* 2008;**14**(6):519–524.

24. Lack LC, Gradisar M, Van Someren EJ, Wright HR, Lushington K. The relationship between insomnia and body temperatures. *Sleep Med Rev.* 2008; **12**(4):307–317.

25. Krauchi K. The human sleep-wake cycle reconsidered from a thermoregulatory point of view. *Physiol Behav.* 2007;**90**(2–3):236–245.

26. Gutierrez E, Vazquez R, Boakes RA. Activity-based anorexia: ambient temperature has been a neglected factor. *Psychon Bull Rev.* 2002;**9**(2):239–249.

27. Nobili L, Baglietto MG, Beelke M, et al. Impairment of the production of delta sleep in anorectic adolescents. *Sleep.* 2004;**27**(8):1553–1559.

28. Obal F Jr, Krueger JM. GHRH and sleep. *Sleep Med Rev.* 2004;**8**(5):367–377.

29. Freeman ME, Kanyicska B, Lerant A, Nagy G. Prolactin: structure, function, and regulation of secretion. *Physiol Rev.* 2000;**80**(4):1523–1631.

30. Van Cauter E, Plat L, Copinschi G. Interrelations between sleep and the somatotropic axis. *Sleep.* 1998; **21**(6):553–566.

31. Roky R, Obal F Jr, Valatx JL, et al. Prolactin and rapid eye movement sleep regulation. *Sleep.* 1995; **18**(7):536–542.

32. Wagner U, Born J. Memory consolidation during sleep: interactive effects of sleep stages and HPA regulation. *Stress.* 2008;**11**(1):28–41.

33. Luboshitzky R. Endocrine activity during sleep. *J Pediatr Endocrinol Metab.* 2000;**13**(1):13–20.

34. Krauchi K, Cajochen C, Pache M, Flammer J, Wirz-Justice A. Thermoregulatory effects of melatonin in relation to sleepiness. *Chronobiol Int.* 2006;**23**(1–2):475–484.

35. Czeisler CA, Klerman EB. Circadian and sleep-dependent regulation of hormone release in humans. *Recent Prog Horm Res.* 1999;**54**:97–130; discussion 130–132.

36. Clark RW, Schmidt HS, Malarkey WB. Disordered growth hormone and prolactin secretion in primary disorders of sleep. *Neurology.* 1979;**29**(6):855–861.

37. Knutson KL, Van Cauter E. Associations between sleep loss and increased risk of obesity and diabetes. *Ann N Y Acad Sci.* 2008;**1129**:287–304.

38. Van Cauter E, Knutson KL. Sleep and the epidemic of obesity in children and adults. *Eur J Endocrinol.* 2008;**159**(Suppl 1):S59–66.

39. Schmidt MH, Schmidt HS. Sleep-related erections: neural mechanisms and clinical significance. *Curr Neurol Neurosci Rep.* 2004;**4**(2):170–178.

40. Morales A, Condra M, Reid K. The role of nocturnal penile tumescence monitoring in the diagnosis of impotence: a review. *J Urol.* 1990;**143**(3):441–446.

41. Abel GG, Murphy WD, Becker JV, Bitar A. Women's vaginal responses during REM Sleep. *J Sex Marital Ther.* 1979;**5**(1):5–14.

42. Berger H. [Uber das Elektrenkephalogramm des Menschen]. *Archiv fur Psychiatrie und Nervenkrankheiten.* 1929;**87**:527–580.

43. Myslobodsky MS, Coppola R, Bar-Ziv J, Weinberger DR. Adequacy of the International 10–20 electrode system for computed neurophysiologic topography. *J Clin Neurophysiol.* 1990;**7**(4):507–518.

44. Ferrarelli F, Huber R, Peterson MJ, et al. Reduced sleep spindle activity in schizophrenia patients. *Am J Psychiatry.* 2007;**164**(3):483–492.

45. Littner M, Hirshkowitz M, Kramer M, et al. Practice parameters for using polysomnography to evaluate insomnia: an update. *Sleep.* 2003;**26**(6):754–760.

46. Kushida CA, Littner MR, Morgenthaler T, et al. Practice parameters for the indications for polysomnography and related procedures: an update for 2005. *Sleep.* 2005;**28**(4):499–521.

47. Bixler EO, Kales A, Soldatos CR, Kales JD, Healey S. Prevalence of sleep disorders in the Los Angeles metropolitan area. *Am J Psychiatry.* 1979;**136**(10):1257–1262.

48. Guilleminault C, Cummiskey J, Dement WC. Sleep apnea syndrome: recent advances. *Adv Intern Med.* 1980;**26**:347–372.

49. Guilleminault C, Dement WC. 235 cases of excessive daytime sleepiness: diagnosis and tentative classification. *J Neurol Sci.* 1977;**31**(1):13–27.

50. Mitler MM, Carskadon MA, Czeisler CA, et al. Catastrophes, sleep, and public policy: consensus report. *Sleep.* 1988;**11**(1):100–109.

51. Hoddes E, Zarcone V, Smythe H, Phillips R, Dement WC. Quantification of sleepiness: a new approach. *Psychophysiology.* 1973;**10**(4):431–436.

52. Johns MW. A new method for measuring daytime sleepiness: the Epworth sleepiness scale. *Sleep.* 1991;**14**(6):540–545.

53. Benca R, Kwapil TR. Sleep disorders measures. In: *Handbook of psychiatric measures.* Washington, DC: American Psychiatric Association; 2000:673–685.

54. Carskadon MA, Dement WC. The multiple sleep latency test: what does it measure? *Sleep.* 1982;**5**(Suppl 2):S67–72.

55. Mitler MM, Gujavarty KS, Browman CP. Maintenance of wakefulness test: a polysomnographic technique for evaluation treatment efficacy in patients with excessive somnolence. *Electroencephalogr Clin Neurophysiol.* 1982;**53**(6):658–661.

56. Carskadon MA, Dement WC, Mitler MM, et al. Guidelines for the multiple sleep latency test (MSLT): a standard measure of sleepiness. *Sleep.* 1986;**9**(4):519–524.

57. Billiard M, Partinen M, Roth T, Shapiro C. Sleep and psychiatric disorders. *J Psychosom Res.* 1994;**38**(Suppl 1):1–2.

58. van den Hoed J, Kraemer H, Guilleminault C, et al. Disorders of excessive daytime somnolence: polygraphic and clinical data for 100 patients. *Sleep.* 1981;**4**(1):23–37.

59. Guilleminault C, Dement WC. Sleep apnea syndromes and related sleep disorders. In: Williams RL, Karacan I, eds. *Sleep disorders: diagnosis and treatment.* New York: John Wiley & Sons; 1978:9–28.

60. Thorpy MJ. The clinical use of the Multiple Sleep Latency Test. The Standards of Practice Committee of the American Sleep Disorders Association. *Sleep.* 1992;**15**(3):268–276.

61. Rosenthal L, Roehrs TA, Rosen A, Roth T. Level of sleepiness and total sleep time following various time in bed conditions. *Sleep*. 1993;**16**(3):226–232.

62. Arand D, Bonnet M, Hurwitz T, et al. The clinical use of the MSLT and MWT. *Sleep*. 2005; **28**(1):123–144.

63. Buysse DJ, Ancoli-Israel S, Edinger JD, Lichstein KL, Morin CM. Recommendations for a standard research assessment of insomnia. *Sleep*. 2006;**29**(9): 1155–1173.

64. Espiritu JR. Aging-related sleep changes. *Clin Geriatr Med*. 2008;**24**(1):1–14, v.

65. Benca RM, Obermeyer WH, Thisted RA, Gillin JC. Sleep and psychiatric disorders: a meta-analysis. *Arch Gen Psychiatry*. 1992;**49**:651–668.

66. Obermeyer WH, Benca RM. Effects of drugs on sleep [Review]. *Neurol Clin North Am*. 1996;**14**(4):827–840.

67. Peirano P, Algarin C, Uauy R. Sleep-wake states and their regulatory mechanisms throughout early human development. *J Pediatr*. 2003;**143**(4 Suppl):S70–79.

68. Davis KF, Parker KP, Montgomery GL. Sleep in infants and young children: Part one: normal sleep. *J Pediatr Health Care*. 2004;**18**(2):65–71.

69. Grigg-Damberger M, Gozal D, Marcus CL, et al. The visual scoring of sleep and arousal in infants and children. *J Clin Sleep Med*. 2007;**3**(2):201–240.

70. Davis KF, Parker KP, Montgomery GL. Sleep in infants and young children: part two: common sleep problems. *J Pediatr Health Care*. 2004;**18**(3): 130–137.

71. Feinberg I, Higgins LM, Khaw WY, Campbell IG. The adolescent decline of NREM delta, an indicator of brain maturation, is linked to age and sex but not to pubertal stage. *Am J Physiol Regul Integr Comp Physiol*. 2006;**291**(6):R1724–1729.

72. Feinberg I. Schizophrenia: caused by a fault in programmed synaptic elimination during adolescence? *J Psychiatr Res*. 1982;**17**(4):319–334.

73. Diaz-Morales JF, Gutierrez Sorroche M. Morningness-eveningness in adolescents. *Span J Psychol*. 2008; **11**(1):201–206.

74. Bliwise DL. Sleep disorders in Alzheimer's disease and other dementias. *Clin Cornerstone*. 2004; **6**(Suppl 1A):S16–28.

75. Krystal AD, Thakur M, Roth T. Sleep disturbance in psychiatric disorders: effects on function and quality of life in mood disorders, alcoholism, and schizophrenia. *Ann Clin Psychiatry*. 2008;**20**(1):39–46.

76. Kupfer DJ. Sleep research in depressive illness: clinical implications – a tasting menu [Review]. *Biol Psychiatry*. 1995;**38**(6):391–403.

77. Kupfer DJ, Reynolds CF III, Ulrich RF, Grochocinski VJ. Comparison of automated REM and slow-wave sleep analysis in young and middle-aged depressed subjects. *Biol Psychiatry*. 1986;**21**:189–200.

78. Hudson JI, Lipinski JF, Keck PE, et al. Polysomnographic characteristics of young manic patients: comparison with unipolar depressed patients and normal control subjects. *Arch Gen Psychiatry*. 1992;**49**:378–383.

79. Mellman TA. Sleep and anxiety disorders. *Psychiatr Clin North Am*. 2006;**29**(4):1047–1058; abstract x.

80. Ross RJ, Ball WA, Dinges DF, et al. Rapid eye movement sleep disturbance in posttraumatic stress disorder. *Biol Psychiatry*. 1994;**35**:195–202.

81. Insel TR, Gillin JC, Moore A, et al. The sleep of patients with obsessive-compulsive disorder. *Arch Gen Psychiatry*. 1982;**39**:1372–1377.

82. Hendrick I. Dream resistance and schizophrenia. *J Am Psychoanal Assoc*. 1958;**6**(4):672–690.

83. Benson KL, Zarcone VP Jr. Low REM latency in schizophrenia. *Sleep Res*. 1985;**14**:124.

84. Hiatt JF, Floyd TC, Katz PH, Feinberg I. Further evidence of abnormal non-rapid-eye-movement sleep in schizophrenia. *Arch Gen Psychiatry*. 1985;**42**:797–802.

85. Monti JM, Monti D. Sleep disturbance in schizophrenia. *Int Rev Psychiatry*. 2005;**17**(4):247–253.

86. Schenck CH, Hurwitz TD, Bundlie SR, Mahowald MW. Sleep-related eating disorders: polysomnographic correlates of a heterogeneous syndrome distinct from daytime eating disorders. *Sleep*. 1991;**14**(5): 419–431.

87. Brower KJ, Aldrich MS, Robinson EA, Zucker RA, Greden JF. Insomnia, self-medication, and relapse to alcoholism. *Am J Psychiatry*. 2001;**158**(3):399–404.

88. Crum RM, Ford DE, Storr CL, Chan YF. Association of sleep disturbance with chronicity and remission of alcohol dependence: data from a population-based prospective study. *Alcohol Clin Exp Res*. 2004; **28**(10):1533–1540.

89. Placidi F, Scalise A, Marciani MG, et al. Effect of antiepileptic drugs on sleep. *Clin Neurophysiol*. 2000;**111**(Suppl 2):S115–119.

90. Bazil CW. Effects of antiepileptic drugs on sleep structure: are all drugs equal? *CNS Drugs*. 2003; **17**(10):719–728.

91. Cohen RM, Pickar D, Garnett D, et al. REM suppression induced by selective monoamine oxidase inhibitors. *Psychopharmacology*. 1982;**78**:137–140.

92. Gervasoni D, Panconi E, Henninot V, et al. Effect of chronic treatment with milnacipran on sleep architecture in rats compared with paroxetine and

imipramine. *Pharmacol Biochem Behav*. 2002;
73(3):557–563.

93. Monaca C, Boutrel B, Hen R, Hamon M, Adrien J. 5-HT 1A/1B receptor-mediated effects of the selective serotonin reuptake inhibitor, citalopram, on sleep: studies in 5-HT 1A and 5-HT 1B knockout mice. *Neuropsychopharmacology*. 2003;**28**(5):850–856.

94. Gillin JC, Jernajczyk W, Valladares-Neto DC, et al. Inhibition of REM sleep by ipsapirone, a 5HT1A agonist, in normal volunteers. *Psychopharmacology (Berl)*. 1994;**116**(4):433–436.

95. Haas H, Panula P. The role of histamine and the tuberomammillary nucleus in the nervous system. *Nat Rev Neurosci*. 2003;**4**(2):121–130.

96. Parent MB, Master S, Kashlub S, Baker GB. Effects of the antidepressant/antipanic drug phenelzine and its putative metabolite phenylethylidenehydrazine on extracellular gamma-aminobutyric acid levels in the striatum. *Biochem Pharmacol*. 2002;**63**(1):57–64.

97. Linnoila M, Erwin CW, Logue PE. Efficacy and side effects of flurazepam and a combination of amobarbital and secobarbital in insomniac patients. *J Clin Pharmacol*. 1980;**20**:117–123.

98. Benca RM. Diagnosis and treatment of chronic insomnia: a review. *Psychiatr Serv*. 2005; **56**(3):332–343.

99. Ebert B, Wafford KA, Deacon S. Treating insomnia: current and investigational pharmacological approaches. *Pharmacol Ther*. 2006; **112**(3):612–629.

100. Taylor SF, Tandon R, Shipley JE, Eiser AS. Effect of neuroleptic treatment on polysomnographic measures in schizophrenia. *Biol Psychiatry*. 1991; **30**(9):904–912.

101. Sharpley AL, Vassallo CM, Cowen PJ. Olanzapine increases slow-wave sleep: evidence for blockade of central 5-HT(2C) receptors in vivo. *Biol Psychiatry*. 2000;**47**(5):468–470.

102. Krystal AD, Goforth HW, Roth T. Effects of antipsychotic medications on sleep in schizophrenia. *Int Clin Psychopharmacol*. 2008;**23**(3):150–160.

103. Benson KL. Sleep in schizophrenia: impairments, correlates, and treatment. *Psychiatr Clin North Am*. 2006;**29**(4):1033–1045; abstract ix–x.

104. Bonnet MH, Balkin TJ, Dinges DF, et al. The use of stimulants to modify performance during sleep loss: a review by the Sleep Deprivation and Stimulant Task Force of the American Academy of Sleep Medicine. *Sleep*. 2005;**28**(9):1163–1187.

105. Mitler MM, Hajdukovic R. Relative efficacy of drugs for the treatment of sleepiness in narcolepsy. *Sleep*. 1991;**14**(3):218–220.

106. Nicholson AN, Stone BM. Heterocyclic amphetamine derivatives and caffeine on sleep in man. *Br J Clin Pharmacol*. 1980;**9**:195–203.

107. McGuire P, Howes OD, Stone J, Fusar-Poli P. Functional neuroimaging in schizophrenia: diagnosis and drug discovery. *Trends Pharmacol Sci*. 2008; **29**(2):91–98.

108. Nofzinger EA. What can neuroimaging findings tell us about sleep disorders? *Sleep Med* 2004; 5(Suppl 1):S16–22.

109. Braun AR, Balkin TJ, Wesenten NJ, et al. Regional cerebral blood flow throughout the sleep-wake cycle. An H2(15)O PET study. *Brain*. 1997;**120**(Pt 7): 1173–1197.

110. Kajimura N, Uchiyama M, Takayama Y, et al. Activity of midbrain reticular formation and neocortex during the progression of human non-rapid eye movement sleep. *J Neurosci*. 1999;**19**(22):10065–10073.

111. Maquet P, Degueldre C, Delfiore G, et al. Functional neuroanatomy of human slow wave sleep. *J Neurosci*. 1997;**17**(8):2807–2812.

112. Andersson JL, Onoe H, Hetta J, et al. Brain networks affected by synchronized sleep visualized by positron emission tomography. *J Cereb Blood Flow Metab*. 1998;**18**(7):701–715.

113. Braun AR, Balkin TJ, Wesensten NJ, et al. Regional cerebral blood flow throughout the sleep-wake cycle. *Brain*. 1997;**120**:1173–1197.

114. Braun AR, Balkin TJ, Wesensten NJ, et al. Dissociated pattern of activity in visual cortices and their projections during human rapid eye movement sleep. *Science*. 1998;**279**(5347):91–95.

115. Dang-Vu TT, Desseilles M, Laureys S, et al. Cerebral correlates of delta waves during non-REM sleep revisited. *Neuroimage*. 2005;**28**(1):14–21.

116. Amzica F, Steriade M. Disconnection of intracortical synaptic linkages disrupts synchronization of a slow oscillation. *J Neurosci*. 1995;**15**(6):4658–4677.

117. Steriade M. The corticothalamic system in sleep. *Front Biosci*. 2003;**8**:D878–899.

118. Cavanna AE. The precuneus and consciousness. *CNS Spectr*. 2007;**12**(7):545–552.

119. Schabus M, Dang-Vu TT, Albouy G, et al. Hemodynamic cerebral correlates of sleep spindles during human non-rapid eye movement sleep. *Proc Natl Acad Sci U S A*. 2007;**104**(32):13164–13169.

120. Steriade M, McCormick DA, Sejnowski TJ. Thalamocortical oscillations in the sleeping and aroused brain. *Science*. 1993;**262**(5134): 679–685.

121. Maquet P, Peters J, Aerts J, et al. Functional neuroanatomy of human rapid-eye-movement sleep and dreaming. *Nature*. 1996;**383**(6596):163–166.

122. Datta S. Neuronal activity in the peribrachial area: relationship to behavioral state control. *Neurosci Biobehav Rev*. 1995;**19**(1):67–84.

123. Marini G, Gritti I, Mancia M. Enhancement of tonic and phasic events of rapid eye movement sleep following bilateral ibotenic acid injections into centralis lateralis thalamic nucleus of cats. *Neuroscience*. 1992;**48**(4):877–888.

124. Jones BE. Basic mechanisms of sleep-wake states. In: Kryger MH, Roth T, Dement WC, eds. *Principles and practice of sleep medicine*, 3rd ed. Philadelphia: WB Saunders Co.; 2000:134–154.

125. Steriade M, Datta S, Pare D, Oakson G, Curro Dossi RC. Neuronal activities in brain-stem cholinergic nuclei related to tonic activation processes in thalamocortical systems. *J Neurosci* 1990; **10**:2541–2559.

126. Calvo JM, Badillo S, Morales-Ramirez M, Palacios-Salas P. The role of the temporal lobe amygdala in ponto-geniculo-occipital activity and sleep organization in cats. *Brain Res*. 1987; **403**(1):22–30.

127. Calvo JM, Simon-Arceo K, Fernandez-Mas R. Prolonged enhancement of REM sleep produced by carbachol microinjection into the amygdala. *Neuroreport*. 1996;**7**(2):577–580.

128. Nofzinger E, Mintun M, Wiseman M, Kupfer D, Moore R. Forebrain activation in REM sleep: an FDG PET study. *Brain Res*. 1997;**770**(1–2):192–201.

129. Maquet P, Peters JM, Aerts J, et al. Functional neuroanatomy of human rapid-eye-movement sleep and dreaming. *Nature*. 1996;**383**:163–166.

130. Maquet P, Ruby P, Maudoux A, et al. Human cognition during REM sleep and the activity profile within frontal and parietal cortices: a reappraisal of functional neuroimaging data. *Prog Brain Res*. 2005;**150**:219–227.

131. Fuller PM, Saper CB, Lu J. The pontine REM switch: past and present. *J Physiol*. 2007;**584**(Pt 3): 735–741.

132. Lovblad KO, Thomas R, Jakob PM, et al. Silent functional magnetic resonance imaging demonstrates focal activation in rapid eye movement sleep. *Neurology*. 1999;**53**(9):2193–2195.

133. Hobson JA, Pace-Schott EF. The cognitive neuroscience of sleep: neuronal systems, consciousness and learning. *Nat Rev Neurosci*. 2002;**3**(9):679–693.

134. Maquet P. The role of sleep in learning and memory. *Science*. 2001;**294**(5544):1048–1052.

135. Maquet P, Laureys S, Peigneux P, et al. Experience-dependent changes in cerebral activation during human REM sleep. *Nat Neurosci*. 2000;**3**(8):831–836.

136. Walker MP, Stickgold R, Alsop D, Gaab N, Schlaug G. Sleep-dependent motor memory plasticity in the human brain. *Neuroscience*. 2005;**133**(4):911–917.

137. Walker MP, Stickgold R, Jolesz FA, Yoo SS. The functional anatomy of sleep-dependent visual skill learning. *Cereb Cortex*. 2005;**15**(11):1666–1675.

138. Huber R, Esser SK, Ferrarelli F, et al. TMS-induced cortical potentiation during wakefulness locally increases slow wave activity during sleep. *PLoS ONE*. 2007;**2**(3):e276.

139. Huber R, Ghilardi MF, Massimini M, et al. Arm immobilization causes cortical plastic changes and locally decreases sleep slow wave activity. *Nat Neurosci*. 2006;**9**(9):1169–1176.

140. Huber R, Ghilardi MF, Massimini M, Tononi G. Local sleep and learning. *Nature*. 2004;**430**(6995):78–81.

141. Walker MP, Stickgold R. Sleep, memory, and plasticity. *Annu Rev Psychol*. 2006;**57**:139–166.

142. Tononi G, Cirelli C. Some considerations on sleep and neural plasticity. *Arch Ital Biol*. 2001;**139**(3):221–241.

143. Horne JA, Reyner LA. Sleep related vehicle accidents. *BMJ*. 1995;**310**(6979):565–567.

144. Lim J, Choo WC, Chee MW. Reproducibility of changes in behaviour and fMRI activation associated with sleep deprivation in a working memory task. *Sleep*. 2007;**30**(1):61–70.

145. Chee MW, Chuah LY, Venkatraman V, et al. Functional imaging of working memory following normal sleep and after 24 and 35 h of sleep deprivation: Correlations of fronto-parietal activation with performance. *Neuroimage*. 2006;**31**(1):419–428.

146. Mu Q, Mishory A, Johnson KA, et al. Decreased brain activation during a working memory task at rested baseline is associated with vulnerability to sleep deprivation. *Sleep*. 2005;**28**(4):433–446.

147. Choo WC, Lee WW, Venkatraman V, Sheu FS, Chee MW. Dissociation of cortical regions modulated by both working memory load and sleep deprivation and by sleep deprivation alone. *Neuroimage*. 2005;**25** (2):579–587.

148. Caldwell JA, Mu Q, Smith JK, et al. Are individual differences in fatigue vulnerability related to baseline differences in cortical activation? *Behav Neurosci*. 2005;**119**(3):694–707.

149. Habeck C, Rakitin BC, Moeller J, et al. An event-related fMRI study of the neurobehavioral impact of sleep deprivation on performance of a delayed-match-to-sample task. *Brain Res Cogn Brain Res*. 2004;**18**(3): 306–321.

150. Bell-McGinty S, Habeck C, Hilton HJ, et al. Identification and differential vulnerability of a neural network in sleep deprivation. *Cereb Cortex*. 2004; **14**(5):496–502.

151. Drummond SP, Bischoff-Grethe A, Dinges DF, et al. The neural basis of the psychomotor vigilance task. *Sleep*. 2005;**28**(9):1059–1068.

152. Thomas M, Sing H, Belenky G, et al. Neural basis of alertness and cognitive performance impairments during sleepiness. I. Effects of 24 h of sleep deprivation on waking human regional brain activity. *J Sleep Res*. 2000;**9**(4):335–352.

153. Wu JC, Gillin JC, Buchsbaum MS, et al. The effect of sleep deprivation on cerebral glucose metabolic rate in normal humans assessed with positron emission tomography. *Sleep*. 1991;**14**(2):155–162.

154. Chuah YM, Venkatraman V, Dinges DF, Chee MW. The neural basis of interindividual variability in inhibitory efficiency after sleep deprivation. *J Neurosci*. 2006;**26**(27):7156–7162.

155. Yoo SS, Gujar N, Hu P, Jolesz FA, Walker MP. The human emotional brain without sleep – a prefrontal amygdala disconnect. *Curr Biol*. 2007; **17**(20):R877–878.

156. Curtis CE, D'Esposito M. Persistent activity in the prefrontal cortex during working memory. *Trends Cogn Sci*. 2003;**7**(9):415–423.

157. Pessoa L, Gutierrez E, Bandettini P, Ungerleider L. Neural correlates of visual working memory: fMRI amplitude predicts task performance. *Neuron*. 2002; **35**(5):975–987.

158. Drummond SP, Brown GG. The effects of total sleep deprivation on cerebral responses to cognitive performance. *Neuropsychopharmacology*. 2001; **25**(5 Suppl):S68–73.

159. Drummond SP, Brown GG, Gillin JC, Stricker JL, Wong EC, Buxton RB. Altered brain response to verbal learning following sleep deprivation [see comments]. *Nature*. 2000;**403**(6770):655–657.

160. Drummond SP, Brown GG, Stricker JL, Buxton RB, Wong EC, Gillin JC. Sleep deprivation-induced reduction in cortical functional response to serial subtraction. *Neuroreport*. 1999;**10**(18):3745–3748.

161. Chee MW, Choo WC. Functional imaging of working memory after 24 hr of total sleep deprivation. *J Neurosci*. 2004;**24**(19):4560–4567.

162. Drummond SP, Gillin JC, Brown GG. Increased cerebral response during a divided attention task following sleep deprivation. *J Sleep Res*. 2001;**10**(2):85–92.

Figure citations (see color plate section)

1. Ferrarelli F, Huber R, Peterson MJ, et al. Reduced sleep spindle activity in schizophrenia patients. *Am J Psychiatry*. 2007;**164**(3):483–492.

2. Braun AR, Balkin TJ, Wesenten NJ, et al. Regional cerebral blood flow throughout the sleep-wake cycle: An H2(15)O PET study. *Brain*. 1997; **120**(Pt 7):1173–1197.

3. Huber R, Ghilardi MF, Massimini M, Tononi G. Local sleep and learning. *Nature*. 2004;**430**(6995): 78–81.

4. Huber R, Ghilardi MF, Massimini M, et al. Arm immobilization causes cortical plastic changes and locally decreases sleep slow wave activity. *Nat Neurosci* 2006;**9**:1169–1176.

5. Huber R, Esser SK, Ferrarelli F, Massimini M, Peterson MJ, Tononi G. TMS-induced cortical potentiation during wakefulness locally increases slow wave activity during sleep. *PLoS ONE*. 2007;**2**(3):e276.

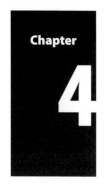

Chapter

4

The function(s) of sleep

Marcos G. Frank

Introduction

In the last few decades, scientists have made extraordinary progress characterizing the neurobiology [1], regulatory mechanisms [2], and genetic underpinnings of mammalian sleep [3]. Yet despite these great advances, the most fundamental question about sleep is still unanswered. *Why animals sleep* remains one of Nature's greatest unsolved mysteries. There are several reasons why this is more than just an embarrassing omission in the field. Far from being a trivial behavior, sleep with a few possible exceptions [4] is abundant in the animal kingdom [5] and comprises about one-third of human existence [6]. When animals sleep, they do so at the expense of clearly adaptive behaviors (eating, mating, defending territory) and put themselves at risk for predation. In humans, sleep is characterized by profound changes in somatic and neural physiology and its disruption is associated with physical and cognitive deficits and disease [7,8,9,10,11]. Therefore, our continued ignorance about sleep function presents a major impediment to our understanding of physiology, neurobiology, animal behavior, and sleep medicine.

In this chapter, I discuss the current status of this central problem in the field of sleep biology. I begin by discussing key concepts and theoretical issues that should be kept in mind when evaluating theories of sleep function. I then critique several categories of sleep function proposed over the last 50 years. As each of these categories can form the basis of an entire review, only selected studies are cited here. I conclude with a synthesis that winnows the thicket of competing ideas to those most likely to be true.

Key concepts in sleep function(s)

Over the years, sleep has been hypothesized to be critical for a dizzying array of somatic and neural

functions. A non-exhaustive list includes: anabolic processes, brain cooling, energy conservation, restoration of brain molecules, removal of neurotoxins, and higher-order functions such as brain maturation, species-specific "programming," and brain plasticity [12,13]. This complicated situation has led some researchers to conclude that sleep has no primary function and instead may serve different purposes in different animals and possibly at different stages of life [4]. This is a valid position, but one that must be critically evaluated because it is also possible that this collection of hypotheses is merely an incomplete description of a deeper, more basic process. Therefore it is useful to consider why scientists have been unable to identify a core function of sleep, and what basic properties of sleep a *unifying* theory of sleep function must explain.

The problem with evolution

Sleep is reported in an impressively wide variety of animals, including terrestrial [14,15] and aquatic invertebrates [16,17], birds [18], reptiles [19], placental, marsupial, and monotrematous mammals [6,20], and even *Caenorhabditis elegans* [21]. While this diversity has yielded valuable clues about the origins of sleep behavior [22], it also paradoxically complicates the search for core sleep functions. This is because sleep in different animals is not the result of a single evolutionary process, but the product of millions of years of complex interactions between different evolutionary forces. For example, shared features of sleep across species (e.g. heightened arousal thresholds, homeostatic regulation [5]) may reflect common ancestral origins, *or* convergent evolution. More specialized features of sleep found only in certain animals (e.g. slow-wave EEG activity in birds

Foundations of Psychiatric Sleep Medicine, ed. John W. Winkelman and David T. Plante. Published by Cambridge University Press.
© Cambridge University Press 2010.

and mammals [18]) may in turn reflect secondary adaptations arising via divergent evolution *or* evolutionary spandrels.

These complex interactions have led to much confusion regarding sleep function. First, not all changes in the brain or the body during sleep may be critically important in a given species. Some may reflect vestigial aspects of sleep that once were adaptive, but during the course of evolution have lost their importance, much like the appendix, or pilo-erection in humans. An example of such a vestigial sleep process may be sleep-related changes in thermoregulation in humans [11]. A reduction in heat production (and associated metabolism) during sleep may have been an adaptive, energy-conservation strategy in our smaller mammalian ancestors (the so-called "energy conservation" theory of sleep) [23,24], but the energy savings obtained in humans is minuscule [6] – and likely offset by the increased brain metabolism of REM sleep [25].

Others may represent what Gould and Lewontin termed evolutionary spandrels, which are characteristics not directly selected for, but appear during evolution as side-effects of adaptation [26]. For example, it is possible that EEG slow-wave activity is a "sleep spandrel" that arose as a by-product of the evolution of mammalian neocortex and related structures in birds [18], but is itself unrelated to sleep function. This may explain why hypnotic drugs that reduce slow-wave activity still produce restorative sleep [27] and do not impair hypothesized functions of sleep (i.e. brain plasticity [28]). Second, if not all observed sleep phenomena have important functions, and this varies across different species, cross-species correlations between sleep parameters and constitutional variables (e.g. brain mass, metabolism) may not be revealing with respect to core functions of sleep. Indeed, several studies employing this approach have reached strikingly different conclusions [6,23,29,30]. Therefore, any unifying theory must reconcile the presence of sleep in diverse species with the very real differences in sleep expression across the animal kingdom. It must also distinguish core functions of sleep from specialized adaptations present only in a given species and vestigial, non-functional remnants due to a shared evolutionary path.

Ontogenetic considerations

A second important consideration is that sleep is not *static* across the life-span. For example, in mammals sleep amounts, brain activity, and sleep regulation undergo dramatic transformations during development [31]. The most prominent changes are in the amounts and types of sleep, with overall sleep amounts (and REM sleep in particular) being much higher in early life than at any other point in the life-span [31]. The regulation of sleep is also quite different in developing mammals. Circadian rhythms in sleep and wake are not observed at birth, even though the states of REM and non-REM (NREM) sleep are present in many species [31]. The classic homeostatic increases in EEG slow-wave activity and REM sleep amounts following sleep deprivation are also absent in neonatal/juvenile rats [32,33] and appear quite abruptly coincident with changes in sleep-deprivation-induced neurotrophins [34]. On the other hand, neonatal sleep time is finely regulated [32], which suggests (see below) that it must serve some purpose for the developing animal. Sleep in developing non-mammalian vertebrates and invertebrates has only been minimally investigated, but similar changes in sleep amounts across the life-span may occur [32,33]. A unifying theory of sleep function should therefore account for these dramatic changes in sleep expression. It should also address whether the presumed function is different in developing animals or preserved in some fashion across the life-span.

Homeostatic regulation

A critical criterion for sleep is that it be homeostatically regulated. This has been best demonstrated in mammals, where a sleep homeostat determines the amount and intensity of sleep based on prior sleep–wake history [35], though similar processes exist in many animal species [5]. In mammals, this homeostatic mechanism can act globally and influence sleep behavior and activity across the brain [36], and it appears that local homeostatic mechanisms can increase sleep intensity within circuits previously active during prior wakefulness [37]. The presence of homeostasis is striking evidence of an important function served by the regulated behavior. Thirst, hunger, and temperature regulation are but a few salient examples of behaviors and/or physiological processes that exhibit homeostatic regulation.

As discussed by Benington [38], the homeostatic regulation of sleep should also be closely associated with its function. According to this argument, for any sleep-dependent process there should be a feedback mechanism that communicates the state of progress of that process to the homeostat if that process is central to sleep expression. A unifying theory of sleep function must therefore indicate how that function communicates with the sleep homeostat.

The primacy of sleep

The most basic requirement of a unifying theory of sleep function is that it explains why sleep, and no other state (e.g. quiet wakefulness) or change in other systems (e.g. increased enzymatic activity), is required for that function. In particular, such a theory should explain why the specific somatic or nervous system changes unique to sleep, such as heightened arousal thresholds, are *necessary and sufficient* for that function. This last criterion is rarely met. As discussed below, there are a number of physiological or neurological processes that, under short-term manipulations of sleep, appear to be enhanced by sleep and more commonly, reduced by sleep deprivation. However, when the manipulation is extended, these changes no longer occur, and/or the observed process begins to exhibit its normal pattern of expression. Thus, in these cases, sufficiency, but not necessity, is demonstrated. In short, a unifying theory of sleep function must explain what makes sleep and no other behavioral state uniquely suited for the proposed function.

Evaluating theories of sleep function

With these points in mind, we can begin our discussion by reviewing classic categories of sleep function. First, we can address whether sleep has evolved in service of the entire organism (*ecological* theories) or in response to some need of the body or the brain (*somatic* vs. *neural* theories). Ecological theories posit that sleep protects animals from being active during times of low food or mate availability and/or times of high predation [23]. These ideas may explain the behavioral context from which sleep evolved in primitive organisms (i.e. circadian rhythms of activity), but otherwise have low explanatory power and are not discussed further here. Somatic theories of sleep function propose that sleep facilitates anabolic processes or restores some bodily function (e.g. organ function, metabolism, etc.) worn down by wakefulness [39–40]. Neural theories, on the other hand, propose that sleep is primarily for the brain, and are further subdivided into *metabolic* and *cognitive* categories. Neuro-

metabolic theories propose that sleep detoxifies substances that accumulate during wake, or restores and repairs neural substrates degraded by wakefulness. Neurocognitive theories propose that sleep serves higher-order functions such as neural development or memory, presumably by promoting brain plasticity [40]. As each of these putative functions of sleep have been extensively reviewed elsewhere [12,38,41,42,43,44,45], only findings from selected studies are discussed below.

Somatic theories of sleep function

Sleep has historically been thought of as a time when our body reverses the wear and tear of wakefulness; but is sleep fundamentally concerned with somatic functions? As reviewed by Akerstedt and Nilsson, mortality rates in short and long sleepers do indicate a link between sleep and physical well-being [46]. Individuals who sleep much more or much less than average have higher mortality rates and greater incidences of myocardial infarction and type 2 diabetes [46]. Sleep also appears to be vital for animals because prolonged sleep deprivation is fatal in rats and fruit flies [47–50]. Although the precise cause of death is not linked to a specific organ or neural pathology in these studies, it does not appear to be due to the stress of the sleep deprivation procedure [48,49,50, 51,52,53,54]. How then, does sleep influence the body and what evidence is there that this is a core function of sleep?

Endocrine systems, metabolism, and sleep

One possible explanation for the link between sleep and physical health is that sleep regulates metabolic/endocrine systems that control energy balance in the body [44,55,56,57,58]. NREM sleep is associated with increases in growth hormone (GH) release, and substances which increase GH concentrations in the brain (in some studies) increase NREM sleep [46,55,56]. NREM sleep is also associated with a suppression of the hypothalamic-pituitary-adrenal (HPA) axis, and it is believed that an interplay between growth hormone-releasing hormone (GHRH) and corticotropin-releasing hormone (CRH) influences the quality of sleep [46,55,56]. More recently, it has been shown that prolonged total sleep deprivation in rodents reduces thyroid hormone levels and the pulsatile release of GH and prolactin that normally occurs during NREM sleep [52]. A very intriguing series of studies also shows that simply curtailing sleep in humans increases the risk for diabetes, and negatively impacts blood glucose metabolism [8]. In addition, anatomical and transgenic studies in rodents have revealed interactions between peptides important in feeding and satiety (ghrelin and leptin, respectively), and areas of the brain that control sleep/wake expression [58]. For example, studies in mice and rats indicate that leptin and ghrelin interact with hypocretin- and melanin-concentrating hormone (MCH)-containing neurons in the lateral hypothalamus, which in turn regulate arousal and sleep (reviewed in [58]).

Despite these findings, it is still unclear if a core function of sleep is to regulate metabolic/endocrine biology. Shorter periods of sleep deprivation (24–72 hours) only modestly affect organ function, athletic performance, and recovery from exercise [59–61]. With respect to interactions between sleep and the endocrine system, the close correlation between GH release and NREM sleep is not universally found in other vertebrates. For example, only faint associations between GH release and sleep are observed in rodents [62]. Non-human primates display strong circadian rhythms in corticosterone release, but no association between GH release and NREM sleep [63,64]. Even in humans the reduction in pulsatile GH release by sleep deprivation can be compensated for by large pulses that occur during wakefulness [65]. The effects of exogenous GH, somatostatin, or blockade of GHRH receptors on mammalian sleep expression are also quite variable, with some studies showing no effects [66–69].

Some of the other changes in human metabolism observed after sleep deprivation appear to be strongly influenced by circadian mechanisms or may reflect side-effects of sleep deprivation rather than sleep *per se*. For example, cortisol release is under circadian control [9], is known to increase after sleep deprivation [70], and has been linked to some of the metabolic disturbances reported after sleep deprivation [71]. Sleep deprivation is also known to reduce cortical metabolism [72], which may contribute to elevated blood glucose following restricted sleep [8]. If indeed the fundamental purpose of sleep is to regulate blood glucose, using the brain as a glucose "sponge" seems a rather inelegant way to do it.

The evidence that sleep is principally concerned with food intake is likewise less than straightforward. As is true for changes in hormones, it is not clear if

the cycling of leptin and ghrelin in humans reflects the influence of sleep, or independent circadian rhythms in the release of these peptides [8]. Studies in rodents have produced mixed results. The putative associations between leptin and ghrelin release and sleep observed in humans do not occur in rats [73]. Constitutive knock-out of leptin (*ob/ob*) [74] or leptin (*db/db*) receptors [75] in mice results in abnormal sleep patterns (increases in NREM sleep, sleep fragmentation), but it is not clear if these changes are secondary to other abnormalities, developmental or otherwise, in these mouse lines. For example, *ob/ob* mice do not thermoregulate normally [74], and *ob/ob* and *db/db* mice both display abnormal levels of motor activity [74,75]; either abnormality would be expected to impact sleep expression, if only indirectly. Ghrelin knock-out mice display even fainter sleep phenotypes, displaying modest increases in NREM sleep time versus wild-type mice both in the baseline and following recovery from sleep deprivation [76]. The effects of knocking out melanin-concentrating hormone (MCH) or the MCH type 1 receptor (MCH R1) are also inconclusive. MCH knock-out mice are hyperactive (with a corresponding reduction in sleep time), but show normal compensatory changes in sleep following sleep deprivation [77]. MCH R1 knock-outs, however, show no hyperactivity, an increase in REM sleep amounts, and a small increase in the homeostatic response to sleep deprivation [78]. As is true for other constitutive knock-out mice, it is unknown how many of these changes are due to developmental compensation or other indirect effects of the absent gene.

Immune function

There appear to be stronger and more direct links between sleep and the immune system [45,56,57]. Bacterial and viral infection in animals and humans are known to increase NREM sleep time via the release of several immune factors (primarily cytokines). Importantly, some of these effects appear to reflect direct modulation of sleep/wake areas of the brain rather than indirect effects of fever [45,56,57]. Exogenous administration of cytokines like tumor necrosis factor (TNF) and interleukin 1B (IL-1B) also increase NREM sleep amounts, while antagonists of these cytokines or their receptors reduce sleep time. In addition, the endogenous release of TNF and IL-1B levels is highest during the normal rest phase in rodents [56,57], and in contrast to molecular deletion of feeding/satiety peptides, knock-out of several immune factors leads to pronounced alterations in sleep/wake expression and sleep homeostasis [79,80].

As is true for endocrine/metabolic and sleep interactions, a number of issues must be resolved before one can conclude that sleep's primary function concerns immune biology. First, it has not been definitively shown that sleep is necessary for a healthy immune system. Some studies indicate that short periods of sleep deprivation or sleep restriction decrease immune function as measured by changes in cytokines, lymphocytes, immune cell activity, and control of microorganisms [81–85]. In other studies, however, sleep deprivation has negligible effects on immunity, and with continued sleep deprivation, markers of normal immune function return to baseline and, in some cases, are heightened [56,86–89]. In addition, during prolonged sleep deprivation rats given antibiotics still die even though their tissues are free from infection; thus the cause of death cannot be ascribed to compromised host defense [51]. The knock-out mouse studies are intriguing, but once again, these are constitutive gene deletions, and the resulting phenotypes reflect a mixture of compensatory effects as well as absence of the targeted gene. In this regard, it is important to point out that some mice lacking immune peptides are underweight and show disturbances in locomotor activity and abnormalities in temperature regulation [79,80].

Neural theories of sleep function

A universal feature of sleep across the animal kingdom is that it involves both behavioral and neural withdrawal from the outside world. Behaviorally, this is manifested by an animal constructing and/or securing an isolated area that is safe from predators and reduces exogenous sensory input. Neurologically, sleep is associated with the activation of inhibitory mechanisms that reduce sensory transmission through the thalamus, and during REM sleep, inhibit motor output [7,90]. In addition, while the effects of sleep loss on somatic function are variable, and possibly restricted to certain mammalian species, the effects on neural functioning appear more conserved [10,91–93]. Generally speaking, sleep loss results in cognitive deficits in animals as diverse as the fruit-fly [93] to man [10]. These findings strongly suggest that the core function of sleep concerns the brain.

Detoxification theories

As originally proposed at the beginning of the twentieth century, the "hypnotoxin" theory of sleep function posited that sleep removes a noxious by-product of the waking brain [94]. Modern versions of this theory propose that sleep reverses or protects against neuronal damage caused by prolonged glutamate release or oxidative processes that occur during wakefulness [95–97]. For example, it is hypothesized that uridine and glutathione accumulate in the brain as a function of waking metabolism and induce sleep by enhancing GABAergic and reducing glutamatergic synaptic transmission, respectively. In addition, glutathione has potent antioxidant properties and is hypothesized to protect cells from oxidative damage [95]. While it is true that exogenous uridine and glutathione induce sleep, and both molecules accumulate in neural tissues of sleep-deprived rats [95,98], the extent to which waking or sleep influences oxidative processes in the brain is controversial. Prolonged REM sleep deprivation in rodents selectively reduced glutathione levels in the hypothalamus and thalamus, but other markers of oxidative stress were not altered [99,100]. These findings were not replicated in a follow-up study from the same group that found signs of oxidative stress only in the hippocampus [101]. Slightly different results were recently reported by a separate group of investigators who found decreased glutathione after REM sleep deprivation in these structures and also the hippocampus, but also signs of reduced oxidative stress in other brain structures, including the cortex [102]. The results of two studies of the effects of extended total sleep deprivation using the same technique are contradictory. Ramanathan et al. reported that 5–11 days of total sleep deprivation reduced levels of the free-radical scavenger superoxide dismutase (SOD) in the hippocampus and brainstem, while other markers of oxidative stress (mitochondrial metabolic activity, glutathione peroxidase) were unchanged [103]. Gopalakrishanan et al., however, found no changes in SOD and little evidence of oxidative stress in brains of rats totally sleep deprived for 3–14 days. There was also no evidence that sleep-deprived brains were less able to respond to an oxidative challenge [104].

There is no evidence that sleep loss produces neural damage as might be expected by unchecked oxidative processes. Ninety-six hours of REM sleep deprivation has no effect on neuronal apoptosis or necrotic markers [105] and total sleep deprivation (hours to days) has inconsistent neuronal effects [47,49]. Even in rats sleep-deprived to death, there was no gross neuronal damage [51]. A more recent study using the same, extended sleep-deprivation techniques in rats reported no changes in markers of neural cell degeneration and no increases in apoptosis gene expression [47]. Eiland et al. found an increase in a more sensitive marker of cell degeneration in the supraoptic nucleus (SON) after total sleep deprivation for more than 45 hours. The significance of this latter finding is unclear since no other signs of neuronal damage were found in the SON [49].

Sleep and neuronal restoration: regeneration

The main evidence for neural regeneration during sleep comes from studies of the effects of normal sleep and wake and sleep deprivation on the synthesis and degradation of a variety of biomolecules (e.g. nucleotides, proteins, and mRNAs). NREM sleep has historically been viewed as the "restorative" sleep state [106]. Though far from conclusive, there are a number of findings which support this view. NREM sleep amounts are positively correlated with cerebral protein synthesis in adult rats, monkeys, and the ovine fetus [107–110]. Studies in rabbits show positive correlations between RNA synthesis in purified nuclear fractions of neocortical neurons and EEG synchronization during sleep [111,112].

Molecular studies show that recovery sleep after total sleep deprivation upregulates cortical and medullary expression of genes that may play a role in protein biogenesis in the endoplasmic reticulum (ER) [113]. Complementary results have been reported after 6 hours of total sleep deprivation in mice, which induces cellular events that decrease protein synthesis [114]. Other studies have found sleep-related increases in several genes implicated in cholesterol synthesis, membrane trafficking, and vesicle maintenance and transport [115–118]. Total sleep deprivation is also reported to reduce cell proliferation in the hippocampus [119–122]. This latter effect does not appear to be simply due to stress accompanying sleep deprivation because it persists even when stress hormones are clamped [123].

In contrast to NREM sleep, the evidence for neural regeneration in REM sleep is comparatively weak. REM sleep deprivation also reduces hippocampal neurogenesis [124], but it has inconsistent effects on protein synthesis, with some investigators reporting no effects [125], and others showing reductions, chiefly in non-cortical structures [126,127]. REM sleep deprivation alters the expression of several genes associated with REM sleep mechanisms, but there is little evidence that REM sleep enhances the expression of genes other than those located in REM sleep circuits [128–130]. Although REM sleep is accompanied by reduced monoaminergic activity [131], the significance of this interaction in terms of neuroregeneration is unclear. For example, short-term REM sleep deprivation (96 hours) has been shown to increase noradrenergic activity and down-regulate beta-adrenergic receptors [132,133], but extended total sleep deprivation or REM sleep deprivation minimally impact monoamine levels and receptor number [48,134–136], and only modestly affect neuronal morphology in cholinergic and noradrenergic neurons [137].

Several studies indicate that REM sleep deprivation increases neuronal excitability, possibly by increasing NA-K ATPase activity, which suggests that REM sleep normally regulates this process [61,138–140]. These effects appear to be regionally dependent since REM sleep deprivation does not increase neuronal excitability in the hippocampus [140,141]. REM sleep deprivation has also been reported to alter neuronal membrane fluidity [142]. Unfortunately, it is difficult to isolate the effects of REM sleep loss from stress and other side-effects of the REM sleep deprivation techniques ("flower-pot" or multiple-platform) in which the animal is kept on a small platform surrounded by water so that it falls off during periods of REM atonia, used in these latter studies. There are also no studies that have conclusively demonstrated neuroregeneration of any kind during naturally occurring REM sleep.

Sleep and neuronal restoration: energy substrates

Several studies have reported interesting relationships between sleep and brain energy [143–145]. Total sleep deprivation, for example, has been shown to reduce cortical metabolism [72,146] and alter lactate synthesis, which suggests that sleep might be important for cerebral energy supplies [147]. Sleep is also associated with increases in the expression of several genes important for neuronal metabolism [116] and following sleep deprivation, may promote the restoration of ATP in the human brain [148].

One of the more influential theories relating brain energy substrates and sleep was proposed by

Benington and Heller [106]. According to the Benington–Heller hypothesis, glial glycogen – which acts as a reserve glucose store for neurons – is depleted during wakefulness and restored during NREM sleep. The depletion of glycogen is mediated by the heightened release of excitatory neurotransmitters during wake, which through enzymatic mechanisms convert glycogen into glucose. The restoration of glycogen is favored by states with lowered excitation, such as NREM sleep. NREM sleep in turn is triggered and maintained by the increased release of neuronal adenosine that occurs as glycogen is mobilized.

The evidence for this theory, while initially promising, now appears quite weak. Karnovsky et al. found transient increases in whole brain glycogen after a few minutes of NREM sleep, but these changes were rapidly reversed after only a short period of wakefulness [149]. A more recent study of glycogen and sleep showed persistent decreases in brain glycogen content following sleep deprivation and increases following recovery sleep [150]. These findings have not been replicated in a series of studies from the Heller laboratory. In one study, total sleep deprivation *increased* cortical glycogen in 59-day-old rats. Shorter periods of total sleep deprivation in younger rats had no effect on cerebral glycogen levels [151]. A second study found no relationship between sleep homeostatic responses and brain glycogen amounts following total sleep deprivation in several strains of mice [152]. A third study in 34-day-old rats found that 6 hours of total sleep deprivation decreased glycogen in the cerebellum and hippocampus of intact rats, and *increased* cortical glycogen in adrenalectomized rats [153]. A study in *Drosophila* also failed to provide convincing evidence for the hypothesis. In this study, 3 hours of sleep deprivation decreased brain glycogen content, but when the sleep deprivation was extended, glycogen synthesis recovered [154]. Therefore, while a role for sleep in restoring some, unidentified, energy store in the brain is still possible [155], the specific theory developed by Benington and Heller is not supported by current data.

Cognitive theories of sleep function: memory, synaptic plasticity, and neurodevelopment

The prevailing view among the general public is that sleep is good for memory and brain plasticity but among sleep scientists this idea has been hotly contested for decades [156–164]. Early critics pointed out that the effects of sleep on various forms of animal learning were inconsistent and confounded by the use of stressful forms of sleep deprivation [61,160]. Nor were the results of early human studies particularly encouraging. Many studies found no effect of sleep loss (generally REM sleep) on verbal learning tasks (e.g. word association), and those that did reported relatively marginal effects [61,160]. Therefore, after a flurry of interest, many scientists concluded that sleep had nothing to do with memory and the search for sleep function shifted elsewhere [61,160].

The idea that sleep promotes memory consolidation has rebounded dramatically in the last decade. Although there remain a handful of naysayers [156,157], there is a growing consensus in the field that sleep promotes memory processing and brain plasticity [43,92,159,165,166]. The majority of animal studies in the last 10 years have shown significant associations between sleep and memory consolidation [13,158,167–173]. In many cases, studies were designed to reduce the likelihood that positive results were due to stress, motivation, fatigue, and other factors that confounded earlier studies (reviewed in [13]). There has also been an accumulation of positive findings in the human literature since the mid 1990s [13,158,164,169]. Several issues need to be resolved; for example, there is little agreement over which sleep state is important for learning (REM vs. NREM) and it is unclear what kind of learning is most affected by sleep (episodic vs. procedural) (reviewed in [13]).

It is unlikely, however, that the debate over sleep's putative role in higher-order functions will ever be resolved by studies that rely solely on measurements of memory. Such studies, no matter how sophisticated they become, are inherently limited because they measure an outcome of a plastic event (i.e. learning or memory) and not the plastic event itself (i.e. the changes in the brain that result from sleep). As pointed out by Rechtschaffen [12], what is needed is a convincing demonstration that sleep directly influences the underlying mechanisms of memory – synaptic plasticity. In the following sections, I summarize three key lines of evidence that in conjunction with behavioral measures in animals and humans, support the hypothesis that a core function of sleep is to promote brain plasticity. These are the effects of sleep and sleep loss on *in vitro* and *in vivo* forms of brain plasticity, sleep-dependent changes in neuronal activity, and state-dependent changes in the expression of proteins and genes in the brain.

Sleep, long-term potentiation (LTP), and long-term depression (LTD): *in vitro* and *in vivo* studies in adult animals

LTP and LTD refer to use-dependent, persistent alterations in synaptic weights that strengthen (LTP) or weaken (LTD) specific synapses, respectively [13,174,175]. Although these effects were originally identified *in vitro* and involved what were at the time considered "non-physiological" stimulus protocols, LTP and LTD can be induced and may occur naturally *in vivo* [174–176]. These and related forms of synaptic plasticity are now widely considered to be cellular correlates of memory [174,175]. To what extent, then, does sleep influence LTP and LTD?

Beginning in the late 1980s several investigators have shown that sleep states influence tetany-induced LTP in animal models (reviewed in [13,177]). Overall, it appears that hippocampal LTP can be induced during REM sleep, whereas similar stimulus protocols during NREM sleep have no effect or produce LTD [178–180]. Subsequent investigations have shown that sleep and sleep loss can affect the induction or maintenance of LTP. Romcy-Pereira and Pavlides [181] found that REM sleep deprivation and total sleep deprivation impair the maintenance of LTP in the dentate gyrus, but enhance this process in the medial prefrontal cortex (mPFC). Marks and Wayner found that sleep disruption also reduces hippocampal LTP in anesthetized rats [182]. Kim et al. also employed the "flower-pot" REM sleep deprivation technique for 5 days in rats, after which tetany was applied to the hippocampus while the animals were awake [183]. In contrast to Marks and Wayner, these investigators report a delayed effect of REM sleep deprivation on LTP; reductions in LTP were observed 24 hours after the termination of REM sleep deprivation. Seven recent studies also show that *in vitro* hippocampal LTP (either the incidence or maintenance) is reduced in rodents that undergo varying amounts of REM sleep deprivation, total sleep deprivation, or sleep restriction [140,183–189]. In some cases, these deficits can be clearly dissociated from changes due to stress [187]. The diminished plasticity may be linked to decrements in NMDA receptor (NMDAR) currents and an internalization of the NR1 and NR2A subunits that form the heterotetrameric NMDAR [186].

Sleep and developmental plasticity

In a variety of mammalian species, sleep amounts are highest during neonatal periods of rapid brain development and synaptic plasticity than at any other time of life [190–192]. Therefore, if sleep contributes to synaptic plasticity one would expect this to be especially true in developing animals. This possibility has been investigated in the maturing visual system that is highly plastic during a critical period of development. The critical period has been traditionally investigated by surgically closing an eye (monocular deprivation (MD)), which alters cortical responses and lateral geniculate nucleus (LGN) morphology in favor of the open eye (reviewed in [193,194]). These changes *in vivo* are temporally associated with a form of an *in vitro* cortical LTP. In this type of LTP, high-frequency white-matter stimulation in cortical slices prepared from post-natal (P) day 28–30 rats produces synaptic potentiation in cortical layers II/III. This form of LTP is not observed in cortical slices from adult rats [195]. In the last decade, several *in vitro* and *in vivo* studies suggested an important role for sleep in these types of plasticity.

REM sleep may play an important role in the developmentally regulated form of LTP [196]. Shaffery et al. [196] reported that 1 week of REM sleep deprivation prolonged the critical period for the developmentally regulated form of LTP. A similar extension of the critical period was not seen in cortical slices from control rats. Conversely, REM sleep deprivation had no effect on a non-developmentally regulated form of LTP evoked by layer IV stimulation. Subsequent studies from these investigators showed that this plasticity could be partially rescued if REM sleep deprivation was administered near (or overlapping) the end of the critical period [197,198].

Sleep also contributes to developmental cortical plasticity *in vivo*. My colleagues and I have shown that as little as 6 hours of sleep significantly enhances the effects of monocular deprivation on cortical neurons; a process which does not occur when animals are instead sleep-deprived [199].The precise mechanisms governing this process are unknown, but several clues have emerged from our studies. First, it appears to be dependent upon NREM sleep because changes in plasticity are positively correlated with NREM sleep [199], and because REM sleep deprivation does not block the normal consolidation of ocular dominance plasticity that occurs after sleep [28,200]. Second, we have determined that the underlying mechanisms require cortical activity [201,202] and the activation of NMDAR-PKA signaling [200], which may in turn trigger CREB-dependent gene transcription and translation [203]. These findings are consistent with previous suggestions that the consolidation of memory and synaptic plasticity involve secondary waves of NMDAR activation that occur after experience [204].

Neurophysiological/molecular changes during sleep and synaptic plasticity

There are a number of neurophysiological events in the sleeping brain that strongly suggest that sleep promotes synaptic remodeling [13]. These include neurophysiological changes in single neurons or neuronal ensembles that suggest "reactivation" of wake-active circuits, and a transmission of information between the cortex and subcortical areas during sleep [205–208]. Thalamocortical spindles and cortical slow waves typical of NREM sleep may also trigger Hebbian (i.e. synaptic efficacy is proportional to the presynaptic cell's stimulation of the post-synaptic cell) and non-Hebbian forms of synaptic plasticity [13,166]. Several genes and proteins known to influence plasticity are also modulated by sleep [209]. These findings have been extensively reviewed elsewhere [13,165,210] and are briefly discussed and updated in the following sections.

Hippocampal–neocortical and thalamocortical interactions

Since the initial findings of Pavlides and Winson [211], several investigators have reported reactivation (or "replay") in circuits during sleep previously active during wake [212–220]. The phenomenon appears quite robust, as it has been found in the rodent hippocampus, ventral striatum and cortex [212–215, 218,221,222], the primate cortex [220], and even in the zebra finch brain [219]. Although the precise function of "replay" is still unclear [13,210], it is possible that it is part of a larger dialog between subcortical brain areas and the cortex necessary for long-term, memory formation [205]. This dialog is conjectured to occur during NREM sleep when activity in the hippocampus is consistent with outflow, rather than inflow [205,206,223]. There are indeed

interesting correlations between ripples and sharp waves (hippocampal events when replay is reported) and thalamocortical spindles and delta waves consistent with this hypothesis [224–226]. In addition, though quite rare, there are instances when hippocampal and cortical replay occur simultaneously [222]. It is unclear, however, if the correlations between hippocampal and cortical activity during sleep reflect an actual transmission of information between these structures [227]. Pelletier et al., for example, found little evidence that signals propagate either to or from the hippocampus (via entorhinal cortices) during NREM sleep [227].

There is stronger evidence of a rich exchange between the thalamus and the cortex during sleep that may promote synaptic plasticity [208,228,229]. For example, in vivo recordings in cats have shown that experimentally induced thalamic volleys (approximating spindles) or anesthesia-induced spindles produce augmenting responses in cortical neurons that persist for several minutes (for review, see [230]). More recent work has shown that simulated sleep rhythms (in anesthetized cats) can depress or potentiate cortical post-synaptic responses, depending on the proportion of excitatory and inhibitory post-synaptic potentials and the level of background firing [231]. Similar plasticity has also been reported in vitro, where experimentally induced "spindles" can produce short-term potentiation (STP), LTP, or LTD in cortical neurons as a function of post-synaptic depolarization and the number of stimulus pulses [232,233].

It has also been proposed that NREM slow-wave activity downscales synaptic strength across the neocortex (a process known as homeostatic plasticity [234]) [166]. According to the "synaptic homeostasis" hypothesis, waking is associated with synaptic strengthening that triggers, possibly through neurotrophin release [235], heightened slow-wave activity during subsequent sleep [166]. Slow-wave activity then globally down-scales synaptic weights throughout the cortical network, which preserves the relative changes in synapses obtained during wake, but allows for further plastic changes after sleep [166]. While there is yet no direct evidence that synapses are actually downscaled during sleep, this hypothesis is supported by several indirect findings, including changes in protein phosphorylation and electrically evoked responses in the cortex in vivo [236].

Cellular and molecular changes during sleep and synaptic plasticity

As discussed above, a number of studies have reported increases in macromolecule synthesis in the sleeping brain [107–109]. While many of these molecules have yet to be identified, several of them are known to influence synaptic plasticity [13]. For example, cortical mRNA transcripts for two genes important for LTD (i.e. calcineurin and CaMKIV) are specifically upregulated by sleep [116,209], and neuronal expression of the LTP-related gene *zif-268* is increased in REM sleep following exposure to enriched environments and LTP *in vivo* [217,237]. In addition, neuronal concentrations of neurogranin, snap25b, NSF, neuromodulin, phosphorylated ERK, and activated MMP9 – all proteins implicated in synaptic plasticity – are decreased by sleep deprivation, suggesting that they are normally synthesized during sleep [117,238,239]. In addition, neuronal decreases in hippocampal ERK and active forms of MMP9 induced by sleep deprivation are associated with learning deficits in rodents, suggesting functional relationships between sleep, the expression of these molecules, and learning.

Discussion

Many clues about sleep function have amassed over the years, but no one theory or even category of theories has adequately answered the question of why we sleep. Nevertheless, some theories are better supported than others and by re-examining these findings in light of our key concepts (*evolution, ontogeny, regulation, and primacy*) some tentative conclusions can be made. The first is that while there are interesting interactions between the body and sleep, it seems unlikely that sleep's principal functions are concerned with somatic physiology. On the other hand, converging lines of evidence strongly suggest that sleep in some way promotes normal neuronal function, which would include brain plasticity. These ideas are discussed in greater detail in the following sections.

Sleep and the body

In terms of the four key issues outlined above (evolution, ontogeny, regulation, and primacy), current somatic theories of sleep function seem to fall short. From an evolutionary point of view, the fact that sleep-related changes in hormone release observed in humans generally do not occur in other animals (even among other primates) suggests that this is a specialized adaptation that occurred late in evolution, rather than a core, conserved function of sleep. There may be stronger, more ancient relationships between the immune system and sleep [88], but it is unclear if this reflects direct effects of peripheral immune molecules on the brain, or cytokine-based signaling that is distinct from peripheral immune response [44]. For example, the immune factor TNFα is also known to mediate brain plasticity (a putative function of sleep) via mechanisms outside of peripheral immune signaling [240].

Ontogenetic considerations are difficult to address as very little is known about the interrelationship between sleep and endocrine biology, energy metabolism, or immune function, in developing humans or animals. However, as discussed by Feinberg, peak GH release and amounts of the deeper NREM sleep stages are *inversely* related across development in human children [241]. One might also expect that if sleep function was tied to GH release, this would be especially true in neonates, as this a period of rapid physical growth. Yet, in both animals and humans, NREM sleep is at its nadir and REM sleep instead predominates in newborns [190,192].

There also appears to be no obvious relationship between the ontogenesis of the immune system and sleep. For example, if sleep expression is intimately related to circulating levels of cytokines and related molecules, then greater amounts of sleep in infancy should also be accompanied by greater blood or lymph levels of these peptides. This general prediction is not borne out [242]. For example, in developing mice there are generally fewer T helper cells (which produce the interleukins and other factors linked to sleep promotion in adults) and the immune response to infection is comparatively blunted [242]. Similar results are also reported in toddlers and children [243].

In terms of regulation, some feeding/satiety peptides, hormone-releasing peptides, and immune molecules can modulate arousal and sleep, which could potentially provide a feedback mechanism between the state of progress of energy balance, or immune function, and sleep expression. However, these relationships are often based on studies where the effects of sleep *per se* are difficult to disentangle from circadian release of peptides and hormones, or indirect effects of sleep deprivation. They also rely heavily on mice studies where genes are deleted from the embryonic period onward, leaving open the possibility that some of the behavioral phenotypes reflect developmental compensation.

With respect to primacy, somatic theories seem wholly inadequate. If we accept that a core feature of sleep is a diminution of consciousness, then why should this be required for the facilitation of endocrine or immune function? These events could just as easily occur during periods of quiet wake when the animal is less subject to predation [60]. Moreover, while there is evidence in some species that sleep is *sufficient* for hormone release or normal changes in immune function, it is not yet clear if sleep is *necessary* for these processes. For example, as discussed earlier, GH release in humans is indeed blunted by sleep deprivation, but this can be compensated for by pulses in waking [65]. Likewise, while a single night of sleep loss can negatively impact some immune molecules [82,83], the clinical significance of these changes are unknown, nor has it been shown that these effects persist during longer sleep deprivations.

Sleep and the brain

As reviewed in the preceding sections, there are several categories of ideas that relate neural function to sleep (metabolic: neurotoxin vs. regeneration, cognitive: brain plasticity and memory). Neurotoxin theories currently have weak experimental support. In contrast, there is strong evidence in favor of one type of neuroregeneration (macromolecule synthesis) and cognitive theories. For example, sleep is associated with cerebral protein synthesis and the upregulation of genes important for neuronal metabolism, membranes, and other structural components. There is also behavioral, electrophysiological, cellular, and molecular evidence to support the hypothesis that sleep promotes higher order functions such as memory consolidation and brain plasticity.

A parsimonious reconciliation of these findings is that sleep is a brain state that promotes structural rearrangements in neurons. This is an energetic process (hence the upregulation of genes and proteins related to neuronal metabolism) that requires macromolecule synthesis. It is also more likely to be intensified under conditions such as brain development and following events that trigger synaptic plasticity. One might also expect there to be a steady-state need for such a brain state, as macromolecules in neurons (as well as neuronal processes such as dendritic

spines) are highly dynamic [244,245]. If indeed this is the core function of sleep, it would account for the two strongest sets of findings we have concerning sleep and the brain, but how does it fare in light of our four key concepts?

In terms of evolution, this theory may account for the ubiquity of the central nervous system changes that occur during sleep in the animal kingdom, and the fact that challenges to the brain that trigger structural changes in synapses are associated with more sleep, or more intense sleep in diverse species [13,21,166,246,247]. In terms of ontogeny, it may explain the abundance of sleep in early life, which is a time of massive synaptic rearrangement [13], and the abrupt appearance of adult forms of sleep homeostasis at ages when plasticity-related peptides (i.e. the neurotrophin BDNF) concentrations sharply increase after sleep deprivation [32,34]. It may also account for the decline in sleep amounts and intensity in senescence [248] when brain plasticity reaches its nadir [249].

What is less clear is the relationship between this process and sleep homeostasis (regulation) and why sleep would be the preferred state for this process to occur (primacy). With respect to regulation, some progress has been made in that plasticity-related molecules (e.g. neurotrophins, TNFα) can increase EEG correlates of sleep intensity [235,250]. We have also shown that astrocytes influence sleep homeostasis and, because they also modulate synaptic plasticity, they represent a cellular link between sleep regulation and structural changes in circuits [251]. However, it is not clear if these relationships exist in animals that lack neocortex, or at earlier stages of life in animals that have neocortex.

In terms of primacy, it is hypothesized that the electrical activity or the neurochemical/molecular milieu of the sleeping brain is especially conducive for structural changes in neurons [13,166]. Yet the precise and complete set of cellular processes promoted by sleep (and not wake) in the brain has not been identified. It would appear, however, that in some cases they are *necessary* and *sufficient* for memory consolidation and brain plasticity because in their absence, these processes do not occur and/or are attenuated [92,199,201].

Concluding remarks

Sleep scientists, for all their advances, remain in the awkward position of not knowing why we sleep. An analogous situation in the sciences is difficult to find.

For example, eating, like sleep, is a complex, regulated behavior governed by specific brain regions, neurotransmitters, and hormones. Eating, like sleep, is ubiquitous in the animal kingdom and undergoes important transformations during ontogeny [252] – yet there is no confusion and debate over why animals eat. The evidence to date strongly suggests that sleep primarily serves the brain rather than the body, and the neural processes most impacted by sleep are cognitive. This does not, however, change the fact that sleep deprivation or restriction negatively impacts somatic function – if perhaps only indirectly. The challenge now is to isolate further the effects of sleep versus other interlocking physiological systems on the body and to determine precisely what sleep provides the brain that wakefulness cannot.

In conclusion, scientists may eventually discover that there are deeper, more fundamental reasons why we sleep, but the idea that sleep promotes structural changes in the brain provides a strong theoretical framework for understanding sleep function. Continued investigation along these lines is therefore useful because it will either elucidate exactly how sleep achieves this function or reveal a more elegant, unifying process.

References

1. Jones BE. Basic mechanisms of sleep-waking states. In: Kryger MH, Roth T, Dement WC, eds. *Principles and practice of sleep medicine*, 4th ed. Philadelphia: WB Saunders; 2005:136–153.

2. Dijk DJ, Lockley SW. Integration of human sleep-wake regulation and circadian rhythmicity. *J Appl Physiol.* 2002;**92**(2):852–862.

3. Shaw PJ, Franken P. Perchance to dream: Solving the mystery of sleep through genetic analysis. *J Neurobiol.* 2003;**54**(1):179–202.

4. Siegel JM. Do all animals sleep? *Trends Neurosci.* 2008;**31**(4):208–213.

5. Tobler I. Phylogeny of sleep regulation. In: Kryger M, Roth T, Dement WC, eds. *Principles and practice of sleep medicine*, 4th ed. Philadelphia: W.B Saunders; 2005:72–90.

6. Zepelin H. Mammalian sleep. In: Kryger M, Roth T, Dement WC, eds. *Principles and practice of sleep medicine*, 4th ed. Philadelphia: WB Saunders; 2005:91–100.

7. Steriade M. Brain electrical activity and sensory processing during waking and sleep states. In: Kryger MH, Roth T, Dement WC, eds. *Principles and practice of sleep medicine*, Vol 4. Philadelphia: WB Saunders; 2005:101–119.

8. Knutson K, Van Cauter E. Associations between sleep loss and increased risk of obesity and diabetes. *Ann NY Acad Sci.* 2008;**1129**:287–304.

9. Van Cauter E. Endocrine physiology. In: Kryger M, Roth T, Dement WC, eds. *Principles and practice of sleep medicine*, 5th ed. Philadelphia: Elsevier; 2005:266–282.

10. Banks S, Dinges DF. Behavioral and physiological consequences of sleep restriction. *J Clin Sleep Med.* 2007;**3**(5):519–528.

11. Glotzbach SF, Heller HC. Temperature regulation. In: Roth C, Kryger M, Dement WC, eds. *Principles and practice of sleep medicine*, 3rd ed. Philadelphia: WB Saunders; 2000:289–304.

12. Rechtschaffen A. Current perspectives on the function of sleep. *Perspect Biol Med.* 1998;**41**(3):359–390.

13. Benington JH, Frank MG. Cellular and molecular connections between sleep and synaptic plasticity. *Progr Neurobiol.* 2003;**69**(2):77–101.

14. Shaw P. Awakening to the behavioral analysis of sleep in Drosophila. *J Biol Rhythms.* 2003;**18**(1):4–11.

15. Eban-Rothschild AD, Bloch G. Differences in the sleep architecture of forager and young honeybees (*Apis mellifera*). *J Exp Biol.* 2008;**211**(15): 2408–2416.

16. Brown ER, Piscopo S, De Stefano R, Giuditta A. Brain and behavioural evidence for rest-activity cycles in *Octopus vulgaris*. *Behav Brain Res.* 2006;**172**(2): 355–359.

17. Ramon F, Hernandez-Falcon J, Nguyen B, Bullock TH. Slow wave sleep in crayfish. *PNAS.* 2004;**101**(32): 11857–11861.

18. Rattenborg NC, Martinez-Gonzalez D, Lesku JA. Avian sleep homeostasis: Convergent evolution of complex brains, cognition and sleep functions in mammals and birds. *Neurosci Biobehav Rev.* 2009;**33**(3):253–270.

19. Ayala-Guerrero F, Mexicano G. Sleep and wakefulness in the green iguanid lizard (*Iguana iguana*). *Comp Biochem Physiol A Mol Integr Physiol.* 2008;**151**(3): 305–312.

20. Siegel JM. Sleep phylogeny: Clues to the evolution and function of sleep. In: Luppi PH, ed. *Sleep: circuits and function.* Boca Raton: CRC Press; 2005:163–176.

21. Raizen DM, Zimmerman JE, Maycock MH, et al. Lethargus is a *Caenorhabditis elegans* sleep-like state. *Nature.* 2008;**451**(7178):569–572.

22. Allada R, Siegel JM. Unearthing the phylogenetic roots of sleep. *Curr Biol.* 2008;**18**(15):R670–R679.

23. Siegel JM. Clues to the functions of mammalian sleep. *Nature.* 2005;**437**(7063):1264–1271.

24. Berger RJ. Energy conservation and sleep. *Behav Brain Res*. 1995;**69**(1–2):65–73.

25. Buchsbaum MS, Hazlett EA, Wu J, Bunney WE Jr. Positron emission tomography with deoxyglucose-F18 imaging of sleep. *Neuropsychopharmacology*. 2001; **25**(5 Suppl):S50–56.

26. Gould SJ, Lewontin RC. The spandrels of San Marco and the Panglossian paradigm: A critique of the adaptionist programme. *Proc R Soc Lond*. 1979;**205**:581–598.

27. Wagner J, Wagner ML. Non-benzodiazepines for the treatment of insomnia. *Sleep Med Rev*. 2000; **4**(6):551–581.

28. Seibt J, Aton S, Jha SK, et al. The non-benzodiazepine hypnotic Zolpidem impairs sleep-dependent cortical plasticity. *Sleep*. 2008;**31**(10):1381–1392.

29. Lesku JA, Roth IITC, Amlaner CJ, Lima SL. A phylogenetic analysis of sleep architecture in mammals: The integration of anatomy, physiology, and ecology. *Am Nat*. 2006;**168**(4):441–453.

30. Lesku JA, Roth TC, Rattenborg NC, Amlaner CJ, Lima SL. Phylogenetics and the correlates of mammalian sleep: A reappraisal. *Sleep Med Rev*. 2008; **12**(3):229–244.

31. Davis FC, Frank MG, Heller HC. Ontogeny of sleep and circadian rhythms. In: Zee PC, Turek FW, eds. *Regulation of sleep and circadian rhythms*, Vol **133**. New York: Marcel Dekker, Inc.; 1999:19–80.

32. Frank MG, Morrissette R, Heller HC. Effects of sleep deprivation in neonatal rats. *Am J Physiol*. 1998;**275** (44):R148–R157.

33. Feng P, Ma Y, Vogel GW. Ontogeny of REM rebound in postnatal rats. *Sleep*. 2001;**24**(6):645–653.

34. Hairston IS, Peyron C, Denning DP, et al. Sleep deprivation effects on growth factor expression in neonatal rats: A potential role for BDNF in the mediation of delta power. *J Neurophysiol*. 2004;**91**(4):1586–1595.

35. Borbely AA, Achermann P. Sleep homeostasis and models of sleep regulation. In: Kryger M, Roth T, Dement WC, eds. *Principles and practice of sleep medicine*, 3rd ed. Philadelphia: WB Saunders; 2000:377–390.

36. Dijk D-J, Edgar DM. Circadian and homeostatic control of wakefulness and sleep. In: Turek FW, Zee PC, eds. *Regulation of sleep and circadian rhythms*, Vol **133**. New York: Marcel Dekker, Inc.; 1999:111–148.

37. Vyazovskiy VV, Tobler I. Handedness leads to interhemispheric EEG asymmetry during sleep in the rat. *J Neurophysiol*. 2008;**99**(2):969–975.

38. Benington J. Sleep homeostasis and the function of sleep. *Sleep*. 2001;**23**(7):959–966.

39. Oswald I. Sleep as a restorative process: Human clues. *Prog Brain Res*. 1980;**53**:279–288.

40. Adam K. Sleep as a restorative process and a theory to explain why. *Prog Brain Res*. 1980;**53**:289–305.

41. Frank MG. Sleep, synaptic plasticity and the developing brain. In: Luppi P-H, ed. *Sleep. Circuits and functions*. Boca Raton: CRC Press; 2004:177–192.

42. Frank MG. The function of sleep. In: Chiong LT, ed. *The encyclopedia of sleep medicine*. Chichester: John Wiley & Sons; 2006:45–48.

43. Frank MG. The mystery of sleep function: current perspectives and future directions. *Rev Neurosci*. 2006; **17**; 375–392.

44. Opp MR. Cytokines and sleep. *Sleep Med Rev*. 2005;**9**(5):355–364.

45. Opp MR. Sleep and psychoneuroimmunology. *Neurol Clin Psychoneuroimmunol*. 2006;**24**(3):493–506.

46. Akerstedt T, Nilsson PM. Sleep as restitution: an introduction. *J Intern Med*. 2003;**254**(1):6–12.

47. Cirelli C, Shaw PJ, Rechtschaffen A, Tononi G. No evidence of brain cell degeneration after long-term sleep deprivation in rats. *Brain Res*. 1999;**840** (1–2):184–193.

48. Rechtschaffen A, Bergmann BM, Everson CA, Kushida CA, Gilliland MA. Sleep deprivation in the rat: X. Integration and discussion of the findings. 1989. *Sleep*. 2002;**25**(1):68–87.

49. Eiland MM, Ramanathan L, Gulyani S, et al. Increases in amino-cupric-silver staining of the supraoptic nucleus after sleep deprivation. *Brain Res*. 2002; **945**(1):1–8.

50. Shaw PJ, Tononi G, Greenspan RJ, Robinson DF. Stress response genes protect against lethal effects of sleep deprivation in *Drosophila*. *Nature*. 2002;**417** (6886):287–291.

51. Rechtschaffen A, Bergmann BM. Sleep deprivation in the rat: an update of the 1989 paper. *Sleep*. 2002; **25**(1):18–24.

52. Everson CA, Crowley WR. Reductions in circulating anabolic hormones induced by sustained sleep deprivation in rats. *Am J Physiol Endocrinol Metab*. 2004;**286**(6):E1060–1070.

53. Everson CA, Laatsch CD, Hogg N. Antioxidant defense responses to sleep loss and sleep recovery. *Am J Physiol Regul Integr Comp Physiol*. 2005;**288**(2):R374–383.

54. Koban M, Swinson KL. Chronic REM-sleep deprivation of rats elevates metabolic rate and increases UCP1 gene expression in brown adipose tissue. *Am J Physiol Endocrinol Metab*. 2005;**289**(1):E68–74.

55. Cauter EV, Spiegel K. Circadian and sleep control of hormonal secretions. In: Zee PC, Turek FW, eds.

Regulation of sleep and circadian rhythms, Vol **133**. New York: Marcel Dekker, Inc.; 1999:397–425.

56. Bryant PA, Trinder J, Curtis N. Sick and tired: Does sleep have a vital role in the immune system? *Nat Rev Immunol.* 2004;**4**(6):457–467.

57. Krueger JM, Majde JA. Humoral links between sleep and the immune system: research issues. *Ann NY Acad Sci.* 2003;**992**(1):9–20.

58. Adamantidis A, de Lecea L. Sleep and metabolism: shared circuits, new connections. *Trends Endocrinol Metab.* 2008;**19**(10):362–370.

59. Bonnet MH. Sleep deprivation. In: Kryger M, Roth T, Dement WC, eds. *Principles and practice of sleep medicine*, 3rd ed. Philadelphia: WB Saunders; 2000:53–71.

60. Horne JA. Sleep function, with particular reference to sleep deprivation. *Ann Clin Res.* 1985;**17**(5):199–208.

61. Ellman SJ, Spielman AJ, Luck D, Steiner SS, Halperin R. REM deprivation: A Review. In: Ellman SJ, Antrobus JS, eds. *The mind in sleep*, 2nd ed. New York: John Wiley & Sons, Inc.; 1991:329–369.

62. Iyer KS, Marks GA, Kastin AJ, McCann SM. Evidence for a role of delta sleep-inducing peptide in slow-wave sleep and sleep-related growth hormone release in the rat. *PNAS.* 1988;**85**(10):3653–3656.

63. Bunner DL, McNamee GA Jr, Dinterman RE, Wannemacher RW Jr. Lack of enhanced nocturnal growth hormone release in tethered cynomolgus monkeys. *Am J Physiol Regul Integr Comp Physiol.* 1982;**243**(3):R213–217.

64. Quabbe HJ, Gregor M, Bumke-Vogt C, Eckhof A, Witt I. Twenty-four-hour pattern of growth hormone secretion in the rhesus monkey: studies including alterations of the sleep/wake and sleep stage cycles. *Endocrinology.* 1981;**109**(2):513–522.

65. Brandenberger G, Weibel L. The 24-h growth hormone rhythm in men: sleep and circadian influences questioned. *J Sleep Res.* 2004;**13**(3):251–255.

66. Van Cauter E, Latta F, Nedeltcheva A, et al. Reciprocal interactions between the GH axis and sleep. *Growth Horm IGF Res.* 2004;**14**(Suppl A):S10–17.

67. Jessup S, Malow B, Symons K, Barkan A. Blockade of endogenous growth hormone-releasing hormone receptors dissociates nocturnal growth hormone secretion and slow-wave sleep. *Eur J Endocrinol.* 2004;**151**(5):561–566.

68. Steiger A, Antonijevic IA, Bohlhalter S, et al. Effects of hormones on sleep. *Horm Res.* 1998;**49**(3–4):125–130.

69. Kern W, Halder R, al-Reda S, et al. Systemic growth hormone does not affect human sleep. *J Clin Endocrinol Metab.* 1993;**76**(6):1428–1432.

70. Tobler I, Murrison R, Ursin R, Ursin H, Borbely AA. The effect of sleep deprivation and recovery sleep on plasma corticosterone in the rat. *Neurosci Lett.* 1983;**35**:297–300.

71. Mujica-Parodi LR, Renelique R, Taylor MK. Higher body fat percentage is associated with increased cortisol reactivity and impaired cognitive resilience in response to acute emotional stress. *Int J Obes.* 2009;**33**:157–165.

72. Wu JC, Gillin JC, Buchsbaum MS, et al. Frontal lobe metabolic decreases with sleep deprivation not totally reversed by recovery sleep. *Neuropsychopharmacology.* 2006;**31**(12):2783–2792.

73. Bodosi B, Gardi J, Hajdu I, et al. Rhythms of ghrelin, leptin, and sleep in rats: effects of the normal diurnal cycle, restricted feeding, and sleep deprivation. *Am J Physiol Regul Integr Comp Physiol.* 2004;**287**(5):R1071–1079.

74. Laposky AD, Shelton J, Bass J, et al. Altered sleep regulation in leptin-deficient mice. *Am J Physiol Regul Integr Comp Physiol.* 2006;**290**(4):R894–903.

75. Laposky AD, Bradley MA, Williams DL, Bass J, Turek FW. Sleep-wake regulation is altered in leptin resistant (db/db) genetically obese and diabetic mice. *Am J Physiol Regul Integr Comp Physiol.* 2008;**295**(6):R2059–R2066.

76. Szentirmai E, Kapas L, Sun Y, Smith RG, Krueger JM. Spontaneous sleep and homeostatic sleep regulation in ghrelin knockout mice. *Am J Physiol Regul Integr Comp Physiol.* 2007;**293**(1):R510–517.

77. Willie JT, Sinton CM, Maratos-Flier E, Yanagisawa M. Abnormal response of melanin-concentrating hormone deficient mice to fasting: hyperactivity and rapid-eye-movement sleep suppression. *Neuroscience.* 2008;**156**:819–829.

78. Adamantidis A, Salvert D, Goutagny R, et al. Sleep architecture of the melanin-concentrating hormone receptor1-knockout mice. *Eur J Neurosci.* 2008;**27**(7):1793–1800.

79. Baracchi F, Opp MR. Sleep-wake behavior and responses to sleep deprivation of mice lacking both interleukin-1[beta] receptor 1 and tumor necrosis factor-[alpha] receptor 1. *Brain Behav Immun.* 2008;**22**(6):982–993.

80. Jhaveri KA, Ramkumar V, Trammell RA, Toth LA. Spontaneous, homeostatic, and inflammation-induced sleep in NF-κB p50 knockout mice. *Am J Physiol Regul Integr Comp Physiol.* 2006;**291**(5):R1516–1526.

81. Everson CA, Toth LA. Systemic bacterial invasion induced by sleep deprivation. *Am J Physiol Regul Integr Comp Physiol.* 2000;**278**(4):R905–916.

82. Benedict C, Dimitrov S, Marshall L, Born J. Sleep enhances serum interleukin-7 concentrations in humans. *Brain Behav Immun.* 2007;**21**(8):1058–1062.

83. Dimitrov S, Lange T, Nohroudi K, Born J. Number and function of circulating human antigen presenting cells regulated by sleep. *Sleep.* 2007;**30**(4):401–411.

84. Hu J, Chen Z, Gorczynski CP, et al. Sleep-deprived mice show altered cytokine production manifest by perturbations in serum IL-1ra, TNFa, and IL-6 levels. *Brain Behav Immun.* 2003;**17**(6):498–504.

85. Zager A, Andersen ML, Ruiz FS, Antunes IB, Tufik S. Effects of acute and chronic sleep loss on immune modulation of rats. *Am J Physiol Regul Integr Comp Physiol.* 2007;**293**(1):R504–509.

86. Reneger KB, Floyd RA, Krueger JM. Effects of short-term sleep deprivation on murine immunity to influenza virus in young adult and senescent mice. *Sleep.* 1998;**21**(3):241–248.

87. Reneger KB, Floyd R, Krueger JM. Effects of sleep deprivation on serum influenza-specific IgG. *Sleep.* 1998;**21**(1):19–24.

88. Williams JA, Sathyanarayanan S, Hendricks JC, Sehgal A. Interactions between sleep and the immune response in *Drosophila*: a role for the NFkappaB relish. *Sleep.* 2007;**1**(30):389–400.

89. Ricardo J, Cartner L, Oliver S, et al. No effect of a 30-h period of sleep deprivation on leukocyte trafficking, neutrophil degranulation and saliva IgA responses to exercise. *Eur J Appl Physiol.* 2009;**105**:499–504.

90. Chase M, Morales FR. Control of motorneurons during sleep. In: Kryger M, Roth T, Dement WC, eds. *Principles and practice of sleep medicine.* Philadelphia: WB Saunders; 2000:155–168.

91. Smith C. Sleep states and learning: A review of the animal literature. *Neurosci Biobehav Rev.* 1985;**9**:157–168.

92. Stickgold R. Sleep-dependent memory consolidation. *Nature.* 2005;**437**(7063):1272–1278.

93. Seugnet L, Suzuki Y, Vine L, Gottschalk L, Shaw PJ. D1 receptor activation in the mushroom bodies rescues sleep-loss-induced learning impairments in *Drosophila. Curr Biol.* 2008;**18**(15):1110–1117.

94. Ishimori K. True cause of sleep: a hypnogenic substance as evidenced in the brain of sleep-deprived animals. *Tokyo Igakkai Zasshi.* 1909;**23**:429–457.

95. Inoue S, Honda K, Komoda Y. Sleep as neuronal detoxification and restitution. *Behav Brain Res.* 1995;**69**:91–96.

96. Reimund E. The free radical theory of sleep. *Medical Hypotheses.* 1994;**43**:231–233.

97. Schulze G. Sleep protects excitatory cortical circuits against oxidative damage. *Medical Hypotheses.* 2004;**63**(2):203–207.

98. Honda K, Komoda Y, Inoue S. Oxidized glutathione regulates physiological sleep in unrestrained rats. *Brain Res.* 1994;**636**:253–258.

99. D'Almeida V, Lobo LL, Hipolide DC, et al. Sleep deprivation induces brain region-specific decreases in glutathione levels. *Neuroreport.* 1998;**9**(12):2853–2856.

100. D'Almeida V, Hipolide DC, Azzalis LA, et al. Absence of oxidative stress following paradoxical sleep deprivation in rats. *Neurosci Lett.* 1997;**235**(1–2):25–28.

101. Silva RH, Abilio VC, Takatsu AL, et al. Role of hippocampal oxidative stress in memory deficits induced by sleep deprivation in mice. *Neuropharmacology.* 2004;**46**(6):895–903.

102. Singh R, Kiloung J, Singh S, Sharma D. Effect of paradoxical sleep deprivation on oxidative stress parameters in brain regions of adult and old rats. *Biogerontology.* 2008;**9**(3):153–162.

103. Ramanathan L, Gulyani S, Nienhuis R, Siegel JM. Sleep deprivation decreases superoxide dismutase activity in rat hippocampus and brainstem. *Neuroreport.* 2002;**13**(11):1387–1390.

104. Gopalakrishnan A, Ji LL, Cirelli C. Sleep deprivation and cellular responses to oxidative stress. *Sleep.* 2004;**27**(1):27–35.

105. Hipolide DC, D'Almeida V, Raymond R, Tufik S, Nobrega JN. Sleep deprivation does not affect indices of necrosis or apoptosis in rat brain. *Int J Neurosci.* 2002;**112**(2):155–166.

106. Benington J, Heller HC. Restoration of brain energy metabolism as the function of sleep. *Progr Neurobiol.* 1995;**45**(4):347–360.

107. Czikk MJ, Sweeley JC, Homan JH, Milley JR, Richardson BS. Cerebral leucine uptake and protein synthesis in the near-term ovine fetus: relation to fetal behavioral state. *Am J Physiol Regul Integr Comp Physiol.* 2003;**284**(1):R200–207.

108. Ramm P, Smith CT. Rates of cerebral protein synthesis are linked to slow-wave sleep in the rat. *Physiol Behav.* 1990;**48**:749–753.

109. Nakanishi H, Sun Y, Nakamura RK, et al. Positive correlations between cerebral protein synthesis rates and deep sleep in *Macaca mulatta. Eur J Neurosci.* 1997;**9**:271–279.

110. Vazquez J, Hall SC, Witkowska HE, Greco MA. Rapid alterations in cortical protein profiles underlie spontaneous sleep and wake bouts. *J Cell Biochem.* 2008;**105**:1472–1484.

111. Giuditta A, Rutigliano B, Vitale-Neugebauer A. Influence of synchronized sleep on the biosynthesis of

RNA in two nuclear classes isolated from rabbit cerebral cortex. *J Neurochem.* 1980;**35**(6):1259–1266.

112. Giuditta A, Rutigliano B, Vitale-Neugebauer A. Influence of synchronized sleep on the biosynthesis of RNA in neuronal and mixed fractions isolated from rabbit cerebral cortex. *J Neurochem.* 1980;**35**(6):1267–1272.

113. Terao A, Steininger TL, Hyder K, et al. Differential increase in the expression of heat shock protein family members during sleep deprivation and during sleep. *Neuroscience.* 2003;**116**(1):187–200.

114. Naidoo N, Giang W, Galante RJ, Pack AI. Sleep deprivation induces the unfolded protein response in mouse cerebral cortex. *J Neurochem.* 2005;**92**(5):1150–1157.

115. Taishi P, Sanchez C, Wang Y, et al. Conditions that affect sleep alter the expression of molecules associated with synaptic plasticity. *Am J Physiol.* 2001;**281**:R839–R845.

116. Cirelli C, Gutierrez CM, Tononi G. Extensive and divergent effects of sleep and wakefulness on brain gene expression. *Neuron.* 2004;**41**(1):35–43.

117. Basheer R, Brown R, Ramesh V, Begum S, McCarley RW. Sleep deprivation-induced protein changes in basal forebrain: Implications for synaptic plasticity. *J Neurosci Res.* 2005;**82**(5):650–658.

118. Mackiewicz M, Shockley KR, Romer MA, et al. Macromolecule biosynthesis: a key function of sleep. *Physiol Genomics.* 2007;**31**(3):441–457.

119. Guzman-Marin R, Suntsova N, Stewart DR, et al. Sleep deprivation reduces proliferation of cells in the dentate gyrus of the hippocampus in rats. *J Physiol (Lond).* 2003;**549**(2):563–571.

120. Tung A, Takase L, Fornal C, Jacobs B. Effects of sleep deprivation and recovery sleep upon cell proliferation in adult rat dentate gyrus. *Neuroscience.* 2005;**134**(3):721–723.

121. Guzman-Marin R, Suntsova N, Methippara M, et al. Sleep deprivation suppresses neurogenesis in the adult hippocampus of rats. *Eur J Neurosci.* 2005;**22**(8):2111–2116.

122. Hairston IS, Little MTM, Scanlon MD, et al. Sleep restriction suppresses neurogenesis induced by hippocampus-dependent learning. *J Neurophysiol.* 2005;**94**(6):4224–4233.

123. Mueller AD, Pollock MS, Lieblich SE, et al. Sleep deprivation can inhibit adult hippocampal neurogenesis independent of adrenal stress hormones. *Am J Physiol Regul Integr Comp Physiol.* 2008;**294**(5): R1693–1703.

124. Guzman-Marin R, Suntsova N, Bashir T, et al. Rapid eye movement sleep deprivation contributes to

125. Bobillier P, Sakai F, Seguin S, Jouvet M. Deprivation of paradoxical sleep and in vitro cerebral protein synthesis in the rat. *Life Sciences.* 1971;**10**(Part II): 1349–1357.

126. Shapiro C, Girdwood P. Protein synthesis in rat brain during sleep. *Neuropharmacology.* 1981; **20**:457–460.

127. Denin NN, Mallikov UM, Rubinskaia NL. Concentration of proteins and RNA in neurons and gliocytes of the rat locus coeruleus during natural sleep and REM-sleep deprivation. *Fiziol ZH SSSR Im I Sechnonovia.* 1980;**66**(11):1626–1631.

128. Maloney KJ, Mainville L, Jones BE. c-Fos expression in dopaminergic and GABAergic neurons of the ventral mesencephalic tegmentum after paradoxical sleep deprivation and recovery. *Eur J Neurosci.* 2002; **15**(4):774–778.

129. Toppila J, Stenberg D, Alanko L, et al. REM sleep deprivation induces galanin gene expression in the rat brain. *Neurosci Lett.* 1995;**183**(3):171–174.

130. Merchant-Nancy H, Vazquez J, Aguilar-Roblero R, Drucker-Colin R. c-fos proto-oncogene changes in relation to REM sleep duration. *Brain Res.* 1992; **579**(2):342–346.

131. Hobson JA. Neural control of sleep. In: Turek FW, Zee PC, eds. *Regulation of sleep and circadian rhythms*, Vol **133**. New York: Marcel Dekker, Inc.; 1999:81–110.

132. Andersen ML, Martins PJF, D'almeida V, Bignotto M, Tufik S. Endocrinological and catecholaminergic alterations during sleep deprivation and recovery in male rats. *J Sleep Res.* 2005;**14**(1):83–90.

133. Pedrazzoli M, Benedito MAC. Rapid eye movement sleep deprivation-induced down-regulation of beta-adrenergic receptors in the rat brainstem and hippocampus. *Pharmacol Biochem Behav.* 2004;**79**(1):31–36.

134. Farooqui SM, Brock JW, Zhou J. Changes in monoamines and their metabolite concentrations in REM sleep-deprived rat forebrain nuclei. *Pharmacol Biochem Behav.* 1996;**54**(2):385–391.

135. Hipolide DC, Tufik S, Raymond R, Nobrega JN. Heterogeneous effects of rapid eye movement sleep deprivation on binding to [alpha]- and [beta]-adrenergic receptor subtypes in rat brain. *Neuroscience.* 1998;**86**(3):977–987.

136. Porrka-Heiskanen T, Smith SE, Taira T, et al. Noradrenergic activity in rat brain during rapid eye movement sleep deprivation and rebound sleep. *Am J Physiol Regul Integr Comp Physiol.* 1995;**268**(37): R1456–R1463.

137. Majumdar S, Mallick BN. Cytomorphometric changes in rat brain neurons after rapid eye movement sleep deprivation. *Neuroscience*. 2005;**135**(3):679–690.

138. Adya HVA, Mallick BN. Comparison of Na-K ATPase activity in rat brain synaptosome under various conditions. *Neurochem Int*. 1998;**33**:283–286.

139. Kaur S, Panchal M, Faisal M, et al. Long term blocking of GABA-A receptor in locus coeruleus by bilateral microinfusion of picrotoxin reduced rapid eye movement sleep and increased brain Na-K ATPase activity in freely moving normally behaving rats. *Behav Brain Res*. 2004;**151**(1–2):185–190.

140. McDermott CM, LaHoste GJ, Chen C, et al. Sleep deprivation causes behavioral, synaptic, and membrane excitability alterations in hippocampal neurons. *J Neurosci*. 2003;**23**(29): 9687–9695.

141. Gorter JA, Kamphuis W, Coenan AM. Paradoxical sleep deprivation does not affect neuronal excitability in the rat hippocampus. *Brain Res*. 1989;**476**(1):16–20.

142. Mallick BN, Thakkar M, Gangabhagirathi R. Rapid eye movement sleep deprivation decreases membrane fluidity in the rat brain. *Neurosci Res*. 1995;**22**:117–122.

143. Karnovsky ML, Reich P. Biochemistry of sleep. *Adv Neurochem*. 1977;**628**(2):213–275.

144. Netchiporouk L, Shram N, Salvert D, Cespuglio R. Brain extracellular glucose assessed by voltammetry throughout the rat sleep-wake cycle. *Eur J Neurosci*. 2001;**13**(7):1429–1434.

145. Shram N, Netchiporouk L, Cespuglio R. Lactate in the brain of the freely moving rat: voltammetric monitoring of the changes related to the sleep-wake states. *Eur J Neurosci*. 2002;**16**(3):461–466.

146. Nofzinger EA. Functional neuroimaging of sleep. *Semin Neurol*. 2005;**25**(1):9–18.

147. Urrila AS, Hakkarainen A, Heikkinen S, et al. Stimulus-induced brain lactate: effects of aging and prolonged wakefulness. *J Sleep Res*. 2004; **13**(2):111–119.

148. Dorsey CM, Lukas SE, Moore CM, et al. Phosphorous31 magnetic resonance spectroscopy after total sleep deprivation in healthy adult men. *Sleep*. 2003;**26**(5):573–577.

149. Karnovsky ML, Reich P, Anchors JM, Burrows BL. Changes in brain glycogen during slow-wave sleep in the rat. *J Neurochem*. 1983;**41**:1498–1501.

150. Kong J, Shepel PN, Holden CP, et al. Brain glycogen decreases with increased periods of wakefulness: implications for homeostatic drive to sleep. *J Neurosci*. 2002;**22**(13):5581–5587.

151. Gip P, Hagiwara G, Ruby NF, Heller HC. Sleep deprivation decreases glycogen in the cerebellum but not in the cortex of young rats. *Am J Physiol Regul Integr Comp Physiol*. 2002;**283**(1):R54–59.

152. Franken P, Gip P, Hagiwara G, Ruby NF, Heller HC. Changes in brain glycogen after sleep deprivation vary with genotype. *Am J Physiol Regul Integr Comp Physiol*. 2003;**285**(2):R413–419.

153. Gip P, Hagiwara G, Sapolsky RM, et al. Glucocorticoids influence brain glycogen levels during sleep deprivation. *Am J Physiol Regul Integr Comp Physiol*. 2004;**286**(6):R1057–1062.

154. Zimmerman JE, Mackiewicz M, Galante RJ, et al. Glycogen in the brain of *Drosophila melanogaster*: diurnal rhythm and the effect of rest deprivation. *J Neurochem*. 2004;**88**(1):32–40.

155. Scharf MT, Naidoo N, Zimmerman JE, Pack AI. The energy hypothesis of sleep revisited. *Progr Neurobiol*. 2008;**86**(3):264–280.

156. Siegel JM. The REM sleep-memory consolidation hypothesis. *Science*. 2001;**294**(5544):1058–1063.

157. Vertes RP, Eastman KE. The case against memory consolidation in REM sleep. *Behav Brain Sci*. 2000;**23**(6):867–876.

158. Stickgold R, Hobson JA, Fosse R, Fosse M. Sleep, learning and dreams: off-line memory reprocessing. *Science*. 2001;**294**:1052–1057.

159. Maquet P. The role of sleep in learning and memory. *Science*. 2001;**294**:1048–1051.

160. Vertes RP. Memory consolidation in sleep: dream or reality. *Neuron*. 2004;**44**(1):135–148.

161. Vertes RP, Siegel JM. Time for the sleep community to take a critical look at the purported role of sleep in memory processing. *Sleep*. 2005;**28**(10):1228–1229.

162. Walker MP, Stickgold R. Sleep-dependent learning and memory consolidation. *Neuron*. 2004;**44**(1):121–133.

163. Walker MP, Stickgold R, Alsop D, Gaab N, Schlaug G. Sleep-dependent motor memory plasticity in the human brain. *Neuroscience*. 2005;**133**(4):911–917.

164. Stickgold R, Walker MP. Sleep and memory: the ongoing debate. *Sleep*. 2005;**28**(10):1225–1227.

165. Frank MG, Benington J. The role of sleep in brain plasticity: dream or reality? *The Neuroscientist*. 2006;**12**(6):477–488.

166. Tononi G, Cirelli C. Sleep function and synaptic homeostasis. *Sleep Med Rev*. 2006;**10**(1):49–62.

167. Smith C. Sleep states and memory processes. *Behav Brain Res*. 1995;**69**:137–145.

168. Datta S, Mavanji V, Ulloor J, Patterson EH. Activation of phasic pontine-wave generator prevents rapid eye movement sleep deprivation-induced learning impairment in the rat: A mechanism for sleep-dependent plasticity. *J. Neurosci*. 2004;**24**(6):1416–1427.

169. Rauchs G, Desgranges B, Foret J, Eustace F. The relationships between memory systems and sleep stages. *J Sleep Res*. 2005;**14**:123–140.

170. Graves LA, Heller EA, Pack AI, Abel T. Sleep deprivation selectively impairs memory consolidation for contextual fear conditioning. *Learn Mem*. 2003;**10**(3):168–176.

171. Ulloor J, Datta S. Spatio-temporal activation of cyclic AMP response element-binding protein, activity-regulated cytoskeletal-associated protein and brain-derived nerve growth factor: a mechanism for pontine-wave generator activation-dependent two-way active-avoidance memory processing in the rat. *J Neurochem*. 2005;**95**(2):418–428.

172. Deregnaucourt S, Mitra PP, Feher O, Pytte C, Tchernichovski O. How sleep affects the developmental learning of bird song. *Nature*. 2005;**433**(7027): 710–716.

173. Datta S. Avoidance task training potentiates phasic pontine-wave density in the rat: A mechanism for sleep-dependent plasticity. *J Neurosci*. 2000; **20**(22):8607–8613.

174. Malenka RC, Bear MF. LTP and LTD: An embarassment of riches. *Neuron*. 2004;**44**:5–21.

175. Bear MF, Malenka RC. Synaptic plasticity: LTP and LTD. *Curr Opin Neurobiol*. 1994;**4**:389–399.

176. Dan Y, Poo M-M. Spike timing-dependent plasticity of neural circuits. *Neuron*. 2004;**44**:23–30.

177. Hennevin E, Huetz C, Edeline J-M. Neural representations during sleep: From sensory processing to memory traces. *Neurobiol Learn Mem*. 2007;**87**(3): 416–440.

178. Leonard BJ, McNaughton BL, Barnes CA. Suppression of hippocampal synaptic plasticity during slow-wave sleep. *Brain Res*. 1987;**425**:174–177.

179. Bramham CR, Srebro B. Synaptic plasticity in the hippocampus is modulated by behavioral state. *Brain Res*. 1989;**493**:74–86.

180. Bramham CR, Maho C, Laroche S. Suppression of long-term potentiation during alert wakefulness but not during 'enhanced' REM sleep after avoidance learning. *Neuroscience*. 1994;**59**:501–509.

181. Romcy-Pereira R, Pavlides C. Distinct modulatory effects of sleep on the maintenance of hippocampal and medial prefrontal cortex LTP. *Eur J Neurosci*. 2004;**20**(12):3453–3462.

182. Marks CA, Wayner MJ. Effects of sleep disruption on rat dentate granule cell LTP in vivo. *Brain Res Bull*. 2005;**66**(2):114–119.

183. Kim E, Mahmoud GS, Grover LM. REM sleep deprivation inhibits LTP in vivo in area CA1 of rat hippocampus. *Neurosci Lett*. 2005;**388**(3):163–167.

184. Campbell IG, Guinan MJ, Horowitz JM. Sleep deprivation impairs long-term potentiation in the rat hippocampal slices. *J Neurophysiol*. 2002;**88**:1073–1076.

185. Davis CJ, Harding JW, Wright JW. REM sleep deprivation-induced deficits in the latency-to-peak induction and maintenance of long-term potentiation within the CA1 region of the hippocampus. *Brain Res*. 2003;**973**(2):293–297.

186. McDermott CM, Hardy MN, Bazan NG, Magee JC. Sleep-deprivation induced alterations in excitatory synaptic transmission in the CA1 region of the rat hippocampus. *J Physiol (Lond)*. 2006;**570**:553–565.

187. Kopp C, Longordo F, Nicholson JR, Luthi A. Insufficient sleep reversibly alters bidirectional synaptic plasticity and NMDA receptor function. *J Neurosci*. 2006;**26**(48):12456–12465.

188. Tartar JL, Ward CP, McKenna JT, et al. Hippocampal synaptic plasticity and spatial learning are impaired in a rat model of sleep fragmentation. *Eur J Neurosci*. 2006;**23**(10):2739–2748.

189. Ishikawa A, Kanayama Y, Matsumura H, et al. Selective rapid eye movement sleep deprivation impairs the maintenance of long-term potentiation in the rat hippocampus. *Eur J Neurosci*. 2006;**24**(1):243–248.

190. Roffwarg HP, Muzio JN, Dement WC. Ontogenetic development of the human sleep-dream cycle. *Science*. 1966(152):604–619.

191. Frank MG, Heller HC. Development of REM and slow wave sleep in the rat. *Am J Physiol*. 1997;**272**: R1792–R1799.

192. Jouvet-Mounier D, Astic L, Lacote D. Ontogenesis of the states of sleep in rat, cat and guinea pig during the first postnatal month. *Dev Psychobiol*. 1970;**2**(4):216–239.

193. Sengpiel F, Godecke I, Stawinski P, et al. Intrinsic and environmental factors in the development of functional maps in cat visual cortex. *Neuropharmacology*. 1998; **37**:607–621.

194. Singer W. Neuronal mechanisms in experience dependent modification of visual cortex function. In: Cuenod M, Kreutzberg GW, Bloom FE, eds. *Development and chemical sensitivity of neurons*, Vol **31**. Amsterdam: Elsevier/North-Holland Biomedical Press; 1979:457–477.

195. Kirkwood A, Lee HK, Bear MF. Co-regulation of long-term potentiation and experience-dependent synaptic plasticity in visual cortex. *Nature*. 1995;**375**:328–331.

196. Shaffery JP, Sinton CM, Bissette G, Roffwarg HP, Marks GA. Rapid eye movement sleep deprivation modifies expression of long-term potentiation in visual cortex of immature rats. *Neuroscience*. 2002; **110**(3):431–443.

197. Shaffery JP, Lopez J, Bissette G, Roffwarg HP. Rapid eye movement sleep deprivation revives a form of developmentally regulated synaptic plasticity in the visual cortex of post-critical period rats. *Neurosci Lett.* 2005;**391**(3):131–135.

198. Shaffery JP, Roffwarg HP. Rapid eye-movement sleep deprivation does not 'rescue' developmentally regulated long-term potentiation in visual cortex of mature rats. *Neurosci Lett.* 2003;**342**(3):196–200.

199. Frank MG, Issa NP, Stryker MP. Sleep enhances plasticity in the developing visual cortex. *Neuron.* 2001;**30**(1):275–287.

200. Aton S, Seibt J, Dumoulin M, et al. Mechanisms of sleep-dependent consolidation of cortical plasticity. *Neuron.* 2009; **61**(3):454–466.

201. Jha SK, Jones BE, Coleman T, et al. Sleep-dependent plasticity requires cortical activity. *J Neurosci.* 2005;**25**(40):9266–9274.

202. Frank MG, Jha SK, Coleman T. Blockade of post-synaptic activity in sleep inhibits developmental plasticity in visual cortex. *NeuroReport.* 2006; **17**:1459–1463.

203. Dadvand L, Stryker MP, Frank MG. Sleep does not enhance the recovery of deprived eye responses in developing visual cortex. *Neuroscience.* 2006;**143**(3):815–826.

204. Wang H, Hu Y, Tsien JZ. Molecular and systems mechanisms of memory consolidation and storage. *Progr Neurobiol.* 2006;**79**(3):123–135.

205. Buzsaki G. The hippocampo-neocortical dialogue. *Cerebral Cortex.* 1996;**6**:81–92.

206. Hasselmo ME. Neuromodulation: acetylcholine and memory consolidation. *Trends Cog Sci.* 1999;**3** (9):351–359.

207. Sejnowski TJ, Destexhe A. Why do we sleep? *Brain Res.* 2000;**886**:208–223.

208. Timofeev I, Grenier F, Bazhenov M, et al. Short- and medium-term plasticity associated with augmenting responses in cortical slabs and spindles in intact cortex of cats in vivo. *J Physiol (Lond).* 2002;**542**(2):583–598.

209. Cirelli C. A molecular window on sleep: changes in gene expression between sleep and wakefulness. *Neuroscientist.* 2005;**11**(1):63–74.

210. Frank MG. Hippocampal dreams, cortical wishes: a closer look at neuronal replay and the hippocampal-neocortical dialogue during sleep. *Cell Sci Rev.* 2007;**3**(4):161–171.

211. Pavlides C, Winson J. Influences of hippocampal place cell firing in the awake state on the activity of these cells during subsequent sleep. *J Neurosci.* 1989; **9**(8):2907–2918.

212. Wilson MA, McNaughton BL. Reactivation of hippocampal ensemble memories during sleep. *Science.* 1994;**265**:676–682.

213. Skaggs WE, McNaughton BL. Replay of neuronal firing sequences in rat hippocampus during sleep following spatial experience. *Science.* 1996;**271**: 1870–1873.

214. Louie K, Wilson MA. Temporally structured replay of awake hippocampal ensemble activity during rapid eye movement sleep. *Neuron.* 2001;**29**:145–156.

215. Kudrimoti HS, Barnes CA, McNaughton BL. Reactivation of hippocampal cell assemblies: Effects of behavioral state, experience and EEG dynamics. *J Neurosci.* 1999;**19**(10):4090–4101.

216. Nadasky Z, Hirase H, Czurko A, Csicsvari J, Buzsaki G. Replay and time compression of recurring spike sequences in the hippocampus. *J Neurosci.* 1999;**19**(21):9497–9507.

217. Ribeiro S, Gervasoni D, Soares ES, et al. Long-lasting novelty-induced neuronal reverberation during slow-wave sleep in multiple forebrain areas. *PLoS Biol.* 2004;**2**(1):E24.

218. Lee AK, Wilson MA. Memory of sequential experience in the hippocampus during slow wave sleep. *Neuron.* 2002;**36**:1183–1194.

219. Dave AS, Margoliash D. Song replay during sleep and computational rules of sensorimotor vocal learning. *Science.* 2000;**290**:812–816.

220. Hoffman KL, McNaughton BL. Coordinated reactivation of distributed memory traces in primate cortex. *Science.* 2002;**297**:2070–2073.

221. Pennartz CMA, Lee E, Verheul J, et al. The ventral striatum in off-line processing: ensemble reactivation during sleep and modulation by hippocampal ripples. *J Neurosci.* 2004;**24**(29):6446–6456.

222. Ji D, Wilson MA. Coordinated memory replay in the visual cortex and hippocampus during sleep. *Nat Neurosci.* 2007;**10**(1):100–106.

223. Graves L, Pack A, Abel T. Sleep and memory: a molecular perspective. *Trends Neurosci.* 2001;**24**(4):237–243.

224. Siapas AG, Wilson MA. Coordinated interactions between hippocampal ripples and cortical spindles during slow-wave sleep. *Neuron.* 1998;**21**:1123–1128.

225. Battaglia FP, Sutherland GR, McNaughton BL. Hippocampal sharp wave bursts coincide with neocortical "up-state" transitions. *Learn Mem.* 2004;**11**(6):697–704.

226. Sirota A, Csicsvari J, Buhl D, Buzsaki G. Communication between neocortex and hippocampus during sleep in rodents. *PNAS.* 2003;**100**(4): 2065–2069.

227. Pelletier JG, Apergis J, Pare D. Low-probability transmission of neocortical and entorhinal impulses through the perirhinal cortex. *J Neurophysiol.* 2004;**91**(5):2079–2089.

228. Steriade M. Corticothalamic resonance, states of vigilance and mentation. *Neuroscience.* 2000;**101**(2):243–276.

229. Steriade M, Amzica F. Coalescence of sleep rhythms and their chronology in corticothalamic networks. *Sleep Res Online.* 1998;**1**(1):1–10.

230. Steriade M, Timofeev I. Neuronal plasticity in thalamocortical networks during sleep and waking oscillations. *Neuron.* 2003;**37**(4):563–576.

231. Crochet S, Fuentealba P, Cisse Y, Timofeev I, Steriade M. Synaptic plasticity in local cortical network in vivo and its modulation by the level of neuronal activity. *Cereb Cortex.* 2006;**16**:618–631.

232. Rosanova M, Ulrich D. Pattern-specific associative long-term potentiation induced by a sleep spindle-related spike train. *J Neurosci.* 2005;**25**(41):9398–9405.

233. Czarnecki A, Birtoli B, Ulrich D. Cellular mechanisms of burst firing-mediated long-term depression in rat neocortical pyramidal cells. *J Physiol (Lond).* 2007;**578**(2):471–479.

234. Turrigiano GG. Homeostatic plasticity in neuronal networks: the more things change, the more they stay the same. *Trends Neurosci.* 1999;**22**(5):221–227.

235. Faraguna U, Vyazovskiy VV, Nelson AB, Tononi G, Cirelli C. A causal role for brain-derived neurotrophic factor in the homeostatic regulation of sleep. *J Neurosci.* 2008;**28**(15):4088–4095.

236. Vyazovskiy VV, Cirelli C, Pfister-Genskow M, Faraguna U, Tononi G. Molecular and electrophysiological evidence for net synaptic potentiation in wake and depression in sleep. *Nat Neurosci.* 2008;**11**(2):200–208.

237. Ribeiro S, Goyal V, Mello CV, Pavlides C. Brain gene expression during REM sleep depends on prior waking experience. *Learn Mem.* 1999;**6**(5):500–508.

238. Neuner-Jehle M, Rhyner TA, Borbely AA. Sleep deprivation differentially affects the mRNA and protein levels of neurogranin in rat brain. *Brain Res.* 1995;**685**:143–153.

239. Guan Z, Peng X, Fang J. Sleep deprivation impairs spatial memory and decreases extracellular signal-regulated kinase phosphorylation in the hippocampus. *Brain Res.* 2004;**1018**(1):38–47.

240. Beattie EC, Stellwagen D, Morishita W, et al. Control of synaptic strength by glial TNFalpha. *Science.* 2002;**295**(5563):2282–2285.

241. Feinberg I. Slow wave sleep and release of growth hormone. *JAMA.* 2000;**284**(21):2717–2718.

242. Adkins B, Leclerc C, Marshall-Clarke S. Neonatal adaptive immunity comes of age. *Nat Rev Immun.* 2004;**4**(7):553–564.

243. Yerkovich ST, Wikstrom ME, Suriyaarachchi D, et al. Postnatal development of monocyte cytokine responses to bacterial lipopolysaccharide. *Pediatr Res.* 2007;**62**(5):547–552.

244. McKinney RA. Physiological roles of spine motility: development, plasticity and disorders. *Biochem Soc Trans.* 2005;**33**(Pt 6):1299–1302.

245. Esteban JA. Intracellular machinery for the transport of AMPA receptors. *Br J Pharmacol.* 2008;**153**(1):S35–S43.

246. von der Ohe CG, Garner CC, Darian-Smith C, Heller HC. Synaptic protein dynamics in hibernation. *J Neurosci.* 2007;**27**(1):84–92.

247. Ganguly-Fitzgerald I, Donlea J, Shaw PJ. Waking experience affects sleep need in drosophila. *Science.* 2006;**313**(5794):1775–1781.

248. Espiritu JRD. Aging-related sleep changes. *Clin Geriatr Mede Sleep Elderly Adults.* 2008;**24**(1):1–14.

249. Mora F, Segovia G, del Arco A. Aging, plasticity and environmental enrichment: Structural changes and neurotransmitter dynamics in several areas of the brain. *Brain Res Rev Intercellr Commun Brain.* 2007;**55**(1):78–88.

250. Churchill L, Rector DM, Yasuda K, et al. Tumor necrosis factor [alpha]: Activity dependent expression and promotion of cortical column sleep in rats. *Neuroscience.* 2008;**156**(1):71–80.

251. Hallasa M, Florian C, Fellin T, et al. Astrocytic modulation of sleep homeostasis and cognitive consequences of sleep loss. *Neuron.* 2009;**61**:213–219.

252. Broberger C. Brain regulation of food intake and appetite: molecules and networks. *J Int Med.* 2005;**258**(4):301–327.

Chapter 5

Dreams

Michael Schredl

Introduction

Mankind has been fascinated with dreaming since the dawn of history. The recorded dreams in the Giglamesh epic or the Old Testament (Joseph interpreting the dreams of the Pharaoh) are examples of this fascination. The first comprehensive dream book was compiled by Artemidorus of Daldis in the second century AD. The "Oneirocritica" included interpretations of a large variety of dream elements like body parts and animals; this work served as basis for dream books that were popular in medieval times [1]. In the scientific realm, three major approaches to the study of dreams can be differentiated: psychoanalytic, neurophysiological, and psychological.

From the psychoanalytic perspective, described initially by Sigmund Freud in his fundamental book "Die Traumdeutung" (The Interpretation of Dreams) published in 1899, the dream is conceptualized as expression of the person's inner life, i.e. "the interpretation of dreams is the royal road to a knowledge of the unconscious activities of the mind" [2]. Although psychoanalysis has brought together a large variety of interesting clinical material and may be helpful to patients on a case-by-case basis, psychoanalytic dream theories remain speculative and they are at least partly not in concordance with recent research findings.

The discovery of REM sleep was the starting point of the neurophysiological approach for studying the dream state. In 1953, Eugene Aserinsky and Nathaniel Kleitman published their finding that in the course of the night the sleeper goes through different sleep stages, among others periods with rapid eye movements [3]. After awakenings from these sleep stages, a vivid and pictorial dream was reported very often. The initial euphoria in hoping to find a direct access to the dream world subsided very quickly, because REM sleep measured by EEG, EOG, and EMG recordings and dreams (elicited by interviews) are two distinct realms (physiological level vs. psychological level) which variably correspond (see Dream content and sleep physiology section) and might not share similar functions (see Functions of dreaming section).

The third approach is based on methods of academic psychology. Although there had been several papers on dreams [4–6], the basic methodology was provided by Calvin S. Hall who published the book "The content analysis of dreams" with his coworker Robert Van de Castle in 1966 [7]. Extensive research carried out since the 1940s led to a comprehensive coding system for dream content analysis and to "norms" which were derived from 1000 dreams of college students. The major advantage of this approach is that specific dream characteristics can be quantified in a reliable fashion so that hypotheses can be tested by using common statistical methods. For example, Hall and Van de Castle [7] have shown that men dream significantly more often of physical aggression and sex than women. Subsequent studies with different samples [8,9] were able to replicate this finding. The psychological approach tries to find answers to a variety of questions: What are dreams like? How are dreams related to waking-life experiences? And how do dreams affect subsequent waking-life?

This chapter reviews the basic methodology and findings of the psychologically oriented research and the collaboration of neurophysiological and psychological approaches which is necessary to investigate the fascinating topic of possible interactions between physiological processes and psychological experiences during REM sleep. In the end, the aim of this kind of paradigm is to answer the question whether dreaming serves a function or several functions independently

Foundations of Psychiatric Sleep Medicine, ed. John W. Winkelman and David T. Plante. Published by Cambridge University Press.
© Cambridge University Press 2010.

from the functions of sleep, especially those formulated for REM sleep.

Definitions and methodological issues

First, a clear definition of dreaming is necessary in order to specify the subject of dream research. The following definition attempts to cover the consensus of the researchers in the field:

> A dream or a dream report is the recollection of mental activity which has occurred during sleep.
>
> ([10], p. 12)

It is important to notice that dreaming as a mental activity during sleep is not directly measurable; two boundaries have to be crossed (sleep–wake transition and time) before the person can report the subjective experiences which occurred during sleep. This leads to the problem of validity, i.e. is the dream report an appropriate account of the actual dream experience (see Dream content analysis section). The second question which has been raised by Maury [11] is whether the dream report reflects mental activity during sleep or is merely produced during the awakening process. Modern research combining physiological approaches with dream content analysis, however, has been able to demonstrate that dream reports are accounts of mental activity during sleep since physiological parameters (e.g. eye movements, heart rate) during REM sleep at least partially match with dream contents elicited upon awakening (cf. [12]). In addition, the incorporation of stimuli applied during sleep into dreams [10,13] corroborates the assumption that dreaming occurs during sleep.

A detailed differentiation of the dream phenomena is given in Table 5.1. The first three dream "types" are related to the different sleep stages. During the initial phase of psychophysiological dream research, REM sleep was considered to be the physiological concomitant of dreaming [14]. However, in 1962, Foulkes showed that dream reports can be elicited after awakening out of all stages of sleep [15]; although a recent review showed recall rates are somewhat lower for NREM awakenings (43.0%) than for REM awakenings (81.9%) [16]. Although Nielsen [16] tried to connect NREM dreaming with REM sleep by postulating that covert REM processes were responsible for dream recall out of NREM sleep, Wittmann and Schredl [17] pointed out the logical errors of this assumption and argued that mental activity is

Table 5.1 Different kinds of dreams

Dream types	Definition
REM dreams	Recollection of mental activity during REM sleep
NREM dreams	Recollection of mental activity during NREM sleep
Sleep-onset dreams	Recollection of mental activity during NREM stage 1
Nightmares	REM dreams with strong negative emotions which cause awakening
Night terrors	Sudden arousal with intense anxiety out of slow-wave sleep; sometimes accompanied by short NREM dreams
Post-traumatic re-enactments	REM or NREM dreams which replay the original traumatic experience in a less distorted way
Lucid dreams	REM dreams in which the dreamer is aware that she or he is dreaming

presumably present continuously during sleep. Dreaming therefore is the psychic correlate of the continuous brain activity, reflecting the (sleep) stage-dependent physiological conditions of the brain. Differences regarding formal characteristics of dreaming and waking cognition as well as between dream reports of different sleep stages can be explained by factors such as cortical activation, blockade of external sensory input, and neuromodulation as described by the AIM-model [18] (see Chapter 1: Sleep medicine and psychiatry: history and significance, for detailed discussion).

Nightmares are a subgroup of REM dreams with strong negative emotions, but whether these actually cause awakening is not yet known (cf. [10]). Night terrors, on the other hand, occur out of NREM sleep and the person often does not remember the incident in the morning (see Chapter 10: Parasomnias, for detailed discussion). The third dream phenomenon associated with fear are called post-traumatic re-enactment or post-traumatic nightmares, which are special since they seem to occur in REM sleep as well as in NREM sleep (cf. [19]). Lucid dreams in which the dreamer is aware that she/he is dreaming offer fascinating opportunities to study the body–mind relationship during sleep because the dreamer can carry out prearranged tasks during the dream and

Table 5.2 Methods of dream collection

Method	Example study
Questionnaire	Domhoff [23]
Interview	Parekh [124]
Dream diary	Schredl [25]
Laboratory awakenings	Strauch & Meier [13]

mark their beginning and end by distinct eye movements which can be measured electrically (cf. [20]).

Naturally, dream recall is a prerequisite for dream content studies. The large amount of research in this area (overview: [21]) showed that personality factors such as "thin boundaries," absorption, openness to experiences, creativity, visual memory, and sleep behavior (frequent nocturnal awakenings) are associated with heightened dream recall. But a recent large-scale study including these factors indicated that the variance explained by these factors is rather small (below 10%) [22]. At present, the reasons for the large interindividual differences or intraindividual fluctuations in dream recall are poorly understood. Sophisticated studies (e.g. applying event-related potential paradigms) investigating the awakening process are necessary.

Several approaches have been used to elicit dream reports (see Table 5.2). The easiest way to collect dream reports from large samples is the so-called "most recent dream" approach (see [23]). The participants are asked to write down (as completely as possible) the last dream they remember. The advantage of this retrospective collecting method is that dreaming is not affected by the method but, on the other hand, depending on how long ago the dream was recalled in the first place, the participant might have problems remembering the dream fully. For example, research has demonstrated that intense, bizarre dreams are more often reported in such settings than mundane dreams [10]. Similar effects have been found for dreams reported during an interview or patients' dreams recorded by the therapist after the therapy session [24]. To minimize recall bias, dream diaries are an appropriate tool [25]. In order to optimize controllability of the experimental situation and enhance the amount of dream material – in addition to measuring physiological parameters – dream reports collected during laboratory awakenings are the "gold standard." The major drawback of this paradigm, however, is

the strong effect of the setting on dream content; i.e. up to 50% of the dreams include laboratory references [26]. Other studies (e.g. [27]) found that aggressive and sexual elements occur in laboratory dreams less often than in home dreams; a finding which is interpreted as an "inhibitory" effect of the laboratory setting (including video taping of the sleeper, technical staff presence, etc.). Some researchers (e.g. [28]) have tried to combine the advantages of the different methods by using ambulatory measurement units to collect dreams and physiological parameters in the home setting.

Dream content analysis

The main goal of dream content analysis is the quantification of specific aspects of the dream (e.g. number of dream persons, types of interactions, settings) in order to perform statistical analyses (cf. [7]). The following fictive example illustrates the procedure. A clinical psychologist formulates the hypothesis that depressed patients dream more often about rejection than healthy persons. The researcher develops a scale measuring rejection (occurrence vs. not present in the dream content). Dream reports are collected from the two groups and ordered randomly so that external judges applying the content scale do not know whether the dream is a patient's dream or a control dream. After the rating procedure, the dream reports are reassigned to the two groups and the difference in percentage of dreams including at least one rejection of the dream can be tested statistically.

Within their book "Dimensions of dreams," Winget and Kramer have compiled 132 scales and rating systems [29]. The most elaborated coding system was published by Hall and Van de Castle [7]. Domhoff [23] presents an overview of the dream content analytic studies and concludes that this coding system is widely used as a research tool. Sometimes, it seems more appropriate to use global rating scales, e.g. for measuring emotional intensity (see below). In some cases, it is also useful to use a self-rating scale applied by the dreamer herself/himself.

The most important methodological issues in dream content analysis are reliability and validity. The interrater reliability designates the agreement between two or more external judges rating the same dream material. High indices indicate that the scale can be applied easily and the findings are not the results of the raters' subjective point of view.

Cut-off points for sufficient interrater reliability have not yet been published. The exact agreements for the Hall and Van de Castle system vary between 61% and 98% [23]; for ordinal rating scales the coefficients are typically between 0.70 and 0.95 [10]. Only one study, however, has systematically studied the effect of training on interrater reliability [30]. The findings indicate that training (coding 100 to 200 dreams and discussing differences) is valuable in improving reliability. In addition to the issue of interrater reliability indicating the quality of the scales, the "normal" reliability problem also has to be considered in dream content research. Schredl [31] reported that up to 20 dream reports per participant are necessary to measure reliably interindividual differences in dream content, which is necessary, for example, if dream characteristics are related to differences in personality measures.

At first glance, the validity issue seems very easy to solve; a scale designed for measuring aggression reflects the amount of aggression within the dream report. But one has to keep in mind that the researcher is genuinely interested in the dream experience itself, i.e. the question arises whether the dream report represents the dream experience sufficiently. The following example that includes the measurement of dream emotions will illustrate this line of thinking. Schredl and Doll [32] applied three different methods of measuring dream emotions: the emotion scales of Hall and Van de Castle [7] measuring only explicitly mentioned emotions; the four-point global rating scales designed by Schredl [10] allowing the coding of emotions when it is obvious from the dream action; and similar four-point scales rated by the dreamer. The dreams were sorted into four groups (see Table 5.3).

Two findings are striking: first, the emotions are markedly underestimated by the external judges; and second, the ratio of positive and negative emotions differs, depending on the measurement technique – a balanced ratio for the self-ratings and predominantly negative for the external ratings [32]. A similar underestimation was found for the number of bizarre elements within the dream [33]. These two studies clearly indicate that some aspects of the dream experiences might not be measured validly if dream content analytic scales were applied to dream reports only. More research is needed to estimate the effect of the validity problem on dream content analytic findings.

Table 5.3 Dream emotions (N = 133 dreams [32])

Category	Self-rating (%)	Rating by judge (%)	Hall & Van de Castle (%)
No emotions	0.8	13.5	57.9
Balanced emotions	12.0	9.0	6.8
Predominantly negative emotions	50.4	56.4	26.3
Predominantly positive emotions	36.8	21.1	9.0

Phenomenology of dreams

In the analysis of large samples of dream reports, different dream aspects like bizarreness, emotions, and perception have been characterized. Over 90% of the dreams included the dream ego, i.e. dreaming is experienced in a similar way to waking-life (with the exception of lucid dreams, which are very rare [10]). About 20% of the laboratory dream reports collected by Strauch and Meier [13] included bizarre elements (30% of diary dreams; [34]), whereas about 30% were realistic (could have happened in the exact same way in waking-life), and 50% were fictional, e.g. possible in real life but unlikely to happen in the dreamer's everyday life. Using a broader definition of bizarreness, e.g. including incongruencies with waking-life (e.g. a street of the home town with a new building), the number of bizarre elements increases drastically [35]. Strauch and Meier [13] and Schredl and Doll [32] found a balance between positive and negative emotions in larger samples of laboratory and home dreams in healthy persons. Studies reporting predominantly negative dreams (e.g. [7]) have to be considered with caution due to methodological problems (see Dream content analysis section).

In Table 5.4, three studies investigating sensory perceptions are presented. Visual perceptions are present in every dream. Auditory perceptions are very common whereas tactile, gustatory, and olfactory perceptions and pain are quite rare. Colors are not very often reported spontaneously (25% of dream reports [39]) but Rechtschaffen and Buchignani [40,41] who instructed their participants to compare their dream images with 129 colored pictures with

Table 5.4 Sensory perceptions in dreams

Modality	Laboratory dreams[1] (%, N = 635)	Laboratory dreams[2] (%, N = 107)	Diary dreams[3] (%, N = 3372)
Visual	100	100	100
Auditory	76	65	53
Vestibular	–	8	–
Tactile	1	1	–
Gustatory	1	1	<1
Olfactory	<1	1	1
Pain	–	–	1

Notes: [1][36];
[2][37];
[3][38].

Table 5.5 Paradigms to study the effect of waking-life experiences on dream content

Research paradigms
Assessing temporal references of dream elements
Experimental manipulation
Field studies
– intraindividual fluctuations
– interindividual differences

different intensities and contrasts found that colors of elements which are prominent in the dream are comparable to the colors experienced in waking-life, solely the colors in the background of dreams are less intense than one would expect in waking-life. Whether this is merely a problem of recall has not been analyzed by these authors.

Factors influencing dream content

The main focus of this section will be the effect of waking-life experiences on subsequent dream content. In Table 5.5, different methodological approaches for studying the relationship between waking-life and dreaming are listed.

The most detailed study regarding temporal references of dream elements were carried out by Strauch and Meier [13]. Fifty dreams stemming from REM awakenings of five subjects included 80 key role characters, 39 extras (person playing a minor role in the dream), 74 settings, and 298 objects. Strauch and Meier [13] not only asked about the last occurrence in waking-life but also when the dream element had appeared in waking thought. Over 50% of the references were from the previous day and less than 10% were older than 1 year. The major drawback of this approach is the limited memory capacity of the subjects; it is difficult to remember completely all waking-life experiences let alone all thoughts occurring during the preceding days. Another problem is that of multiple correspondences, e.g. if the mother was present in the dream, it could not easily

be determined whether this refers to a childhood experience or a recent telephone conversation.

The experimental approach manipulates the pre-sleep situation, most often by showing an exciting film (e.g. [42]). Dreams in the night after such a film will be compared to a control condition (e.g. neutral film). Interestingly, the effect of films (even if they are strongly negatively toned) on subsequent dreams is quite small (for overview see [10]). The effect of "real" stress like intense psychotherapy or awaiting a major surgery is much stronger [43]. The strong effect of traumata such as war experiences [44], kidnapping [45], or sexual abuse [46] on dreams, even years later, also indicates that the emotional intensity affects the incorporation rate of waking-life events into dreams.

Another approach for investigating the effects of waking-life on dreams is to look at differences in dreams of specific groups of persons who differ in particular aspects of their waking-life. Gender differences in dream content, e.g. heightened physical aggression in male dreams, are paralleled by similar differences in waking-life behavior found in meta-analyses [9].

The last paradigm presented in this section uses the method of correlating waking-life parameters with dream content variables. For example, the amount of time spent with a particular waking-life activity (e.g. driving a car, reading, spending time with the partner, etc.) was positively correlated with the number of occurrences of these elements within dreams [47].

In Table 5.6, the factors which might affect the continuity between waking-life and dreaming and, thus, are of importance for a mathematical model (see next section), have been compiled from the literature by Schredl [48].

Many studies (e.g. [13,49]) have shown an exponential decrease of the incorporation rate of waking-life experiences into dreams with elapsed time between experience and the subsequent dream. Also, the differences in effects of experimental stress and "real" stress and trauma research (see above) indicate that emotional involvement affects the incorporation rate. Three studies [47,50,51] have shown that focused thinking activity (reading, working with a computer) during dreams occurs less frequently than unfocused activities such as talking with friends, etc. These results also indicate that the type of activity is of importance for the continuity between waking-life and dreaming. The time of the night or the time interval between sleep onset and dream onset has affected the incorporation rate of waking-life experiences in two studies [52,53]; dreams of the second part of the night comprise more elements of the distant past while dreams of the first part of the night incorporate mostly recent daytime experiences (cf. [54,55]). The last factor, which has been studied rarely, is the interaction between personality traits and incorporation of waking-life experiences. It seems plausible that personality dimensions such as field dependence (this concept describes how people are influenced by inner (field-independent) or environmental (field-dependent) cues in orienting themselves

in space and the extent to which they select information within the environment [56]) or thin boundaries [57] moderate the magnitude of continuity between waking and dreaming.

The "continuity hypothesis" of dreaming

Many researchers (e.g. [10,13,23]) are advocating the so-called "continuity hypothesis" of dreaming which simply states that dreams reflect waking-life experiences. However, for deriving specific hypotheses the continuity hypothesis in its general formulation is too imprecise. In order to advance the research in this field, Schredl [48] postulated a mathematical model that is based on the published findings and seems to be promising for further empirical testing (see Figure 5.1). The multiplying factor includes the effects of emotional involvement (EI), type of waking-life experience (TYPE), and the interaction between personality traits and incorporation rates (PERS). The relationships between these factors should be determined by future studies. The slope of the exponential function may be moderated by the time interval between sleep onset and dream onset (time of the night; TN).

Dreams and psychopathology

Two motives have stimulated investigating the relationship between dreaming and mental disorders. First, the dream state itself was conceptualized by several theorists (e.g. [58]) as a mental disorder and, in reverse, hallucinations of schizophrenic patients have been thought of as breakthroughs of dreams into the waking state (e.g. [59]). Second, many clinicians since Freud have attempted to use dreams in the diagnosis and treatment of their patients (e.g. [60]). The basic assumption for this research is the so-called continuity hypothesis [48]

Table 5.6 Factors which affect the continuity between waking-life and dreaming

Factors
• Exponential decrease with time
• Emotional involvement
• Type of waking-life experience
• Personality traits
• Time of the night (time interval between sleep onset and dream onset)

Incorporation rate = a (EI, TYPE, PERS) $\cdot$ e$^{-b(TN)\cdot t}$ + Constant	
a (EI, TYPE, PERS)	multiplying factor which is a function of emotional involvement (EI), type of the waking-life experience (TYPE), and the interaction between experience and personality traits (PERS)
b (TN)	Slope of the exponential function which is itself a function of the time interval between sleep onset and dream onset (TN)
t	Time interval between waking-life experience and occurrence of the dream incorporation

Figure 5.1 Mathematical model for the continuity between waking-life and dreaming.

which predicts that for patients with mental disorders, it should thus be possible to detect the specific waking symptomatology within their dreams.

The literature reviews showed that the majority of empirical studies support the continuity hypothesis [61–63]. On the one hand, it was found that hallucinations of schizophrenic patients are not dreams experienced during the waking state (e.g. [64]) and that the concept of dreaming as a mental disorder is not very helpful (cf. [65]). On the other hand, dreams of schizophrenic patients are typical for this disorder, i.e. the dreams are more bizarre [65] and are characterized by aggression and negative emotions [61]. For depressive patients, Beck and Hurvich [66] and Beck and Ward [67] have found an increased amount of "masochistic" themes in their dreams. Subsequent studies (overview: [68]) confirmed that dreams of depressive patients are more negatively toned and include unpleasant experiences more often (definitions of "masochistic" dream content according to Beck & Hurvich [66]) than healthy controls. Schredl and Engelhardt [65] were able to demonstrate that severity of depressive symptomatology was directly correlated with the intensity of negative dream emotions, irrespective of the patients' diagnoses, supporting a dimensional and not categorical relationship between waking-life symptoms and dream content. In addition, severely depressed patients dreamed more often about aggression and death [65].

Regarding dream recall, many studies failed to show marked differences among various diagnostic groups, such as schizophrenia, eating disorders, etc., and healthy controls [61]. An exception is depression where patients have a reduced dream recall frequency [69,70]; the reduction was again related to symptom severity [71]. The explanations for the reduced dream recall in depressed patients, however, remain unclear. The question of whether the typical sleep architecture of depressive patients (decreased latency to REM sleep), cognitive impairment often found in severely disturbed patients, or intrinsic alterations related to depression is responsible has yet to be answered.

Dreams and sleep disorders

This section will focus on several sleep disorders which have been studied in relation to dreaming: insomnia, sleep apnea syndrome, narcolepsy, and restless legs syndrome. For other diagnoses, like idiopathic hypersomnia, or NREM parasomnias, such as sleepwalking or night terrors, systematic dream content analytic studies are lacking. However, extensive reviews are available for nightmares [72], REM sleep behavior disorder (see Chapter 10: Parasomnias), and dreaming in post-traumatic stress disorder [19].

Schredl et al. [73] found an elevated dream recall frequency in insomnia patients in contrast to healthy controls; a finding which was no longer significant if number of nocturnal awakenings (self-report measure) was statistically controlled. This parallels the correlation between nocturnal awakenings and increased dream recall in healthy persons [22]. Percentage of dream recall after REM awakenings carried out in the laboratory did not differ between insomnia patients and controls [74]. Ermann [75] and Schredl et al. [73] found more negatively toned dreams in patients with insomnia. In addition, occurrence of problems within the dream was directly correlated with the number of waking-life problems the patients reported in the questionnaire. Therefore, dreams might reflect the topics which are at least partially responsible for the development and maintenance of the primary insomnia.

In sleep apnea, the findings regarding the dream recall frequency are inconsistent (cf. [76]). In the nineteenth century, nightmares were thought to be due to decreased flow of oxygen (e.g. due to pillow blocking of the mouth and nose; see [77]). However, parameters like minimal oxygen saturation nadir or respiratory disturbance index do not correlate with dream recall frequency [78]. Furthermore, a heightened nightmare frequency in sleep apnea patients has not been found [76]. Only very few dream reports include the massive physiological apnea processes:

> During the dream I felt tied up or chained. I saw thick ropes around my arms and was not able to move.
> I experienced the fear of suffocation without being able to cope with the situation. Powerlessness and also resignation came up.
>
> (Patient with sleep apnea, male, 39 years, respiratory disturbance index (RDI): 68.1 apneas per hour, maximal drop of blood oxygen saturation: 43%).
>
> ([79], p. 295)

Overall, the low incidence of breathing-related dream topics might be explained by adaptation, i.e. the increase of number and severity of sleep apneas over months and years might explain why this stimuli is rarely incorporated into dreams whereas external stimuli are at least sometimes incorporated into dreams [76]. It would be intriguing to conduct a systematic study where the sleeper wears a mask which would allow transient occlusion of airflow and, thus, would allow testing of whether a "novel" apnea is more often incorporated into dreams.

Narcolepsy is a sleep disorder characterized by a disinhibition of the REM sleep regulations systems, and, therefore, the findings of increased dream recall frequency [80] and higher occurrence of nightmares [81] are not astonishing. In addition, dream content is more bizarre [80] and more negatively toned [82], whereas dream reports of the first REM period were longer in patients compared to healthy controls [83]. Asking for dreams while taking a sleep history of the patient might, in theory, help to differentiate narcolepsy from other forms of hypersomnia, such as idiopathic hypersomnia.

Lastly, Schredl [84] found a negative correlation between number of periodic limb movements associated with arousals and dream recall frequency in a sample of 131 restless legs patients. Taken together with the fact that high respiratory disturbance indices are related to less bizarre dreams in sleep apnea patients [85], one might hypothesize that frequent microarousal might interfere with the dreaming process itself. Systematic studies in this area, however, are lacking.

Dream content and sleep physiology

The combination of neurophysiological sleep research and dream research has shed light on the body/mind interaction, i.e. how and to what extent are physiological processes related to specific dream characteristics?

First of all, researchers were interested in whether the typical eye movements of REM sleep are related to gaze shifts within the dream. The studies yielded inconsistent results (for a review see [12]), but Herman et al. [86] who carried out the most sophisticated study concluded that there is a small but substantial relationship, i.e. some eye movements correspond to dream content and some do not. For deliberately carried out gaze shifts during lucid dreams, the results are more clear. Proficient lucid dreamers can carry out prearranged eye movements while dreaming, e.g. right-left-right-left. These patterns can be identified in the EOG pattern with high reliability (see [87]). Previous studies investigated the relationship between other peripheral parameters, like EMG, heart rate, respiratory rate, and sexual excitement (cf. [12]). Wolpert [88], for example, found that dreams which included many dreamed movements are associated

with elevated EMG activity in arms and legs. For lucid dreaming, Erlacher and Schredl [89] were able to demonstrate that squats performed within the dream are associated with an increase in heart rate; comparable to the findings regarding imagined motor activities.

Even though the findings regarding peripheral parameters and dream content implicate a relatively close interaction between the physiological level and the psychological level (mind–body interaction) during dreaming, the fundamental question is whether specific dream content is related to specific brain activation. The findings of imaging studies of REM sleep have been linked to specific dream features, e.g. high limbic activity, especially in the amygdala, reflecting reported intense dream emotions, and reduced prefrontal activation might account for the fact that the dreamer is not aware of his/her state (for an overview see [90]). The activation–synthesis hypothesis formulated by Hobson and McCarley [91] postulated that ponto-geniculo-occipital (PGO) waves might be linked to bizarre elements and/or scene shift within the dreams. The AIM model formulated by Hobson et al. [18], expanding the activation–synthesis hypothesis, assumes that the cholinergic neurotransmission which is more active during REM sleep than during NREM sleep and the waking state is responsible for the bizarre features of REM dreams. Although these theories are highly interesting and plausible, they remain largely speculative because studies directly linking brain activity to specific dream features or contents are still very sparse. Hong et al. [92], for example, reported a significant relationship between talking and listening during the dream and activation of Broca's and Wernicke's areas (responsible for speech processing) measured by EEG (activation paralleled a decrease in alpha power). For lucid dreams, Erlacher and coworkers [93] found correlations between motor cortex activity and hand clenching performed within the dream. It seems to be very promising to use imaging techniques, especially fMRI because of its good time resolution [94], in dream research, to study the relationship between brain activation patterns and dream content.

Effect of dreams on waking-life

Whereas the amount of studies investigating the effect of waking-life on dreams is considerable, research looking into the effect of dreams on waking-life is encountered quite rarely. Three major topics have been studied: (1) effect of nightmares on daytime mood, (2) creative inspiration by dreams, and (3) dreams and psychotherapy.

Schredl's [95] finding that "dreams affect the mood of the following day" is the effect most often reported of dreams on waking-life. Carrying out a carefully designed diary study, Köthe and Pietrowsky [96] reported that days after experiencing a nightmare are rated much lower on scales of anxiety, concentration, and self-esteem than days after non-nightmare nights. The hypothesis of Belicki [97] that the effects of nightmares on waking-life are overestimated by persons with high neuroticism scores were not supported by the findings of Schredl et al. [98]. The major factor contributing to nightmare distress is nightmare frequency, which is best explained by current stress and personality factors (neuroticism, thin boundaries, etc.; see [99]). In addition, the fact that anxiety phenomena can be perpetuated by avoidance behaviors [99] is very important regarding the therapy of nightmares.

The most effective treatment strategy for reducing nightmare frequency and their effects on waking-life is imagery rehearsal therapy (IRT), developed by Barry Krakow and coworkers [100]. Patients write down a recent (less intense) nightmare and they are asked to change the dream in any way they wish and to write down the altered version. Lastly, they are instructed to rehearse the new "dream" once a day over a 2-week period. Five randomized controlled trials of IRT performed with chronic nightmare sufferers (e.g. [101]) showed the efficiency of confronting the nightmare anxiety (by writing down the dream) and coping with this anxiety by creating a new action pattern. Long-term follow-ups have shown stable treatment effects over time [102].

Many examples of creative inspiration from dreams have been reported over the years (for overviews see [1,103]): "Wild strawberries" (a film by Ingmar Bergman), the story of Dr. Jekyll and Mr. Hyde by Robert Louis Stevenson, the pop song "Yesterday" by Paul McCartney, and the paintings of Salvador Dali all provide excellent examples. Kuiken and Sikora [104] and Schredl [95] found that 20% and 28% of the participants (student samples), respectively, reported creative inspirations from dreams at least twice a year. In a large-scale study with over 1000 participants [105], about 7.8% of the recalled dreams included a creative aspect. Reported were dreams stimulating art, giving an impulse to try something new (approaching a person, traveling, etc.), or helping to solve a problem (e.g. mathematical problems, etc.). The factors that are associated with the frequency of creative dreams in this study were dream recall frequency itself, the "thin boundaries" personality dimension, a positive attitude towards creative activities, and visual imagination.

Dreams and psychotherapy

Although dream work is quite common in modern psychotherapy [106,107] and despite the extensive literature on case reports since Freud's "The interpretation of dreams," systematic research on the efficiency of dream work is limited to the research efforts of one group. For over 10 years, Clara Hill and her coworkers carried out studies to measure the effectiveness of single dream interpretation sessions [108], dream groups over 6 weeks [109], or dream interpretation within short-term psychotherapy [110]. The basis for their work is a cognitive-experiential model of dream interpretation that includes the three stages: exploration, insight, and action [111]. Reviewing the research, Hill and Goates [112] cited three sources of evidence for the beneficial effects of dream work: (a) Clients have reported on post-session measures that they gained insight, (b) judges rated clients' levels of insight in written dream interpretations as higher after dream sessions than before, and (c) clients identified gaining awareness or insight as the most helpful component of dream sessions. Similar studies for other therapeutic approaches to dream work are overdue.

Functions of dreaming

Prior to reviewing the major theories regarding dream function, two very important issues have to be discussed. First, it is crucial to differentiate between the physiological level (REM sleep) and the psychological level (dreaming). This was not clarified in one of the first publications on REM sleep deprivation [113]. Since dreaming as subjective experience which is recallable after awakening does not reflect the total brain activity during REM sleep or other sleep stages, the functions of sleep and particularly REM sleep must not parallel the functions of dreaming. REM sleep, for example, is important for memory consolidation, especially procedural and emotional memory (cf. [114]), but whether dreams are related to this memory consolidation has not been studied systematically; only a pilot study [115] reported a correlation between overnight improvement in a procedural task and incorporation of task-related topics into dreams. Walker [116] pointed out that memory consolidation might happen on a cellular level without any consciousness involved.

The second problem is a methodological one, namely, how to measure a possible beneficial effect of dreams on subsequent waking-life. Cartwright et al. [117], for example, found that divorcing women dreaming about their ex-husband are more psychologically adapted than women who dreamed about other topics. The authors concluded that working through the divorce issue within the dream serves an adaptive function. But one might argue that the women who reported the ex-husband dreams began to think about the dream and, therefore, were able to cope better with the stressful divorce. From this viewpoint, the yet unsolvable problem is that one cannot differentiate between the effect of the dreamed dream and the effect of the recalled, reported dream (necessarily processed by the waking mind), i.e. we do not know and might never know whether unremembered dreams serve any function.

Despite these problems, a variety of researchers have proposed different functions of dreaming which are listed in Table 5.7. Flanagan [118], for example, put forward the idea that dreams are a pure epiphenomenon of sleep, especially REM sleep, and did not have any additional functions to the well-documented functions of sleep and REM sleep, e.g. memory consolidation. Jouvet [119] postulates that the function of REM sleep is to periodically reinforce genetic programs to restore our individuality and diversity within our species, despite a changing environment. In his model dreams are the software deployed on the hardware (the brain). Freud [2] termed dreams as the guardian of sleep because they allow the catharsis of unconscious id impulses which would have awakened the sleeper otherwise. Based on C. G. Jung's analytical psychology, the dream serves as a compensatory mechanism for the single-minded waking consciousness, i.e. dreams incorporate aspects of the dreamer which are neglected during waking-life.

The reverse learning theory assumes that the human memory can be modelled as a neural network. During the process of learning, many parasite (unnecessary) modes will be learned in addition to the useful material. The random stimulation (PGO waves; see activation-synthesis theory [91]) then

Table 5.7 Functions of dreaming

Theories
• Dreams as epiphenomenon
• Iterative programming
• Guardian of sleep
• Compensation
• Reverse learning hypothesis
• Mastery hypothesis
• Mood regulation
• Systematic desensitization
• Threat simulation theory

activates these parasite modes and unlearns them. Therefore, proponents of reverse learning theory suggest that the bizarre and illogical associations often occurring in dreams are the material we should forget.

The mastery hypothesis was formulated by Wright and Koulack [120]. Their basic assumption is that dreaming serves a similar function like waking thought, which is problem solving. The idea is supported by paralleling basic problem solving processes with dreaming, e.g. combining old information of the dreamer's past with current waking-life issues and playing through different possibilities in order to evaluate the outcome. The function that dreams regulate mood was proposed by Kramer [121] based on his findings that more extreme emotions in the evening and during the night are evened out in the morning. The extreme low muscle tone during REM sleep was the key for the theory of Perlis and Nielsen [122]. They hypothesized that REM sleep is the ideal modus for anxiety extinction, i.e. experiencing anxiety while deeply relaxed helps to unlearn the anxiety; this is a common technique applied in cognitive behavioral therapy. The threat simulation theory postulates that simulation of threats during dreaming enhances survival and reproductive success because humans will avoid dangerous situations and places (in the ancestral environment long ago) by rehearsing this information during sleep [123].

To summarize, dreaming might serve one or more functions (cf. [104]) but due to immanent methodological issues (see above) we still do not know whether dreaming itself has a beneficial effect. This does not mean that working with dreams during waking-life is not beneficial; there is support for this approach (see Dreams and psychotherapy section).

Summary

Dreams have been studied from different perspectives: psychoanalysis, academic psychology, and neurosciences. After presenting the definition of dreaming and the methodological tools of dream research, the major findings regarding the phenomenology of dreaming and the factors influencing dream content have been reviewed. The so-called continuity hypothesis stating that dreams reflect waking-life experiences is supported by studies investigating the dreams of psychiatric patients and patients with sleep disorders, i.e. their daytime symptoms and problems are reflected in their dreams. Dreams also play an important role in psychotherapy; the efficiency of nightmare treatment strategies in particular has been demonstrated in randomized controlled trials. The question about the functions of dreaming is still unanswered and open to future research.

References

1. Van de Castle RL. *Our dreaming mind*. New York: Ballentine; 1994.

2. Freud S. *Die Traumdeutung (1900)*. Frankfurt: Fischer Taschenbuch; 1987.

3. Aserinsky E, Kleitman N. Regularly occuring periods of eye motility and concomitant phenomena during sleep. *Science*, 1953;**118**:273–274.

4. Calkins MW. Statistics of dream. *Am J Psychol*. 1893; **5**:311–343.

5. Weed SC, Hallam FM. A study of the dream consciousness. *Am J Psychol*. 1896;**7**:405–411.

6. Bentley M. The study of dreams. *Am J Psychol* 1915;**26**:196–210.

7. Hall CS, Van de Castle RL. *The content analysis of dreams*. New York: Appleton-Century-Crofts; 1966.

8. Hall CS, Domhoff GW, Blick KA, Weesner KE. The dreams of college men and women in 1959 and 1980: a comparison of dream contents and sex differences. *Sleep*. 1982;**5**:188–194.

9. Schredl M, Sahin V, Schäfer G. Gender differences in dreams: Do they reflect gender differences in waking-life? *Personality and Individual Differences*. 1998;**25**:433–442.

10. Schredl, M. *Die nächtliche Traumwelt: Einführung in die psychologische Traumforschung*. Stuttgart: Kohlhammer; 1999.

11. Maury A. *Le sommeil et les reves*. Paris: Didier; 1861.

12. Schredl M. Body-mind interaction: dream content and REM sleep physiology. *N Am J Psychol*. 2000;**2**:59–70.

13. Strauch I, Meier B. *Den Träumen auf der Spur: Zugang zur modernen Traumforschung*. Bern: Huber; 2004.

14. Dement WC, Kleitman N. The relation of eye movements during sleep to dream activity: an objective method for the study of dreaming. *J Exp Psychol*. 1957;**53**:339–346.

15. Foulkes D. Dream reports from different stages of sleep. *J Abnorm Social Psychol*. 1962;**65**:14–25.

16. Nielsen TA. A review of mentation in REM and NREM sleep: "covert" REM sleep as a possible reconciliation of two opposing models. *Behav Brain Sci*. 2000;**23**:851–866.

17. Wittmann L, Schredl M. Does the mind sleep? An answer to "What is a dream generator?" *Sleep and Hypnosis*. 2004;**6**:177–178.

18. Hobson JA, Pace-Schott EF, Stickgold R. Dreaming and the brain: toward a cognitive neuroscience of conscious states. *Behav Brain Sci*. 2000;**23**:793–842.

19. Wittmann L, Schredl M, Kramer M. The role of dreaming in posttraumatic stress disorder. *Psychother Psychosom*. 2007;**76**:25–39.

20. LaBerge S. *Lucid dreaming*. Los Angeles: Jeremy P. Tarcher; 1985.

21. Schredl M. Dream recall: models and empirical data. In: Barrett D, McNamara P, eds. *The new science of dreaming – Volume 2: Content, recall, and personality correlates*. Westport: Praeger, S; 2007:79–114.

22. Schredl M, Wittmann L, Ciric P, Götz S. Factors of home dream recall: a structural equation model. *J Sleep Res*. 2003;**12**:133–141.

23. Domhoff GW. *Finding meaning in dreams: a quantitative approach*. New York: Plenum Press; 1996.

24. Hopf HH. [Wie "objektiv" sind unsere Notizen? Ein Vergleich von Patiententraumprotokollen mit von Therapeuten niedergeschriebenen Protokollen]. *Kind und Umwelt*. 1989;**63**:42–52.

25. Schredl M. Questionnaires and diaries as research instruments in dream research: methodological issues. *Dreaming*. 2002;**12**:17–26.

26. Schredl M. Laboratory references in dreams: Methodological problem and/or evidence for the continuity hypothesis of dreaming? *Int J Dream Res*. 2008;**1**:3–6.

27. Weisz R, Foulkes, D. Home and laboratory dreams collected under uniform sampling conditions. *Psychophysiology*. 1970;**6**:588–596.

28. Hobson JA, Stickgold R. Dreaming: a neurocognitive approach. *Consciousness and Cognition*, 1994;**3**:1–15.

29. Winget C, Kramer M. *Dimensions of dreams.* Gainesville: University of Florida Press; 1979.

30. Schredl M, Burchert N, Gabatin Y. The effect of training on interrater reliability in dream content analysis. *Sleep and Hypnosis.* 2004;**6**:139–144.

31. Schredl M. The stability and variability of dream content. *Percept Mot Skills.* 1998; **86**:733–734.

32. Schredl M, Doll E. Emotions in diary dreams. *Conscious Cogn.* 1998;7:634–646.

33. Schredl M, Erlacher D. The problem of dream content analysis validity as shown by a bizarreness scale. *Sleep and Hypnosis.* 2003;**5**:129–135.

34. Schredl M, Schäfer G, Hofmann F, Jacob S. Dream content and personality: thick vs. thin boundaries. *Dreaming.* 1999;**9**:257–263.

35. Hobson JA, Hoffman SA, Helfand R, Kostner D. Dream bizarreness and the activation-synthesis hypothesis. *Hum Neurobiol.* 1987;**6**:157–164.

36. Snyder F. The phenomenology of dreaming. In: Madow L, Snow LH, eds. *The psychodynamic implications of the physiological studies on dreams.* Springfield: Charles C. Thomas; 1970:124–151.

37. McCarley RW, Hoffman E. REM sleep dreams and the activation-synthesis hypothesis. *Am J Psychiatry.* 1981;**138**:904–912.

38. Zadra AL, Nielsen TA, Donderi DC. The prevalence of auditory, olfactory, gustatory and pain experiences in 3372 home dreams. *Sleep Res.* 1997;**26**:281.

39. Kahn E, Dement W, Fisher C, Barmack JE. Incidence of color in immediately recalled dreams. *Science.* 1962;**137**:1054–1055.

40. Rechtschaffen A, Buchignani C. Visual dimensions and correlates of dream images. *Sleep Res.* 1983; **12**:189.

41. Rechtschaffen A, Buchignani C. The visual appearance of dreams. In: Antrobus JS, Bertini M, eds. *The neuropsychology of sleep and dreaming.* Hillsdale: Lawrence Erlbaum; 1992:143–155.

42. Foulkes D, Rechtschaffen A. Presleep determinants of dream content. *Percept Mot Skills.* 1964;**19**: 983–1005.

43. Breger L, Hunter I, Lane RW. *The effect of stress on dreams.* New York: International Universities Press; 1971.

44. Schreuder BJ, Kleijn WC, Rooijmans HG. Nocturnal re-experiencing more than forty years after war trauma. *J Trauma Stress.* 2000;**13**:453–463.

45. Terr LC. Psychic trauma in children: Observations following the Chowchilla schoolbus kidnapping. *Am J Psychiatry.* 1981;**138**:14–19.

46. Krakow B, Tandberg D, Barey M, Scriggins L. Nightmares and sleep disturbance in sexually assaulted women. *Dreaming.* 1995;**5**:199–206.

47. Schredl M, Hofmann F. Continuity between waking activities and dream activities. *Conscious Cogn.* 2003;**12**:298–308.

48. Schredl M. Continuity between waking and dreaming: A proposal for a mathematical model. *Sleep and Hypnosis.* 2003;**5**:38–52.

49. Botman HI, Crovitz HF. Dream reports and autobiographical memory. *Imagination, Cognition and Personality.* 1989–90;**9**:213–224.

50. Hartmann E. We do not dream of the 3 R's: implications for the nature of dream mentation. *Dreaming.* 2000;**10**:103–110.

51. Schredl M. Continuity between waking life and dreaming: are all waking activities reflected equally often in dreams? *Percept Mot Skills.* 2000;**90**: 844–846.

52. Verdone P. Temporal reference of manifest dream content. *Percept Mot Skills.* 1965;**20**:1253–1268.

53. Roussy F, Raymond I, Gonthier I, Grenier J, De Koninck J. Temporal references in manifest dream content: confirmation of increased remoteness as the night progresses. *Sleep Supplement.* 1998;**21**:285.

54. Roffwarg HP, Herman JS, Bowe-Anders C, Tauber ES. The effects of sustained alterations of waking visual input on dream content. In: Arkin AM, Antrobus JS, Ellman SJ, eds. *The mind in sleep: psychology and psychophysiology.* Hillsdale, New Jersey: Lawrence Erlbaum; 1978:295–349.

55. Lauer C, Riemann D, Lund R, Berger M. Shortened REM latency: a consequence of psychological strain? *Psychophysiology.* 1987;**24**:263–271.

56. Baekeland F, Resch R, Katz D. Presleep mentation and dream reports: I. Cognitive style, contiguity to sleep and time of the night. *Arch Gen Psychiatry.* 1968;**19**:300–311.

57. Schredl M, Kleinferchner P, Gell T. Dreaming and personality: thick vs. thin boundaries. *Dreaming.* 1996;**6**:219–223.

58. Hobson JA. Dreaming as delirium: a mental status examination of our nightly madness. *Sem Neurol.* 1997;**17**:121–128.

59. Noble D. A study of dreams in schizophrenia and allied states. *Am J Psychiatry.* 1950;**107**: 612–616.

60. Whitman RM, Kramer M, Ornstein PH, Baldridge BJ. The varying uses of the dream in clinical psychiatry. In: Madow L, Snow LH, eds. *The psychodynamic implications of the physiological studies on dreams.* Springfield: Charles C. Thomas; 1970:24–46.

61. Kramer M, Roth T. Dreams in psychopathologic patient groups. In: Williams RL, Karacan I, eds. *Sleep disorders: diagnosis and treatment*. New York: John Wiley & Sons; 1978:323–349.

62. Mellen RR, Duffey TH, Craig SM. Manifest content in the dreams of clinical populations. *J Mental Health Counseling*. 1993;**15**:170–183.

63. Kramer M. Dreams and psychopathology. In: Kryger MH, Roth T, Dement WC, eds. *Principles and practice of sleep medicine*. Philadelphia: WB Saunders; 2000:511–519.

64. Fischman LG. Dreams, hallucinogenic drug states and schizophrenia: a psychological and biological comparison. *Schizophr Bull*. 1983;**9**:73–94.

65. Schredl M, Engelhardt H. Dreaming and psychopathology: Dream recall and dream content of psychiatric inpatients. *Sleep and Hypnosis*. 2001;**3**:44–54.

66. Beck AT, Hurvich MS. Psychological correlates of depression: I. Frequency of "masochistic" dream content in a private practice sample. *Psychosom Med*. 1959;**1**:50–55.

67. Beck AT, Ward CH. Dreams of depressed patients. *Arch Gen Psychiatry*. 1961;**5**:462–467.

68. Schredl M, Schnitzler M. [Träume und Depression: Eine Literaturübersicht]. *Psycho*. 1999;**25**:693–696.

69. Riemann D, Löw H, Schredl M, et al. Investigations of morning and laboratory dream recall and content in depressive patients during baseline conditions and under antidepressive treatment with trimipramine. *Psychiatric Journal of the University of Ottawa*. 1990;**15**:93–99.

70. Armitage R, Rochlen A, Fitch T, Trivedi M, Rush AJ. Dream recall and major depression: a preliminary report. *Dreaming*. 1995;**5**:189–198.

71. Schredl M. [Traumerinnerung bei depressiven Patienten]. *Psychother Psychosom Med Psychol*. 1995;**45**:414–417.

72. Levin R, Nielson TA. Disturbed dreaming, posttraumatic stress disorder, and affect distress: a review and neurocognitive model. *Psychol Bull*. 2007;**133**:482–528.

73. Schredl M, Schäfer G, Weber B, Heuser I. Dreaming and insomnia: Dream recall and dream content of patients with insomnia. *J Sleep Res*. 1998;**7**:191–198.

74. Ermann M, Peichl J, Pohl H, Schneider MM, Winkelmann Y. [Spontanerwachen und Träume bei Patienten mit psychovegetativen Schlafstörungen]. *Psychother Psychosom Med Psychol*. 1993; **43**:333–340.

75. Ermann M. [Die Traumerinnerung bei Patienten mit psychogenen Schlafstörungen: Empirische Befunde und einige Folgerungen für das Verständnis des Träumens]. In: Leuschner W & Hau S, eds. *Traum und Gedächtnis: Neue Ergebnisse aus psychologischer, psychoanalytischer und neurophysiologischer Forschung*. Münster: LIT Verlag; 1995: 165–186.

76. Schredl M. Dreams in patients with sleep disorders. *Sleep Med Rev*. 2009;**13**:215–221.

77. Boerner, J. *Das Alpdrücken: Seine Begründung und Verhütung*. Würzburg: Carl Joseph Becker; 1855.

78. Schredl M, Schmitt J, Hein G, et al. Nightmares and oxygen desaturations: is sleep apnea related to heightened nightmare frequency? *Sleep and Breathing*. 2006;**10**:203–209.

79. Schredl M. *Träume und Schlafstörungen: Empirische Studie zur Traumerinnerungshäufigkeit und zum Trauminhalt von schlafgestörten PatientInnen*. Marburg: Tectum; 1998.

80. Schredl M. Dream content in narcoleptic patients: preliminary findings. *Dreaming*. 1998;**8**:103–107.

81. Mayer G, Kesper K, Peter H, et al. [Untersuchung zur Komorbidität bei Narkolepsiepatienten]. *Dtsch Med Wochenschr*. 2002;**127**:1942–1946.

82. Fosse R, Stickgold R, Hobson JA. Emotional experience during rapid-eye-movement sleep in narcolepsy. *Sleep*. 2002;**25**:724–732.

83. Cipolli C, Bellucci C, Mattarozzi K, et al. Story-like organization of REM-dreams in patients with narcolepsy-cataplexy. *Brain Res Bull*. 2008; **77**:206–213.

84. Schredl M. Dream recall frequency of patients with restless legs syndrome. *Eur J Neurol*. 2001;**8**:185–189.

85. Schredl M, Kraft-Schneider B, Kröger H, Heuser I. Dream content of patients with sleep apnea. *Somnologie*. 1999;**3**:319–323.

86. Herman JH, Erman M, Boys R, et al. Evidence for a directional correspondence between eye movements and dream imagery in REM sleep. *Sleep*. 1984;**7**: 52–63.

87. Erlacher D, Schredl M. Do REM (lucid) dreamed and executed actions share the same neural substrate? *Int J Dream Res*. 2008;**1**:7–14.

88. Wolpert EA. Studies in psychophysiology of dreams: II. An electromyographic study of dreaming. *Arch Gen Psychiatry*. 1960;**2**:231–241.

89. Erlacher D, Schredl M. Physiological response to "physical" activity during REM lucid dreaming. *Dreaming*. 2008;**18**:112–121.

90. Dang-Vu TT, Desseilles M, Petit D, et al. Neuroimaging in sleep medicine. *Sleep Med*. 2007;**8**:349–372.

91. Hobson JA, McCarley RW. The brain as a dream state generator: an activation-synthesis hypothesis of the dream process. *Am J Psychiatry*. 1977;**134**: 1335–1348.

92. Hong CC, Jin Y, Potkin S, et al. Language in dreaming and regional EEG alpha power. *Sleep*. 1996; **19**:232–235.

93. Erlacher D, Schredl M, LaBerge S. Motor area activation during dreamed hand clenching: a pilot study on EEG alpha band. *Sleep and Hypnosis*. 2003;**5**:182–187.

94. Czisch M, Wehrle R, Kaufmann C, et al. Functional MRI during sleep: BOLD signal decreases and their electrophysiological correlates. *Eur J Neurosci*. 2004;**20**:566–574.

95. Schredl M. The effect of dreams on waking life. *Sleep and Hypnosis*. 2000;**2**:120–124.

96. Köthe M, Pietrowsky R. Behavioral effects of nightmares and their correlations to personality patterns. *Dreaming*. 2001;**11**:43–52.

97. Belicki K. Nightmare frequency versus nightmare distress: Relation to psychopathology and cognitive style. *J Abnorm Psychol*. 1992; **101**:592–597.

98. Schredl M, Landgraf C, Zeiler O. Nightmare frequency, nightmare distress and neuroticism. *N Am J Psychol*. 2003;**5**:345–350.

99. Schredl M. Effects of state and trait factors on nightmare frequency. *Eur Arch Psychiatry Clin Neurosci*. 2003;**253**:241–247.

100. Krakow B, Zadra A. Clinical management of chronic nightmares: Imagery Rehearsal Therapy. *Behav Sleep Med*. 2006;**4**:45–70.

101. Krakow B, Hollifield M, Johnston L, et al. Imagery rehearsal therapy for chronic nightmares in sexual assault survivors with posttraumatic stress disorder: a randomized controlled trial. *JAMA*. 2001;**286**:537–545.

102. Krakow B, Kellner R, Neidhardt J, Pathak D, Lambert L. Imagery rehearsal treatment of chronic nightmares: with a thirty month follow-up. *J Behav Ther Exp Psychiatry*. 1993;**24**:325–330.

103. Barrett D. *The committee of sleep: How artists, scientists, and athletes use dreams for creative problem-solving – and how you can too*. New York: Crown; 2001.

104. Kuiken D, Sikora S. The impact of dreams on waking thoughts and feelings. In: Moffitt A, Kramer M, Hoffmann R, eds. *The functions of dreaming*. Albany: State University of New York Press; 1993:419–476.

105. Schredl M, Erlacher D. Self-reported effects of dreams on waking-life creativity: An empirical study. *J Psychol*. 2007;**141**:35–46.

106. Schredl M, Bohusch C, Mader A, Somesan A. The use of dreams in psycho-therapy: a survey of psychotherapists in private practice. *J Psychother: Pract Res*. 2000;**9**:81–87.

107. Crook RE, Hill CE. Working with dreams in psychotherapy: the therapists's perspective. *Dreaming*. 2003;**13**:83–93.

108. Hill CE, Diemer R, Hess S, Hillyer A, Seeman R. Are the effects of dream interpretation on session quality, insight and emotion due to the dream itself, to projection or to the interpretation process? *Dreaming*. 1993;**3**:269–280.

109. Falk DR, Hill CE. The effectiveness of dream interpretation groups for women undergoing a divorce transition. *Dreaming*. 1995;**5**:29–42.

110. Diemer RA, Lobell LK, Vivino BL, Hill CE. Comparison of dream interpretation, event interpretation, and unstructured sessions in brief therapy. *J Consult Psychol*. 1996;**43**:99–112.

111. Hill CE. *Dream work in therapy: facilitating exploration, insight, and action*. Washington, DC: American Psychological Association; 2004.

112. Hill CE, Goates MK. Research on the Hill cognitive-experiential dream model. In: Hill CE, ed. *Dream work in therapy: facilitating exploration, insight, and action*. Washington, DC: American Psychological Association; 2004:245–288.

113. Dement WC. The effect of dream deprivation. *Science*. 1960;**131**:1705–1707.

114. Wagner U, Born J. Memory consolidation during sleep: interactive effects of sleep stages and HPA regulation. *Stress*. 2008;**11**:28–41.

115. De Koninck J, Prevost F, Lortie-Lussier M. Vertical inversion of the visual field and REM sleep mentation. *J Sleep Res*. 1996;**5**:16–20.

116. Walker MP. A refined model of sleep and the time course of memory formation. *Behav Brain Sci*. 2005;**28**:51–64.

117. Cartwright RD, Lloyd S, Knight S, Trenholm I. Broken dreams: a study of the effects of divorce and depression on dream content. *Psychiatry*. 1984;**47**:251–259.

118. Flanagan O. Deconstructing dreams: The spandrels of sleep. In: Hameroff SR, Kaszniak AW, Scott AC, eds. *Toward a science of consciousness: The first Tucson discussions and debates – Complex adaptive systems*. Cambridge: MIT Press; 1996:67–88.

119. Jouvet M. *Die Nachtseite des Bewußtseins – Warum wir träumen*. Reinbek: Rowohlt; 1994.

120. Wright J, Koulack D. Dreams and contemporary stress: a disruption-avoidance-adaptation model. *Sleep*. 1987;**10**:172–179.

121. Kramer M. *The dream experience: a systematic exploration*. New York: Routledge; 2007.

122. Perlis ML, Nielsen TA. Mood regulation, dreaming and nightmares: evaluation of a desensitization function for REM sleep. *Dreaming*. 1993; **3**:243–257.

123. Revonsuo A. The reinterpretation of dreams: an evolutionary hypothesis of the function of dreaming. *Behav Brain Sci*. 2000;**23**:877–901.

124. Parekh H. *Träume der "Gesunden" – Inhaltsanalyse von manifesten Traumtexten aus einer Zufallsstichprobe einer Großstadtpopulation*. Universität Heidelberg: Dissertation für Klinische Medizin Mannheim; 1988.

6

Taking a sleep history

Karl Doghramji and Dani Choufani

Introduction

The history and examination are the cornerstones of an evaluation of the patient who has sleep-related complaints. Various guidelines have been proposed for history-taking in sleep disorders, yet differences between these guidelines have not been systematically explored. Additionally, proposed history-gathering methods do not address issues that are specific to the evaluation of sleep disorders in the psychiatric context. In this chapter, we will present our recommendations regarding a systematic approach to the psychiatric patient with sleep-related complaints. To a large extent, these are consistent with recommendations of major publications in the field [1,2,3,4].

The first step in gathering the history is identification of the chief complaint, which determines, in large part, the specific questions and areas of exploration. The cardinal complaints indicating the presence of a sleep disorder are insomnia, excessive daytime sleepiness, and parasomnias. Each of these complaints will be discussed in the following sections with a focus on specific components of the history that are pertinent to each of these problems. The reader will also be directed to other chapters in this volume for further details regarding specific sleep disorders and/or sleep complaints in psychiatric disorders, as a detailed account of these is beyond the scope of this chapter.

Although a focused history is often of greatest clinical utility, there are components of a sleep history that should be ascertained in all patients with any sleep-related complaint. These parameters encompass core features of sleep–wake patterns and are listed in Table 6.1. We have found it helpful to organize clinical history-taking of the sleep complaint around these key elements to construct a "typical" 24-hour pattern. For example, beginning with the time and

Table 6.1 Key sleep parameters that must be obtained in all patients with sleep-related complaints

Bedtime

Sleep latency (time to fall asleep after lights out)

Nocturnal awakenings; number and duration

Time of final morning awakening

Rising time (i.e. time out of bed)

Number, time, and duration of daytime naps

Daytime symptoms including levels of sleepiness and fatigue over the course of the day

activities occurring before a patient prepares for bed, followed by bedtime, sleep latency, occurrences during the night, wake-time, time out of bed, daytime symptoms, patterns, and activities (including naps), then concluding back at the time at which the inquiry began. Once "typical" patterns are established, deviations from these patterns (e.g. sleeping in late on the weekends) can also be determined.

In addition to these principal elements of the sleep history, after discussing history-taking of specific sleep complaints (insomnia, excessive sleepiness (ES), and parasomnias), we will detail other components of the evaluation that are crucial to the development of a differential diagnosis of the sleep complaint. These include collecting collateral information, and ascertainment of other elements of the patient's history including: medical and psychiatric history, medications, family history, and social/occupational history. We will also discuss how a focused physical exam may suggest increased likelihood of specific sleep disorders such as obstructive sleep apnea syndrome (OSA). We will conclude by discussing diagnostic testing

Foundations of Psychiatric Sleep Medicine, ed. John W. Winkelman and David T. Plante. Published by Cambridge University Press.
© Cambridge University Press 2010.

modalities available to clinicians that can aid in determining the final diagnosis.

Before we discuss specifics of sleep-related complaints, we feel it is important to acknowledge that, in the office, it can seem a daunting task to collect all the pertinent information to make an accurate diagnosis. Most medical and mental health providers are not provided with formal instruction on taking a sleep history during their training, and thus may feel uncomfortable with doing so within the scope of their practice. It can be particularly challenging when evaluating sleep-related complaints in psychiatric patients as the details and longitudinal course of the psychiatric history must be considered in concert with the sleep history, and, at times, the details of the history may be unclear (e.g. if the patient has a cognitive or thought disorder). However daunting it may be, it is important to ask key questions about a sleep complaint and to build a differential diagnosis to guide appropriate treatment, rather than treat symptoms without assessment. The concern is that a psychiatric patient may complain of insomnia and be prescribed a sedative-hypnotic, or ES and be prescribed a stimulant, without adequate consideration of the disorders that may underlie the complaint. In so doing, common sleep disorders (e.g. restless legs syndrome (RLS), OSA, narcolepsy, etc.) can be missed, and opportunities for non-pharmacological interventions (e.g. use of cognitive behavioral techniques for insomnia, use of positive airway pressure devices for sleep apnea, etc.) may be overlooked. Therefore, one goal of this chapter is to provide clinicians with tools to feel more confident in evaluating and treating sleep complaints themselves, and recognize symptoms and signs that may suggest referral to a sleep medicine specialist is indicated.

Insomnia: history of the chief complaint

Insomnia is a repeated difficulty with sleep initiation, duration, consolidation, or quality that occurs despite adequate opportunity for sleep and results in some form of daytime impairment [5]. Stated in another way, an insomnia complaint can involve difficulty in initiating sleep, multiple nocturnal awakenings, a difficulty in reinitiating sleep, early morning awakening, or a combination of these. From the standpoint of diagnosis and treatment, it is important to identify the portions of sleep that are affected.

The time of onset and duration of symptoms also should be determined. Insomnias of long duration

are thought to have greater impact on daytime functioning. Although such beliefs seem to be clinically supported, they have yet to be confirmed by systematic studies. Additionally, there is considerable variability in the definition of the time course for acute and long-term insomnia, with minimum durations for chronic insomnia ranging from 30 days to as long as 6 months [6].

The longitudinal pattern of insomnia is also an important component of the history. Symptoms of insomnia typically change over time, as a complaint of initial insomnia, for example, can progress into one of a difficulty in sleep maintenance. In one study, the nature of symptoms changed in over half of insomniacs over the course of 4 months [7]. The temporal relationship between insomnia and co-morbid illnesses can also indicate what factors may have caused insomnia, and provide a basis for treatment. It should be borne in mind, however, that this relationship can be complex, especially in the case of psychiatric illness. For example, the presence and persistence of insomnia predicts the future onset of new psychiatric disorders, especially depression [8]. Insomnia can temporally precede, follow, or occur in concurrence with, the onset of a major depressive episode [9]. Insomnia can, therefore, be a harbinger of affective disease, and a residual symptom following treatment.

The severity of symptoms is also typically not static; bouts of insomnia tend to recur episodically over time, and insomniacs remain symptomatic to variable degrees between episodes. The frequency of nights affected per week or month during each episode can be a useful indicator of severity. In a national survey [10], 36% of 1000 adults reported a current sleep problem, of which 27% indicated that sleep problems occurred occasionally and 9% reported difficulty sleeping on a frequent basis; insomnia episodes typically lasted 4.7 days. Chronic insomniacs reported that sleep problems affected over half of the nights in an average month (16.4 days).

Precipitants of the insomnia complaint also should be determined. Common precipitants include job loss, engaging in shift work or travel across time zones, breaches in relationships or loss of relatives, onset of medical and psychiatric illness, and introduction of new medications or changes in dosages and times of administration of existing medications, among others. Medications likely to precipitate insomnia in psychiatric practice are antidepressants and stimulants, among others. Perpetuating factors of insomnia should also be identified. Following the onset of insomnia, these factors can transform insomnia into a chronic disorder. They include the development of poor sleep hygiene practices and of anticipatory anxiety with the approach of bedtime. From the standpoint of future treatment, it is additionally useful to understand the type of interventions that have already been attempted for insomnia and the effectiveness and side-effects of each of these.

Daytime symptoms

An assessment of daytime symptoms is useful in understanding the impact of insomnia on an individual's functioning. Additionally, the correction of daytime impairment is an important measure of treatment efficacy. Typically, the severity of daytime symptoms in insomnia co-varies with the degree of impairment in the quality and quantity in nocturnal sleep. At times, however, despite minimal apparent difficulty with sleep latency or nocturnal awakenings, patients can complain that sleep is unproductive and non-restorative. It is, therefore, important to independently explore daytime symptoms.

As a group, insomniacs obtain less sleep than non-complaining individuals. Interestingly, however, they are generally not excessively sleepy during the course of the day, where sleepiness is defined as the tendency to fall asleep. In fact, most complain that they are unable to fall asleep during attempts at napping. This is supported by objective evidence that insomniacs are less prone to falling asleep compared to normal sleepers during multiple sleep latency testing [11,12]. The finding of decreased daytime sleepiness despite disturbed nocturnal sleep may be the result of hyperarousal, during sleep and wakefulness, in multiple biological and psychological systems including cognition, the hypothalamic-pituitary axis, sympathetic nervous system, metabolic rate, and electroencephalographic frequency [13]. Insomnia represents the inability to sleep or sleep well despite adequate opportunity. In contrast, in individuals whose opportunity for sleep is reduced (i.e. those undergoing sleep curtailment or deprivation), decrements in nocturnal sleep duration are directly related to the tendency to fall asleep during the day (i.e. the level of daytime sleepiness).

Insomniacs do, however, more frequently report a variety of daytime psychological symptoms, including feeling depressed, hopeless, helpless, worried, tense, anxious, irritable, lonely, and lacking in self-confidence, than control subjects [14]. Individuals with insomnia also report feeling tired, physically fatigued, anergic, and unmotivated. They also report cognitive difficulties such as memory impairment, difficulty with focus and attention, and mental slowing. Interestingly, these subjective complaints are evident on objective testing, as impaired psychomotor performance (reaction time) has recently been demonstrated in insomniacs [12]. Insomniacs can also report impairments in coping, accomplishing tasks, and in family and social relationships and occupational function [15].

Inventories can assist in the quantification of the severity of insomnia; although many are available, the insomnia severity index (ISI; Figure 6.1) is one of the few that have been subjected to empirical validation [16,17]. ISI takes into account subjective symptoms and consequences of insomnia and the degree of concern or distress caused by the disturbance. It is a useful clinical and research tool for measuring treatment outcome.

Daytime habits and behaviors

Daytime behaviors can adversely affect nocturnal sleep and aggravate insomnia. The patient's daytime activities and their timing should, therefore, be systematically explored. Intense exercise too close to bedtime can disrupt sleep [18]. Long periods of bed rest, inactivity, and excessive napping can foment circadian rhythm disturbances and aggravate insomnia. Exposure to bright light can be helpful in establishing circadian cycling and, conversely, lack of sufficient light exposure during the morning hours can disrupt sleep timing. Frequent travel and shift work can also disrupt sleep and contribute to both insomnia and daytime sleepiness. It is useful to understand the patient's preferred social and occupational activities as this information can be helpful in devising a daily structure that promotes consistent sleep scheduling.

Sleep-related habits and behaviors

Although not typically explored in the routine psychiatric evaluation, the behaviors in which the patient engages during the few hours prior to bedtime, during bedtime hours, and just after morning awakening can cause or significantly intensify existing insomnia. These are listed in Table 6.2. Although

Name: _____ Date: _____

1. Please rate the current (i.e., last 2 weeks) **SEVERITY** of your insomnia problem(s).

	None	Mild	Moderate	Severe	Very
Difficulty falling asleep:	0	1	2	3	4
Difficulty staying asleep:	0	1	2	3	4
Problem waking up too early:	0	1	2	3	4

2. How **SATISFIED**/dissatisfied are you with your current sleep pattern?

Very Satisfied				Very Dissatisfied
0	1	2	3	4

3. To what extent do you consider your sleep problem to **INTERFERE** with your daily functioning (e.g. daytime fatigue, ability to function at work/daily chores, concentration, memory, mood, etc.).

Not at all Interfering	A Little	Somewhat	Much	Very Much Interfering
0	1	2	3	4

4. How **NOTICEABLE** to others do you think your sleeping problem is in terms of impairing the quality of your life?

Not at all Noticeable	Barely	Somewhat	Much	Very Much Noticeable
0	1	2	3	4

5. How **WORRIED**/distressed are you about your current sleep problem?

Not at all	A Little	Somewhat	Much	Very Much
0	1	2	3	4

Guidelines for Scoring/Interpretation:

Add scores for all seven items (1a+1b+1c+ 2+3+4+5)   = _____
Total score ranges from 0-28
0-7	= No clinically significant insomnia
8-14	= Subthreshold insomnia
15-21	= Clinical insomnia (moderate severity)
22-28	= Clinical insomnia (severe)

Figure 6.1 The insomnia severity index. Reprinted, with permission, from [17]. Copyright Charles M. Morin, 1993.

these factors are seldom the lone cause of an insomnia complaint, a lack of awareness of them can lead to a failure in other treatment modalities.

Similarly, the patient's attitude towards their insomnia can itself have an important influence on the ability to sleep. In particular, the extent of dysfunctional beliefs and attitudes as well as sleep-related anxiety as bedtime approaches and during the bedtime hours provide the clinician with important insights into the role these processes play in perpetuating or exacerbating the insomnia. Therefore, information about the dysfunctional cognitions of

Table 6.2 Sleep-related habits and behaviors that can disrupt sleep

Caffeine and alcohol prior to bedtime
Nicotine (both smoking and cessation)
Large meals or excessive fluid intake within 3 hours of bedtime
Exercising within 3 hours of bedtime
Utilizing the bed for non-sleep activities (work, telephone, internet)
Staying in bed while awake for extended periods of time
Activating behaviors up to the point of bedtime
Excessive worrying at bedtime
Clock-watching prior to sleep onset or during nocturnal awakenings
Exposure to bright light prior to bedtime or during awakenings
Keeping the bedroom too hot or too cold
Noise
Behaviors of a bed partner (e.g. snoring, leg movements)

the insomniac such as catastrophic attributions of the effects of insomnia, the time of day that the insomniac begins to worry about sleep, and the state of mind of the insomniac during time awake during the night should all be solicited.

Sleep patterns

Although the assessment of bedtime and sleep patterns is important in the evaluation of any sleep-related complaint, it is a particularly essential component of the evaluation of insomnia (Table 6.1). Patients should be asked regarding these parameters on initial and follow-up visits. These patterns can also be assessed by utilizing patient-completed sleep logs or diaries that track sleep–wake patterns over time (Figure 6.2). Sleep logs and diaries may be more useful than subjective summaries since insomniacs tend to underestimate total sleep time and overestimate sleep latency, possibly resulting from a preferential recall bias for particularly bad nights of sleep that do not reflect the longitudinal course of their complaints [19].

Ideally, individuals retire and emerge from bed at consistent times day to day, including weekends. The time spent in bed between retiring and falling asleep

would preferably be less than 20 minutes, and individuals would emerge from bed soon after awakening in the morning. Additionally, awakenings in good sleepers are typically limited to one or two, and time spent in bed following awakenings kept to a minimum (i.e. less than 15 minutes). Of note, these variables may be affected by age [20]. Patients with insomnia can have large discrepancies from these norms, and patterns may emerge that suggest specific underlying causes of insomnia and/or help guide treatment.

Characteristic disturbances in sleep–wake patterns can point to circadian rhythm disturbances such as delayed sleep phase disorder, in which the time of falling asleep and the time of awakening are consistently delayed, and advanced sleep phase disorder, in which these times are consistently advanced, relative to the desired night/day schedule (see Chapter 11: Circadian rhythm disorders). Multiple nocturnal awakenings and prolonged sleep latencies are not specific for any one disorder, yet keeping track of these parameters can help to quantify the severity of insomnia and determine the effectiveness of treatment measures. Determining these patterns can also suggest the utility of certain behavioral interventions to improve sleep, such as restriction of overall time spent in bed. It is also useful to ascertain each of these parameters not only for the "average" day, but also for a sequence of days, as such a temporal record can demonstrate variability in sleep patterns over time which can, in turn, contribute to poor sleep. The assessment of variability between workdays/schooldays, weekends, and vacations can also be useful. Insomniacs characteristically do not maintain rigorous sleep/wake schedules, and introducing such regularity into their lives is one of the primary elements of sleep hygiene education and other cognitive behavioral techniques (see Chapter 14: Cognitive behavioral therapy for insomnia).

Excessive sleepiness (ES): history of the chief complaint

Sleepiness, the tendency to fall asleep, is a normal phenomenon when it occurs at the desired time of the day. ES is the tendency to fall asleep at inappropriate times or settings [4]. ES should be distinguished from fatigue, which is classically defined as the inability to sustain performance over time and is typically associated with subjective reports of tiredness,

TWO WEEK SLEEP DIARY

INSTRUCTIONS:
1. Write the date, day of the week, and type of day: Work, School, Day Off, or Vacation.
2. Put the letter "C" in the box when you have coffee, cola or tea. Put "M" when you take any medicine. Put "A" when you drink alcohol. Put "E" when you exercise.
3. Put a line (I) to show when you go to bed. Shade in the box that shows when you think you fell asleep.
4. Shade in all the boxes that show when you are asleep at night or when you take a nap during the day.
5. Leave boxes unshaded to show when you wake up at night and when you are awake during the day.

SAMPLE ENTRY BELOW: On a Monday when I worked, I jogged on my lunch break at 1 PM, had a glass of wine with dinner at 6 PM, fell asleep watching TV from 7 to 8 PM, went to bed at 10:30 PM, fell asleep around Midnight, woke up and couldn't got back to sleep at about 4 AM, went back to sleep from 5 to 7 AM, and had coffee and medicine at 7:00 in the morning.

Today's Date	Day of the week	Type of Day Work, School, Off, Vacation	Noon	1PM	2	3	4	5	6PM	7	8	9	10	11PM	Midnight	1AM	2	3	4	5	6AM	7	8	9	10	11AM
sample	Mon.	Work		E					A						I							C M				

Figure 6.2 Sleep log. Reproduced, with permission, from [5]. Copyright American Academy of Sleep Medicine, 2005.

weariness, exhaustion, and lack of energy [21]. Even though fatigued patients can perceive themselves as being excessively sleepy, in its pure form, fatigue does not result in an increased propensity to fall asleep. Fatigue is a symptom of a wide variety of medical, psychiatric, and neurological disorders and less specific for sleep disorders than is ES. It has been most widely examined in the context of multiple sclerosis, autoimmune disorders, and psychiatric conditions (Figure 6.3). Also, a complaint of ES may co-occur with that of hypersomnia, which is an abnormal increase in time spent asleep or trying to sleep. In this section, we will limit our discussion primarily to ES.

The time of onset, temporal pattern, duration, and daily pattern of ES should be determined. ES onset in early life is more consistent with narcolepsy, whereas onset in middle age is more consistent with OSA. ES that is episodic over time is consistent with periods of sleep restriction due to social and occupational needs.

However, ES that is constant and unremitting may be more consistent with narcolepsy, OSA, or potentially affective disorders. ES that is most prominent in the morning hours, especially when accompanied by a prolonged sleep latency and complaint of initiation insomnia, can be due to delayed sleep phase syndrome, whereas ES that is most prominent in the late evening hours and associated with early morning awakening can be due to advanced sleep phase syndrome. ES that is most prominent in the morning hours and gradually resolves as the day progresses is also consistent with the carryover effects of a sedating bedtime medication. Afternoon sleepiness is commonly associated with disturbances of the quality and quantity of nocturnal sleep, and the extent of sleepiness in the afternoon is proportional to the extent of these disturbances.

The severity of ES should be quantified. Direct questioning regarding how sleepy an individual feels

Statement*
1. My motivation is lower when I am fatigued.
2. Exercise brings on my fatigue.
3. I am easily fatigued.
4. Fatigue interferes with my physical functioning.
5. Fatigue causes frequent problems for me.
6. My fatigue prevents sustained physical functioning.
7. Fatigue interferes with carrying out certain duties and responsibilities.
8. Fatigue is among my three most disabling symptoms.
9. Fatigue interferes with my work, family, or social life.

Figure 6.3 The fatigue severity scale. Copyright 1989, American Medical Association.

*Patients are instructed to choose a number from 1 to 7 (1 = "strongly disagree" and 7 = "strongly agree") that indicates their degree of agreement with each statement. Reprinted with permission from Krupp et al. *Arch Neurol.* 1989; **46**:1121–1123. Copyright 1989, American Medical Association. All rights reserved.

is generally not a highly useful measure of the degree of sleepiness, since patients can over-report or under-report the *sensation* of sleepiness, compared to their behavioral tendency to nod off or fall asleep during activities of daily life. Individuals who are exposed to long periods of sleep deprivation are especially prone to under-recognize the severity of their sleepiness, possibly owing to their becoming accustomed to this state. Therefore, behavioral assessments of ES may be more useful. Behavioral indicators of ES include yawning, ptosis, reduced activity, lapses in attention, and head nodding. The patient can also be questioned about his/her tendency to fall asleep in situations of everyday life; milder levels of daytime sleepiness result in falling asleep in passive situations such as while reading, watching television, and attending meetings. In severe cases, individuals fall asleep while actively engaged in complex tasks such as driving, speaking, writing, or even eating. Highly sleepy patients may also experience sleep attacks, episodes of sleep that strike without warning, whose occurrence mandates rapid clinical intervention, in part due to significantly increased risk of motor vehicle accidents. However, all patients with a complaint of ES should be cautioned about the risks of drowsy driving.

A validated inventory for the quantification of the tendency to fall asleep is the Epworth sleepiness scale (ESS) [22]. It is widely utilized for the assessment of the severity of ES and for the determination of treatment effects over time (Figure 6.4). The scores for individual items are added, and the total score is reported. A score of 10 or above is considered to represent an abnormally high level of daytime sleepiness.

Related symptoms

Patients with ES may also complain of the many consequences of ES. In the evaluation of the sleepy patient, an exploration of these related complaints may be helpful in understanding the effects of ES on the patient's daily life. These consequences also represent symptoms that should be followed clinically to ensure that ES has been adequately managed.

Napping in patients with ES is common. If naps are reported, the possibility that they are related to narcolepsy should be examined by determining whether they are refreshing, brief in duration, or accompanied by dreams. Naps are also refreshing in individuals who are sleep deprived. In contrast, they tend to not be refreshing in OSA and idiopathic hypersomnia. The timing of naps should also be determined as this may alert the physician to the possibility of circadian rhythm disorders.

Most of the sequelae of ES that have been examined have fallen in the realm of psychomotor and attentional behaviors. These include slower response times, cognitive slowing, performance errors, decline in both short-term recall and working memory, reduced learning of new tasks, increased response perseveration on ineffective solutions, increased neglect of non-essential activities (loss of situational awareness), increased compensatory effort to maintain the same performance, and diminished insight into subtle meanings [23]. ES can also contribute to depressed mood [24].

ES is associated with an increased risk for accidents at work and while driving [25] and has been

---

THE EPWORTH SLEEPINESS SCALE

Name: _____

Today's date: _____ Your age (years):_____

Your sex (male = M; female = F): _____

How likely are you to doze off or fall asleep in the following situations, in contrast to feeling just tired? This refers to your usual way of life in recent times. Even if you have not done some of these things recently try to work out how they would have affected you. Use the following scale to choose the *most appropriate number* for each situation:

    0 = would *never* doze
    1 = *slight* chance of dozing
    2 = *moderate* chance of dozing
    3 = *high* chance of dozing

Situation	Chance of dozing
Sitting and reading	_____
Watching TV	_____
Sitting, inactive in a public place (e.g. a theater or a meeting)	_____
As a passenger in a car for an hour without a break	_____
Lying down to rest in the afternoon when circumstances permit	_____
Sitting and talking to someone	_____
Sitting quietly after a lunch without alcohol	_____
In a car, while stopped for a few minutes in the traffic	_____

Thank you for your cooperation

Figure 6.4 The Epworth sleepiness scale. Reprinted with permission from [22].

implicated as a factor in many catastrophes such as the meltdown of the Three Mile Island nuclear reactor in 1979, the erroneous launch of the Challenger spacecraft in 1986, and the grounding of the Exxon Valdez oil tanker in 1989 [26]. Daytime sleepiness peaks during the mid-afternoon hours, and the consequences of sleepiness, such as traffic accidents, errors in performance, and lapses in attention, are most apparent during these times [27].

Other components in the history-taking of ES are described in the section on insomnia; these include daytime habits and behaviors, sleep-related habits and behaviors, and sleep patterns.

Parasomnias: history of the chief complaint

Parasomnias are undesirable physical events or experiences that occur during entry into sleep, within sleep, or during arousals from sleep [5] (See Chapter 10: Parasomnias). Most of the parasomnias are defined by their specific behavioral features. Therefore, the characteristics of the disturbance should be carefully determined. The time of night that they occur, whether the patient remembers the event, whether there is associated dreaming, and age of onset should be evaluated. For example, disorders of arousal such as sleepwalking and night terrors usually occur during the first third of night since they arise from slow-wave sleep, are associated with amnesia for the event or a vague sense of imminent danger, are not associated with reports of dreaming, are common in childhood, and decrease in incidence with increasing age. On the other hand, REM sleep behavior disorder (RBD) is more likely to occur in the latter portions of the night since it arises from REM sleep, is often associated with intense dreaming and later memory of the dream and associated behaviors, and is more common in middle and older age [28]. A good approximation of the frequency of the episodes and their potential danger or other consequences (e.g. daytime sleepiness) is helpful, as this will help guide the necessity of treatment. Parasomnias are associated with an increased risk of harm to self and others; for example, RBD sufferers may strike out in response to dreams and injure themselves or a bed partner. Therefore, an understanding of the extent of such injurious behavior in the past can be important in determining the urgency of treatment and the implementation of safety precautions.

Collateral information from bed partners and family members

Many of the symptoms and behaviors that are necessary for the completion of the history occur during sleep, or during periods of extreme sleepiness, making the patient's own account unreliable. Therefore, it is helpful to obtain this information from bed partners and family members. Examples of symptoms patients may underreport include:

1. Snoring
2. Breathing pauses during sleep
3. Unusual behaviors during sleep such as walking, talking, thrashing, headbanging, body rocking, and limb movements
4. The tendency to fall asleep unintentionally during the day
5. The extent and frequency of naps
6. Cognitive and behavioral disturbances associated with insomnia and ES, such as diminished social contact, slow mannerisms, decrement in mood, lapses in memory, etc.

Past medical, psychiatric, and surgical history

Co-morbid disorders should be reviewed, along with their dates of onset, types of treatment, and results of treatment. Surgeries and hospitalizations should also be evaluated. Major medical disorders can affect sleep by virtue of their psychological impact, through pain and discomfort, as well as direct effects on sleep and wakefulness. It is important to note that myriad psychiatric illnesses are associated with sleep disturbance, and careful evaluation of the timing of the sleep complaint in relation to psychiatric symptoms may be of high value in patients with psychiatric illness. For a review of psychiatric disorders and their effects on sleep, please see Section VI of this book.

Additionally, the patient may have a history of a primary sleep disorder, and review of prior documentation including results of polysomnographic studies

and other laboratory tests may be extremely helpful. For a review of primary sleep disorders, please see Section IV of this volume.

Medications

A history of current and prior medications is an integral part of the history. The list should include not only prescribed medications, but over-the-counter agents, nutraceuticals, herbal substances, dietary supplements, and even foods. Their effects, side-effects, dosages or quantities, and timing of administration should be recorded. If the use of a medication correlates temporally with the onset of the sleep complaint, a medication-induced sleep disorder should be suspected. Medications can also have secondary effects by virtue of their exacerbation of underlying conditions. For example, weight gain associated with medication use can lead to the development of symptoms of OSA, such as ES, snoring, and breathing pauses during sleep. Allergies to medications should also be recorded. The effects of commonly used medications on sleep are reviewed in Chapter 3: Neurophysiology and neuroimaging of human sleep.

Substances

Insomnia, ES, and parasomnias can be related to substance use. Chronic and excessive use of substances may lead to substance use disorders, which are characterized by either abuse or dependence. Stimulants such as caffeine, amphetamines, and cocaine classically disrupt sleep. Sedatives such as opiates and analgesics cause ES. Alcohol, at low dosages, can help with sleep initiation, yet chronic and excessive use can lead to disturbed sleep and the complaint of insomnia [29]. The effects of substances on sleep are reviewed in greater detail in Chapter 19: Sleep in substance use disorders.

Family history

Certain sleep disorders, such as RLS, can have a hereditary component, in which 50% of primary cases have a positive family history [30]. The incidence of certain parasomnias of arousal such as sleepwalking and sleep terrors is ten times greater in first degree relatives than in the general population [31]. OSA may have a familial basis.

Social and occupational history

Several social or occupational factors can contribute to sleep-related complaints, necessitating evaluation. For example, ES and insomnia are common in shift workers and individuals whose occupations require frequent travel across time zones. Exposure to industrial toxins and chemicals can also produce sleep/wake symptoms. Job loss and retirement can result in the loss of regularity in daily schedule, which is important in maintaining circadian rhythm consistency in some individuals, leading to erratic sleep/wake hours and the complaints of insomnia and ES. Disruption in interpersonal relationships, family, job, and hobbies can cause anxiety and subsequent insomnia.

Differential diagnosis

Table 6.3 outlines some of the more commonly encountered sleep disorders that are related to insomnia and ES. The differential diagnosis of the parasomnias is discussed in Chapter 10: Parasomnias.

Several disorders may present with either insomnia and/or ES, which may complicate the differential diagnosis. Thus, it is important for the practicing clinician to be familiar with some common symptoms

Table 6.3 Differential diagnosis of insomnia and ES

Disorder	Insomnia	ES
Inadequate sleep hygiene	*	*
Sleep restriction		*
Adjustment sleep disorder	*	
Psychophysiological insomnia	*	
Obstructive sleep apnea syndrome	*	*
Central sleep apnea syndrome	*	*
Narcolepsy		*
Periodic limb movement disorder	*	*
Idiopathic hypersomnia		*
Restless legs syndrome	*	*
Drug-dependent and drug-induced sleep disorders	*	*
Circadian rhythm sleep disorders	*	*
Medical/psychiatric sleep disorders	*	*

of sleep disorders, to aid in the evaluation and management of sleep complaints.

Symptoms of specific disorders

The existence of certain symptoms in addition to insomnia and/or ES can indicate the presence of specific disorders as a cause of these complaints. Defining symptoms for a selected list of sleep disorders are listed in Table 6.4. Defining symptoms for the parasomnias is discussed in Chapter 10: Parasomnias. These symptoms should be systematically explored to refine the diagnostic possibilities. Readers are referred to Sections IV and VI of this book for a more detailed discussion of each disorder and its hallmark symptoms.

Physical examination

The physical examination can contribute essential information to the process of understanding the etiology of the sleep complaint. Vital signs should include the measurement of neck circumference; a thick and/or muscular neck, as well as a neck circumference of 16 inches or greater in women and 17 inches or greater in men, are associated with an increased risk for sleep-related breathing disorders [33]. Body habitus should be inspected; obesity with fat distribution around the neck or midriff suggests the diagnosis of OSA. Other contributors to sleep-related breathing disorders include nasal obstruction, mandibular hypoplasia, and retrognathia. Oropharyngeal abnormalities can also be involved, including enlarged tonsils and tongue, an elongated uvula and soft palate, diminished pharyngeal patency, and redundant pharyngeal mucosa. The Mallampati airway classification score should be determined (Figure 6.5), which is useful in assessing the risk for OSA. On average, for every 1-point increase in the Mallampati score, the odds of having OSA increases more than two fold [34]. The chest examination should be scrutinized for expiratory wheezes and kyphoscoliosis, indicative of, among others, asthma and restrictive lung disease, respectively, which, in turn, can be associated with the complaint of insomnia. Signs of right heart failure should be noted; heart failure can cause abnormalities of breathing during sleep, which, in turn, can be associated with the complaint of frequent nocturnal awakenings and unrefreshing sleep. A basic neurological examination should be performed to rule out neurological disorders that may mimic certain sleep disorders or which may co-exist with them. For

Table 6.4 Defining symptoms for selected disorders

Disorder	Symptoms
Psychophysiological insomnia	"Trying" to fall asleep Difficulty falling asleep at desired bedtime Frequent nocturnal awakenings Anxiety regarding sleeplessness
Restless legs syndrome[1]	Irresistible urge to move the extremities Limb paresthesiae Onset of symptoms during periods of rest and in the evening or at bedtime Relief of symptoms with movement
Periodic limb movement disorder	Repetitive involuntary movements of the extremities during sleep or just prior to falling asleep
Narcolepsy	Excessive daytime sleepiness Cataplexy Sleep paralysis Hypnopompic and hypnagogic hallucinations
Obstructive sleep apnea syndrome	Snoring Breathing pauses during sleep Choking Gasping Morning dry mouth
Chronic obstructive pulmonary disease	Dyspnea
Gastroesophageal reflux	Epigastric pain or burning Laryngospasm Acid taste in mouth Sudden nocturnal awakenings
Prostatic hypertrophy	Frequent nocturia
Nocturnal seizures	Thrashing in bed Loss of bladder or bowel control
Nocturnal panic attacks	Sudden surges of anxiety Tachycardia Diaphoresis Choking Laryngospasm
Post-traumatic stress disorder	Recurring, vivid dreams and nightmares Anxiety and hypervigilance in sleep environment
Delayed sleep phase syndrome	Inability to fall asleep at desired time Inability to awaken at desired time
Advanced sleep phase syndrome	Inability to stay awake until the desired bedtime Inability to remain asleep until the desired awakening time

Note: [1] The URGE mnemonic has been proposed as a convenient way to recall most of the symptoms of RLS [32]. It includes the following: Urge to move; Rest induced; Gets better with activity; Evening and night accentuation.

example, the presence of increased resting muscle tone, cogwheel rigidity, and tremor can indicate the presence of Parkinson's disease, which can share some of the behavioral and sensory disturbances of REM behavior disorder. The mental status examination should include an evaluation of affect, anxiety, psychomotor agitation

Physical Findings Mallampati Scale

On average, the odds of having OSA increase more than 2-fold for every 1-point increase in Mallampati Scale.

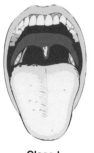 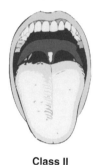 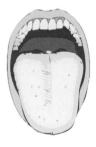 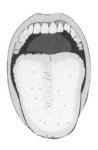

Class I
Tonsil visible

Class II
Upper half of tonsil fossa visible

Class III
Soft and hard palate visible

Class IV
Only hard palate visible

Figure 6.5 Mallampati airway classification. During assessment the patient is instructed to open his or her mouth as wide as possible, while protruding the tongue as far as possible. Patients are instructed to not emit sounds during the assessment. Class I: soft palate and entire uvula visible; Class II: soft palate and portion of uvula visible; Class III: soft palate visible (may include base of uvula); Class IV: soft palate not visible. Reproduced with permission from [34].

or slowing, cognition, the possibility of reduced alertness and slurred speech, and perceptual disturbances.

Scales and inventories

A few of the more commonly utilized inventories have already been described, including the insomnia severity index, the fatigue severity scale, the Epworth sleepiness scale, sleep diaries, and the Mallampati airway classification. The STOP-bang scoring model [35] is a method that was recently introduced, which strives to predict the risk of OSA without the use of polysomnography, the gold-standard procedure for the diagnosis of the disorder (Figure 6.6). It includes elements of the history and physical examination, and was validated in preoperative patients. "Yes" answers to three or more questions place the patient at high risk for OSA. The questionnaire was validated in a mixed group of preoperative patients against in-lab polysomnography. Sensitivities and specificities of the questionnaire are, respectively, as follows: for mild OSA (apnea-hypopnea index, or AHI, between 6 and 15), 83.6% and 56.4%; for moderate OSA (AHI between 16 and 29), 92.9% and 43.0%; for severe OSA (AHI greater than 30), 100% and 37%.

Tests and consultations

Serum laboratory tests have not been systematically explored in the evaluation of insomnia and ES. However, it seems reasonable that, providing they have not been performed in the past 6 months to 1 year, general serum laboratory tests including thyroid function

1. *Snoring*
   Do you snore loudly (louder than talking or loud enough to be heard through closed doors)?
   Yes   No
2. *Tired*
   Do you often feel tired, fatigued, or sleepy during daytime?
   Yes   No
3. *Observed*
   Has anyone observed you stop breathing during your sleep?
   Yes   No
4. *Blood pressure*
   Do you have or are you being treated for high blood pressure?
   Yes   No
5. *BMI*
   BMI more than 35 kg/m^2?
   Yes   No
6. *Age*
   Age over 50 yr old?
   Yes   No
7. *Neck circumference*
   Neck circumference greater than 40 cm?
   Yes   No
8. *Gender*
   Gender male?
   Yes   No

High risk of OSA: answering yes to three or more items
Low risk of OSA: answering yes to less than three items

Figure 6.6 The STOP-bang scoring model. Reproduced with permission from [35].

studies should be considered. RLS is more common in iron deficiency states and conditions associated with iron deficiency such as pregnancy and anemia [36]. The level of serum ferritin, an important indicator of iron deficiency, is inversely correlated with severity of RLS symptoms and iron supplementation has been shown to reduce RLS symptoms. Therefore, serum ferritin should be obtained in patients presenting with insomnia or ES and associated RLS symptoms, and a level of 50 µg/L or less is considered significant.

Actigraphy utilizes small, wristwatch-like devices to record movement. It assumes that lack of movement is equivalent to sleep, and is not, therefore, useful to measure exact sleep times. Although it is not appropriate for the routine diagnosis of sleep disorders, it can be useful as an adjunct to other procedures for the assessment of sleep–wake patterns when such information is not reliably available by other means such as sleep logs. It can be appropriate for the documentation of changes in sleep patterns over prolonged diagnosis and treatment periods; for the assessment of whether an insomniac follows certain sleep hygiene advice (e.g. to curtail time in bed or to regularize wake-up times) and of improvement in sleep following behavioral treatment; and for the assessment of daytime and night-time sleep and daytime somnolence in ES disorders [37].

Polysomnography (PSG) is the technique of monitoring multiple physiological measures during sleep, including brain waves, eye movements, heart rate, respirations, oxyhemoglobin saturation, and muscle tone and activity. Video recording may be used to identify abnormal movements during sleep. This test is typically performed in a sleep laboratory. Polysomnography is appropriate to establish the diagnosis when the office-based evaluation raises the possibility of a sleep-related breathing disorder (SRBD). It is also appropriate for a determination of the appropriate treatment settings during continuous positive airway pressure (CPAP) titration, and for the assessment of SRDB treatment results. With multiple sleep latency testing (see below), it is utilized for the diagnosis of narcolepsy. PSG is also utilized for the evaluation of the parasomnias which feature sleep-related behaviors that are violent or potentially injurious to the patient or others, to assist in the diagnosis of paroxysmal arousals or other sleep disruptions thought to be seizure related, and in a presumed parasomnia or sleep-related seizure disorder that does not respond to conventional therapy. It is also utilized for the diagnosis of periodic limb movement disorder [38].

The *multiple sleep latency test* (MSLT) is a daytime polysomnographic test which measures the extent of ES by assessing the speed of onset of sleep in five daytime nap opportunities, beginning 1.5 to 3 hours after awakening, and each separated by 2 hours. The patient lies down in a darkened room and is asked to not resist the urge to fall asleep. The onset and stage of sleep (including REM) are monitored. This test is used if the diagnosis of narcolepsy or idiopathic hypersomnia is suspected. A variation on the MSLT is the *maintenance of wakefulness test* (MWT), in which the patient is asked to stay awake while sitting in a dimly lit bedroom. It is considered by many to be a more accurate measure of sleep tendency in situations of everyday living, where individuals are trying to stay awake, rather than fall asleep, during the day. It is utilized for the assessment of individuals in whom the inability to remain awake constitutes a safety issue, and in patients with narcolepsy or idiopathic hypersomnia to assess response to treatment with medications [39].

There are several situations in which *sleep medicine consultations* may be useful following the office-based evaluation. These include: when the diagnosis is in doubt, seeming adequate treatment of the presumed disorder does not result in the alleviation of symptoms, or PSG/MSLT/MWT testing with follow-up treatment is desired.

Conclusions and recommendations

Insomnia, ES, and parasomnias are commonly encountered in psychiatric practice. They are the hallmark symptoms of a variety of sleep disorders, many of which will be discussed in greater detail in the ensuing chapters. This chapter has focused on the critical first steps in bridging symptom with disorder, namely the history and examination. These represent the cornerstones of the evaluation process. Below are some key recommendations that emerge from this chapter:

1. Develop a systematic process to address sleep-related complaints
2. Organize the clinical history around a typical 24-hour sleep/wake pattern beginning with bedtime and ending back at the time at which the inquiry began and determine deviations from normal patterns
3. Obtain the nocturnal or diurnal pattern, onset and longitudinal course, and severity of the chief complaint
4. Understand the temporal relationship between the chief complaint and potential precipitants such as psychosocial disruption, co-morbid illnesses, and prior treatments
5. Systematically explore sleep-related habits and behaviors and maladaptive psychological reactions and cognitions that may foment and perpetuate sleep/wake disturbances

6. Appreciate the nature and extent of consequences of the chief complaint on daytime functioning
7. Obtain collateral information from bed partners
8. Ask for symptoms of specific sleep disorders
9. Complete the essential elements of a general medical and psychiatric history gathering process and examination
10. Utilize inventories, tests, and consultations to complete the diagnostic picture
11. Arrive at a diagnostic formulation prior to resorting to treatment

References

1. Sateia MJ, Doghramji K, Hauri PJ, Morin CM. Evaluation of chronic insomnia. An American Academy of Sleep Medicine review. *Sleep.* 2000; 23(2):243–308.

2. Morgenthaler TI, Lee-Chiong T, Alessi C, et al. Practice parameters for the clinical evaluation and treatment of circadian rhythm sleep disorders. An American Academy of Sleep Medicine report. *Sleep.* 2007;**30** (11):1445–1459.

3. Schutte-Rodin S, Broch L, Buysse D, Dorsey C, Sateia M. Clinical guideline for the evaluation and management of chronic insomnia in adults. *J Clin Sleep Med.* 2008;4(5):487–504.

4. Vaughn BV, O'Neill DF. Cardinal manifestations of sleep disorders. In: Kryger M, Roth T, Dement WC, eds. *Principles and practice of sleep medicine,* 4th ed. Philadelphia: Elsevier; 2005:589.

5. American Academy of Sleep Medicine. *International classification of sleep disorders,* 2nd ed. Westchester, IL: American Academy of Sleep Medicine; 2005.

6. National Institutes of Health. National Institutes of Health state of the science conference statement on manifestations and management of chronic insomnia in adults, june 13–15, 2005. *Sleep.* 2005; 28(9):1049–1057.

7. Hohagen F, Rink K, Kappler C, et al. Prevalence and treatment of insomnia in general practice: a longitudinal study. *Eur Arch Psychiatry Clin Neurosci.* 1993;**242**(6):329–336.

8. Ford DE, Kamerow DB. Epidemiologic study of sleep disturbances and psychiatric disorders. an opportunity for prevention? *JAMA.* 1989;**262**(11): 1479–1484.

9. Ohayon MM, Roth T. Place of chronic insomnia in the course of depressive and anxiety disorders. *J Psychiatr Res.* 2003;**37**(1):9–15.

10. Ancoli-Israel S, Roth T. Characteristics of insomnia in the United States: Results of the 1991 National Sleep Foundation survey. I. *Sleep.* 1999;**22**(Suppl 2): S347–353.

11. Stepanski E, Zorick F, Roehrs T, Young D, Roth T. Daytime alertness in patients with chronic insomnia compared with asymptomatic control subjects. *Sleep.* 1988;**11**(1):54–60.

12. Edinger JD, Means MK, Carney CE, Krystal AD. Psychomotor performance deficits and their relation to prior nights' sleep among individuals with primary insomnia. *Sleep.* 2008;**31**(5):599–607.

13. Buysse DJ, Germaine A, Moul D, Nofzinger EA. Insomnia. In: Buysse DJ, ed. *Sleep disorders and psychiatry.* Arlington, VA: American Psychiatric Publishing, Inc.; 2005:31–84.

14. Kales JD, Kales A, Bixler EO, et al. Biopsychobehavioral correlates of insomnia, V: Clinical characteristics and behavioral correlates. *Am J Psychiatry.* 1984; **141**(11):1371–1376.

15. Kuppermann M, Lubeck DP, Mazonson PD, et al. Sleep problems and their correlates in a working population. *J Gen Intern Med.* 1995; **10**(1):25–32.

16. Bastien CH, Vallieres A, Morin CM. Validation of the insomnia severity index as an outcome measure for insomnia research. *Sleep Med.* 2001;**2**(4):297–307.

17. Morin CM. *Insomnia: psychological assessment and management.* New York: Guilford Press; 1993.

18. Stepanski EJ, Wyatt JK. Use of sleep hygiene in the treatment of insomnia. *Sleep Med Rev.* 2003;7(3): 215–225.

19. Carskadon MA, Dement WC, Mitler MM, et al. Self-reports versus sleep laboratory findings in 122 drug-free subjects with complaints of chronic insomnia. *Am J Psychiatry.* 1976;**133**(12):1382–1388.

20. Cooke JR, Ancoli-Israel S. Sleep and its disorders in older adults. *Psychiatr Clin North Am.* 2006;**29**(4): 1077–1093; abstract x–xi.

21. Krupp LB, LaRocca NG, Muir-Nash J, Steinberg AD. The fatigue severity scale. Application to patients with multiple sclerosis and systemic lupus erythematosus. *Arch Neurol.* 1989;**46**(10):1121–1123.

22. Johns MW. A new method for measuring daytime sleepiness: The Epworth sleepiness scale. *Sleep.* 1991; **14**(6):540–545.

23. Wagner U, Gais S, Haider H, Verleger R, Born J. Sleep inspires insight. *Nature.* 2004;**427**(6972): 352–355.

24. Blagrove M, Alexander C, Horne JA. The effects of chronic sleep reduction on the performance of

cognitive tasks sensitive to sleep deprivation. *Appl Cogn Psychol*. 1995;**9**:21–40.

25. Broughton R, Ghanem Q, Hishikawa Y, et al. Life effects of narcolepsy in 180 patients from North America, Asia and Europe compared to matched controls. *Can J Neurol Sci*. 1981; **8**(4):299–304.

26. National Commission on Sleep Disorders Research. *Wake up America: A national sleep alert – Report of the National Commission on Sleep Disorders Research*. Washington, DC: Department of Health and Human Services, Superintendent of Documents, U.S. Government Printing Office; 1992;92.

27. Mitler MM, Carskadon MA, Czeisler CA, et al. Catastrophes, sleep, and public policy: Consensus report. *Sleep*. 1988;**11**(1):100–109.

28. Mahowald MW, Schenck CH. REM sleep parasomnias. In: Kryger MH, Roth T, Dement WC, eds. *Priniciples and practice of sleep medicine*, 4th ed. Philadelphia: Elsevier; 2005:897–916.

29. Roehrs T, Roth T. Sleep, sleepiness and alcohol use. *Alcohol Res Health*. 2001;**25**(2):101–109.

30. Montplaisir J, Allen R, Walters A, Ferini-Strambi L. Restless legs syndrome and periodic limb movements in sleep. In: Kryger M, Roth T, Dement W, eds. 4th ed. Philadelphia: Elsevier; 2005:839–852.

31. Kales A, Soldatos CR, Bixler EO, et al. Hereditary factors in sleepwalking and night terrors. *Br J Psychiatry*. 1980;**137**:111–118.

32. Hening W, Allen RP, Tenzer P, Winkelman JW. Restless legs syndrome: Demographics, presentation, and differential diagnosis. *Geriatrics*. 2007;**62**(9): 26–29.

33. Millman RP, Carlisle CC, McGarvey ST, Eveloff SE, Levinson PD. Body fat distribution and sleep apnea severity in women. *Chest*. 1995;**107**(2):362–366.

34. Nuckton TJ, Glidden DV, Browner WS, Claman DM. Physical examination: Mallampati score as an independent predictor of obstructive sleep apnea. *Sleep*. 2006;**29**(7):903–908.

35. Chung F, Yegneswaran B, Liao P, et al. STOP questionnaire: A tool to screen patients for obstructive sleep apnea. *Anesthesiology*. 2008; **108**(5):812–821.

36. Sun ER, Chen CA, Ho G, Earley CJ, Allen RP. Iron and the restless legs syndrome. *Sleep*. 1998;**21**(4): A371–377.

37. Sadeh A, Hauri PJ, Kripke DF, Lavie P. The role of actigraphy in the evaluation of sleep disorders. *Sleep*. 1995;**18**(4):288–302.

38. Kushida CA, Littner MR, Morgenthaler T, et al. Practice parameters for the indications for polysomnography and related procedures: An update for 2005. *Sleep*. 2005;**28**(4):499–521.

39. Littner MR, Kushida C, Wise M, et al. Practice parameters for clinical use of the multiple sleep latency test and the maintenance of wakefulness test. *Sleep*. 2005;**28**(1):113–121.

7

Sleep-related breathing disorders

In-Soo Lee and Joel E. Dimsdale

Introduction

Although the historical description of obstructive sleep apnea goes back to at least the time of Charles Dickens' *Pickwick Papers*, the first real case report was published roughly 50 years ago in the *American Journal of Medicine*. It is interesting to read this rich case report and to note the powerful confluence of psychiatric and cardiopulmonary symptoms in sleep apnea. The case describes a sleepy, obese patient who was a middle-aged business executive, troubled by anxieties and simmering frustrations, who did not request medical attention, despite severe fatigue and functional limitations. He didn't request evaluation, that is, until a sentinel event occurred in his life. He was a life-long poker player and when he fell asleep after having been dealt a "full house," he decided something needed to be done [1].

That setting of admixture of fatigue, forgetfulness, anxiety, and depressive symptoms is quite common in patients with obstructive sleep apnea (OSA). This chapter reviews the association between sleep-related breathing disorders (SRBDs) and cognitive functioning, depression, and anxiety. We also briefly review the effects of psychotropic medications that may be particularly important to consider in a setting of SRBD.

Sleep-related breathing disorders

Sleep-related breathing disorders are characterized by disturbed respiration during sleep. These respiratory events may range from recurrent mild upper airway constriction (called upper airway resistance syndrome) to recurrent total obstruction. SRBDs are subdivided into those with obstruction (obstructive sleep apnea) and those with diminished or absent respiratory effort (central sleep apnea). In addition, there may be a mixture of these components (mixed type). Within these categories, there is a continuum in the degree of obstruction and in the frequency of these obstructive or central events. A great deal of work has gone into defining the epidemiology of these disturbances and their associated risks and pathophysiologies. Obstructive sleep apnea (OSA) is a chronic condition characterized by repetitive upper airway obstruction during sleep leading to apneic episodes, hypoxemia, and recurrent arousals from sleep [2]. It has been estimated that 2% to 4% of middle-aged men and 1% to 2% of middle-aged women suffer from OSA [3]. OSA is particularly prevalent in later life [4], and in obese men [5,6], although its existence in women [7], as well as in lean individuals, is increasingly recognized [3].

Risk factors for OSA include obesity and craniofacial or upper airway soft tissue abnormalities. Common craniofacial or upper airway soft tissue abnormalities that increase the risk of OSA include alterations in mandibular or maxillary size and position, narrowed nasal cavities, as well as tonsillar hypertrophy [8]. The Mallampati classification is a useful tool for assessing the probability of sleep disordered breathing. The Mallampati classification is based on the structures visualized with maximal mouth opening and tongue protrusion. The original goal of this classification was to assess whether the upper airway could be readily visualized during tracheal intubation [9] (see Figure 7.1). However, Liistro and colleagues showed that a high Mallampati score (stage 3 or 4) and nasal obstruction are associated risk factors for OSA [10].

Obesity is the most important reversible risk factor for OSA [11]. The prevalence of OSA among morbidly obese patients is 12- to 30-fold higher than in the general population [12]. Other risk factors for

Foundations of Psychiatric Sleep Medicine, ed. John W. Winkelman and David T. Plante. Published by Cambridge University Press.

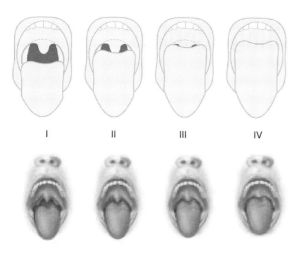

I   II   III   IV

Figure 7.1 The Mallampati classification. The class is determined by looking at the oral cavity as the patient protrudes the tongue, and tongue size is described relative to oropharyngeal size. The subsequent classification is based on the pharyngeal structures that are visible. Class 1: full visibility of tonsils, uvula, and soft palate; Class 2: visibility of hard and soft palate, upper portion of tonsils, and uvula; Class 3: soft and hard palate and base of the uvula are visible; Class 4: only hard palate visible. Modified after Mallampati SR, Gatt SP, Gugino LD, et al. A clinical sign to predict difficult tracheal intubation: a prospective study. Can Anaesth Soc J. 1985;32:429–434. Reprinted from [167].

OSA include genetic factors, smoking, menopause, and alcohol use [13].

The cardinal symptom of OSA is excessive daytime sleepiness, which appears to be related to recurrent arousals from sleep associated with obstructive events [14]. Other associated signs and symptoms include snoring, unrefreshing sleep, nocturnal choking (or dreams about choking or drowning), witnessed apneas, nocturia, morning headaches, mild cognitive impairment, and reduced libido [2]. Diagnosis is confirmed by assessment of sleep, typically via polysomnography. While exact cut points are arbitrary, a mean of 5–15 obstructive events per hour of sleep represents mild dysfunction, 15–30 events per hour represents moderate dysfunction, and >30 events per hour represents severe dysfunction [15]. Treatment options for OSA include weight loss, including discontinuation of weight-increasing medications, positional therapy, continuous positive airway pressure (CPAP), and mandibular advancement devices or surgery for clearly identifiable causes of upper airway obstruction [14]. The first line of therapy is CPAP, but its efficacy can be limited partially because adherence may be poor [5,16]. Weaver and colleagues

suggested "good" adherence should be defined as at least 6 hours a night [17].

OSA is associated with considerable morbidity and mortality, particularly from hypertension, cardiovascular disease, and insulin resistance [16]. Furthermore, the excessive daytime sleepiness associated with OSA can result in decreased quality of life [18] and increased risk for automobile accidents [19] or serious industrial accidents [20].

Psychiatric presentations of OSA

OSA patients complain of various neuropsychiatric symptoms. Cognitive impairment [21] and affective disorders such as depression are frequently encountered in OSA. In addition, a high prevalence of other psychiatric symptoms such as anxiety, somatization, ADHD-type, and obsessive-compulsive symptoms have been reported in these patients [22,23]. Clinicians can also encounter nocturnal panic attacks, diverse parasomnias, delirium, psychosis, personality change, and violent outbursts in some OSA patients [24–30]. Therefore, practicing psychiatrists and psychologists must consider OSA in the differential diagnosis of a large number of psychiatric presentations.

Cognitive and performance impairments in OSA

Approximately 80% of OSA patients complain of both excessive daytime sleepiness and cognitive impairments, and half report personality changes [31]. In addition to significant negative consequences on quality of life and auto vehicle safety, the neuropsychological effects of OSA can aggravate scholastic and occupational achievement as well as contribute to relationship problems.

Considerable research has examined neuropsychological deficits associated with OSA. Beebe and colleagues conducted a meta-analysis of 25 recent studies (involving >2000 patients) to examine patterns of neuropsychological deficits in OSA. They found impairments in vigilance, executive function, and motor coordination but no effect of OSA on general intelligence and verbal ability. The effects of OSA on visual and motor skill and memory functioning were inconsistent [32]. In a separate review, Aloia and colleagues reported that 60% of reviewed studies found deficits in attention and vigilance, executive functioning, and memory impairment, and 80% of reviewed studies found visuoconstruction and psychomotor functioning impairments [33]. Below, we review selected studies to give a sense for the types of neuropsychological probes that have been applied in this area.

Sustained attention or vigilance

Sustained attention is one of the most commonly affected cognitive problems for OSA patients [34–39]. It is assessed by tests such as the psychomotor vigilance task (PVT). OSA patients initially perform comparably to normal controls during short-duration tasks, but performance degrades with longer duration tasks, where one sees increased response time, lapses or failure to respond, and false responses [40,41]. Operating a motor vehicle requires sustained vigilance, and impairments in this cognitive function may contribute to elevated rate of car accidents. OSA patients with excessive daytime sleepiness are 6 to 10 times more likely to have an accident than non-sleepy controls [42]. The reaction time of patients with mild to moderate sleep disordered breathing is worse than that found in healthy, non-sleepy subjects with blood alcohol levels of 0.080 g/dL (the typical legal limit for intoxicated driving in the USA) [43].

Memory

There is less consistency in studies of short-term and long-term memory functioning in OSA patients [32,34,44,45]. Bedard and colleagues described diminished performance on short-term memory in patients with moderate and severe sleep apnea, although only the severe group demonstrated evidence of impairment in delayed recall. These memory disturbances were associated with a decrease in vigilance [34]. Others have reported short- and long-term memory problems [38,46–49]. On the other hand, Greenberg and colleagues found no differences between patients with OSA and controls on subscales of the Wechsler memory scale (in either immediate or delayed conditions) [37].

Differences in samples such as level of disease severity, clinic versus population-based studies, or the use of normal controls versus norm-referenced comparisons may account for the inconsistencies. These inconsistencies may also reflect impairment in organization and retrieval caused by different levels of executive function deficits in OSA patients [32].

Executive functions

Executive function refers to a set of higher cognitive abilities that control and regulate other basic abilities like attention, memory, and motor skills. Executive functions may involve the ability to engage in goal-directed behaviors and abstract thinking. Executive function impairments can be measured by assessing diverse domains such as planning, sequencing, self-monitoring, set-shifting, verbal fluency, abstract reasoning, working memory, visual–spatial organization, and memory [50–52].

Many studies have examined disturbances in executive function in OSA, demonstrating impairment in several domains. For example, Bedard and colleagues reported widespread deficits in various executive functions (verbal fluency, planning, sequential thinking, and constructional ability), with extent of impairment related to severity of the breathing abnormality [34,53].

Etiology and mechanism of cognitive and performance impairments

The pathogenesis of cognitive deficits in OSA is controversial and most likely multifactorial. The two most commonly implicated etiological mechanisms are repetitive sleep fragmentation and nocturnal hypoxemia. However, the evidence is as yet tenuous linking either measure of OSA severity and any cognitive domain [33].

Researchers have assumed that neuropsychological tests reflect abnormalities in specific brain regions. The evidence of disturbance in executive functions has led to the suggestion that OSA may be associated with frontal lobe dysfunction [34,36]. In this context, the prefrontal model has been proposed as a conceptual framework for the relationship between sleep disruption and nocturnal hypoxemia and primarily frontal deficits in OSA. This model hypothesizes that OSA-related sleep disruption and intermittent hypoxemia as well as hypercarbia alter the brain's restorative processes, thereby inducing a variety of cellular and biochemical stresses that disrupt functional homeostasis as well as neuronal and glial viability within the prefrontal cortex [54] (see Figure 7.2).

Animal studies demonstrate that intermittent exposure to low O_2 damages hippocampal CA1 regions and frontal cortex. Such damage has been correlated with cognitive deficits [55], especially learning and

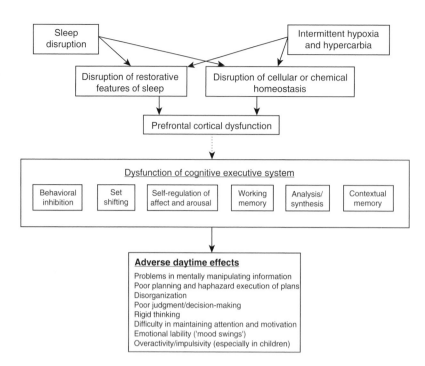

Figure 7.2 The proposed prefrontal model. In this model, OSA-related sleep disruption and intermittent hypoxemia and hypercarbia alter the efficacy of restorative processes occurring during sleep, and disrupt the functional homeostasis and neuronal and glial viability within particular brain regions. Subsequent dysfunction of prefrontal cortical regions is manifested by dysfunction of the cognitive "executive system," which alters cognitive abilities, thereby resulting in maladaptive daytime behaviors. Adapted from [54], with permission.

memory alterations which are similar to cognitive defects found in OSA patients [56].

Volumetric studies in OSA patients also show diminished gray matter in the hippocampus, nearby cerebral cortex, and cerebellar cortex and deep nuclei [57]. The cerebellar damage in OSA may contribute to loss of coordination of upper airway muscle activity (hypotonia of upper airway muscles), failure to regulate sympathetic tone, and further disruption of higher-order cognitive processes [58].

Recently, functional neuroimaging studies have begun to investigate the cerebral substrates of cognitive function in OSA. In an fMRI study, Thomas and colleagues reported that untreated OSA patients showed reduced performance on a 2-back working memory task, as well as reduced activation within anterior cingulate, dorsolateral prefrontal, and posterior parietal cortices. They suggested that the fragmented sleep contributed to these deficits more than the nocturnal hypoxia [59].

In another fMRI study, Ayalon and colleagues examined the cerebral response to a verbal learning task in OSA patients. They found that verbal learning performance was similar in both the OSA and control groups, but OSA patients showed increased brain activation in several brain regions (bilateral inferior frontal and middle frontal gyri, cingulate gyrus, areas

at the junction of the inferior parietal and superior temporal lobes, thalamus, and cerebellum). The recruitment of additional brain areas during tasks in OSA patients was felt to reflect an adaptive compensatory recruitment response [60].

Effect of treatment on cognitive and performance impairments

Many studies have examined cognitive functioning after treatment for OSA has been initiated [61]. Treatment effects have been inconsistent for sustained attention, memory, executive functioning, and psychomotor function. However, treatment was noted to improve attention/vigilance in most studies but did not improve constructional abilities or psychomotor functioning [33]. Aloia and colleagues found deficits in fine motor coordination more resistant to effects of treatment. They suggested that brain regions serving fine motor coordination (such as basal ganglia, subcortical gray matter, and cerebellum) may be particularly vulnerable to hypoxemia resulting from OSA [33].

Because neuropsychological testing improves upon retesting, pre- and post-studies of treatment effects are difficult to interpret unless appropriate controls have been used. Unfortunately controlled studies in this area are still rare. In uncontrolled studies, CPAP treatment had a moderate to large effect on cognitive processing, memory, sustained attention, and executive functions [38]. However, other studies show persistent cognitive deficits despite treatment [62,63].

The majority of controlled clinical trials evaluating the efficacy of CPAP treatment have enrolled predominantly moderate to severe OSA patients. In mild OSA patients, the only improvement in quality of life after 8 weeks of CPAP treatment was in vitality [64]. Some studies suggest that beneficial CPAP treatment effects for cognition might be attributable to changes in the underlying level of daytime sleepiness [64,65].

Bardwell and colleagues evaluated the effectiveness of 1-week CPAP treatment versus placebo-CPAP (i.e. CPAP administered at subtherapeutic pressure) on cognitive functioning in patients with OSA. Although CPAP improved overall cognitive functioning, no beneficial effects in any specific domain were found. But, only 1 of the 22 neuropsychological test scores (Digit Vigilance–Time, a measure of speed of information processing, vigilance, or sustained attention and alertness) showed significant changes specific to CPAP treatment [66]. In their replication study with 2 weeks of CPAP treatment, two-thirds of neuropsychological test scores improved with time regardless of treatment; however, once again only Digit Vigilance–Time showed significant improvement specific to CPAP treatment. They concluded that Digit Vigilance–Time might be the most sensitive neuropsychological test for measuring the effects of CPAP. Furthermore, 2 weeks of CPAP treatment might be sufficient to improve speed of information processing, vigilance, as well as sustained attention and alertness [67].

Evaluating the evidence for the efficacy of treatment on the cognitive and performance impairments in OSA is challenging because of differences in length of treatment, adherence to treatment, type of control, and placebo employed. It is as yet unclear how long treatment should be provided in order to document efficacy. What is the time course of response? What cognitive functions respond first? Are there certain cognitive functions that improve only after weeks of treatment? Future research is required to clarify these issues.

Clinical implications of cognitive impairments in OSA

Beebe and colleagues recommended that sleep clinicians should routinely assess cognitive symptoms of OSA patients. If residual deficits are suspected following treatment, cognitive evaluations of vigilance, executive functioning, and motor functioning should be undertaken. They also suggest interestingly that undiagnosed sleep disordered breathing should be suspected in individuals who display evidence of poor vigilance, or executive dysfunction [32].

Depression in OSA

Depression is the most commonly encountered affective disorder associated with OSA [68]. The prevalence of depression in OSA has ranged from 7% to 63% [69]. Early investigations by Guilleminault and colleagues reported that 24% of male patients with OSA had previously seen a psychiatrist for anxiety and depression [70]. A recent epidemiological study of 18 980 subjects representative of the general population in the UK, Germany, Italy, Portugal, and Spain found that 17.6% of subjects with a *Diagnostic and Statistical Manual of Mental Disorders IV* (DSM-IV) breathing-related sleep disorder diagnosis (by history, without sleep study) have major depressive disorder (MDD) [71]. Thus, some co-morbidity between SRBD and depression has long been observed. The variations in the prevalence of depression are thought to be affected by sampling characteristics, mood assessment methods, and diagnostic difficulty due to an overlap of symptoms across depression and OSA.

A number of studies, using varied designs, report an association between OSA and depression, based on elevated co-morbidity of OSA and MDD [30,70,72–74], as well as increased levels of depressive symptoms [75–80] that do not necessarily reflect a major depressive episode [73]. Other studies observe a correlation between apnea-hypopnea index (AHI; number of apneas and hypopneas per hour of sleep) and depression [81], with increased depressive symptoms found in association with more severe SRBD [82], and improvement of depressive symptoms after treatment with CPAP, uvulopalatopharyngoplasty, or tracheostomy [74,76,77,79,83]. Peppard and colleagues found a dose–response association between SRBD severity (AHI) and depression in their population-based, longitudinal investigation (see Figure 7.3). Figure 7.3 compares the rates of depression found amongst individuals with differing levels of respiratory disturbance. Depression was defined as a score of 50 or higher on the Zung depression scale in individuals who were not receiving antidepressant

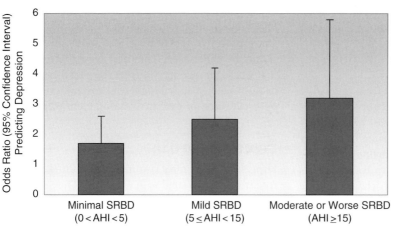

Figure 7.3 Association between depression and SRBD as compared with participants with no SRBD. Depression was defined as a score of 50 or higher on the Zung depression scale. Antidepressant users were excluded in this model. AHI, apnea-hypopnea index; SRBD, sleep-related breathing disorder. Adapted from [82], with permission.

medication. The prevalence of depression was increased with increasing severity of SRBD (minimal SRBD: OR, 1.7, 95% CI: 1.1–2.6; mild SRBD: 2.5, 1.5–4.2; moderate or worse SRBD: 3.2, 1.8–5.8) [82]. These dose–response observations suggest a strong link between depression and SRBD.

However, the association between OSA and depression remains controversial, as a number of studies have found no correlation between the two disorders. For instance, Pillar and Lavie found that neither the existence nor the severity of sleep apnea syndrome was associated with depression in a large male population (N=1977) [84]. Other researchers reported that patients with sleep apnea do not show clinically significant levels of depression, nor do they have levels of depressive symptoms higher than normal controls [85–87]. As discussed later in this chapter, other researchers have examined if treatment for SRBD improved depressive symptoms, but the evidence is far from compelling (see Table 7.1).

This inconsistency of the association between OSA and depression may stem from the complexity in assessing depression in OSA and from confounding factors related to characteristics of the sampled population. Diagnostic limitations are one of the fundamental difficulties. For example, SRBD can be diagnosed by nocturnal polysomnography (PSG), the standard diagnostic test for sleep apnea. Upper airway resistance syndrome (UARS) is an important phenomenon that is also related to excessive daytime sleepiness and depressive mood [88]. However, recognition of UARS is complicated because it is not detected by standard nocturnal polysomnography. The gold standard in the diagnosis

of UARS is nocturnal esophageal manometry, but this invasive method is not tolerated by every patient and needs extra equipment and expertise. There is need for development of alternative accurate and non-invasive methods for diagnosing this particular form of sleep disordered breathing [89,90].

In addition, OSA and depression share common symptoms such as fatigue and sleepiness, multiple awakenings, psychomotor retardation, poor concentration and memory, low sexual drive, and irritability. So it is often difficult to clinically distinguish these two disorders. Unfortunately, diagnostic evaluations for depression in OSA are not standardized. Researchers have used various measurement scales, cut-points, or psychiatric interviews. This can lead to different diagnoses and also can confound the association between OSA and depression.

Because OSA is widely distributed in the population, over a wide range of age and medical co-morbidities, association studies can be limited by confounding factors related to population sampled. Bardwell and colleagues suggested that depression in OSA patients may be determined by confounding factors such as age, body mass, and hypertension rather than OSA *per se* [91]. They also demonstrated that depression may account for the fatigue seen in OSA, after controlling for OSA severity [92]. To understand this area, it seems reasonable to include several potentially confounding variables such as: (1) specific age–gender distribution in OSA (e.g. high SRBD prevalence in post-menopausal women) [93]; (2) role of antihypertensive medication in depression; (3) hypertensive patients' own psychological characteristics [94,95]; (4) diabetes; (5) obesity;

Table 7.1 The effect of CPAP treatment on depression and anxiety in patients with obstructive sleep apnea

Reference (year)	Number of subjects	Study design	CPAP treatment time	Effect on mood
Borak et al. (1996) [22]	20	Prospective, uncontrolled study	3 months and 12 months	No improvements in emotional status after 3 and 12 months
Engleman et al. (1997) [168]	16	Prospective, placebo-controlled, randomized, crossover study	4 weeks	Significant decline in HAD-depression
Engleman et al. (1998) [169]	23	Prospective, randomized, single blind, placebo controlled, crossover study	4 weeks	No changes in HAD
Jokic et al. (1998) [170]	10	Prospective, controlled, single blind crossover study	4 weeks	Use of CPAP was associated with a decrease in HAD-anxiety scores
Redline et al. (1998) [64]	97	Randomized, controlled study	8 weeks	CPAP showed beneficial effect over mechanical nasal ventilator in POMS and PANAS scores
Engleman et al. (1999) [171]	34	Randomized, placebo controlled, crossover study	4 weeks	Compared with placebo, CPAP improved depression score in HAD
Kingshott et al. (2000) [182]	62	Prospective, uncontrolled study	6 months	Significant decline in HAD-depression and anxiety
Munoz et al. (2000) [114]	80	Prospective, controlled study	12 months	CPAP failed to modify anxiety and depression in Beck tests
Yamamoto et al. (2000) [172]	47	Prospective, uncontrolled study	2 years	Significant decrease in SDS
Sanchez et al. (2001) [122]	51	Prospective, uncontrolled study	1 month and 3 months	Significant decrease in BDI and STAI (depression and anxiety-trait) after both 1 month and 3 months
Barnes et al. (2002) [173]	28	Randomized, controlled, crossover study	8 weeks	No benefit of CPAP on BDI and POMS scores
Doherty et al. (2003) [174]	45	Prospective, uncontrolled study	8 weeks	Significant decline in HAD-depression and anxiety
Means et al. (2003) [83]	39	Prospective, uncontrolled study	3 months	Significant decrease in BDI
Svaldi et al. (2003) [175]	54	Prospective, uncontrolled study	6–9 weeks	Significant decrease in BDI
Barnes et al. (2004) [176]	114	Randomized, controlled, crossover study	3 months	Improvements of depression were no better than placebo effect
Mackinger et al. (2004) [177]	54	Prospective, controlled study	2 months	Significant decrease in BDI in patients with previous depression
Goncalves et al. (2005) [178]	34	Prospective, controlled study	4 weeks	Significant decrease in BDI
Schwartz et al. (2005) [179]	50	Prospective, uncontrolled study	4–6 weeks	Significant decrease in BDI

Table 7.1 (cont.)

Reference (year)	Number of subjects	Study design	CPAP treatment time	Effect on mood
Schwartz et al. (2007) [180]	50	Prospective, uncontrolled study	1 year	Significant decrease in BDI
Wells et al. (2007) [181]	54	Prospective, uncontrolled study	30 days	Significant decrease in BDI, but, improvements were not associated with CPAP use

Notes: Tabled studies examined treatment time ≥4 weeks.
BDI, the Beck depression inventory; HAD, hospital anxiety and depression scale; MADRS, Montgomery Asberg depression rating scale; PANAS, the positive and negative affects scale; POMS, profile of moods states; SDS, the self-related depression scale; STAI, the state-trait anxiety inventory.
Adapted from [69] and updated.

and (6) apnea patients' other psychological characteristics such as irritability [75,77,80], anxiety [70,76–78, 96], and fatigue [76,79,85,97]. Future studies addressing these diagnostic and methodological issues are needed to examine bidirectional effects between SRBD and depression.

Possible mechanisms underlying the association between depression and OSA

As with cognitive impairment, sleep fragmentation and hypoxemia during sleep are suspected to be responsible for depressive symptoms in OSA. Sleep fragmentation certainly contributes to the excessive daytime sleepiness (EDS) in OSA patients. Several studies have supported positive correlation between EDS as measured by the Epworth sleepiness scale and depressive symptoms [23,98].

Hypoxemia provides another mechanism linking SRBD to depression. Recent imaging studies in OSA report cerebral metabolic impairment resulting from recurrent nocturnal hypoxemia [99–101]. Aloia and colleagues reported that more subcortical white matter hyperintensities were found on MRI in patients with severe OSA as compared to mild OSA. In the same study, they reported a trend for a positive correlation between the subcortical hyperintensities and depression scores on the Hamilton depression scale [33].

The high co-morbidity of OSA and depression also suggests that both disorders may share a common neurobiological risk factor. On the neurotransmitter level, the serotonergic system is involved in the regulation of sleep and wakefulness (see Chapter 2:

Neuroanatomy and neurobiology of sleep and wakefulness). Its activity is higher during wakefulness than in sleep [102]. The production of rapid eye movement (REM) sleep depends on the decrease of serotonergic tone in brainstem structures. Patients with OSA have a central deficiency of serotonin activity [103], and it is interesting that depression is also associated with a decreased serotonergic neurotransmission [104].

Cytokine and metabolic-related hormone studies

There is a growing literature suggesting that the links between depressive symptoms and OSA may be associated with obesity and the metabolic syndrome. Although both OSA and depression have independently been shown to be associated with metabolic syndrome and cardiovascular disease [105,106], it is still poorly understood how these risk factors interact with each other.

It has been suggested that some of the psychological symptoms experienced by OSA patients may be related to high levels of proinflammatory cytokines. Vgontzas and colleagues reported that the inflammatory cytokines tumor necrosis factor-α (TNF-α) and interleukin-6 (IL-6), which produce sleepiness and fatigue, are elevated in sleep apnea and obesity and might play a role in the pathogenesis and pathological sequelae of both disorders [107]. Haensel and colleagues found that elevated levels of the soluble tumor necrosis factor receptor 1 (sTNF-R1) were significantly correlated with cognitive dysfunction in untreated OSA patients. They suggest that inflammation in OSA may be an important factor to

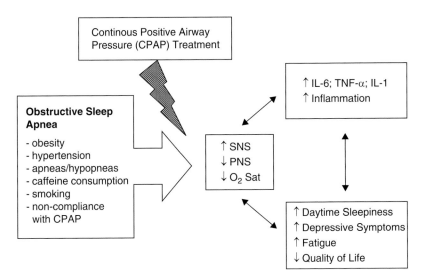

Figure 7.4 A schematic summary of a research model using obstructive sleep apnea (OSA) for studying sleep and cytokines. CPAP, continuous positive airway pressure; SNS, sympathetic nervous system; PNS, parasympathetic nervous system; O$_2$ Sat, oxygen saturation. Reprinted from [112], with permission.

consider in understanding cognitive functioning in these patients [108].

Leptin (an adipocyte-derived hormone) is a crucial mediator of energy homeostasis. Several studies have shown that higher levels of leptin are associated with sleep apnea [109]. Recent studies also suggested the novel function of leptin as a possible explanation of mood disorders. Low levels of leptin have been found to be associated with depressive behaviors in rodents and humans. Pharmacological studies indicate that leptin has antidepressant-like efficacy. Both leptin insufficiency and leptin resistance may contribute to alterations of affective status [110,111].

In order to integrate these complicated relationships, Mills and Dimsdale suggested a research model regarding the relationship between neuroimmune interactions, mood changes, as well as behavioral aspects in OSA [112]. Figure 7.4 provides a schematic summary of this model. Because of its many relevant characteristics, including neuroimmune interactions, mood changes (such as fatigue and depression), as well as behaviors that directly affect the course of the disorder (such as excessive caffeine consumption, smoking, diet, and difficulties with adherence to treatment), OSA presents researchers with a unique opportunity to tease apart the many complex and interwoven components of sleep that are relevant to cytokines and psychoneuroimmunology.

Treatment effects on depression in OSA

Studies of CPAP's treatment effect on depressive mood are not consistent. Table 7.1 summarizes studies reporting the impact of CPAP treatment (for over 1 month of treatment) on depression and anxiety. Many studies reported that depressive symptoms were ameliorated by CPAP treatment. It is gratifying to see that this field is attracting careful study. At the risk of merely counting positive versus negative studies, it appears that more studies (i.e. 14 studies) report positive effects of CPAP on mood as compared to non-significant effects on mood (i.e. 6 studies). Differences in experimental design such as sample size, the nature of depressive symptoms, CPAP compliance, and co-morbid medical conditions need further exploration.

In some negative studies, baseline depressive symptoms were not particularly high, and one could speculate that the lack of a treatment effect on depression was due to a "floor effect" [22]. Millman and colleagues found that OSA patients with more severe depressive symptoms responded better to CPAP treatment, whereas patients with less severe or no mood symptoms actually had less benefit from CPAP therapy [74]. Although CPAP is a very effective treatment for OSA, compliance may be problematic, and better CPAP compliance has been predicted by lower pretreatment depressive symptomatology [113]. Munoz and colleagues found that anxious and depressive symptoms may develop despite effective treatment because of the patients' disappointment with chronic CPAP treatment [114]. Patients' personality characteristics and coping strategies certainly contribute to mood symptoms during CPAP treatment [115]. In the future, long-term follow-up studies in

OSA patients with a broader range of depressive symptoms are required to examine whether CPAP has a positive effect on mood in depressed OSA patients and how CPAP adherence can be improved in patients with depression.

Obesity has a major negative impact on both physical and mental components of health-related quality of life in OSA. Redline and colleagues found that CPAP was beneficial (in terms of mood, fatigue, and functional status) for OSA patients without sinus problems, and that OSA patients with higher body mass indices were more likely to improve than were subjects with less obesity [64]. Weight reduction is important in the treatment of overweight patients with OSA. Some studies show that weight loss is associated with major improvements in sleep disturbance and OSA severity in obese subjects [116,117]. Recently, Dixon and colleagues reported weight reduction reduced not only daytime sleepiness but also depressive mood in 25 severely obese OSA patients [118].

Clinical implication: depression in OSA

Clinicians should suspect OSA particularly in depressed patients who present with symptoms such as snoring and excessive daytime fatigue [119]. Moreover, undiagnosed OSA should be considered when depressed patients do not respond to antidepressant treatment. In this sense, depression refractory to treatment may be akin to hypertension refractory to treatment, with both instances possibly denoting occult OSA [120].

OSA lurking behind depression is important, because some pharmacological treatments of depression may exacerbate OSA. Some sedative antidepressants and benzodiazepine hypnotics have the potential to exacerbate OSA by either increasing weight gain or causing oversedation. Oversedation may precipitate an excessively drowsy state during sleep that could inhibit sleep arousals, which are important for resumption of breathing effort.

Anxiety and SRBD

In a meta-analysis, Saunamaki and colleagues found that while reports of anxiety in the context of OSA are less common than depression, anxiety in OSA is not unusual, with the prevalence of anxiety ranging from 11% to 70% in OSA patients [69]. There is considerable disagreement with respect to the relationship of anxiety to OSA. Some studies found higher levels of anxiety in OSA [76,77,121–123], but others failed to find a relationship between any sleep variables and anxiety [91].

Borak and colleagues reported an association between anxiety and OSA, but CPAP treatment did not improve patients' anxiety scores [22]. Several researchers found that high anxiety or depression contribute to non-compliance with CPAP treatment [124–127]. Such symptoms may leave patients less tolerant of the equipment. Some patients express claustrophobic anxiety when wearing a CPAP mask [128,129]. Hence, treatment of their anxiety symptoms as well as patient trial of diverse types of CPAP masks may be necessary to insure improved compliance with CPAP treatment.

ADHD and OSA

Attention-deficit/hyperactivity disorder (ADHD) is a common childhood illness with prevalence between 3% and 16%. It is characterized by hyperactivity, impulsiveness, impairment in academic, social, and occupational functioning, and short attention span. OSA is also a common medical problem in children with a prevalence rate of 2% in general pediatric populations [130]. Several studies have reported a relationship between ADHD and sleep problems [131,132]. Parents of children with ADHD report decreased nocturnal sleep efficiency and sleep fragmentation in their children as compared to parents of healthy controls [133]. Experimental sleep restriction, leading to daytime somnolence, is associated with ADHD-like behavior and poor cognitive functioning. Golan and colleagues found that children with ADHD had a high prevalence of primary sleep disorders and objective daytime somnolence [134]. Thus, in evaluating children with ADHD symptoms, it is wise to consider the possibility that undiagnosed OSA may be contributing to the child's behavioral symptoms (see Chapter 21: Sleep in attention-deficit/hyperactivity disorder (ADHD)).

Effects of psychiatric medications on SRBD

In OSA, any sedative agent can aggravate or precipitate an excessively drowsy state that could inhibit sleep arousals that are critical to the resumption of breathing. Atypical antipsychotics (such as olanzapine or clozapine), mood-stabilizing medications, or antiepileptic drugs (such as valproic acid and carbamazepine), antidepressants (such as tricyclic antidepressants), and benzodiazepine hypnotics have the potential to exacerbate OSA by either increasing weight gain or causing oversedation.

Antipsychotics

Patients taking chronic antipsychotic medications may gain 15–75 lb (6.8–33.8 kg) over the first 2 years of treatment, and 35–50% of such patients may become clinically obese [135]. Winkelman reported that obesity, male gender, and chronic neuroleptic administration are risk factors for OSA in psychiatric patients. He also reported that OSA in schizophrenic patients was severe, with a mean respiratory disturbance index (RDI) of 64.8 events per hour [136]. Since patients with schizophrenia are often on long-term neuroleptic treatment, they may have high rates of OSA, aggravated by the weight gain produced by such medications.

Although OSA in schizophrenics might contribute to cardiovascular disease and increased mortality, the condition is underdiagnosed, partially because of confusion between daytime sleepiness and negative symptoms or medication side-effects.

Antidepressants

Several animal studies suggest that serotonin is important in the maintenance of upper airway patency. Serotonergic neurons (mediated predominantly via $5-HT_{2A}$ and $5-HT_{2C}$ receptor subtypes) exert an excitatory effect on upper airway dilator motor neurons [137,138]. When serotonin delivery is reduced to upper airway dilator motor neurons in sleep, this contributes to reductions in dilator muscle activity and upper airway obstruction.

Administration of paroxetine increased activity of upper airway dilator muscle during wakefulness in normal subjects [139] and during non-REM sleep in patients with OSA [140], which suggested that the SSRI may be effective in treating OSA. However, in clinical studies, serotonergic drugs such as protriptyline, fluoxetine, paroxetine, and mirtazapine have been tested as treatments for OSA, with limited improvement and significant side-effects [141,142]. Administration of the serotonin precursor, L-tryptophan, was reported to be effective in decreasing obstructive apneas in non-REM sleep in an uncontrolled study of 12 patients with OSA [143]. However, L-tryptophan was previously withdrawn from the market as a result of reports linking tryptophan use with eosinophilic myalgia syndrome and life-threatening pulmonary hypertension. The serotonin option for treatment of OSA remains an intriguing, novel theoretical approach, but one that has not yet been proven effective.

SSRIs are widely used to treat depressive mood and anxiety in OSA patients. Moreover, SSRIs may be at least partially (and theoretically) effective in OSA by virtue of their REM sleep suppression (as OSA tends to worsen during REM sleep when muscle tone is lowest and the upper airway is most prone to obstruct) and/or augmentation of upper airway dilator muscle activity. While SSRIs are relatively tolerable in OSA, antidepressants with side-effects of sedation or weight gain (such as antidepressants with H1 receptor blockade property) may exacerbate OSA.

Sedative hypnotics

Experts recommend caution in prescribing hypnotics to patients with severe OSA, especially those with daytime hypoventilation or hypercapneic chronic obstructive pulmonary disease (COPD), unless such patients are simultaneously effectively treated with CPAP. Benzodiazepines can decrease respiratory effort, upper airway muscle tone, and blunt arousal responses to hypoxia/hypercapnia [144,145]. They may thus worsen sleep apnea [146]. Long-acting benzodiazepines such as flurazepam [146] and nitrazepam [147] produce the most marked respiratory depression. Thus, it is recommended that benzodiazepine hypnotics be used cautiously in OSA patients with compromised respiratory function [148]. If sedative hypnotic therapy is needed in patients with OSA, it is very important for clinicians to ensure CPAP adherence by periodic monitoring of compliance. Berry and colleagues reported that triazolam 0.25 mg increases the arousal threshold to airway occlusion, but this results in only modest prolongation of event duration and modestly increased desaturation in severe sleep apnea patients [149].

Non-benzodiazepine hypnotics (such as zolpidem, zopiclone, and zaleplon) generally produce fewer effects on respiratory depression in patients with OSA [150]. Many previous studies demonstrated that zolpidem does not considerably affect respiratory parameters in patients with COPD [151–154] or OSA [155,156]. Zopiclone and eszopiclone also did not cause deterioration in respiratory parameters (SaO_2, apnea index) in patients with UARS [157,158] or with mild to moderate

OSA [159]. Zaleplon's effect on respiratory function was not significantly different from placebo in mild to moderate OSA [156]. However, some studies reported that zolpidem reduces oxygen desaturation and increases the apnea index in patients with OSA [155,160]. Although we can generally assume that non-benzodiazepine hypnotics are safer in these patient populations, given the small number of studies, further investigation is required and one should be cautious when administering any type of non-benzodiazepine hypnotic to patients with OSA.

Alcohol

Alcohol is known to exacerbate OSA. Alcohol induces oropharyngeal muscle hypotonia and depression of arousal mechanisms as well as weight gain [161]. Thus, OSA patients should reduce or abstain from alcohol intake, particularly during night-time.

Modafinil

Medications can be used as an adjunctive treatment in OSA. Approximately 40% of patients do not tolerate CPAP, and patients with OSA treated with CPAP may still have daytime sleepiness. If CPAP treatment is being used optimally and daytime sleepiness persists, wakefulness-promoting medications (such as modafinil, amphetamines, and methylphenidate) may improve sleepiness and quality of life.

Modafinil (Provigil®) is approved by the US Food and Drug Administration for residual excessive sleepiness in patients with obstructive sleep apnea syndrome after the CPAP regimen is optimized [162]. Modafinil is not approved for use in pediatric patients. In OSA, a concerted effort to treat with CPAP for an adequate period of time should be made prior to initiating modafinil or other wakefulness-promoting medications. If modafinil is used adjunctively with CPAP, encouragement and periodic assessment of CPAP compliance is necessary.

Previous studies reported that modafinil (either with or without CPAP treatment) may improve not only wakefulness but also cognitive performance and memory without affecting night-time sleep, blood pressure, or heart rate [163,164]. Given the long and bitter history of abuse of stimulant medications, the use of modafinil as adjunctive therapy in treating depression and fatigue is being considered carefully, and more research is needed to determine its role in these settings [165,166].

Conclusion

In the last 50 years we have made enormous strides in our understanding of the epidemiology of SRBD as well as their treatment. We have also come to realize that OSA is commonly accompanied by various neuropsychological impairments and is associated with depressive symptoms and, to a lesser extent, anxiety symptoms. The principal treatment of OSA–CPAP may be difficult to tolerate, and compliance may be lower in those with co-morbid psychiatric symptoms, underscoring the need to improve adherence in those with severe mental illness. Treatment of an underlying psychiatric disorder may lead to OSA via weight gain in response to psychotropic medication. On the other hand, psychiatric disorders that are refractory to treatment may be associated with occult OSA.

References

1. Burwell CS, Robin ED, Whaley RD, Bickelmann AG. Extreme obesity with alveolar hypoventilation: a Pickwickian syndrome. *Am J Med.* 1956; **21**:811–818.

2. Gibson GJ. Obstructive sleep apnoea syndrome: underestimated and undertreated. *Br Med Bull.* 2004;**72**:49–65.

3. Young T, Peppard PE, Gottlieb DJ. Epidemiology of obstructive sleep apnea: a population health perspective. *Am J Respir Crit Care Med.* 2002;**165**(9): 1217–1239.

4. Ancoli-Israel S, Kripke DF, Klauber MR, et al. Sleep-disordered breathing in community-dwelling elderly. *Sleep.* 1991;**14**(6):486–495.

5. Vgontzas AN, Kales A. Sleep and its disorders. *Annu Rev Med.* 1999;**50**:387–400.

6. Young T, Palta M, Dempsey J, et al. The occurrence of sleep-disordered breathing among middle-aged adults. *N Engl J Med.* 1993;**328**(17):1230–1235.

7. Bixler EO, Vgontzas AN, Lin HM, et al. Prevalence of sleep-disordered breathing in women: effects of gender. *Am J Respir Crit Care Med.* 2001;**163** (3 Pt 1):608–613.

8. Riley RW, Powell NB, Li KK, Troell RJ, Guilleminault C. Surgery and obstructive sleep apnea: long-term clinical outcomes. *Otolaryngol Head Neck Surg.* 2000;**122**(3):415–421.

9. Mallampati SR, Gatt SP, Gugino LD, et al. A clinical sign to predict difficult tracheal intubation: a prospective study. *Can Anaesth Soc J.* 1985;**32** (4):429–434.

10. Liistro G, Rombaux P, Belge C, et al. High Mallampati score and nasal obstruction are associated risk factors

for obstructive sleep apnoea. *Eur Respir J.* 2003;**21**(2):248–252.

11. Malhotra A, White DP. Obstructive sleep apnoea. *Lancet.* 2002;**360**(9328):237–245.

12. Peiser J, Lavie P, Ovnat A, Charuzi I. Sleep apnea syndrome in the morbidly obese as an indication for weight reduction surgery. *Ann Surg.* 1984;**199**(1):112–115.

13. Young T, Skatrud J, Peppard PE. Risk factors for obstructive sleep apnea in adults. *JAMA.* 2004;**291**(16): 2013–2016.

14. Caples SM, Gami AS, Somers VK. Obstructive sleep apnea. *Ann Intern Med.* 2005;**142**(3):187–197.

15. American Academy of Sleep Medicine. Sleep-related breathing disorders in adults: recommendations for syndrome definition and measurement techniques in clinical research: The Report of a Task Force. *Sleep.* 1999;**22**(5):667–689.

16. Pack AI. Advances in sleep-disordered breathing. *Am J Respir Crit Care Med.* 2006;**173**(1):7–15.

17. Weaver TE, Kribbs NB, Pack AI, et al. Night-to-night variability in CPAP use over the first three months of treatment. *Sleep.* 1997;**20**(4):278–283.

18. Jenkinson C, Stradling J, Petersen S. Comparison of three measures of quality of life outcome in the evaluation of continuous positive airways pressure therapy for sleep apnoea. *J Sleep Res.* 1997;**6**(3):199–204.

19. George CF, Nickerson PW, Hanly PJ, Millar TW, Kryger MH: Sleep apnoea patients have more automobile accidents. *Lancet.* 1987;**2**(8556):447.

20. Dinges DF. An overview of sleepiness and accidents. *J Sleep Res.* 1995;**4**(S2):4–14.

21. Kezirian EJ, Harrison SL, Ancoli-Israel S, et al. Behavioral correlates of sleep-disordered breathing in older women. *Sleep.* 2007;**30**(9):1181–1188.

22. Borak J, Cieslicki JK, Koziej M, Matuszewski A, Zielinski J. Effects of CPAP treatment on psychological status in patients with severe obstructive sleep apnoea. *J Sleep Res.* 1996;**5**(2):123–127.

23. Yue W, Hao W, Liu P, et al. A case-control study on psychological symptoms in sleep apnea-hypopnea syndrome. *Can J Psychiatry.* 2003;**48**(5):318–323.

24. Edlund MJ, McNamara ME, Millman RP. Sleep apnea and panic attacks. *Compr Psychiatry.* 1991;**32**(2):130–132.

25. Enns MW, Stein M, Kryger M. Successful treatment of comorbid panic disorder and sleep apnea with continuous positive airway pressure. *Psychosomatics.* 1995;**36**(6):585–586.

26. Whitney JF, Gannon DE. Obstructive sleep apnea presenting as acute delirium. *Am J Emerg Med.* 1996;**14**(3): 270–271.

27. Lee JW. Recurrent delirium associated with obstructive sleep apnea. *Gen Hosp Psychiatry.* 1998;**20**(2):120–122.

28. Berrettini WH. Paranoid psychosis and sleep apnea syndrome. *Am J Psychiatry.* 1980;**137**(4):493–494.

29. Lee S, Chiu HF, Chen CN. Psychosis in sleep apnoea. *Aust N Z J Psychiatry.* 1989;**23**(4):571–573.

30. Sharafkhaneh A, Giray N, Richardson P, Young T, Hirshkowitz M. Association of psychiatric disorders and sleep apnea in a large cohort. *Sleep.* 2005;**28**(11): 1405–1411.

31. Guilleminault C, Hoed, JVD, Mitler M. *Clinical overview of sleep apnea syndromes.* New York: Allan R Liss; 1978.

32. Beebe DW, Groesz L, Wells C, Nichols A, McGee K. The neuropsychological effects of obstructive sleep apnea: a meta-analysis of norm-referenced and case-controlled data. *Sleep.* 2003;**26**(3):298–307.

33. Aloia MS, Arnedt JT, Davis JD, Riggs RL, Byrd D. Neuropsychological sequelae of obstructive sleep apnea-hypopnea syndrome: a critical review. *J Int Neuropsychol Soc.* 2004;**10**(5):772–785.

34. Bedard MA, Montplaisir J, Richer F, Rouleau I, Malo J. Obstructive sleep apnea syndrome: pathogenesis of neuropsychological deficits. *J Clin Exp Neuropsychol.* 1991;**13**(6):950–964.

35. Bedard MA, Montplaisir J, Malo J, Richer F, Rouleau I. Persistent neuropsychological deficits and vigilance impairment in sleep apnea syndrome after treatment with continuous positive airways pressure (CPAP). *J Clin Exp Neuropsychol.* 1993;**15**(2):330–341.

36. Feuerstein C, Naegele B, Pepin JL, Levy P. Frontal lobe-related cognitive functions in patients with sleep apnea syndrome before and after treatment. *Acta Neurol Belg.* 1997;**97**(2):96–107.

37. Greenberg GD, Watson RK, Deptula D. Neuropsychological dysfunction in sleep apnea. *Sleep.* 1987;**10**(3):254–262.

38. Naegele B, Thouvard V, Pepin JL, et al. Deficits of cognitive executive functions in patients with sleep apnea syndrome. *Sleep.* 1995;**18**(1):43–52.

39. Redline S, Tishler PV, Hans MG, et al. Racial differences in sleep-disordered breathing in African-Americans and Caucasians. *Am J Respir Crit Care Med.* 1997;**155**(1):186–192.

40. Chugh D, Dinges D. Mechanisms of sleepiness. In: Pack A, ed. *Sleep apnea: pathogenesis, diagnosis, and treatment.* New York: Marcel Dekker; 2002.

41. Weaver TE. Outcome measurement in sleep medicine practice and research. Part 2: Assessment of neurobehavioral performance and mood. *Sleep Med Rev.* 2001;**5**(3):223–236.

42. George CF. Driving simulators in clinical practice. *Sleep Med Rev.* 2003;7(4):311–320.

43. Powell NB, Riley RW, Schechtman KB, et al. A comparative model: reaction time performance in sleep-disordered breathing versus alcohol-impaired controls. *Laryngoscope.* 1999;**109**(10):1648–1654.

44. Rouleau I, Decary A, Chicoine AJ, Montplaisir J. Procedural skill learning in obstructive sleep apnea syndrome. *Sleep.* 2002;**25**(4):401–411.

45. Engleman HM, Kingshott RN, Martin SE, Douglas NJ. Cognitive function in the sleep apnea/hypopnea syndrome (SAHS). *Sleep.* 2000;**23**(Suppl 4):S102–108.

46. Findley LJ, Barth JT, Powers DC, **et al**. Cognitive impairment in patients with obstructive sleep apnea and associated hypoxemia. *Chest.* 1986;**90**(5):686–690.

47. Salorio CF, White DA, Piccirillo J, Duntley SP, Uhles ML. Learning, memory, and executive control in individuals with obstructive sleep apnea syndrome. *J Clin Exp Neuropsychol.* 2002;**24**(1):93–100.

48. Roehrs T, Merrion M, Pedrosi B, et al. Neuropsychological function in obstructive sleep apnea syndrome (OSAS) compared to chronic obstructive pulmonary disease (COPD). *Sleep.* 1995;**18**(5):382–388.

49. Telakivi T, Kajaste S, Partinen M, et al. Cognitive function in middle-aged snorers and controls: role of excessive daytime somnolence and sleep-related hypoxic events. *Sleep.* 1988;**11**(5):454–462.

50. Lezak MD. *Neuropsychological assessment.* New York: Oxford University Press; 1995.

51. Eslinger PJ. *Conceptualizing, describing, and measuring components of executive function: a summary.* Baltimore, MD: Paul H. Brookes Publishing; 1996.

52. Goldberg E. *The executive brain: frontal lobes and the civilized mind.* Oxford: Oxford University Press; 2001.

53. Sateia MJ. Neuropsychological impairment and quality of life in obstructive sleep apnea. *Clin Chest Med.* 2003;**24**(2):249–259.

54. Beebe DW, Gozal D. Obstructive sleep apnea and the prefrontal cortex: towards a comprehensive model linking nocturnal upper airway obstruction to daytime cognitive and behavioral deficits. *J Sleep Res.* 2002;**11**(1):1–16.

55. Row BW, Kheirandish L, Neville JJ, Gozal D. Impaired spatial learning and hyperactivity in developing rats exposed to intermittent hypoxia. *Pediatr Res.* 2002;**52**(3):449–453.

56. Naegele B, Pepin JL, Levy P, et al. Cognitive executive dysfunction in patients with obstructive sleep apnea syndrome (OSAS) after CPAP treatment. *Sleep.* 1998;**21**(4):392–397.

57. Macey PM, Henderson LA, Macey KE, et al. Brain morphology associated with obstructive sleep apnea. *Am J Respir Crit Care Med.* 2002;**166**(10):1382–1387.

58. Schmahmann JD. Rediscovery of an early concept. *Int Rev Neurobiol.* 1997;**41**:3–27.

59. Thomas RJ, Rosen BR, Stern CE, Weiss JW, Kwong KK. Functional imaging of working memory in obstructive sleep-disordered breathing. *J Appl Physiol.* 2005;**98**(6):2226–2234.

60. Ayalon L, Ancoli-Israel S, Klemfuss Z, Shalauta MD, Drummond SP. Increased brain activation during verbal learning in obstructive sleep apnea. *Neuroimage.* 2006;**31**(4):1817–1825.

61. Ancoli-Israel S, Palmer BW, Cooke JR, et al. Effect of treating sleep disordered breathing on cognitive functioning in patients with Alzheimer's disease: a randomized controlled trial. *J Am Geriatr Soc.* 2008;**56**(11):2076–2081.

62. Valencia-Flores M, Bliwise DL, Guilleminault C, Cilveti R, Clerk A. Cognitive function in patients with sleep apnea after acute nocturnal nasal continuous positive airway pressure (CPAP) treatment: sleepiness and hypoxemia effects. *J Clin Exp Neuropsychol.* 1996;**18**(2):197–210.

63. Kotterba S, Rasche K, Widdig W, et al. Neuropsychological investigations and event-related potentials in obstructive sleep apnea syndrome before and during CPAP-therapy. *J Neurol Sci.* 1998;**159**(1):45–50.

64. Redline S, Adams N, Strauss ME, et al. Improvement of mild sleep-disordered breathing with CPAP compared with conservative therapy. *Am J Respir Crit Care Med.* 1998;**157**(3 Pt 1):858–865.

65. Barbe F, Mayoralas LR, Duran J, et al. Treatment with continuous positive airway pressure is not effective in patients with sleep apnea but no daytime sleepiness: a randomized, controlled trial. *Ann Intern Med.* 2001;**134**(11):1015–1023.

66. Bardwell WA, Ancoli-Israel S, Berry CC, Dimsdale JE. Neuropsychological effects of one-week continuous positive airway pressure treatment in patients with obstructive sleep apnea: a placebo-controlled study. *Psychosom Med.* 2001;**63**(4):579–584.

67. Lim W, Bardwell WA, Loredo JS, et al. Neuropsychological effects of 2-week continuous positive airway pressure treatment and supplemental oxygen in patients with obstructive sleep apnea: a randomized placebo-controlled study. *J Clin Sleep Med.* 2007;**3**(4):380–386.

68. Andrews JG, Oei TP. The roles of depression and anxiety in the understanding and treatment of Obstructive Sleep Apnea Syndrome. *Clin Psychol Rev.* 2004;**24**(8):1031–1049.

69. Saunamaki T, Jehkonen M. Depression and anxiety in obstructive sleep apnea syndrome: a review. *Acta Neurol Scand.* 2007;**116**(5):277–288.

70. Guilleminault C, Eldridge FL, Tilkian A, Simmons FB, Dement WC. Sleep apnea syndrome due to upper airway obstruction: a review of 25 cases. *Arch Intern Med.* 1977;**137**(3):296–300.

71. Ohayon MM. The effects of breathing-related sleep disorders on mood disturbances in the general population. *J Clin Psychiatry.* 2003;**64**(10):1195–1200; quiz: 1274–1276.

72. Deldin PJ, Phillips LK, Thomas RJ. A preliminary study of sleep-disordered breathing in major depressive disorder. *Sleep Med.* 2006; 7(2):131–139.

73. Reynolds CF 3rd, Kupfer DJ, McEachran AB, et al. Depressive psychopathology in male sleep apneics. *J Clin Psychiatry.* 1984;**45**(7):287–290.

74. Millman RP, Fogel BS, McNamara ME, Carlisle CC. Depression as a manifestation of obstructive sleep apnea: reversal with nasal continuous positive airway pressure. *J Clin Psychiatry.* 1989;**50**(9):348–351.

75. Flemons WW, Tsai W. Quality of life consequences of sleep-disordered breathing. *J Allergy Clin Immunol.* 1997;**99**(2):S750–756.

76. Engleman HM, Martin SE, Deary IJ, Douglas NJ. Effect of continuous positive airway pressure treatment on daytime function in sleep apnoea/hypopnoea syndrome. *Lancet.* 1994;**343**(8897):572–575.

77. Borak J, Cieslicki J, Szelenberger W, et al. Psychopathological characteristics of the consequences of obstructive sleep apnea prior to and three months after CPAP. *Psychiatr Pol.* 1994;**28**(3 Suppl):33–44.

78. Ramos Platon MJ, Espinar Sierra J. Changes in psychopathological symptoms in sleep apnea patients after treatment with nasal continuous positive airway pressure. *Int J Neurosci.* 1992;**62**(3–4):173–195.

79. Derderian SS, Bridenbaugh RH, Rajagopal KR. Neuropsychologic symptoms in obstructive sleep apnea improve after treatment with nasal continuous positive airway pressure. *Chest.* 1988;**94**(5):1023–1027.

80. Kales A, Caldwell AB, Cadieux RJ, et al. Severe obstructive sleep apnea–II: Associated psychopathology and psychosocial consequences. *J Chronic Dis.* 1985;**38**(5):427–434.

81. Pochat MD, Ferber C, Lemoine P. Depressive symptomatology and sleep apnea syndrome. *Encephale.* 1993;**19**(6):601–607.

82. Peppard PE, Szklo-Coxe M, Hla KM, Young T. Longitudinal association of sleep-related breathing disorder and depression. *Arch Intern Med.* 2006;**166**(16):1709–1715.

83. Means MK, Lichstein KL, Edinger JD, et al. Changes in depressive symptoms after continuous positive airway pressure treatment for obstructive sleep apnea. *Sleep Breath.* 2003;**7**(1):31–42.

84. Pillar G, Lavie P. Psychiatric symptoms in sleep apnea syndrome: effects of gender and respiratory disturbance index. *Chest.* 1998;**114**(3):697–703.

85. Gall R, Isaac L, Kryger M. Quality of life in mild obstructive sleep apnea. *Sleep.* 1993;**16**(8 Suppl): S59–61.

86. Lee S. Depression in sleep apnea: a different view. *J Clin Psychiatry.* 1990;**51**(7):309–310.

87. Flemons WW, Whitelaw WA, Brant R, Remmers JE. Likelihood ratios for a sleep apnea clinical prediction rule. *Am J Respir Crit Care Med.* 1994; **150** (5 Pt 1):1279–1285.

88. Guilleminault C, Kirisoglu C, Poyares D, et al. Upper airway resistance syndrome: a long-term outcome study. *J Psychiatr Res.* 2006; **40**(3):273–279.

89. Kerl J, Köhler D, Schönhofer B. The application of nasal and oronasal cannulas in detection of respiratory disturbances during sleep: A review. *Somnologie – Schlafforschung und Schlafmedizin.* 2002; 6(4):169–172.

90. Loube DI, Andrada T, Howard RS. Accuracy of respiratory inductive plethysmography for the diagnosis of upper airway resistance syndrome. *Chest.* 1999;**115**(5):1333–1337.

91. Bardwell WA, Berry CC, Ancoli-Israel S, Dimsdale JE. Psychological correlates of sleep apnea. *J Psychosom Res.* 1999;**47**(6):583–596.

92. Bardwell WA, Moore P, Ancoli-Israel S, Dimsdale JE. Fatigue in obstructive sleep apnea: driven by depressive symptoms instead of apnea severity? *Am J Psychiatry.* 2003;**160**(2):350–355.

93. Guilleminault C, Palombini L, Poyares D, Chowdhuri S. Chronic insomnia, postmenopausal women, and sleep disordered breathing: part 1. Frequency of sleep disordered breathing in a cohort. *J Psychosom Res.* 2002;**53**(1):611–615.

94. Diamond EL. The role of anger and hostility in essential hypertension and coronary heart disease. *Psychol Bull.* 1982;**92**(2):410–433.

95. Dimsdale JE, Pierce C, Schoenfeld D, Brown A, Zusman R, Graham R. Suppressed anger and blood pressure: the effects of race, sex, social class, obesity, and age. *Psychosom Med.* 1986;**48**(6):430–436.

96. Cheshire K, Engleman H, Deary I, Shapiro C, Douglas NJ. Factors impairing daytime performance in patients with sleep apnea/hypopnea syndrome. *Arch Intern Med.* 1992;**152**(3):538–541.

97. Brown LK. Sleep apnea syndromes: overview and diagnostic approach. *Mt Sinai J Med.* 1994;**61**(2):99–112.

98. Sforza E, de Saint Hilaire Z, Pelissolo A, Rochat T, Ibanez V. Personality, anxiety and mood traits in patients with sleep-related breathing disorders: effect of reduced daytime alertness. *Sleep Med.* 2002;**3**(2): 139–145.

99. Kamba M, Suto Y, Ohta Y, Inoue Y, Matsuda E. Cerebral metabolism in sleep apnea. Evaluation by magnetic resonance spectroscopy. *Am J Respir Crit Care Med.* 1997;**156**(1):296–298.

100. Kamba M, Inoue Y, Higami S, et al. Cerebral metabolic impairment in patients with obstructive sleep apnoea: an independent association of obstructive sleep apnoea with white matter change. *J Neurol Neurosurg Psychiatry.* 2001; **71**(3):334–339.

101. McGown AD, Makker H, Elwell C, et al. Measurement of changes in cytochrome oxidase redox state during obstructive sleep apnea using near-infrared spectroscopy. *Sleep.* 2003;**26**(6):710–716.

102. Portas CM, Bjorvatn B, Ursin R. Serotonin and the sleep/wake cycle: special emphasis on microdialysis studies. *Prog Neurobiol.* 2000;**60**(1):13–35.

103. Hudgel DW, Gordon EA, Meltzer HY. Abnormal serotonergic stimulation of cortisol production in obstructive sleep apnea. *Am J Respir Crit Care Med.* 1995;**152**(1):186–192.

104. Adrien J. Neurobiological bases for the relation between sleep and depression. *Sleep Med Rev.* 2002; **6**(5):341–351.

105. Gami AS, Somers VK. Obstructive sleep apnoea, metabolic syndrome, and cardiovascular outcomes. *Eur Heart J.* 2004;**25**(9):709–711.

106. Lett HS, Blumenthal JA, Babyak MA, et al. Depression as a risk factor for coronary artery disease: evidence, mechanisms, and treatment. *Psychosom Med.* 2004; **66**(3):305–315.

107. Vgontzas AN, Papanicolaou DA, Bixler EO, et al. Elevation of plasma cytokines in disorders of excessive daytime sleepiness: role of sleep disturbance and obesity. *J Clin Endocrinol Metab.* 1997;**82**(5): 1313–1316.

108. Haensel A, Bardwell WA, Mills PJ, et al. Relationship between inflammation and cognitive function in obstructive sleep apnea. *Sleep Breath.* 2009;**13**:35–41.

109. Vgontzas AN, Papanicolaou DA, Bixler EO, et al. Sleep apnea and daytime sleepiness and fatigue: relation to visceral obesity, insulin resistance, and hypercytokinemia. *J Clin Endocrinol Metab.* 2000; **85**(3):1151–1158.

110. Lu XY, Kim CS, Frazer A, Zhang W. Leptin: a potential novel antidepressant. *Proc Natl Acad Sci U S A.* 2006;**103**(5):1593–1598.

111. Lu XY. The leptin hypothesis of depression: a potential link between mood disorders and obesity? *Curr Opin Pharmacol.* 2007;**7**(6):648–652.

112. Mills PJ, Dimsdale JE. Sleep apnea: a model for studying cytokines, sleep, and sleep disruption. *Brain Behav Immun.* 2004;**18**(4):298–303.

113. Edinger JD, Carwile S, Miller P, Hope V, Mayti C. Psychological status, syndromatic measures, and compliance with nasal CPAP therapy for sleep apnea. *Percept Mot Skills.* 1994;**78**(3 Pt 2):1116–1118.

114. Munoz A, Mayoralas LR, Barbe F, Pericas J, Agusti AG. Long-term effects of CPAP on daytime functioning in patients with sleep apnoea syndrome. *Eur Respir J.* 2000;**15**(4):676–681.

115. Bardwell WA, Ancoli-Israel S, Dimsdale JE. Types of coping strategies are associated with increased depressive symptoms in patients with obstructive sleep apnea. *Sleep* 2001; **24**(8):905–909.

116. Kansanen M, Vanninen E, Tuunainen A, et al. The effect of a very low-calorie diet-induced weight loss on the severity of obstructive sleep apnoea and autonomic nervous function in obese patients with obstructive sleep apnoea syndrome. *Clin Physiol.* 1998;**18**(4): 377–385.

117. Pasquali R, Colella P, Cirignotta F, et al. Treatment of obese patients with obstructive sleep apnea syndrome (OSAS): effect of weight loss and interference of otorhinolaryngoiatric pathology. *Int J Obes.* 1990; **14**(3):207–217.

118. Dixon JB, Schachter LM, O'Brien PE. Polysomnography before and after weight loss in obese patients with severe sleep apnea. *Int J Obes (Lond).* 2005;**29**(9):1048–1054.

119. Kaplan R. Obstructive sleep apnoea and depression: diagnostic and treatment implications. *Aust N Z J Psychiatry.* 1992;**26**(4):586–591.

120. Farney RJ, Lugo A, Jensen RL, Walker JM, Cloward TV. Simultaneous use of antidepressant and antihypertensive medications increases likelihood of diagnosis of obstructive sleep apnea syndrome. *Chest.* 2004;**125**(4):1279–1285.

121. Aikens JE, Mendelson WB, Baehr EK. Replicability of psychometric differences between obstructive sleep apnea, primary snoring, and periodic limb movement disorder. *Sleep and Hypnosis* 1999; **4**: 212–216.

122. Sanchez AI, Buela-Casal G, Bermudez MP, Casas-Maldonado F. The effects of continuous positive air pressure treatment on anxiety and depression levels in

apnea patients. *Psychiatry Clin Neurosci.* 2001;**55**(6):641–646.

123. Kaplan R. Sleep fragmentation presenting with mood changes. *Aust N Z J Psychiatry.* 1995;**29**(1):159.

124. Kjelsberg FN, Ruud EA, Stavem K. Predictors of symptoms of anxiety and depression in obstructive sleep apnea. *Sleep Med.* 2005;**6**(4):341–346.

125. Chasens ER, Pack AI, Maislin G, Dinges DF, Weaver TE. Claustrophobia and adherence to CPAP treatment. *West J Nurs Res.* 2005;**27**(3):307–321.

126. Brostrom A, Stromberg A, Martensson J, et al. Association of Type D personality to perceived side effects and adherence in CPAP-treated patients with OSAS. *J Sleep Res.* 2007;**16**(4):439–447.

127. Ayalon L, Ancoli-Israel S, Stepnowsky C, et al. Adherence in patients with Alzheimer's disease and obstructive sleep apnea. *Am J Geriatr Psychiatry* 2006;**14**(2):176–180.

128. Grunstein RR. Sleep-related breathing disorders. 5. Nasal continuous positive airway pressure treatment for obstructive sleep apnoea. *Thorax.* 1995;**50**(10):1106–1113.

129. Kribbs NB, Pack AI, Kline LR, et al. Effects of one night without nasal CPAP treatment on sleep and sleepiness in patients with obstructive sleep apnea. *Am Rev Respir Dis.* 1993;**147**(5):1162–1168.

130. Rosen CL, Larkin EK, Kirchner HL, et al. Prevalence and risk factors for sleep-disordered breathing in 8- to 11-year-old children: association with race and prematurity. *J Pediatr.* 2003;**142**(4):383–389.

131. Picchietti DL, England SJ, Walters AS, Willis K, Verrico T. Periodic limb movement disorder and restless legs syndrome in children with attention-deficit hyperactivity disorder. *J Child Neurol.* 1998;**13**(12):588–594.

132. Corkum P, Tannock R, Moldofsky H. Sleep disturbances in children with attention-deficit/hyperactivity disorder. *J Am Acad Child Adolesc Psychiatry.* 1998;**37**(6):637–646.

133. Marcotte AC, Thacher PV, Butters M, et al. Parental report of sleep problems in children with attentional and learning disorders. *J Dev Behav Pediatr.* 1998;**19**(3):178–186.

134. Golan N, Pillar G. The relationship between attention deficit hyperactivity disorder and sleep-alertness problems. *Harefuah.* 2004;**143**(9):676–680, 693.

135. Silverstone T, Smith G, Goodall E. Prevalence of obesity in patients receiving depot antipsychotics. *Br J Psychiatry.* 1988;**153**:214–217.

136. Winkelman JW. Schizophrenia, obesity, and obstructive sleep apnea. *J Clin Psychiatry.* 2001;**62**(1):8–11.

137. Berger AJ, Bayliss DA, Viana F. Modulation of neonatal rat hypoglossal motoneuron excitability by serotonin. *Neurosci Lett.* 1992;**143**(1–2):164–168.

138. Fenik P, Veasey SC. Pharmacological characterization of serotonergic receptor activity in the hypoglossal nucleus. *Am J Respir Crit Care Med.* 2003;**167**(4):563–569.

139. Sunderram J, Parisi RA, Strobel RJ. Serotonergic stimulation of the genioglossus and the response to nasal continuous positive airway pressure. *Am J Respir Crit Care Med.* 2000;**162**(3 Pt 1):925–929.

140. Berry RB, Yamaura EM, Gill K, Reist C. Acute effects of paroxetine on genioglossus activity in obstructive sleep apnea. *Sleep.* 1999; **22**(8):1087–1092.

141. Veasey SC. Serotonin agonists and antagonists in obstructive sleep apnea: therapeutic potential. *Am J Respir Med.* 2003;**2**(1):21–29.

142. Marshall NS, Yee BJ, Desai AV, et al. Two randomized placebo-controlled trials to evaluate the efficacy and tolerability of mirtazapine for the treatment of obstructive sleep apnea. *Sleep.* 2008;**31**(6):824–831.

143. Schmidt HS. L-tryptophan in the treatment of impaired respiration in sleep. *Bull Eur Physiopathol Respir.* 1983;**19**(6):625–629.

144. Cohn MA. Hypnotics and the control of breathing: a review. *Br J Clin Pharmacol.* 1983;**16**(Suppl 2):S245–S250.

145. Guilleminault C. Benzodiazepines, breathing, and sleep. *Am J Med.* 1990;**88**(3A):25S–28S.

146. Mendelson WB, Garnett D, Gillin JC. Flurazepam-induced sleep apnea syndrome in a patient with insomnia and mild sleep-related respiratory changes. *J Nerv Ment Dis.* 1981;**169**(4):261–264.

147. Model DG. Nitrazepam induced respiratory depression in chronic obstructive lung disease. *Br J Dis Chest.* 1973;**67**(2):128–130

148. Maczaj M. Pharmacological treatment of insomnia. *Drugs.* 1993;**45**(1):44–55.

149. Berry RB, Kouchi K, Bower J, Prosise G, Light RW. Triazolam in patients with obstructive sleep apnea. *Am J Respir Crit Care Med.* 1995;**151**(2 Pt 1):450–454.

150. Wagner J, Wagner ML. Non-benzodiazepines for the treatment of insomnia. *Sleep Med Rev.* 2000; **4**(6):551–581.

151. Murciano D, Armengaud MH, Cramer PH, et al. Acute effects of zolpidem, triazolam and flunitrazepam on arterial blood gases and control of breathing in severe COPD. *Eur Respir J.* 1993;**6**(5):625–629.

152. Murciano D, Aubier M, Palacios S, Pariente R. Comparison of zolpidem (Z), triazolam (T), and

flunitrazepam (F) effects on arterial blood gases and control of breathing in patients with severe chronic obstructive pulmonary disease (COPD). *Chest*. 1990;**97** (3 Suppl):S51–S52.

153. Girault C, Muir JF, Mihaltan F, et al. Effects of repeated administration of zolpidem on sleep, diurnal and nocturnal respiratory function, vigilance, and physical performance in patients with COPD. *Chest*. 1996;**110**(5):1203–1211.

154. Steens RD, Pouliot Z, Millar TW, Kryger MH, George CF. Effects of zolpidem and triazolam on sleep and respiration in mild to moderate chronic obstructive pulmonary disease. *Sleep*. 1993;**16**(4):318–326.

155. Cirignotta F, Mondini S, Zucconi M, et al. Zolpidem-polysomnographic study of the effect of a new hypnotic drug in sleep apnea syndrome. *Pharmacol Biochem Behav*. 1988;**29**(4):807–809.

156. George CF. Perspectives on the management of insomnia in patients with chronic respiratory disorders. *Sleep*. 2000;**23**(Suppl 1):S31–35; discussion S36–38.

157. Lofaso F, Goldenberg F, Thebault C, Janus C, Harf A. Effect of zopiclone on sleep, night-time ventilation, and daytime vigilance in upper airway resistance syndrome. *Eur Respir J*. 1997;**10**(11):2573–2577.

158. Lettieri CJ, Quast TN, Eliasson AH, Andrada T. Eszopiclone improves overnight polysomnography and continuous positive airway pressure titration: a prospective, randomized, placebo-controlled trial. *Sleep*. 2008;**31**(9):1310–1316.

159. Rosenberg R, Roach JM, Scharf M, Amato DA. A pilot study evaluating acute use of eszopiclone in patients with mild to moderate obstructive sleep apnea syndrome. *Sleep Med*. 2007;**8**(5):464–470.

160. Quera-Salva MA, McCann C, Boudet J et al. Effects of zolpidem on sleep architecture, night time ventilation, daytime vigilance and performance in heavy snorers. *Br J Clin Pharmacol*. 1994;**37**(6):539–543.

161. Issa FG, Sullivan CE. Alcohol, snoring and sleep apnea. *J Neurol Neurosurg Psychiatry*. 1982;**45**(4):353–359.

162. Morgenthaler TI, Kapen S, Lee-Chiong T, et al. Practice parameters for the medical therapy of obstructive sleep apnea. *Sleep*. 2006;**29**(8):1031–1035.

163. Kingshott RN, Vennelle M, Coleman EL, et al. Randomized, double-blind, placebo-controlled crossover trial of modafinil in the treatment of residual excessive daytime sleepiness in the sleep apnea/hypopnea syndrome. *Am J Respir Crit Care Med*. 2001;**163**(4):918–923.

164. Dinges DF, Weaver TE. Effects of modafinil on sustained attention performance and quality of life in OSA patients with residual sleepiness while

being treated with nCPAP. *Sleep Med*. 2003;**4**(5): 393–402.

165. DeBattista C, Doghramji K, Menza MA, Rosenthal MH, Fieve RR. Adjunct modafinil for the short-term treatment of fatigue and sleepiness in patients with major depressive disorder: a preliminary double-blind, placebo-controlled study. *J Clin Psychiatry*. 2003;**64** (9):1057–1064.

166. Ninan PT, Hassman HA, Glass SJ, McManus FC. Adjunctive modafinil at initiation of treatment with a selective serotonin reuptake inhibitor enhances the degree and onset of therapeutic effects in patients with major depressive disorder and fatigue. *J Clin Psychiatry*. 2004;**65**(3):414–420.

167. Panossian L, Avidan, AY. Movement disorders of sleep and sleep-disordered breathing. *US Neurol Dis*. 2007;**2**:63–68.

168. Engleman HM, Martin SE, Deary IJ, Douglas NJ. Effect of CPAP therapy on daytime function in patients with mild sleep apnoea/hypopnoea syndrome. *Thorax*. 1997;**52**(2):114–119.

169. Engleman HM, Martin SE, Kingshott RN, et al. Randomised placebo controlled trial of daytime function after continuous positive airway pressure (CPAP) therapy for the sleep apnoea/hypopnoea syndrome. *Thorax*. 1998;**53**(5):341–345.

170. Jokic R, Klimaszewski A, Sridhar G, Fitzpatrick MF. Continuous positive airway pressure requirement during the first month of treatment in patients with severe obstructive sleep apnea. *Chest*. 1998;**114**(4): 1061–1069.

171. Engleman HM, Kingshott RN, Wraith PK, et al. Randomized placebo-controlled crossover trial of continuous positive airway pressure for mild sleep apnea/hypopnea syndrome. *Am J Respir Crit Care Med*. 1999;**159**(2):461–467.

172. Yamamoto H, Akashiba T, Kosaka N, Ito D, Horie T. Long-term effects of nasal continuous positive airway pressure on daytime sleepiness, mood and traffic accidents in patients with obstructive sleep apnoea. *Respir Med*. 2000;**94**(1):87–90.

173. Barnes M, Houston D, Worsnop CJ, et al. A randomized controlled trial of continuous positive airway pressure in mild obstructive sleep apnea. *Am J Respir Crit Care Med*. 2002;**165**(6):773–780.

174. Doherty LS, Kiely JL, Lawless G, McNicholas WT. Impact of nasal continuous positive airway pressure therapy on the quality of life of bed partners of patients with obstructive sleep apnea syndrome. *Chest*. 2003;**124**(6):2209–2214.

175. Svaldi JJ, Mackinger HF. Obstructive sleep apnea syndrome: autobiographical memory predicts the

course of depressive affect after nCPAP therapy. *Scand J Psychol*. 2003;**44**(1):31–37.

176. Barnes M, McEvoy RD, Banks S, et al. Efficacy of positive airway pressure and oral appliance in mild to moderate obstructive sleep apnea. *Am J Respir Crit Care Med*. 2004;**170**(6):656–664.

177. Mackinger HF, Svaldi JJ. Autobiographical memory predicts cognitive but not somatic change in sleep apnea patients vulnerable for affective disorder. *J Affect Disord*. 2004;**81**(1):17–22.

178. Goncalves MA, Guilleminault C, Ramos E, Palha A, Paiva T. Erectile dysfunction, obstructive sleep apnea syndrome and nasal CPAP treatment. *Sleep Med*. 2005;**6**(4):333–339.

179. Schwartz DJ, Kohler WC, Karatinos G. Symptoms of depression in individuals with obstructive sleep apnea may be amenable to treatment with continuous positive airway pressure. *Chest*. 2005;**128**(3):1304–1349.

180. Schwartz DJ, Karatinos G. For individuals with obstructive sleep apnea, institution of CPAP therapy is associated with an amelioration of symptoms of depression which is sustained long term. *J Clin Sleep Med*. 2007;**3**(6):631–635.

181. Wells RD, Freedland KE, Carney RM, Duntley SP, Stepanski EJ. Adherence, reports of benefits, and depression among patients treated with continuous positive airway pressure. *Psychosom Med*. 2007;**69**(5):449–454.

182. Kingshott RN, Vennelle M, Hoy CJ, et al. Predictors of improvements in daytime function outcomes with CPAP therapy. *Am J Respir Crit Care Med*. 2000;**161**(3 Pt 1):866–871.

Sleep-related movement disorders

Marta Novak, Andras Szentkiralyi and Magdolna Hornyak

Introduction

Restless legs syndrome (RLS) and periodic limb movement disorder (PLMD) are prevalent disorders in the general population. RLS is considered to be the most common sleep-related movement disorder. Parasomnias and sleep-related epileptic seizures also involve movements during sleep, however are not considered as sleep-related movement disorders *per se* and are discussed in a separate chapter (see Chapter 10: Parasomnias). Both RLS and PLMD have a high impact on sleep quality and daily performance but are often unrecognized or misdiagnosed. In a study conducted from 2002 to 2003, general physicians correctly diagnosed RLS in less than 10% of cases [1]. Despite growing knowledge about the disorder, RLS is still often referred to as "the most common disorder you have never heard of." Inappropriate treatments, such as the use of neuroleptics or other dopamine antagonists, can aggravate RLS or PLMD symptoms. Therefore, accurate diagnosis and treatment of these disorders may substantially improve the quality of sleep and life in patients who suffer from them. In this chapter, we summarize recent knowledge regarding the diagnosis, epidemiology, pathophysiology, and treatment of RLS and PLMD, and their relevance in psychiatric clinical practice.

Diagnosis of restless legs syndrome and periodic limb movement disorder

RLS is a clinical diagnosis and is based on the patient's description. Diagnostic criteria and clinical characteristics of the disorder were outlined by the International Restless Legs Syndrome Study Group in 1995 [2]. Later, at a National Institutes of Health (NIH)

consensus meeting, diagnostic criteria were modified according to clinical experience and the available scientific research [3] (see also Table 8.1). RLS typically presents with an urge to move the extremities, mostly the legs, caused or accompanied by unpleasant sensations (paresthesias) in the affected limbs. Many patients state they have difficulty describing the sensations, except as uncomfortable and deep inside the legs, while other patients report sensations like "tearing," "burning," "electric current," or "pain." Other required features of the disorder are the appearance of symptoms at rest and an increase in severity of symptoms in the evening or during the night compared to the daytime, though some patients may also develop symptoms during the day as RLS progresses. These essential diagnostic criteria for RLS are easily recalled by the practicing clinician using the mnemonic **U-R-G-E** (Urge to move the legs; Rest-induced; Gets better with movement; Evening predominance).

Due to the nocturnal worsening of symptoms, RLS has its greatest impact on sleep. Sleep disturbance is the most frequent reason that patients with RLS seek medical help [3]. Patients with RLS may suffer from severely disrupted sleep, which mostly presents as initial insomnia. Polysomnography, although not routinely indicated for the evaluation of RLS, reveals an elevated number of periodic leg movements during sleep (PLMS) in 80–90% of RLS cases [4]. PLMS are a sleep-related phenomenon that manifest with periodic episodes of repetitive, stereotyped leg movements [5,6]. These periodic movements are characterized by the extension of the big toe in combination with flexion of the ankle, knee, and sometimes the hip. Most RLS patients also will demonstrate periodic leg movements during wakefulness (PLMW) during

Foundations of Psychiatric Sleep Medicine, ed. John W. Winkelman and David T. Plante. Published by Cambridge University Press.
© Cambridge University Press 2010.

Table 8.1 Diagnostic criteria for RLS [3] (all four essential criteria are necessary for the diagnosis; the supportive criteria can help resolve any diagnostic uncertainty)

Essential criteria

1. An urge to move the legs, usually accompanied or caused by uncomfortable and unpleasant sensations in the legs. (Sometimes the urge to move is present without the uncomfortable sensations and sometimes the arms or other body parts are involved in addition to the legs.)

2. The urge to move or unpleasant sensations begin or worsen during periods of rest or inactivity such as lying or sitting

3. The urge to move or unpleasant sensations are partially or totally relieved by movement, such as walking or stretching, at least as long as the activity continues

4. The urge to move or unpleasant sensations are worse in the evening or night than during the day or only occur in the evening or night. (When symptoms are very severe, the worsening at night may not be noticeable but must have been previously present.)

Supportive clinical features of RLS

1. Positive family history of RLS

2. Response to dopaminergic therapy

   Nearly all people with RLS show at least an initial positive therapeutic response to either L-dopa or a dopamine receptor agonist. This initial response is not, however, universally maintained

3. Periodic limb movements (during wakefulness or sleep)

Associated features of RLS

1. Natural clinical course

   The clinical course of the disorder varies considerably

2. Sleep disturbance

   Disturbed sleep is a common major morbidity for RLS and deserves special consideration in planning treatment

3. Medical evaluation/physical examination

   The physical examination is generally normal and does not contribute to the diagnosis except for those conditions that may be co-morbid or secondary causes of RLS

polysomnographic recordings while awake [6]. PLMS are not specific to RLS and may frequently occur in other sleep disorders such as narcolepsy, obstructive sleep apnea syndrome, or REM sleep behavior disorder. PLMS were found also in various medical and neurological disorders that do not primarily affect sleep [7]. An elevated number of PLMS with complaints of insomnia (particularly restless or non-restorative sleep) and/or excessive daytime sleepiness, but without symptoms of RLS or related sleep disorders, has been defined by the International Classification of Sleep Disorders (ICSD) as periodic limb movement disorder (PLMD) [8]. The frequency of PLMS needed to diagnose PLMD is somewhat controversial because of overlap between symptomatic and asymptomatic individuals; however, a cutoff PLMS index of 15 per hour in adults and 5 per hour in children is generally accepted [8]. Unlike the diagnosis of RLS (described below), the diagnosis of PLMD requires polysomnographic confirmation and is based on the exclusion of other causes of sleep disturbance [8].

The diagnosis of RLS is based on clinical history, and thus can be challenging in patients who have difficulty giving a cogent description of symptoms. Even otherwise healthy patients often have difficulties describing RLS sensations except to say that they are uncomfortable and/or deep inside their legs. The verbal expression of bodily sensations may be particularly disturbed in patients with severe psychiatric symptoms such as psychosis or cognitive impairment. However, the observation of patient behavior such as rubbing the legs or excessive motor activity may be a physical expression of paresthesias and urge to move. Therefore, it has been proposed to apply the diagnostic criteria for RLS in a modified form in patients with cognitive deterioration. The revised criteria [3] emphasize behavioral indicators and supportive features within the diagnostic framework (Table 8.2).

There are several conditions that mimic RLS which should be differentiated when possible. Painful states such as arthritis involving the lower limbs can be distinguished from RLS, as they are not characterized by a circadian rhythm with an increase of severity in the evening or during the night. Symptoms of peripheral neuropathy are commonly worse at night, however the accompanying pain typically does not improve with movement. Unlike RLS, nocturnal leg cramps arise precipitously from sleep, involve sustained contraction of the affected muscle, and are not associated with an urge to move the

Table 8.2 Diagnostic criteria for the diagnosis of probable restless legs syndrome in the cognitively impaired based on Allen et al. [3]

Essential criteria, all five are necessary for the diagnosis
Signs of leg discomfort such as rubbing or kneading the legs and groaning while holding the lower extremities are present
Excessive motor activity in the lower extremities such as pacing, fidgeting, repetitive kicking, tossing and turning in bed, slapping the legs on the mattress, cycling movements of the lower limbs, repetitive foot tapping, rubbing the feet together, and the inability to remain seated are present
Signs of leg discomfort are exclusively present or worsen during periods of rest or inactivity
Signs of leg discomfort are diminished with activity
Criteria 1 and 2 occur only in the evening or at night or are worse at those times than during the day
Supportive or suggestive criteria for the diagnosis of probable restless legs syndrome in the cognitively impaired elderly
Dopaminergic responsiveness
Patient's past history – as reported by a family member, caregiver, or friend – is suggestive of RLS
A first-degree, biological relative (sibling, child, or parent) has RLS
Observed periodic limb movements while awake or during sleep
Periodic limb movements of sleep recorded by polysomnography or actigraphy
Significant sleep-onset problems
Better quality sleep in the day than at night
The use of restraints at night (for institutionalized patients)
Low serum ferritin level
End-stage renal disease
Diabetes
Clinical, electromyographic, or nerve-conduction evidence of peripheral neuropathy or radiculopathy

legs, but do improve with movement (i.e. stretching). Other causes of nocturnal leg discomfort can include pruritus or venous insufficiency of the legs, which are mostly accompanied by skin manifestations and tend to be described as more superficial sensations than RLS. Neuroleptic-induced akathisia is more typically characterized by a continuous urge to move the legs, body-rocking, and a history of dopaminergic antagonist use. It is not as "focal" as RLS, occurs independently of body position, and does not typically affect sleep [9].

Epidemiology of restless legs syndrome and periodic limb movement disorder

RLS is generally divided into primary (idiopathic) and secondary forms, the latter of which will be discussed later in the chapter. Several studies have shown that the overall prevalence of RLS is roughly 5–10% of the general population (e.g. [10]), though the prevalence of persons in which medical treatment is indicated is estimated to be one-fifth to one-third of affected individuals [11]. Population studies have revealed two potential subtypes of primary RLS. One RLS subtype is characterized by onset of symptoms in early life, with a significantly higher prevalence of affected relatives [12]. These patients are believed to have a relatively low rate of small-fiber neuropathy [13], compared to those with a later age at symptom onset. A second subtype consists of patients without a family history of the disease, have a later age of symptom onset, higher incidence of neuropathy [14], and lower serum ferritin levels [15,16]. One study found that patients with a later onset of RLS are more likely to complain of insomnia than patients with earlier onset of RLS, the latter tending to report hypersomnic complaints such as daytime sleepiness [17]. However, it is not clear if these subtypes of primary RLS reflect different pathophysiology and there is no indication that they significantly affect response to various treatments.

Usually, symptoms of RLS are mild or absent in early adulthood and progress with advancing age. Treatment is generally not sought until the fourth decade of life [18]. Surveys investigating the age distribution of RLS reveal a strong increase in the prevalence in those over age 65, though there may also be a further decline in prevalence over age 80. Additionally, most epidemiological studies find the prevalence of RLS in women to be approximately twice that of men [10]. One study found that the increased prevalence in women was associated with the number of births [19]. Although RLS can occur in people of any background, prevalence tends to vary by ethnic group, with highest rates observed in those of northern European ancestry.

PLMS *per se* are not a diagnosis but a polysomnographic finding which is observed during sleep studies in various diseases and even in the healthy elderly. In fact, the prevalence of PLMS increases with advancing age (for review see also [20]). It is critical to note that PLMS and PLMD are not synonymous, the latter implying a sleep disturbance that is caused independently by PLMS. The largest epidemiological study on PLMD to date documented a 3.9% prevalence in 18 980 subjects aged from 15 to 100 years in the general population using the International Classification of Sleep Disorders (ICSD) criteria in a telephone interview survey [21]. Furthermore, the study identified several factors associated with PLMD, such as female gender, coffee intake, sleep apnea syndrome or snoring, stress, and the presence of mental disorders [21]. However, this study did not employ sleep studies but was based on self-reported leg movements, and thus its findings should be considered preliminary.

Epidemiology of restless legs syndrome and periodic limb movement disorder in children

RLS is often considered to be a disease of middle to older age. However, the onset of RLS symptoms during childhood is commonly reported retrospectively by adult patients [4,18]. In fact, recent studies demonstrate that symptoms often start in childhood and early adolescence [22,23]. According to a recent large pediatric population-based study using consensus criteria developed at an NIH workshop [3] (Table 8.3), the prevalence of RLS was 1.9% of 8- to 11-year-olds and 2% of 12- to 17-year-olds, without significant gender differences [24]. One-quarter to half of those affected within this population reported moderate to severe symptoms. Some pediatric studies have indicated lower than normal serum ferritin levels in those with RLS [22,24], supporting the role of iron deficiency in some childhood RLS cases.

There is less data regarding pediatric PLMS/PLMD than pediatric RLS. The prevalence of pediatric PLMD was reported to be 11.9% in a community-based survey and 8.4% in a sleep-referral population [25]. Normative data suggest that PLMS greater than 5/hour are uncommon in children and adolescents [25–27].

Poor sleep may impair cognitive functions, attention, and memory in children. Several studies have reported an association between RLS, PLMD, and

Table 8.3 Criteria for the diagnosis of RLS in children (according to Allen et al. [3])

Criteria for the diagnosis of definite RLS in children

1. The child meets all four essential adult criteria for RLS and

2. The child relates a description in his or her own words that is consistent with leg discomfort. (The child may use terms such as oowies, tickle, spiders, boo-boos, want to run, and a lot of energy in my legs to describe symptoms. Age-appropriate descriptors are encouraged.)

Or

1. The child meets all four essential adult criteria for RLS and

2. Two of three following supportive criteria are present (see below). Supportive criteria for the diagnosis of definite RLS in children:

   a. Sleep disturbance for age

   b. A biological parent or sibling has definite RLS

   c. The child has a polysomnographically documented periodic limb movement index of 5 or more per hour of sleep

Criteria for the diagnosis of probable RLS in children

1. The child meets all essential adult criteria for RLS, except criterion 4 (the urge to move or sensations are worse in the evening or at night than during the day) and

2. The child has a biological parent or sibling with definite RLS

Or[1]

1. The child is observed to have behavior manifestations of lower extremity discomfort when sitting or lying, accompanied by motor movement of the affected limbs, the discomfort has characteristics of adult criteria 2, 3, and 4 (i.e. is worse during rest and inactivity, relieved by movement, and worse during the evening and at night) and

2. The child has a biological parent or sibling with definite RLS

Note: [1] This last probable category is intended for young children or cognitively impaired children, who do not have sufficient language to describe the sensory component of RLS.

ADHD among children and adolescents [26–28], as well as adults [29]. It is possible that RLS leads to symptoms of ADHD through sleep disruption and increased daytime sleepiness. However, these

133

disorders may share a common pathology of the central nervous system, like iron deficiency [30] or dopaminergic hypofunction. Sleep disruption associated with RLS may also be related to the development of mood and anxiety disorders in childhood. A recent pediatric survey found a co-morbid anxiety and/or depression in nearly 50% of RLS cases, which always developed following the historical onset of clinical sleep disturbance [24].

Pathophysiology of idiopathic restless legs syndrome

The pathophysiology of RLS is still not completely understood; however, in the last few years considerable progress in a number of areas has been made.

Genetics

Roughly half of RLS patients have relatives who also have RLS. In comparison to non-familial cases, familial RLS usually has a younger age at onset and has a more slowly progressive course [12]. The symptom severity within an RLS family can be variable. Linkage studies in RLS families have revealed eight loci of interest in RLS. Based on the assumption that the disease follows a recessive mode of inheritance, linkage to chromosome 12q (RLS1) was identified in a French-Canadian family. Further studies showed linkage to chromosome 14q (RLS2), 9p (RLS3), 20p (RLS4), and 2q (RLS5). Two loci were identified in a single RLS family on chromosome 4q and 17p (for recent overview see [31]). Two recent studies used a large-scale genome-wide approach to identify single nucleotide polymorphisms associated with RLS/PLMS [32,33]. In the study of Winkelmann et al. [33], conducted in German and Canadian populations, three genomic regions were identified encoding the genes MEIS1, BTBD9, and a third region containing MAP2K5 and LBXCOR1. In the study of Stefansson and colleagues [32], conducted in Icelandic and US populations, an association was found with the identical variant in BTBD9. Both studies used different methods of assessment of the phenotype. Although the mechanism through which these genes may confer risk for RLS remains unknown, these recent findings suggest RLS may be a developmental disorder of the central nervous system. In such a paradigm, RLS is a neurological disorder in which the disease manifests when a genetic "inborn error"

confers increased susceptibility to alterations of various neural structures, resulting in the observed clinical symptoms and associated sleep disturbance.

Dopaminergic system

Multiple etiologies likely impact the dopamine system in RLS. The primary evidence for this comes from use of dopaminergic agents over the past 20 years. Most RLS symptoms (and PLMS) respond to treatment with dopaminergic agents, and, conversely, the use of dopamine receptor antagonists exacerbates the RLS symptoms. However, a clear understanding of any defect in the metabolism or signaling in the dopamine system remains elusive. Post-mortem and imaging studies have not provided clear evidence of dysfunction in the dopamine system. The results of SPECT and PET studies are inconclusive or conflict with one another (for overview see also [34] and [35]).

Iron

Conditions associated with reduced body iron content such as late stage pregnancy, advanced renal failure, and blood loss from frequent blood donations appear to precipitate RLS [36,37]. However, only 20–25% of patients with iron deficiency exhibit symptoms of RLS. Studies of cerebrospinal fluid, magnetic resonance imaging of the brain, and post-mortem tissue all demonstrate CNS iron deficiency in RLS. Recent therapeutic trials of oral and intravenously administered iron [38,39] have shown positive effects on the course of RLS in patients with iron deficiency or serum ferritin levels ≤ 45 µg/L. Contrasting findings were reported by Earley and coworkers [40] in a placebo-controlled study of high-dose intravenous iron sucrose in idiopathic RLS and normal iron status (serum ferritin ≥ 45 µg/L). Explanations for the discrepant results may include the type of iron formulation used, the dosing regimen, patient characteristics, or, importantly, the peripheral iron status with or without significant iron store depletion.

Neurophysiological testing

Routine clinical studies of electromyography and nerve conduction velocity and evoked potentials are typically normal in patients with RLS. Research evidence from studies seeking to identify the generator of the periodic movements and sensations of RLS has been mixed. However, experimental studies repeatedly demonstrate disinhibition of the descending cerebrospinal pathways in RLS. Similarly, pain thresholds, H-reflex testing, and quantitative sensory testing are abnormal in small populations of patients with RLS (for overview see also [34]). However, these findings are neither specific nor directive in the diagnostic workup.

Restless legs syndrome secondary to or associated with another disease

RLS may manifest as a secondary disorder due to an underlying primary medical, neurological, or mental disease (Table 8.4). Anemia and iron deficiency have particular relevance, as conditions associated with reduced body iron content appear to precipitate RLS [3]. Furthermore, augmentation, defined as the reappearance and worsening of RLS complaints after a prolonged period of dopamine-induced symptom control, has been associated with low ferritin levels [41]. Prevalence of RLS is also increased in the last trimester of pregnancy, when iron deficiency is common. Folate deficiency and elevated estradiol levels may also contribute to the increased occurrence of RLS in pregnant women [42]. End-stage renal disease is known to be associated with RLS and may occur both in younger and older patients. RLS is especially frequent among patients on dialysis treatment [43,44]. Restless legs syndrome usually improves after kidney transplantation; the prevalence of RLS is not elevated in patients with functioning transplants [43]. Neuropathies and radiculopathies may often co-occur with RLS, and have been implicated as possible underlying causes of RLS, though there is limited data to support this, and it does not appear that there is a higher prevalence of RLS in those with neuropathy [45]. Rheumatoid (but not osteo-) arthritis has an elevated prevalence of RLS, and a high prevalence of RLS was reported in other rheumatological conditions such as fibromyalgia, Sjögren syndrome, and scleroderma [46], suggesting a possible inflammatory cause of RLS in such individuals.

Further, possibly causally related conditions include among others diabetes mellitus, liver disease, and malignancies. A recent study found RLS in 54 out of 121 patients (45%) with type 2 diabetes [47]. Patients with type 2 diabetes and co-morbid RLS had more co-morbidities, worse sleep quality, took more medications to help them sleep, and were more impaired in daytime functioning. As sleep disturbance may affect long-term health outcomes, the evaluation of

this frequent co-morbidity is important to consider in the management of diabetic patients. Chronic liver disease may be a further risk factor for RLS: RLS has been reported in up to 62% of patients in hepatology clinics [48], and interferon-alpha treatment of hepatitis may lead to RLS in this population [49]. Leg restlessness appears to be one of the most common reasons for sleep disturbances in malignant diseases. Davidson et al. [50]. reported the symptom "restless legs" in 41% of a large population of cancer patients. Iron deficiency may have been the underlying cause of this association.

An elevated prevalence of RLS was observed in patients after organ transplantation: one-third of 45 patients with heart transplantation had PLMS and 45% of these patients also had RLS [51], and nearly 50% of lung transplant recipients were affected by RLS [52]. However, in a large study of kidney-transplanted patients the prevalence of RLS was 5%, which is a similar frequency to that found in the general population [43].

RLS can also occur in several neurological disorders, including neurodegenerative disorders such as Parkinson's disease, multiple system atrophy, spinocerebellar ataxia (for overview see [53]), and sclerosis multiplex [54]. Spinal cord injuries [55,56] and ischemic stroke may also be associated with RLS [57]. Recently, a 15–30% prevalence of RLS was found among subjects with migraine [58,59]. Most of the studies investigating co-morbid RLS did not control for underlying causes of RLS such as iron or folate deficiency and the use of medications known to aggravate RLS. If treatment of the underlying disorder is not possible, RLS in secondary cases is treated identically to that in primary RLS.

Drug-induced RLS/PLMS

Drug-induced RLS is a common, though often unrecognized, reason for sleep disturbance. This is particularly important for the practicing psychopharmacologist, as many agents that cause RLS are psychotropic drugs. Several antidepressants, antipsychotics (including atypical antipsychotics like risperidone, olanzapine, and quetiapine), and lithium can induce or exacerbate RLS and PLMS (for overview see [60,61]). Of note, leg restlessness is also a common complaint among those undergoing opiate withdrawal [62]. Systematic or controlled studies evaluating drug-induced RLS still do not exist. Antidepressants, especially mirtazapine, as well as selective serotonin

Table 8.4 Most common secondary forms of RLS* (prevalence data are based on accepted diagnostic criteria [2,3])

Medical condition	Prevalence (%)
Iron deficiency	Association with serum ferritin level
End-stage renal disease	7–62
Pregnancy	26
Parkinson's disease	8–21
Sarcoidosis	52
Charcot-Marie-Tooth Disease, Type 2	37
Rheumatoid arthritis	15–25
Fibromyalgia	31
Polyneuropathy	1–36
Multiple sclerosis	36
HIV	30

Note: *References are available from the corresponding author (Dr. Hornyak).

Table 8.5 Dopaminergic medications for the treatment of RLS

Medication	Daily dose range	Possible side-effects
Levodopa/ dopa- decarboxylase inhibitor	100/25–400/ 100 mg	Diarrhea, nausea, dyspepsia, reduced general drive, muscle weakness, somnolence, headache
Pramipexole	0.125–0.75 mg	Nausea, dizziness, fatigue, somnolence, headache, orthostatic hypotension
Ropinirole	0.25–4.0 mg	Nausea, dizziness, fatigue, somnolence, headache, orthostatic hypotension
Rotigotine (transdermal patches)	1–3 mg	Nausea, dizziness, fatigue, skin reactions at the patch site, orthostatic hypotension
Cabergoline*	0.5–2.0 mg	Nausea, dizziness, fatigue, somnolence, headache, orthostatic hypotension, cardiac valvular disease
Pergolide*	0.25–0.75 mg	Nausea, dizziness, fatigue, somnolence, headache, orthostatic hypotension, cardiac valvular disease

Note: *Pergolide and cabergoline are ergoline dopamine agonists. Recently, an increased risk of valvular fibrosis during treatment with these substances has been reported in patients with Parkinson's disease [69]. Therefore, the use of this group of dopamine agonists is considered today as a third line treatment option.

reuptake inhibitors (SSRIs), serotonin-norepinephrine reuptake inhibitors (SNRIs; e.g. venlafaxine), and some tetracyclic antidepressants may trigger or exacerbate RLS [63]. Similarly, PLMS may be induced by antidepressants, as reported by Yang et al. [64] investigating PLMS in patients referred for polysomnography. In this study, antidepressants with serotonergic activity (SSRIs, venlafaxine) but not bupropion were associated with higher PLMS indices than in those not on an antidepressant [64].

Treatment of restless legs syndrome and periodic limb movement disorder

General considerations

Patients with sporadic or only mild RLS symptoms without significant impairment in daily life are likely not to need pharmacological treatment. No data is yet available on the prevalence of RLS requiring pharmacological treatment. It is estimated that approximately 2–3% of the population have RLS leading to reduced quality of life [10]. A recent epidemiological study in Germany reported an 8.8% prevalence of RLS, and 1.6% of the whole study population had a wish for treatment [11]. Before starting pharmacological treatment, sleep hygiene measures should be recommended and all causes of secondary RLS, such as iron deficiency, should be excluded. The treatment of RLS is guided by clinical symptoms, and it usually results in improvement of RLS and the RLS-related sleep disturbances. Dopaminergic agents (in particular the dopamine agonists ropinirole, pramipexole, and rotigotine) are considered to be the treatment of choice in RLS and PLMD; however, their exact mechanism of action is not understood [65,66] (see also Table 8.5). The dosage of dopamine agonists used in RLS is usually much lower than in the treatment of Parkinson's disease. Contrary to the treatment of Parkinson's disease, medication is usually given only in the evening hours, to suppress RLS symptoms during the night, corresponding to the circadian rhythm of RLS symptoms. However, some patients may also need medication during the day. In those cases, the dosage during the day is usually lower than the dosage given in the evening [3,31]. Pharmacological treatment should begin at the lowest dose needed to control symptoms, as dosage increases over the course of years when using monotherapy are common [31].

Levodopa and dopamine agonists

Levodopa is a short-acting medication. Levodopa combined with the DOPA decarboxylase inhibitor benserazide is approved by regulatory authorities for the treatment of RLS in Germany and Austria, but not in the USA. Treatment trials have investigated dosage ranges between 100 and 300 mg. Levodopa is usually given as a single dose at bedtime, either with a second dose 3 hours after bedtime or in combination with a sustained-release formulation. Levodopa reduces both PLMS and the sensory symptoms of RLS [67]. Patients have reported better quality of life with improved severity of RLS using levodopa (for review see [68]).

The benefit of dopaminergic agonists in RLS has been proven in several studies. The ergot-dopamine agonists, pergolide and cabergoline, have also been investigated in large populations for the treatment of RLS. Both pergolide and cabergoline have shown efficacy in controlling PLMS and sensory symptoms of RLS (for overview see [66]). Cabergoline has the longest half life among the dopamine agonists and covers RLS symptoms over 24 hours when given once a day in the evening. However, recent reports on valvular fibrosis during ergoline dopamine agonist treatment in patients with Parkinson's disease led to a restrictive usage of ergoline dopamine agonists (for review see [69]). This side-effect has been associated with 5-HT$_{2B}$ agonist properties of this group of medications.

Three non-ergot dopamine agonists have been investigated in large-scale clinical trials: ropinirole, pramipexole, and rotigotine. These agents are widely considered first-line agents for RLS. Ropinirole was investigated in seven clinical trials to date including more than 1000 patients with moderate or severe RLS (e.g. [70]). The mean effective daily dose was 2 mg. Ropinirole was effective in reducing RLS symptoms over 4-week and 12-week trial durations. Also polysomnographic parameters and subjective sleep quality improved during ropinirole treatment. Pramipexole has been investigated in three large-scale trials and in a large-scale polysomnography study. Pramipexole was effective in all trials, with improvement in motor and sensory symptoms of RLS (e.g. [71]). The mean dosage of pramipexole used in these clinical trials was 0.25–1.0 mg (corresponds to 0.18–0.70 mg pramipexole base). Ropinirole and pramipexole have similar side-effects: dizziness, nausea, and somnolence. Sleep attacks were not observed in RLS trials, contrary to prior reports in Parkinson's disease. A rotigotine transdermal matrix patch has also been investigated in RLS patients. The lowest efficient dosage was 1 mg/day [72]. In the dose finding study, the 4 mg/day patch did not demonstrate any advantage over the 3 mg/day patch [73]. Local side-effects such as erythema were common and usually did not result in trial discontinuation by participating subjects.

An important longer-term side-effect of dopamine agonists in treating RLS is the development of augmentation [74], which may necessitate a dose increase or switch to another drug. In the treatment of RLS, augmentation is characterized by one or more of the following: earlier time of RLS symptom onset during the day, anatomical extension of RLS symptoms (e.g. encompassing trunk or arms in addition to legs), a shorter latency to symptoms when at rest, an increased severity of the symptoms when they occur, loss of efficacy of dopaminergic medication, and/or a paradoxical response to changes in medication dose [75]. Although consensus guidelines to define augmentation continue to evolve, the quantitative data available suggest optimal augmentation criteria might be defined as either a 4-hour advance in usual starting time for RLS symptoms or a combination of the occurrence of other features. Clinically important is that low serum ferritin levels may enhance the symptoms of augmentation [41]. Dopamine agonists are usually well tolerated; their use, however, may be limited due to possible interactions with multiple other medications and co-morbidities. Dopamine agonists may trigger psychosis, especially in the elderly, and have recently been reported to complicate therapy in Parkinson's disease and RLS by reversibly inducing impulse control disorders [76]. Studies investigating long-term efficacy of dopamine agonists as well as the prevalence and risk factors for augmentation are rare and should be a focus of future research.

Opioids and antiepileptics

If treatment of RLS with a dopamine agonist is unsuccessful or contraindicated, there are several other agents that can be used. Opioids are clinically effective in RLS, however are regarded as second-line treatment in RLS as controlled studies are still lacking. The one double-blind randomized trial with oxycodone revealed a mean dosage of 15 mg reduced sensory and motor symptoms and was well tolerated [77]. In an observational study, tramadol was effective in RLS at a dosage of 50–150 mg/day [78]. Opioids seem to have a long-term efficacy in the treatment of RLS and are generally well tolerated [79]. Clinical or polysomnographic monitoring for the development of sleep apnea is, however, recommended in patients on long-term opioid therapy [80].

Antiepileptic medications may also be second-line agents in the treatment of RLS. Patients with painful paresthesias may respond positively to anticonvulsants like gabapentin [81,82]. Studies have been performed with a mean dosage of 1800 mg and have proven to be effective. Carbamazepine and valproic acid have also demonstrated significant effects in small groups of patients (for overview see also [66]).

Further therapies

Benzodiazepines and benzodiazepine receptor agonist hypnotics such as zopiclone or zolpidem are reported to be helpful as supportive measures in the treatment of RLS-related insomnia, but are not first-line agents in treating RLS and typically do not address the core symptoms of the disorder [83]. In addition to pharmacological treatment, improvement of coping skills may lead to further reduction of

RLS symptoms and a better quality of life for RLS patients [84].

Quality of life and co-morbidities in patients with restless legs syndrome

RLS symptoms do not lead to life-threatening complications but they usually persist chronically and therefore impair the patient's quality of life to a large extent [10,85]. Disrupted sleep and uncomfortable sensations in the leg(s) are the most undesirable symptoms according to patients with RLS [1,10,86]. Up to 40% of patients with RLS report that the symptoms profoundly limit their daily activities, occupational performance, and social life [87].

Several authors found that patients with RLS have impaired quality of life compared to the general population [1,88,89] or to patients with either cardiovascular disease or type 2 diabetes [90] primarily in the physical, but also some mental health domains (e.g. social functioning, role limitation due to emotional reasons). RLS also appears to be associated with unfavorable lifestyle behaviors, adverse effects on daytime functioning [91], and a high incidence of psychosocial impairment [10,19,90]. Severe sleep deprivation might be responsible for diminished daytime functioning. However, the uncomfortable, often painful sensations render activities associated with sitting quietly (e.g. working on a computer, resting, watching a movie or play, long travel, etc.) extremely challenging. Consequently, patients with serious symptoms may be forced to alter their lifestyle and social life in order to avoid these situations.

Recent studies indicate that RLS, in addition to significantly diminishing quality of life in its sufferers, is an important health concern and may be associated with other life-threatening co-morbid diseases such as cardiovascular disorders [92]. Some authors have reported that the presence of RLS predicts mortality in the general population [93] and in patients with end-stage renal disease [94,95].

Affective disorders in RLS

The relationship of RLS to mood disorders is of particular relevance to mental health clinicians. An association of RLS symptoms and depressed mood was first noted nearly half a century ago [96]. Recent epidemiological studies have repeatedly demonstrated an association of RLS and mood disorders (for overview see [61]). Current epidemiological surveys applying validated diagnostic criteria for RLS found self-reported decrease of mental health [88] and self-reported depressed mood and social isolation in RLS patients [86]. Up to now, two studies used a structured diagnostic interview to evaluate the prevalence of co-morbid depression in RLS. Winkelmann and coworkers found a 12-month prevalence of depressive episodes according to DSM-IV criteria in 17.7% (lifetime prevalence 36.9%) and dysthymia in 5.3% (lifetime prevalence 5.3%) in RLS [97]. In this study, the majority of interviewed RLS patients (82%) received pharmacological treatment for RLS. Another study that examined data from the Baltimore epidemiologic catchment area (ECA) study found that the risk of MDD was roughly five times higher amongst those with RLS than those without [98]. An earlier study that examined data from the Wisconsin Sleep Cohort study demonstrated a positive association between RLS symptom frequency and self-reported depression, with individuals with daily RLS symptoms substantially more likely to have depression (based upon a Zung score above 50 or antidepressant administration) than those who experienced non-daily RLS symptoms (1–6 times per week) [99].

There are limited data that indicate RLS may be additionally associated with anxiety disorders. Winkelmann and colleagues [97] found an elevated 12-month risk of panic disorder and generalized anxiety disorder in RLS patients compared to a population-based control group. In the Wisconsin sleep cohort epidemiological study, individuals with daily RLS symptoms were three times more likely to have an anxiety disorder than those without RLS even after adjustment for several potential confounding factors [99]. Saletu et al. [100] used quantitative EEG brain mapping to demonstrate that EEG maps of RLS patients had characteristics similar to major depression, while EEG maps of patients with PLMD were reminiscent of generalized anxiety disorder.

Sustained sleep disturbances in RLS may have particular relevance in the development of affective disorders, especially depression. RLS symptoms appear in a circadian manner with maximum severity between midnight and 4 a.m. and disturb sleep in patients with moderate to severe symptoms, and as such are likely to cause insomnia symtoms. There is a strong relationship between insomnia and depression and studies have shown that subjects with chronic insomnia are at a high risk of developing major depressive disorder (MDD) later in life [101,102]. On the other hand, sleep disruption might not exclusively account for the relationship

between RLS and depression; in a large cohort of patients with chronic kidney disease, the presence of RLS was significantly associated with depressive symptoms independent of insomnia as well as other relevant socio-demographic and clinical factors [103].

Only a few studies have investigated specific depressive symptom profiles in RLS. In a study evaluating depressive symptoms in untreated RLS patients using the Beck depression inventory (BDI), sleep loss-related complaints such as "reduced sleep," "loss of energy," and "irritability" were encountered more frequently than complaints typical for cognitive-affective symptoms such as "feelings of failure," "guilt," "feelings of punishment," "self-contempt," and "self-reproach" [104]. Another study investigating patients with MDD associated with or without RLS co-morbidity found no differences in characteristics of depressive symptoms not related to sleep impairment (e.g. depressed mood, appetite change, guilt, anhedonia, and suicidal thoughts) [98]. The relationship of RLS symptom and depressive symptom severity was also evaluated in the Wisconsin Sleep Cohort epidemiological study, with the authors reporting a dose–effect relationship between RLS symptom frequency and depression severity [99].

The treatment of co-morbid depression and RLS has some unique aspects of which practicing clinicians should be aware. First, several medications used in the treatment of depression or for the treatment of insomnia including antihistaminic agents, low-dose sedating antidepressants, and neuroleptic drugs can trigger or worsen RLS (see Table 8.6). Second, depressed mood in RLS is strongly related to the presence of insomnia, and it is therefore not always clear whether treatment should be targeted towards depressive symptoms, insomnia symptoms, or both simultaneously. Third, no study to date has been published on the course of depression during dopaminergic treatment in RLS, although antidepressant effects of dopamine agonists have been reported in depression [105].

Treatment of depression with antidepressants has the real possibility of either inducing or exacerbating RLS symptoms, with several cases of triggering or worsening of RLS due to antidepressant drugs reported in the literature (Table 8.6). A systematic observational evaluation of the use of second-generation antidepressants and their effect on RLS in 271 patients has recently been published by Rottach et al. [63]. In 9% of patients in this study, RLS was recorded as a side-effect related to the administration of an antidepressant: mirtazapine provoked or

Table 8.6 Antidepressants triggering RLS, reported in case reports or small case series [61]

Tetracyclic antidepressants	
Mianserine	Markkula et al. (1997)
	Paik et al. (1989)
Mirtazapine	Agargun et al. (2002)
	Bahk et al. (1996)
	Bonin et al. (2000)
	Chang et al. (1996)
	Pae et al. (2004)
	Teive et al. (2002)
Selective serotonin reuptake inhibitor	
Citalopram	Perroud et al. (2007)
Fluoxetine	Bakshi et al. (2000)
	Dorsey et al. (1996)
	Prospero-Garcia et al. (2006)
Paroxetine	Sanz-Fuentenebro et al. (1996)
Sertraline	Hargrave et al. (1998)
Serotonin-norepinephrine reuptake inhibitor	
Venlafaxine	Salin-Pascual et al. (1997)

Note: *References are available from the corresponding author.

exacerbated RLS in 28% of patients who received this drug; both in the group of selective serotonin reuptake inhibitors (SSRIs) (which included citalopram, escitalopram, sertraline, paroxetine, and fluoxetine) and in the group of serotonin-norepinephrine reuptake inhibitors (SNRIs) (duloxetine and venlafaxine) the average frequency of drug-induced RLS was approximately 5%. No cases of drug-induced RLS occurred with reboxetine, a specific norepinephrine reuptake inhibitor. In this study, antidepressant drug-induced RLS usually occurred within the first few days of treatment (mean 2.5 days). Of note, bupropion, a selective noradrenaline and dopamine reuptake inhibitor, was not assessed as it was not licensed until 2007 in Germany. A similar positive relationship between antidepressant use and occurrence of RLS was previously reported in work by Lee et al. [98]. In contrast to these studies, a retrospective chart review of 200 patients with insomnia reported no association between RLS and antidepressant use [106]. A possible explanation for the discrepancy in these studies may be that patients developing RLS due to antidepressants either discontinued or switched the medication at an early stage of therapy.

Unlike serotonergic antidepressants, bupropion was found to have neutral or positive effects on RLS [107,108]. Similarly, Yang et al. [64] evaluated the relationship of antidepressant medication and PLMS in an observational study of 274 consecutive patients with antidepressants and 69 control subjects not taking antidepressants referred for overnight diagnostic polysomnography. The odds of having an elevated PLMS index (>20/hour of sleep) was roughly five times greater for both the SSRI group and the venlafaxine group compared with the controls. However, frequency of PLMS did not differ significantly between bupropion and controls. The authors hypothesized that the increase of PLMS during venlafaxine and SSRI treatment might be the result of the enhanced serotonergic availability and/or secondarily decreased dopaminergic effects. Given these findings, unless contraindicated, bupropion is often considered the antidepressant of choice in the treatment of MDD with co-morbid RLS.

There are no evidence-based guidelines for the treatment of co-morbid depression and RLS. An expert-based therapy algorithm was presented by Picchietti and Winkelman [109]. They proposed a differential approach depending on whether RLS/insomnia or other depressive symptoms dominate. In cases of minor depression, they recommended treating RLS first, noting that treatment of RLS may by itself lead to an improvement in sleep continuity and depressive symptoms. In more severe cases of depression, treatment of MDD with noradrenergic antidepressants is preferred because of the potential worsening of RLS by the use of serotonergic drugs [109]. In addition to pharmacotherapy, education of patients with RLS about potential depression-inducing behavioral patterns such as social isolation, dysfunctional cognitions, and raised stress levels may prevent the development of co-morbid depression. In a recent study on non-depressive RLS patients, disorder-specific group therapy with eight sessions resulted in the improvement of RLS-related quality of life; however, such group techniques have not been applied to RLS groups with co-morbid depression [84].

Other sleep-related movement disorders

Other simple sleep-related movement disorders include hypnagogic foot tremor (HFT) and alternating leg muscle activation (ALMA). Additionally, sleep-related rhythmic movement disorder occurs in early childhood, when the children repetitively bang their head against the pillow or rock back and forth from side to side while in bed. The etiology of these disorders is unknown, and they are generally considered benign requiring no specific treatment [8].

Nocturnal leg cramps are characterized by painful sensations in the leg or foot associated with sudden muscle contraction during the sleep period [8]. The pain is relieved by a forceful stretching of the affected muscle. Nocturnal leg cramps may occur at any age, though their frequency increases with age, reaching a prevalence of 6% in those above 60 years of age.

Sleep-related bruxism is the grinding or clenching of teeth during sleep, which may lead to abnormal wear of the teeth, jaw muscle discomfort, temporomandibular disorder, insomnia, orofacial pain, and hypertrophy of the masseter muscle. The tooth-grinding sound may also disrupt the sleep of the bed partner. The prevalence of bruxism is reported to be around 8% and declines with age [110]. The etiology is unknown, though anxiety and stress are generally regarded as potential predisposing factors. Serotonin may be involved in its development, since SSRIs have been reported to exacerbate sleep-related bruxism [111,112].

Conclusion

The most common sleep-related movement disorder is RLS, which is associated with, but not synonymous with, PLMS. The interaction of RLS and psychiatric disorders is complex, as patients with RLS have increased odds of co-occurring affective and anxiety disorders. Furthermore, psychopharmacological agents like antipsychotics or certain antidepressants may trigger or worsen RLS. The specific aspects of diagnosis and treatment of psychiatric disorders in patients with RLS should be carefully considered to avoid exacerbation of RLS and subsequent worsening of sleep-related complaints, and possibly the underlying psychiatric disorder itself.

Acknowledgments

The research of M.N. and A.Sz. has been supported by grants from the National Research Fund (OTKA) (T-048767, TS-049785, F-68841), ETT (100/2006), the Hungarian Kidney Foundation, and the Foundation for Prevention in Medicine, as well as the Center for Integrative Mood Research, Toronto, Canada. This work was also supported by the János Bolyai Research Scholarship of the Hungarian Academy of Sciences (MN).

Financial disclosure

This is not an industry-supported study. The authors have no financial conflict of interest to declare regarding the present review.

Conflict of interest

Dr. Hornyak received lecture fees and honoraria from Hoffmann La-Roche, Böhringer-Ingelheim, Glaxo-Smith-Kline, and Pfizer. Drs. Novak and Szentkiralyi have no conflict of interest to declare.

References

1. Hening W, Walters AS, Allen RP, et al. Impact, diagnosis and treatment of restless legs syndrome (RLS) in a primary care population: the REST (RLS epidemiology, symptoms, and treatment) primary care study. *Sleep Med.* 2004;5:237–246.

2. Walters AS. Toward a better definition of the restless legs syndrome. The International Restless Legs Syndrome Study Group. *Mov Disord.* 1995; **10**:634–642.

3. Allen RP, Picchietti D, Hening WA, et al. Restless legs syndrome: diagnostic criteria, special considerations, and epidemiology: a report from the restless legs syndrome diagnosis and epidemiology workshop at the National Institutes of Health. *Sleep Med.* 2003; 4:101–119.

4. Montplaisir J, Boucher S, Poirier G, et al. Clinical, polysomnographic, and genetic characteristics of restless legs syndrome: a study of 133 patients diagnosed with new standard criteria. *Mov Disord.* 1997;**12**:61–65.

5. American Sleep Disorders Association. Recording and scoring leg movements: The Atlas Task Force. *Sleep.* 1993;**16**:748–759.

6. Zucconi M, Ferri R, Allen RP, et al. The official World Association of Sleep Medicine (WASM) standards for recording and scoring periodic leg movements in sleep (PLMS) and wakefulness (PLMW) developed in collaboration with a task force from the International Restless Legs Syndrome Study Group (IRLSSG). *Sleep Med.* 2006; 7:175–183.

7. Hornyak M, Feige B, Riemann D, Voderholzer U. Periodic leg movements in sleep and periodic limb movement disorder: prevalence, clinical significance and treatment. *Sleep Med Rev.* 2006;**10**(3): 169–177.

8. American Academy of Sleep Medicine. *International classification of sleep disorders. 2nd Edition: Diagnostic and coding manual.* Westchester, Illinois: American Academy of Sleep Medicine; 2005.

9. Walters AS, Hening W, Rubinstein M, Chokroverty S. A clinical and polysomnographic comparison of neuroleptic-induced akathisia and the idiopathic restless legs syndrome. *Sleep.* 1991;**14**(4):339–345.

10. Allen RP, Walters AS, Montplaisir J, et al. Restless legs syndrome prevalence and impact: REST general population study. *Arch Intern Med.* 2005; **165**:1286–1292.

11. Happe S, Vennemann M, Evers S, Berger K. Treatment wish of individuals with known and unknown restless legs syndrome in the community. *J Neurol.* 2008;**255**:1365–1371.

12. Allen RP, Earley CJ. Defining the phenotype of the restless legs syndrome (RLS) using age-of-symptom onset. *Sleep Med.* 2000;**1**:11–19.

13. Polydefkis M, Allen RP, Hauer P, et al. Subclinical sensory neuropathy in late-onset restless legs syndrome. *Neurology.* 2000;**55**:1115–1121.

14. Ondo WG, Vuong KD, Wang Q. Restless legs syndrome in monozygotic twins: clinical correlates. *Neurology.* 2000;**55**:1404–1406.

15. Berger K, von Eckardstein A, Trenkwalder C, et al. Iron metabolism and the risk of restless legs syndrome in an elderly general population – the MEMO-Study. *J Neurol.* 2002;**249**:1195–1199.

16. O'Keeffe ST. Secondary causes of restless legs syndrome in older people. *Age Ageing.* 2005; **34**:349–352.

17. Bassetti CL, Mauerhofer D, Gugger M, Mattis J, Hess CW. Restless legs syndrome: a clinical study of 55 patients. *Eur Neurol.* 2001;**45**:67–74.

18. Walters AS, Hickey K, Maltzman J, et al. A questionnaire study of 138 patients with restless legs syndrome: the 'Night-Walkers' survey. *Neurology.* 1996;**46**:92–95.

19. Berger K, Luedemann J, Trenkwalder C, John U, Kessler C. Sex and the risk of restless legs syndrome in the general population. *Arch Intern Med.* 2004; **164**:196–202.

20. Hornyak M, Voderholzer U, Riemann D. Treatment of depression in patients with restless legs syndrome: what is evidence-based? *Sleep Med.* 2006; 7:301–302; author reply 303–304.

21. Ohayon MM, Roth T. Prevalence of restless legs syndrome and periodic limb movement disorder in the general population. *J Psychosom Res.* 2002;**53**:547–554.

22. Kotagal S, Silber MH. Childhood-onset restless legs syndrome. *Ann Neurol.* 2004:**56**:803–807.

23. Muhle H, Neumann A, Lohmann-Hedrich K, et al. Childhood-onset restless legs syndrome: clinical and genetic features of 22 families. *Mov Disord.* 2008;**23**:1113–1121; quiz 1203.

24. Picchietti DL, Stevens HE. Early manifestations of restless legs syndrome in childhood and adolescence. *Sleep Med.* 2008;**9**:770–781.

25. Crabtree VM, Ivanenko A, O'Brien LM, Gozal D. Periodic limb movement disorder of sleep in children. *J Sleep Res.* 2003;**12**:73–81.

26. Picchietti DL, England SJ, Walters AS, Willis KK, Verrico T. Periodic limb movement disorder and restless legs syndrome in children with attention-deficit hyperactivity disorder. *J Child Neurol.* 1998;**13**:588–594.

27. Picchietti DL, Underwood DJ, Farris WA, et al. Further studies on periodic limb movement disorder and restless legs syndrome in children with attention-deficit hyperactivity disorder. *Mov Disord.* 1999;**14**:1000–1007.

28. Chervin RD, Archbold KH, Dillon JE, et al. Associations between symptoms of inattention, hyperactivity, restless legs, and periodic leg movements. *Sleep.* 2002;**25**:213–218.

29. Wagner ML, Walters AS, Fisher BC. Symptoms of attention-deficit/hyperactivity disorder in adults with restless legs syndrome. *Sleep.* 2004;**27**:1499–1504.

30. Oner P, Dirik EB, Taner Y, Caykoylu A, Anlar O. Association between low serum ferritin and restless legs syndrome in patients with attention deficit hyperactivity disorder. *Tohoku J Exp Med.* 2007;**213**:269–276.

31. Trenkwalder C, Högl B, Winkelmann J. Recent advances in the diagnosis, genetics and treatment of restless legs syndrome. *J Neurol.* 2009;**256**: 539–553.

32. Stefansson H, Rye DB, Hicks A, et al. A genetic risk factor for periodic limb movements in sleep. *N Engl J Med.* 2007;**357**:639–647.

33. Winkelmann J, Schormair B, Lichtner P, et al. Genome-wide association study of restless legs syndrome identifies common variants in three genomic regions. *Nat Genet.* 2007;**39**: 1000–1006.

34. Paulus W, Dowling P, Rijsman R, Stiasny-Kolster K, Trenkwalder C. Update of the pathophysiology of the restless legs syndrome. *Mov Disord.* 2007; **22**(Suppl 18):S431–S439.

35. Satija P, Ondo WG. Restless legs syndrome: pathophysiology, diagnosis and treatment. *CNS Drugs.* 2008;**22**(6):497–518.

36. Bordelon YM, Smith M. Movement disorders in pregnancy. *Semin Neurol.* 2007;**27**(5):467–475.

37. Ulfberg J, Nystrom B. Restless legs syndrome in blood donors. *Sleep Med.* 2004;**5**:15–18.

38. Grote L, Leissner L, Hedner J, Ulfberg J. A randomized, double-blind, placebo controlled, multi-center study of intravenous iron sucrose and placebo in the treatment of restless legs syndrome. *Mov Disord.* 2009;**24**(10):1445–1452.

39. Wang J, O'Reilly B, Venkataraman R, Mysliwiec V, Mysliwiec A. Efficacy of oral iron in patients with restless legs syndrome and a low-normal ferritin: A randomized, double-blind, placebo-controlled study. *Sleep Med.* 2009; Feb 16 [Epub ahead of print].

40. Earley CJ, Horská A, Mohamed MA, et al. A randomized, double-blind, placebo-controlled trial of intravenous iron sucrose in restless legs syndrome. *Sleep Med.* 2009;**10**(2):206–211.

41. Frauscher B, Gschliesser V, Brandauer E, et al. The severity range of restless legs syndrome (RLS) and augmentation in a prospective patient cohort: association with ferritin levels. *Sleep Med.* 2009; **10**(6):611–615.

42. Dzaja A, Wehrle R, Lancel M, Pollmächer T. Elevated estradiol plasma levels in women with restless legs during pregnancy. *Sleep.* 2009;**32**(2):169–174.

43. Molnar MZ, Novak M, Ambrus C, et al. Restless Legs Syndrome in patients after renal transplantation. *Am J Kidney Dis.* 2005;**45**:388–396.

44. Mucsi I, Molnar MZ, Ambrus C, et al. Restless legs syndrome, insomnia and quality of life in patients on maintenance dialysis. *Nephrol Dial Transplant.* 2005;**20**:571–577.

45. Hattan E, Chalk C, Postuma RB. Is there a higher risk of restless legs syndrome in peripheral neuropathy? *Neurology.* 2009;**72**(11):955–960.

46. Hening WA, Caivano CK. Restless legs syndrome: a common disorder in patients with rheumatologic conditions. *Semin Arthritis Rheum.* 2008;**38**:55–62.

47. Cuellar NG, Ratcliffe SJ. Restless legs syndrome in type 2 diabetes: implications to diabetes educators. *Diabetes Educ.* 2008;**34**:218–234.

48. Franco RA, Ashwathnarayan R, Deshpandee A, et al. The high prevalence of restless legs syndrome symptoms in liver disease in an academic-based hepatology practice. *J Clin Sleep Med.* 2008;**4**: 45–49.

49. LaRochelle JS, Karp BI. Restless legs syndrome due to interferon-alpha. *Mov Disord.* 2004;**19**:730–731.

50. Davidson JR, MacLean AW, Brundage MD, Schulze K. Sleep disturbance in cancer patients. *Soc Sci Med.* 2002;**54**:1309–1321.

51. Javaheri S, Abraham WT, Brown C, et al. Prevalence of obstructive sleep apnoea and periodic limb movement in 45 subjects with heart transplantation. *Eur Heart J.* 2004;**25**, 260–266.

52. Minai OA, Golish JA, Yataco JC, et al. Restless legs syndrome in lung transplant recipients. *J Heart Lung Transplant.* 2007; **26**:24–29.

53. Iranzo A, Comella CL, Santamaria J, Oertel W. Restless legs syndrome in Parkinson's disease and other neurodegenerative diseases of the central nervous system. *Mov Disord.* 2007;**22**(Suppl 18): S424–S430.

54. Manconi M, Ferini-Strambi L, Filippi M, et al. Multicenter case-control study on restless legs syndrome in multiple sclerosis: the REMS study. *Sleep.* 2008;**31**:944–952.

55. Brown LK, Heffner JE, Obbens EA. Transverse myelitis associated with restless legs syndrome and periodic movements of sleep responsive to an oral dopaminergic agent but not to intrathecal baclofen. *Sleep.* 2000;**23**:591–594.

56. Abele M, Burk K, Laccone F, Dichgans J, Klockgether T. Restless legs syndrome in spinocerebellar ataxia types 1, 2, and 3. *J Neurol.* 2001;**248**:311–314.

57. Lee SJ, Kim JS, Song IU, et al. Poststroke restless legs syndrome and lesion location: anatomical considerations. *Mov Disord.* 2009;**24**:77–84.

58. Rhode AM, Hosing VG, Happe S, et al. Comorbidity of migraine and restless legs syndrome: a case-control study. *Cephalalgia.* 2007;**27**:1255–1260.

59. d'Onofrio F, Bussone G, Cologno D, et al. Restless legs syndrome and primary headaches: a clinical study. *Neurol Sci.* 2008;**29**(Suppl 1):S169–S172.

60. Cohrs S. Sleep disturbances in patients with schizophrenia: impact and effect of antipsychotics. *CNS Drugs.* 2008;**22**:939–962.

61. Hornyak M. Mood disorders in individuals with restless legs syndrome: epidemiology, pathophysiology and management. *CNS Drugs.* 2010;**24**(2):89–98.

62. Scherbaum N, Stüper B, Bonnet U, Gastpar M. Transient restless legs-like syndrome as a complication of opiate withrawal. *Pharmacopsychiatry.* 2003; **36**(2):70–72.

63. Rottach KG, Schaner BM, Kirch MH, et al. Restless legs syndrome as side effect of second generation antidepressants. *J Psychiatr Res.* 2008;**43**:70–75.

64. Yang C, White DP, Winkelman JW. Antidepressants and periodic leg movements of sleep. *Biol Psychiatry.* 2005;**58**:510–514.

65. Vignatelli L, Billiard M, Clarenbach P, et al. EFNS guidelines on management of restless legs syndrome and periodic limb movement disorder in sleep. *Eur J Neurol.* 2006;**13**:1049–1065.

66. Trenkwalder C, Hening WA, Montagna P, et al. Treatment of restless legs syndrome: an evidence-based review and implications for clinical practice. *Mov Disord*. 2008;**23**:2267–2302.

67. Trenkwalder C, Stiasny K, Pollmächer T, et al. L-dopa therapy of uremic and idiopathic restless legs syndrome: a double-blind, crossover trial. *Sleep*. 1995;**18**(8):681–688.

68. Conti CF, de Oliveira MM, Andriolo RB, et al. Levodopa for idiopathic restless legs syndrome: evidence-based review. *Mov Disord*. 2007; **22**(13):1943–1951.

69. Antonini A, Poewe W. Fibrotic heart-valve reactions to dopamine-agonist treatment in Parkinson's disease. *Lancet Neurol*. 2007;**6**(9):826–829.

70. Bogan RK, Fry JM, Schmidt MH, Carson SW, Ritchie SY. Ropinirole in the treatment of patients with restless legs syndrome: a US-based randomized, double-blind, placebo-controlled clinical trial. *Mayo Clin Proc*. 2006;**81**:17–27.

71. Winkelman JW, Sethi KD, Kushida CA, et al. Efficacy and safety of pramipexole in restless legs syndrome. *Neurology*. 2006;**67**:1034–1039.

72. Trenkwalder C, Benes H, Poewe W, et al. Efficacy of rotigotine for treatment of moderate-to-severe restless legs syndrome: a randomised, double-blind, placebo-controlled trial. *Lancet Neurol*. 2008;**7**(7):595–604.

73. Stiasny-Kolster K, Kohnen R, Schollmayer E, Möller JC, Oertel WH. Rotigotine Sp 666 Study Group. Patch application of the dopamine agonist rotigotine to patients with moderate to advanced stages of restless legs syndrome: a double-blind, placebo-controlled pilot study. *Mov Disord*. 2004;**19**(12): 1432–1438.

74. Paulus W, Trenkwalder C. Less is more: pathophysiology of dopaminergic-therapy-related augmentation in restless legs syndrome. *Lancet Neurol*. 2006:**5**:878–886.

75. García-Borreguero D, Allen RP, Kohnen R, et al. Diagnostic standards for dopaminergic augmentation of restless legs syndrome: report from a World Association of Sleep Medicine-International Restless Legs Syndrome Study Group consensus conference at the Max Planck Institute. *Sleep Med*. 2007; **8**(5):520–530.

76. Tippmann-Peikert M, Park JG, Boeve BF, Shepard JW, Silber MH. Pathologic gambling in patients with restless legs syndrome treated with dopaminergic agonists. *Neurology*. 2007;**68**(4):301–303.

77. Walters AS, Wagner ML, Hening WA, et al. Successful treatment of the idiopathic restless legs syndrome in a randomized double-blind trial of oxycodone versus placebo. *Sleep*. 1993;**16**(4):327–332.

78. Lauerma H, Markkula J. Treatment of restless legs syndrome with tramadol: an open study. *J Clin Psychiatry*. 1999;**60**(4):241–244.

79. Walters AS, Winkelman J, Trenkwalder C, et al. Long-term follow-up on restless legs syndrome patients treated with opioids. *Mov Disord*. 2001;**16**:1105–1109.

80. Farney RJ, Walker JM, Cloward TV, Rhondeau S. Sleep-disordered breathing associated with long-term opioid therapy. *Chest*. 2003;**123**(2):632–639.

81. Happe S, Klosch G, Saletu B, Zeitlhofer J. Treatment of idiopathic restless legs syndrome (RLS) with gabapentin. *Neurology*. 2001;**57**:1717–1719.

82. Garcia-Borreguero D, Larrosa O, de la Llave Y, et al. Treatment of restless legs syndrome with gabapentin: a double-blind, cross-over study. *Neurology*. 2002;**59**:1573–1579.

83. Bezerra M, Martinez J. Zolpidem in restless legs syndrome. *Eur Neurol*. 2002;**48**:180–181.

84. Hornyak M, Grossmann C, Kohnen R, et al. Cognitive behavioural group therapy to improve patients' strategies for coping with restless legs syndrome: a proof-of-concept trial. *J Neurol Neurosurg Psychiatry*. 2008;**79**:823–825.

85. Happe S, Reese JP, Stiasny-Kolster K, et al. Assessing health-related quality of life in patients with restless legs syndrome. *Sleep Med*. 2009;**10**(3):295–305.

86. Ulfberg J, Nystrom B, Carter N, Edling C. Prevalence of restless legs syndrome among men aged 18 to 64 years: an association with somatic disease and neuropsychiatric symptoms. *Mov Disord*. 2001;**16**:1159–1163.

87. Garcia-Borreguero D. Time to REST: epidemiology and burden. *Eur J Neurol*. 2006;**13**(Suppl 3):15–20.

88. Phillips B, Young T, Finn L, et al. Epidemiology of restless legs symptoms in adults. *Arch Intern Med*. 2000;**160**:2137–2141.

89. McCrink L, Allen RP, Wolowacz S, et al. Predictors of health-related quality of life in sufferers with restless legs syndrome: a multi-national study. *Sleep Med*. 2007;**8**:73–83.

90. Abetz L, Allen RP, Follet A, et al. Evaluating the quality of life of patients with restless legs syndrome. *Clin Ther*. 2004;**26**:925–935.

91. Phillips B, Hening W, Britz P, Mannino D. Prevalence and correlates of restless legs syndrome: results from the 2005 National Sleep Foundation Poll. *Chest*. 2006;**129**:76–80.

92. Winkelman JW, Shahar E, Sharief I, Gottlieb DJ. Association of restless legs syndrome and cardiovascular disease in the Sleep Heart Health Study. *Neurology*. 2008;**70**(1):35–42.

93. Mallon L, Broman JE, Hetta J. Restless legs symptoms with sleepiness in relation to mortality: 20-year follow-up study of a middle-aged Swedish population. *Psychiatry Clin Neurosci*. 2008;**62**:457–463.

94. Unruh ML, Levey AS, D'Ambrosio C, et al. Restless legs symptoms among incident dialysis patients: association with lower quality of life and shorter survival. *Am J Kidney Dis*. 2004;**43**:900–909.

95. Molnar MZ, Szentkiralyi A, Lindner A, et al. Restless legs syndrome and mortality in kidney transplant recipients. *Am J Kidney Dis*. 2007;**50**:813–820.

96. Gorman CA, Dyck PJ, Pearson JS. Symptom of restless legs. *Arch Intern Med*. 1965;**115**:155–160.

97. Winkelmann J, Prager M, Lieb R, et al. "Anxietas tibiarum": Depression and anxiety disorders in patients with restless legs syndrome. *J Neurol*. 2005;**252**:67–71.

98. Lee HB, Hening WA, Allen RP, et al. Restless legs syndrome is associated with DSM-IV major depressive disorder and panic disorder in the community. *J Neuropsychiatry Clin Neurosci*. 2008;**20**:101–105.

99. Winkelman JW, Finn L, Young T. Prevalence and correlates of restless legs syndrome symptoms in the Wisconsin Sleep Cohort. *Sleep Med*. 2006;**7**:545–552.

100. Saletu M, Anderer P, Saletu B, et al. EEG mapping in patients with restless legs syndrome as compared with normal controls. *Psychiatry Res*. 2002;**115**(1–2):49–61.

101. Ford DE, Kamerow DB. Epidemiologic study of sleep disturbances and psychiatric disorders: An opportunity for prevention? *JAMA*. 1989;**262**:1479–1484.

102. Riemann D, Voderholzer U. Primary insomnia: a risk factor to develop depression? *J Affect Disord*. 2003;**76**:255–259.

103. Szentkiralyi A, Molnar MZ, Czira ME, et al. Association between restless legs syndrome and depression in patients with chronic kidney disease. *J Psychosom Res*. 2009;**67**(2):173–180.

104. Hornyak M, Kopasz M, Berger M, Riemann D, Voderholzer U. Impact of sleep-related complaints on depressive symptoms in patients with restless legs syndrome. *J Clin Psychiatry*. 2005;**66**:1139–1145.

105. Corrigan MH, Denahan AQ, Wright CE, Ragual RJ, Evans DL. Comparison of pramipexole, fluoxetine, and placebo in patients with major depression. *Depress Anxiety*. 2000;**11**(2):58–65.

106. Brown LK, Dedrick DL, Doggett JW, Guido PS. Antidepressant medication use and restless legs syndrome in patients presenting with insomnia. *Sleep Med*. 2005;**6**:443–450.

107. Kim SW, Shin IS, Kim, JM, et al. Bupropion may improve restless legs syndrome: a report of three cases. *Clin Neuropharmacol*. 2005;**28**:298–301.

108. Perroud N, Lazignac C, Baleydier B, et al. Restless legs syndrome induced by citalopram: a psychiatric emergency? *Gen Hosp Psychiatry*. 2007;**29**:72–74.

109. Picchietti D, Winkelman JW. Restless legs syndrome, periodic limb movements in sleep, and depression. *Sleep*. 2005;**28**:891–898.

110. Lavigne GJ, Khoury S, Abe S, Yamaguchi T, Raphael K. Bruxism physiology and pathology: an overview for clinicians. *J Oral Rehabil*. 2008;**35**:476–494.

111. Romanelli F, Adler DA, Bungay KM. Possible paroxetine-induced bruxism. *Ann Pharmacother*. 1996;**30**:1246–1248.

112. Wise M. Citalopram-induced bruxism. *Br J Psychiatry*. 2001;**178**:182.

Hypersomnias of central origin

Chad C. Hagen and Jed E. Black

Synopsis

Excessive daytime sleepiness (EDS), hypersomnolence, or "pathological sleepiness" is a complaint of increased sleep propensity occurring at inappropriate times that adversely affects vigilance, performance, and daytime function. Psychiatric, medical, or primary sleep disorders and medications can all produce complaints of EDS or fatigue. Insufficient sleep is by far the most common cause of EDS in the general population. Fatigue will not be addressed specifically in this chapter as it is a broader symptom relating to a variety of conditions of tiredness or mental or physical exhaustion and is often independent of sleepiness. This chapter summarizes the clinical presentation, diagnostic criteria, and initial treatment options for the specific subtype of EDS known as hypersomnias of central origin.

Introduction

Daytime sleepiness is a common complaint in both general and psychiatric patient populations. Patients who experience inappropriately timed sleepiness that adversely affects their daytime functioning are said to have pathological sleepiness or EDS. Lack of knowledge about the hypersomnias of central origin may lead to their being misdiagnosed or overlooked, and at times results in gross mismanagement (e.g. the use of antipsychotic medications for narcolepsy-related hypnagogic hallucinations or the initiation of antidepressant therapy in individuals complaining of hypersomnolence misdiagnosed as depression). The American Academy of Sleep Medicine defines EDS in the International Classification of Sleep Disorders (ICSD-2) as the "complaint of difficulty in maintaining desired wakefulness or a complaint of excessive amount of sleep"[1]. The ICSD-2 notes that excessive sleepiness or somnolence is a subjective report of difficulty maintaining the alert awake state, usually accompanied by a rapid entrance into sleep when the person is sedentary [1].

A substantial portion of the general population complains of sleepiness and the reported prevalence figures for EDS vary widely. The largest and most comprehensive representative population survey [2] was performed across four Western European countries (UK, Germany, Spain, and Italy). Substantial EDS, defined as meeting three parameters of marked sleepiness for 3 or more days per week, was reported in 15% of this combined population. In the USA, smaller population surveys have been conducted. Recent polls suggest that 15–16% of the US population 18 years of age and older may experience EDS that interferes with daily activities a few days a week or more [3]. These polls did not differentiate between causes of EDS.

Primary sleep disorders may co-exist with underlying psychiatric illness, complicating the diagnostic workup and treatment of each. Syndromes involving sleep fragmentation (periodic limb movement disorder, upper airway resistance syndrome, or obstructive sleep apnea-hypopnea syndrome) and disorders imposing inadequate sleep duration or quality (such as circadian rhythm disorders, insomnia, or parasomnias) may produce complaints of EDS. An understanding of these disorders and a thorough evaluation to exclude them is a requisite process in the diagnosis of hypersomnias of central origin. These alternate sources of EDS are generally more common than the hypersomnias of central origin and are reviewed in their respective chapters in this volume.

Foundations of Psychiatric Sleep Medicine, ed. John W. Winkelman and David T. Plante. Published by Cambridge University Press.
© Cambridge University Press 2010.

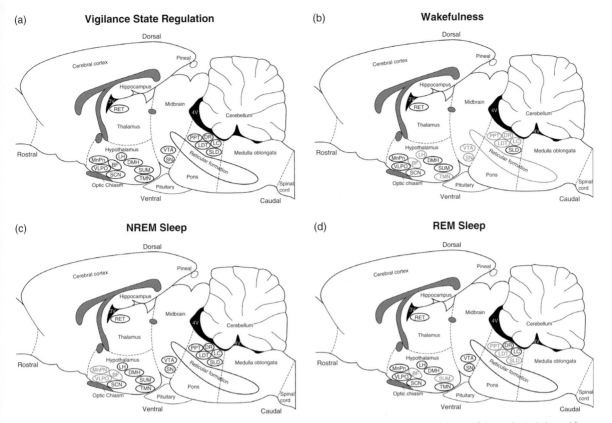

Figure 2.1 A schematic overview of the neural systems involved in vigilance state regulation. (a) Sagittal view of the rat brain (adapted from [3]) depicts nuclei and brain regions involved in vigilance state regulation (wakefulness, NREM sleep, and REM sleep) and circadian rhythmicity. In Figures 1b–d, active regions during the vigilance states are highlighted in red. (b) Nuclei that promote wakefulness, as well as regions activated during wakefulness, include: basal forebrain (BF) cholinergic, GABAergic, and putatively glutamatergic; dorsal raphe (DR) serotonergic; lateral hypothalamus (LH) orexinergic; locus coeruleus (LC) noradrenergic; pedunculopontine/laterodorsal tegmental (PPT/LDT) cholinergic; reticular formation glutamatergic; substantia nigra (SN) dopaminergic; tuberomammillary (TMN) histaminergic; and ventral tegmental area (VTA) dopaminergic nuclei. Thalamocortical and basal forebrain activity produces the EEG profile indicative of wakefulness. (c) Nuclei that promote NREM sleep include GABAergic neurons in the ventrolateral preoptic (VLPO) and median preoptic (MnPN) nuclei. Furthermore, the homeostatic sleep regulator adenosine acts to inhibit wake-promoting BF neurons. The reticular nucleus of the thalamus (RET) is responsible for NREM sleep phenomena such as sleep spindles. (d) Nuclei that promote REM sleep include the pedunculopontine/laterodorsal tegmental nuclei (PPT/LDT), where unique "REM-on" neurons are located. The sublaterodorsal nucleus (SLD) also promotes REM sleep phenomena, including muscle atonia, by means of circuitry involving the spinal cord. The supramammillary nucleus (SUM) and medial septum of the basal forebrain (BF) are part of the circuitry responsible for theta rhythmicity in the hippocampus, which is indicative of REM sleep. Abbreviations: 3V, third ventricle; 4V, fourth ventricle; DMH, dorsomedial nucleus of the hypothalamus; SCN, suprachiasmatic nucleus.

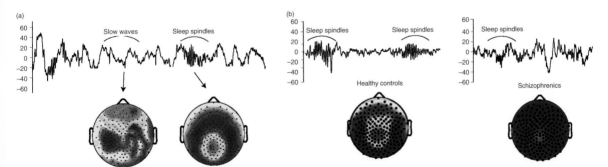

Figure 3.2 (a) NREM sleep EEG traces and topographies of slow waves and sleep spindles in a healthy control. (b) Topographic analysis of sleep spindles revealed that schizophrenics had reduced spindle activity localized in a centroparietal area (adapted from [1]).

(a)

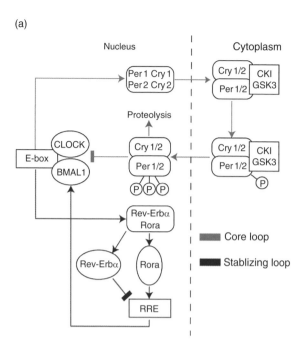

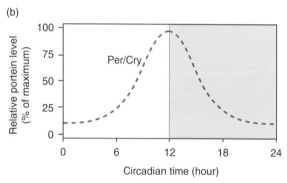

Figure 2.7 Schematic representation of the interaction of mammalian clock genes contributing to cellular circadian oscillations, adapted from [170]. (a) As described in the core feedback loop (depicted in red), a heterodimeric transcription factor, including CLOCK and BMAL1, by acting on the E-box DNA control element, initiates the expression of the negative regulators PER1 and PER2 (period proteins), as well as CRY1 and CRY 2 (cryptochromes). PER and CRY accumulate as the day progresses, multimerize in the cytoplasm, and are phosphorylated by the enzymes casein kinase I (CKI) and glycogen synthase kinase-3 (GSK3). The PER/CRY complex is then translocated to the nucleus, and represses CLOCK/BMAL1 expression. PER and CRY proteins are then degraded at the end of the circadian cycle (CKI dependent), disinhibiting CLOCK and BMAL1 transcription. As described in the stabilizing feedback loop (depicted in blue), BMAL1 transcription can activate the orphan nuclear receptors Rora and Rev-Erbα, which suppress and activate BMAL1 expression respectively through the intermediary ROR-response element (RRE). (b) Graphic depiction of Per/Cry protein levels in the suprachiasmatic nucleus across the 24-hour day, adapted from [168]. Circadian time 0 is the beginning of the subjective day/light period for humans. Abbreviations: P, phosphate.

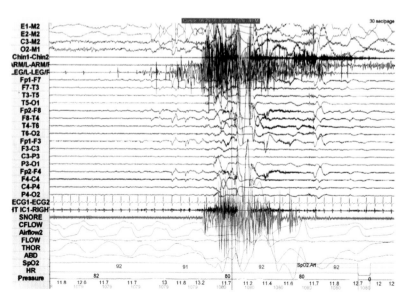

Figure 10.3 Polysomnogram of 72-year-old man with REM sleep behavior disorder. Although the rapid eye movements are typical of REM sleep and the EEG is characteristically desynchronized, chin muscle atonia is incomplete during this burst of phasic eye movements, and there is prominent electromyographic activation of muscles of upper and lower extremities movements with corresponding movement. Patient yelled out during this event and, retrospectively, recalled dreaming of fighting.

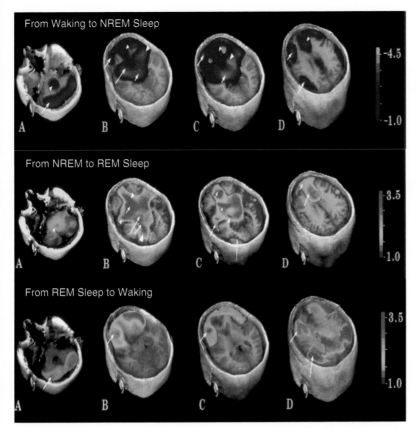

Figure 3.4 Brain maps showing changes in rCBF from waking to NREM (top), NREM to REM (middle), and REM to waking (bottom), measured with H$^2_{15}$O PET. *Top panel*: brain regions with decreased rCBF during NREM sleep compared with presleep wakefulness. The reduction is expressed in Z scores, ranging from −1 (light purple) to −4.5 (deep purple). Significant rCBF reductions were observed in the pons (A, arrowhead), midbrain (B, short arrow), basal ganglia (B, long arrow; C, medium arrowhead), thalamus (C, short arrow), caudal orbital cortex (B, small arrowhead), and cerebellum (A, arrow). Similar rCBF decreases were found in the anterior insula (B, medium arrowhead), anterior cingulate (C and D, small arrowheads), as well as in the orbital (B, medium arrow), dorsolateral prefrontal (C, medium arrow; D, small arrow), and inferior parietal lobes (D, medium arrow). *Middle panel*: brain regions with increased rCBF during REM sleep compared with NREM sleep. Z-scores values range from 1 (green) to 3.5 (red). Significant increases in rCBF during REM sleep were observed in the pons (A, arrowhead), midbrain (B, long arrow), basal ganglia (B, short arrow; C, small arrowhead), thalamus (C, medium arrowhead), and caudal orbital cortex (B, medium arrowhead). Increases were also found in anterior insula (B, small arrowhead), anterior cingulate (C, small arrow; D, medium arrow), mesial temporal (parahippocampal) (B, medium arrow), fusiform–inferotemporal (B, large arrowhead), lateral occipital (C, long arrow), auditory association (C, medium arrow), and medial prefrontal cortices (D, small arrow). *Bottom panel*: brain regions with rCBF increase during post-sleep wakefulness compared to REM sleep. Z-scores values are from 1 (green) to 3.5 (red). Significant increases in rCBF occurred in the orbital (B, small arrow), dorsolateral prefrontal (C and D, small arrows), and inferior parietal lobes (D, medium arrow), as well as in the cerebellar hemispheres (A, small arrow). Reproduced, with permission, from [2].

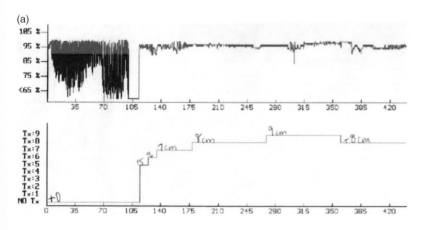

Figure 10.2 (a) Oximetry tracing from an obese 38-year-old woman showing frequent desaturations of oxyhemoglobin, reaching a nadir of <60% during polysomnographically documented non-REM sleep, secondary to obstructive sleep apnea. Apnea and hypopnea events occurred at a rate of 80 per hour of sleep. Each desaturation is accompanied by evidence of arousal from sleep on the corresponding polysomnogram. She had complained of frequent spells of SW, which included eating foods from her cupboards and refrigerator. She responded well to CPAP at 8–9 cmH$_2$O pressure, with resolution of obstructive sleep apnea and SW.

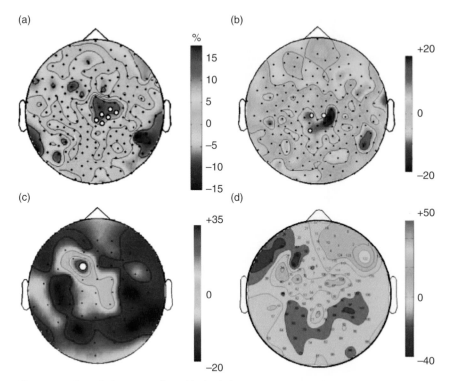

Figure 3.5 Cortical plasticity is reflected by local changes in SWA. In each panel regions with SWA increase are in red, while in blue are regions with SWA decrease. White circles indicate electrodes with significant SWA activity change. (a) Increased SWA after a rotation learning task. Six electrodes with significant differences from baseline located in the right sensorimotor area were found [3]. (b) Decreased SWA following left arm immobilization for one day was found in three electrodes in the right sensorimotor cortex [4]. (c) Increased SWA following rTMS of the left premotor cortex [5]. (d) Increased SWA at the right inferior frontal gyrus, symmetrical to Broca's area, in a stroke patient with expressive aphasia following 4 hours of speech therapy.

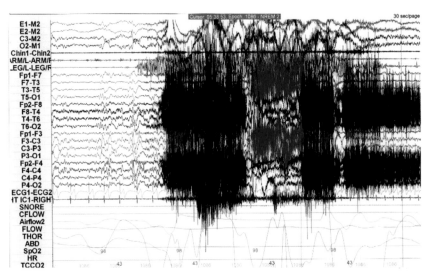

Figure 10.1 Nocturnal polysomnogram of 32-year-old man with history of SW/ST demonstrating an abrupt spontaneous arousal from non-REM stage N2 sleep as the record becomes suddenly obscured by muscular movement artifact. Tachycardia develops later during the arousal and the man subsequently left the bed and later reported dream recall of being in his son's house in a living room filled with red furniture and becoming convinced that "some disaster like a fire" was about to occur. He dreamed that he attempted to warn his wife when he, in fact, bolted from his bed and subsequently only slowly was convinced by the technologist that there was no real imminent danger. There is no epileptiform activity in the EEG.

Evaluation of the patient with EDS

A detailed history and physical examination are of key importance in evaluating the patient complaining of EDS. Important points of the sleep history that the clinician should document include, but are not limited to, total daily 24-hour sleep time, nightly and daily sleep and nap patterns, time to initial sleep onset, and number and duration of nocturnal awakenings. A sleep log in either narrative or graphical form may be used to characterize a patient's sleep further.

When reviewing a patient's sleep log in the workup of EDS, special attention is paid to the quantity, consistency, and continuity of reported sleep. The consistency of sleep–wake times provides insight into circadian and social pressures on the timing of sleep and may help identify causes of insufficient sleep. If the patient is unable to give a reliable history or nightly sleep times are in question, monitoring for several days with actigraphy (a wristwatch-like device that registers movement by the patient) may be useful in evaluating patterns of waking and sleep.

Thorough screening for primary sleep disorders includes assessment of the presence of snoring, witnessed apneas, symptoms of restless legs syndrome, periodic limb movements, and restless sleep or non-refreshing sleep. Medical conditions and alcohol or drug use can be significant contributors to EDS; if any of these are suspected, appropriate evaluation should ensue. Any chronic sedating medications should also be noted.

If a thorough history and physical examination raises suspicion of disorders such as periodic limb movements, obstructive sleep apnea, nocturnal seizure, or parasomnia, then nocturnal polysomnography (PSG) – overnight sleep study – may be indicated to either rule out sleep disturbances or to quantify their severity. This is typically related to sleep disorders that produce sleep fragmentation or sleep inefficiency including sleep-related breathing disorders, periodic limb movement disorder, REM sleep behavior disorder, other sleep-related movement disorders, parasomnias, or nocturnal seizures.

Several questionnaires have been developed to help clinicians screen for and evaluate patients for sleepiness and its impact on daily living. These questionnaires include, among others, the Epworth sleepiness scale (ESS) [4], the Stanford sleepiness scale [5], and the sleep–wake activity inventory [6]. The ESS is the most commonly used questionnaire because of its ease of use and its well-documented validity as a clinically relevant measure of sleepiness in conditions of pathological EDS [7–9].

Although ESS scores are not necessarily representative of true levels of sleepiness and the questionnaire is neither highly specific nor sensitive for the existence of pathological sleepiness, the ESS serves as a useful screen for patients who are severely sleepy [10]. In our experience it has also been a simple, quick, and low-cost method for following patient response to treatment. Given its ease of use and the high prevalence of sleepiness among the general population, we recommend administering the ESS in patients with complaints of excessive sleepiness [4].

The multiple sleep latency test (MSLT) provides a more objective quantification of sleepiness than questionnaires by objectively measuring the propensity to fall asleep. Please see Chapter 3: Neurophysiology and neuroimaging of human sleep for a more detailed review of this procedure. Essentially, this test measures the capacity to fall asleep and propensity for both early sleep onset and early rapid eye movement sleep (REM) onset. The MSLT has specificity limitations due to the variety of conditions that can produce an abnormal result. Nevertheless, following a thorough clinical evaluation, the MSLT is the primary tool for confirming some of the hypersomnias [1,11]. The MSLT consists of four or five 20-minute polysomnographically monitored daytime nap opportunities separated by 2-hour intervals; for the nap opportunities, the patient is reclined in a sleep laboratory bed in a dark room with instructions to fall asleep. The primary assessments made by the MSLT are the rapidity of sleep onset, which correlates to degree of sleepiness, and the occurrence of REM sleep if sleep occurs during the nap opportunity. REM sleep episodes (a period of sleep during which dreams occur) at or close to sleep onset are known as sleep-onset REM periods (SOREMPs). Sleep latencies in normal adults are often between 10 and 20 minutes; pathological sleepiness is manifested by a latency of less than 8 minutes [11,12]. The MSLT should be performed only after the patient has received an adequate amount of nocturnal sleep (approximately 8 hours per night for the typical adult) for a period of at least 2 weeks and immediately following a nocturnal polysomnogram to exclude other causes of EDS due to either sleep fragmentation or insufficient sleep. If the polysomnogram is positive for other causes of EDS, these conditions must be adequately treated before an evaluation of EDS with MSLT is pursued. Practicing clinicians should also be aware that commonly pre-scribed antidepressants can have profound effects on the MSLT by suppressing potential SOREMPs. There-fore, the decision regarding whether such medications should be tapered prior to MSLT should be made cooperatively with the patient, and include the risks of potentially worsening the psychiatric illness versus a confounded MSLT.

The maintenance of wakefulness test (MWT) is another diagnostic test in the sleep laboratory. Rather than evaluating the propensity to fall asleep (like the MSLT), the MWT assesses the capacity to maintain wakefulness while sedentary in a setting conducive to sleep during the patient's regular waking hours. This test is not generally used in the evaluation of hyper-somnias of central origin, rather it is used for safety assessment to evaluate the impact of treatment for sleep disorder-related EDS in specific occupations such as heavy equipment operators or airline pilots.

Behaviorally induced insufficient sleep

Insufficient sleep is the most common cause of EDS in Western culture. Although the exact prevalence is unclear, in the 2002 Sleep in America Poll conducted by the National Sleep Foundation [3], 37% of adults reported sleeping less than 7 hours a night on week-nights and 68% reported sleeping less than 8 hours. Of employed respondents to the 2008 Sleep in Amer-ica Poll, 44% reported sleeping less than 7 hours on work nights [13]. Although sleep requirements vary among individuals, these polls find that weeknight sleep is 2 hours less than that obtained on weekends for 18% of respondents. Of subjects describing this pattern across the week, 24% endorsed sleepiness impairing their performance at least a few days per week, and 40% with this pattern admitted driving when drowsy at least once per month for the previous year. This discrepancy between weeknight and week-end sleep times implies ongoing voluntary sleep restriction during the week with attempted sleep com-pensation on the weekends.

The number of hours of experimental sleep loss in normal volunteers is directly proportional to the degree of increased daytime sleepiness as assessed by the MSLT [14]. The effects of sleep deprivation may be cumulative [8], but this accumulated sleep debt may be countered by extending sleep time over sev-eral days [15]. Insufficient sleep may be due to

voluntary lifestyle choices, job or school demands, shift work, or poor sleep hygiene.

As much as 16% of the US workforce is engaged in shift work [16]. Some research has suggested that despite subjectively experiencing adequate sleep, shift workers sleep approximately 5 to 7 hours less per week when compared with diurnal workers [17]. Studies have consistently shown that workers who regularly work night shifts experience more disrupted sleep as well as sleepiness during waking hours, com-pared with day workers [18,19]. Moreover, the ten-dency to feel sleepy or to doze may be as great for a worker during the night shift as for a person with untreated narcolepsy [20].

Although insufficient sleep might be expected to lead to frank EDS, a constellation of other subject-ive complaints are more commonly seen, including tiredness, lack of energy, or fatigue. Decrements in attention, learning capacity, short-term memory, and psychomotor performance, with or without EDS, also may be present. Moreover, irritability, poor impulse control, or other forms of mood instability may exist alone or in combination with these features in individuals with insufficient sleep. While it is obvi-ous that complete sleep deprivation compromises performance and well-being, until the last decade an erroneous belief has persisted that people adapt to chronic sleep loss without significant compromise. This is being challenged by a rapidly expanding lit-erature suggesting a wide range of adverse medical, cognitive, and socioeconomic effects of sleep loss and untreated sleep disorders [21]. The effects of chronic-ally restricted sleep are often insidious and may be unrecognized by many patients. It has been demon-strated that reducing sleep duration to 6 hours per night for 2 weeks produces detriments in vigilance, attention, and concentration that are equivalent to 2 nights of complete sleep deprivation [22]. Interest-ingly, subjective ratings of sleepiness in this study increased acutely in response to sleep restriction, but minimal additional change was reported on subse-quent days, suggesting that subjects were unaware of their deteriorating neurobehavioral functioning, per-haps explaining why the impact of chronic sleep restriction is misperceived as relatively benign.

While it may seem obvious, education and coun-seling regarding good sleep habits is the first-line treatment for insufficient sleep (Box 9.1). Many patients with behaviorally induced insufficient sleep are surprised to hear that they should be sleeping 7.5

Box 9.1 Healthy sleep habits for people with behaviorally induced insufficient sleep

1. Stay in bed for 8 hours per night
2. Maintain a dark, quiet, comfortable sleep environment (without television or music during sleep)
3. Go to bed and wake up at the same time 7 nights per week
4. Optimize bright light exposure in first few hours of the morning
5. Avoid bright light and stimulating activities (stressful activities, computer use, television, video games, etc.) in the few hours before bedtime
6. Use the bedroom for sleep and sex only
7. Obtain regular exercise, but complete it 3 hours or more before bedtime
8. Avoid caffeine for 5 hours before bedtime
9. Avoid nicotine and alcohol for 3 hours before bedtime

---

to 8 hours per night or more. Many struggle with competing social obligations and may be under tremendous pressure to sleep an inadequate duration. Despite presenting with a complaint of excessive sleepiness, some may argue or resist recommendations to increase sleep time and improve consistency in the timing of sleep. Others need only to be reminded that sleep is essential to well-being and it needs to be prioritized more highly among their other obligations. Shift workers with unavoidable insufficient sleep and concomitant EDS may benefit from modafinil, which has been approved by the Food and Drug Administration (FDA) for treatment of EDS in shift work sleep disorder.

Narcolepsy

Narcolepsy is the most clearly understood of the central hypersomnia syndromes. It is characterized by profound EDS and is associated with cataplexy, sleep paralysis, hypnopompic or hypnagogic hallucinations, automatic behavior, and disrupted sleep. Narcolepsy is rare in all populations with reported prevalences ranging from 0.02% to 0.18% with lower prevalence in Israel and higher reported prevalence in Japan [1]. Symptoms usually arise in adolescence or young adulthood and rarely as early as age 5, although symptom onset can be delayed until the 6th or 7th decade of life.

Narcolepsy results from dysfunction within the hypothalamic hypocretin (orexin) system in both animal models and humans. While mice and canine models of narcolepsy are associated with hypocretin ligand knockout or receptor gene mutations [23,24], genetic abnormalities in the hypocretin system are extremely rare in humans. About 90% of patients with unequivocal narcolepsy with cataplexy have low or undetectable levels of hypocretin in their cerebrospinal fluid – a finding which is quite specific to narcolepsy [25,26]. Human leukocyte antigen (HLA) subtype DQB1*0602 has a strong, but non-specific association with narcolepsy with cataplexy. Nearly all patients with cataplexy have this subtype, while it is found in 12–38% of the general population, across various races. These and other immunological associations along with the age of onset and finding of postmortem destruction of hypothalamic hypocretin-producing cells have led to the theory that narcolepsy may arise from an autoimmune process.

The routine diagnosis of narcolepsy is based on a clinical history of excessive daytime sleepiness occurring almost daily for more than 3 months with a formal workup that excludes other potential etiologies for EDS and a mean sleep latency of less than 8 minutes with two or more sleep onset REM periods on the MSLT. Narcolepsy is categorized as either with cataplexy or without cataplexy. Cataplexy is defined as a discrete episode of sudden and transient bilateral loss of voluntary muscle tone triggered by emotion [1].

Low CSF hypocretin is far more specific than the MSLT for the diagnosis of narcolepsy [27]. HLA subtyping is less invasive and more readily available, but grossly non-specific given the prevalence of this subtype in the general population. The clinical utility of HLA DQB1*0602 subtyping is limited to the fact that in the absence of cataplexy, a negative result very strongly suggests normal hypocretin function and obviates the need for CSF hypocretin evaluation. Currently these assays are not considered standard in the diagnosis of narcolepsy, but ongoing efforts are clarifying their potential clinical utility.

Excessive sleepiness

EDS in narcoleptic patients manifests as an increased propensity to fall asleep in relaxed or sedentary situations or a struggle to avoid sleeping in these situations. These so-called "sleep attacks" are often mistakenly believed to be unique to narcolepsy, but

Table 9.1 Average multiple sleep latency test (MSLT) results by disorder

	Mean Sleep Latency (Minutes)	Number of naps with REM sleep
Narcolepsy	3.1	2 or more
Idiopathic hypersomnia	6.2	<2
Obstructive sleep apnea	10.6	0
Normal controls	11*	0

Note: *30% of normal controls have a mean sleep latency less than 8 minutes.
Source: Adapted from ICSD-2 [1] and AASM MSLT [11] practice guidelines.

actually represent sleepiness that is identical to that of other sleep disorders such as untreated obstructive sleep apnea or sleep deprivation [17]. Epworth sleepiness scale scores of ≥15 are common in untreated patients [4,17,20]. The irresistible urge to sleep commonly occurs in inappropriate or dangerous situations and thus produces significant social and occupational dysfunction. While the ICSD-2 specifies an MSLT mean sleep latency of less than 8 minutes as support for the diagnosis of narcolepsy, narcolepsy patients commonly evidence much shorter mean sleep latencies of less than 5 minutes (Table 9.1).

Cataplexy

Cataplexy is a partial or complete transient bilateral weakness in voluntary muscles in response to strong emotion. This often manifests as bilateral ptosis, head drooping, slurred speech, or dropping things from the hand. It less commonly results in total body paralysis or collapse and injuries are rare as effort and time usually permit successful redirection or protection of oneself. Cataplexy may be associated with a variety of emotions, but is most reliably associated with humorous thoughts, laughing, or joking [17]. Events last from a few seconds up to 3 minutes but occasionally continue longer [28]. Although alert and oriented during the event, if unable to move or speak during an episode of cataplexy, some patients may ultimately lapse into sleep given the narcoleptic's propensity to sleep in sedentary situations. Unlike the other features of narcolepsy, cataplexy is very specific to narcolepsy.

The first experience of cataplexy is usually within a few months of the onset of excessive sleepiness, but the onset of cataplexy can occur many years after the initial onset of sleepiness [28]. Additionally, cataplexy severity can increase over time.

Hypnagogic or hypnopompic hallucinations

These phenomena may be visual, tactile, auditory, or multi-sensory events, usually brief but occasionally continuing for a few minutes, that occur at the transition from wakefulness to sleep (hypnagogic) or from sleep to wakefulness (hypnopompic). Hallucinations may contain elements of dream sleep and consciousness combined and are often bizarre or disturbing to patients. As with excessive sleepiness, these hallucinatory experiences are not specific to narcolepsy, and can be seen with other conditions of excessive sleepiness. Additionally, these phenomena are not necessarily pathological, are common in the general population, and may be reported more frequently in individuals with mood, anxiety, or psychotic illness [29].

Sleep paralysis

Sleep paralysis is the inability to move, lasting from a few seconds to minutes, during the transition from sleep to wakefulness or from wakefulness to sleep. Episodes of sleep paralysis may alarm patients, particularly those who experience the sensation of being unable to breathe. This occurs because accessory respiratory muscles may not be active during these episodes; however, diaphragmatic activity continues and air exchange remains adequate. Sleep paralysis, like excessive sleepiness and hypnagogic and hypnopompic hallucinations, is not specific to narcolepsy and is often seen with various disorders that cause excessive sleepiness (sleep apnea or chronic sleep deprivation). Additionally, sleep paralysis is not necessarily indicative of pathology, but may be more common in patients with mood and anxiety disorders [30].

Treatment of narcolepsy

The most significant impact on the treatment of narcolepsy in recent history has been the characterization of the effect of sodium oxybate (the sodium salt of γ-hydroxybutyrate) on cataplexy, daytime sleepiness, and nocturnal sleep fragmentation. Sodium oxybate's sleep-promoting effect appears to be largely mediated via gamma-aminobutyric acid (GABA) receptor subtype B agonism, but the mechanism by which it improves cataplexy and EDS is unknown. Although the use of low-dose sodium oxybate in treating narcolepsy has been studied for 35 years, it has only been in the past 10 years that thorough investigations in the form of multi-center trials have been conducted. These trials have extensively characterized the dose–response impact of sodium oxybate on the enhancement of nocturnal sleep, improvement of cataplexy, and improvement of EDS [31,32]. These findings support the view that sodium oxybate may be the optimal first-line agent for the treatment of narcolepsy with cataplexy.

While sodium oxybate has demonstrated its efficacy in treating all symptoms of narcolepsy, alerting agents provide a critical adjunctive component in the treatment of patients with narcolepsy, specifically for the treatment of EDS. Sodium oxybate is a controlled substance and distribution is restricted to a single central pharmacy. Appropriate patient selection and monitoring are essential as side-effects include central nervous system depression, and potential for diversion or abuse.

Although stimulants remain the first-line agents for the treatment of EDS in patients with narcolepsy, in our clinical practice they are now considered a useful addition to sodium oxybate in patients who have narcolepsy with cataplexy. Common practice is to combine two agents when one agent does not adequately ameliorate symptoms. The use of modafinil as an adjunct to sodium oxybate has been shown to provide significantly greater improvement in measures of EDS symptoms than either agent alone [33]. Some patients may wish to avoid medications and attempt to take extra naps during the day, but napping alone is rarely successful in alleviating EDS enough to function at or near normal capacity. While alerting agents may not eliminate daytime symptoms, they have been shown to produce substantial improvement in EDS associated with narcolepsy [34].

Modafinil is a novel alerting agent that promotes wakefulness primarily via its dopaminergic effect [35]. Similar to traditional stimulants, modafinil appears to function as a dopamine transporter inhibitor, but unlike the amphetamines, it has a reduced receptor affinity and it does not induce dopamine release. This difference in activity may account for the improved tolerability of modafinil over traditional stimulants as well as its diminished

potential for street use, abuse, and addiction by illicit users [36].

In addition to modafinil, commonly used stimulants include methylphenidate, dextro-amphetamine, and methamphetamine. Side-effects are not uncommon with any stimulant or alerting agent. Agitation, anxiety, tremor, and palpitations are just a few of the commonly reported side-effects associated with traditional stimulants. Some patients may report a rebound hypersomnia as the dose wears off, and tolerance may occur with time. Traditional stimulants are still an important resource in the arsenal of medications for the treatment of narcolepsy, but in our clinical practice they have become second-line agents behind sodium oxybate and/or modafinil for treatment of EDS associated with narcolepsy (see Table 9.2).

While modafinil and traditional stimulants can ameliorate EDS, these agents impart no beneficial impact on cataplexy. However, drugs other than sodium oxybate can be used effectively to treat cataplexy. While not rigorously studied in controlled trials, agents which exhibit affinity for CNS norepinephrine receptors have been in common use for decades as anticataplectic agents. Specifically, tricyclic antidepressants, mixed serotonin-norepinephrine reuptake inhibitors, and more selective serotonin reuptake inhibitors with parent compound or active metabolite affinity for noradrenergic receptors (e.g. fluoxetine) can be effective in the treatment of cataplexy. Frequently patients with narcolepsy experience EDS many months in advance of the development of cataplexy. At this early stage of disease development the patient may present to a physician with a complaint of "tiredness" coupled with diminished motivation and reduced energy and therefore be misdiagnosed with an atypical form of depression. Treating such a patient with antidepressants for presumed depression bears the risk of masking the later development of cataplexy, due to the anticataplectic effect of the antidepressant, and delaying (potentially substantially) the accurate diagnosis of narcolepsy.

Idiopathic hypersomnia

Idiopathic hypersomnia (previously labeled "idiopathic CNS hypersomnia") is a primary disorder of EDS that has historically been given as a diagnosis of exclusion to individuals who complain of EDS when other disorders that cause hypersomnolence have not been found or clearly characterized. There are

Table 9.2 Common alerting agents for the treatment of EDS

Agent	Receptor	Half life t½ (hours)	tmax (hours)	Dose	Side-effects
Modafinil	Dopamine agonist	15	2–4	100–400 mg once daily or divided	Headache, nausea, anxiety, irritability
Amphetamines	Dopamine agonist	10 SR: 15	2 SR: 8–10	5–60 mg divided	Headache, anxiety, irritability, hypertension, palpitations, appetite suppression, tremor, insomnia
Methylphenidate	Dopamine agonist	4 SR: 8–10	2 SR: 5	5–60 mg divided	
Pemoline*	Dopamine agonist	12	2–4	18.75–112.5 mg, daily or divided	As above, but milder. Potentially hepatotoxic – frequent liver function monitoring required
Gamma-hydroxybutyrate	Impact on sleep mediated by GABA-B receptor agonist effect	2	1	6–9 g divided nightly	Sedation, nausea

SR = sustained release.
Note: *Due to hepatotoxicity, pemoline is unavailable in many markets.

numerous documented cases of patients having been misdiagnosed as having idiopathic hypersomnia when in fact they suffered from other disorders that cause EDS, such as narcolepsy without cataplexy, delayed sleep phase syndrome, and upper airway resistance syndrome [37].

True idiopathic hypersomnia is believed to be less common than narcolepsy, but estimating prevalence is difficult because there had been no strict diagnostic criteria and there continue to be no specific biological markers. The first symptoms tend to occur in late adolescence or early adulthood. No cause for idiopathic hypersomnia has been clearly identified, but viral illnesses, including those that may lead to Guillain-Barré syndrome, hepatitis, mononucleosis, and atypical viral pneumonia, may be related to the onset of EDS in a subset of patients [27]. EDS may occur as part of the acute illness but persist after the other symptoms subside. HLA-Cw2 and HLA-DR11 have been noted to occur with increased frequency in some rare familial cases [38].

Most patients with idiopathic hypersomnia have neither a family history nor an obvious associated viral illness. Autonomic nervous system dysfunction has been associated with some of these cases, including orthostatic hypotension, syncope, vascular headaches, and peripheral vascular complaints. Little is known

about the pathophysiology of idiopathic hypersomnia, and no animal model is available for study. Neurochemical studies using CSF have suggested that patients with idiopathic hypersomnia may have altered noradrenergic system function [39–41].

Clinically, the presentation of idiopathic hypersomnia varies among individuals. It is not uncommon for idiopathic hypersomnia to be mistaken for narcolepsy. Because the predominant symptom in both disorders is EDS and age at onset is similar for the two diseases, it is understandable that one may be mistaken for the other. However, with careful history-taking and diagnostic testing, essential differences between the disorders become apparent. Patients with idiopathic hypersomnia present with EDS but without cataplexy or significant nocturnal sleep disruption [42]. The sleepiness they complain of typically interferes with normal daily activities, and occupational and social functioning may be severely affected by sleepiness. Nocturnal sleep tends to be long and unrefreshing, and patients are usually difficult to awaken in the morning. They may become irritable or even abusive in response to others' efforts to rouse them. In some patients, this difficulty may be substantial and include confusion, disorientation, and poor motor coordination, a condition called "sleep drunkenness" or excessive sleep inertia [43]. These patients often take naps, which may be prolonged but usually are unrefreshing, in contrast to classically refreshing naps in narcolepsy. No amount of sleep ameliorates the EDS. "Micro-sleeps," with or without automatic behavior, may occur throughout the day. This diagnosis is distinctly different from that of major depression, as patients with idiopathic hypersomnia lack the generalized anhedonia associated with a major depressive episode and are much sleepier on objective testing than the patient with an atypical depression (see Section VI: Sleep disturbance in psychiatric illness).

Polysomnographic studies of patients with idiopathic CNS hypersomnia usually reveal shortened initial sleep latency, increased total sleep time, high sleep efficiency, and normal sleep architecture. By the ICSD-2 definition, mean sleep latency on the MSLT is less than 8 minutes. Unlike narcolepsy, this shortened sleep latency is associated with less than two sleep-onset REM periods [1]. Idiopathic hypersomnia is subcategorized as being associated either "with long sleep time" or "without long sleep time." Patients with habitual sleep time of greater than 10 hours in a 24-hour period are considered in the former category and those with less than 10 hours in the latter. As with narcolepsy, other disorders that produce EDS (such as insufficient sleep, sleep-related breathing disorders, periodic limb movement disorder, other sleep fragmenting disorders, circadian rhythm disorders, and psychiatric illnesses) must be ruled out before the diagnosis of idiopathic hypersomnia is made.

Lifestyle and behavioral modifications, including good sleep hygiene, are appropriate first steps. As with narcolepsy, treatment with traditional stimulants or modafinil is usually necessary and often provides some benefit. Unfortunately, response to these treatments is often unsatisfactory. None of these medications are FDA approved for the treatment of idiopathic hypersomnia.

Recurrent hypersomnias
Kleine-Levin syndrome

The Kleine-Levin syndrome is a form of recurrent hypersomnia that occurs primarily in adolescents [44], with a 4:1 male predominance [45]. It is characterized by discrete episodes of EDS associated with a striking change in mentation and behavior that typically includes hyperphagia, aggressiveness, and hyper-sexuality. These episodes may last days to weeks and may be separated by asymptomatic periods of weeks or months. During asymptomatic periods patients are completely without EDS or the associated behavioral abnormalities. During symptomatic periods, afflicted individuals sleep up to 18 hours per day and are usually profoundly drowsy (often to the degree of stupor), confused, and irritable when they are awake. During these episodes, polysomnographic studies show long total sleep time with high sleep efficiency and decreased slow-wave sleep. MSLT studies demonstrate short sleep latencies and sleep-onset REM periods [46].

The etiology of this syndrome remains obscure. Symptomatic cases of Kleine-Levin syndrome associated with structural brain lesions have been reported, but most cases are idiopathic. Single photon emission computed tomography has demonstrated hypoperfusion in the thalamus in one patient and in the non-dominant frontal lobe in another [47]. Treatment with stimulant medication may improve alertness, but does little for the striking and more problematic neuropsychological symptoms. Neuroleptics and anti-depressants are not effective [45]. The effects of treatment with lithium, valproic acid, and carbamazepine have been variable and generally unsatisfactory and randomized controlled trials are absent [45]. Arguably, family and patient education is the single most important treatment to provide for KLS sufferers at this time. Fortunately, in most cases, episodes become less frequent over time and eventually subside.

Menstrual-related hypersomnia

Another form of recurrent hypersomnia is menstrual-related periodic hypersomnia, in which EDS occurs during the week preceding menstruation then abruptly abates with the onset of menses [48,49]. The prevalence of this syndrome has not been well characterized and very little research has been conducted thus far. The etiology is not known, but presumably the symptoms are related to hormonal changes. Sustained resolution has been reported by blocking ovulation with estrogen and progesterone (birth control pills) [50].

Idiopathic recurring stupor

Another less commonly seen form of the recurring hypersomnias is idiopathic recurring stupor. Numerous cases have been reported in which, in the absence of obvious cause, individuals are subject to stuporous episodes lasting from hours to days. This syndrome affects predominantly middle-aged males.

The individuals experience normal levels of alertness between episodes, and the episodes occur unpredictably. Elevated plasma and CSF levels of endozepine-4, an endogenous ligand with affinity for the benzodiazepine recognition site at the GABA-A receptor, have been found in several of these patients [51]. EEG data collected during symptomatic episodes have shown fast background activity in the 13–16 Hz range. Administration of flumazenil, a benzodiazepine antagonist, has produced transient awakening with normalization of the EEG [52]. In some cases, the episodes resolved spontaneously after several years. Similar cases have been reported in children [53].

Other hypersomnias of central origin
Nervous system disorders

Patients with disorders of the central or peripheral nervous system often complain of EDS. In some chronic diseases of neurological origin, EDS may be the predominant complaint. EDS may be a dominant clinical feature in many toxic or metabolic encephalopathic processes. Structural brain lesions, including strokes, tumors, cysts, abscesses, hematomas, vascular malformations, hydrocephalus, and multiple sclerosis plaques, are known to produce EDS. It appears that somnolence may result either from direct involvement of discrete brain regions or as a consequence of impaired sleep continuity (for example, nocturnal seizure activity or secondary sleep-related breathing disorder).

Head trauma and encephalitis

Patients who experience head trauma or have been afflicted with encephalitis may have EDS as a chronic sequela. Victims of "encephalitis lethargica" with associated EDS, described by von Economo in the early twentieth century, were found to have lesions at the junction of the midbrain and the diencephalon. Additionally, post-traumatic narcolepsy with cataplexy is well documented [54]. EDS may be seen in patients with epilepsy, due to medication effects or nocturnal seizure activity [55]. EDS may be associated with numerous infectious agents affecting the CNS, including bacteria, viruses, fungi, and parasites. Perhaps the best known is trypanosomiasis, which is called "sleeping sickness" because of the prominent hypersomnia. Certain inflammatory mediators have been shown to cause sleepiness. These agents have been hypothesized to be the origin of EDS in acute

infectious illness, in which EDS occurs without direct invasion of the CNS. These mediators include cytokines, interferon, interleukins, and tumor necrosis factor [56]. EDS may also persist chronically after certain viral infections [57].

Neurodegenerative disorders

Various neurodegenerative disorders, including Parkinson's disease, Alzheimer's disease, other dementias of varied causes, and multiple system atrophy, all commonly have sleep disruption and EDS as manifestations [58–60]. Patients with neuromuscular disorders or peripheral neuropathies have an increased incidence of sleep-related breathing disorders (central or obstructive apnea), pain, and PLMS, and may develop EDS as a result of disrupted sleep from these associated conditions [61]. Patients with myotonic dystrophy often suffer from EDS, even in the absence of sleep-related breathing disorders [62].

Chronic medical conditions and EDS
Fibromyalgia and rheumatoid diseases

Chronic medical conditions may also cause significant sleep disturbance and manifest clinically as either EDS or fatigue. Patients with fibromyalgia frequently characterize their sleep as being restless, light, and unrefreshing [63]. These patients often have an alpha-frequency EEG coincident with delta-frequency sleep, or "alpha-delta" sleep [64]. Alpha activity is characteristic of the EEG pattern seen during quiet wakefulness with the eyes closed and does not typically occur during deep sleep (when delta activity occurs) in normal subjects. This EEG finding has also been reported to occur in rheumatoid arthritis and chronic fatigue syndrome [65,66]. Researchers have found a positive correlation between the frequency of alpha-delta sleep and severity of overnight pain in patients with fibromyalgia, and an inverse correlation between frequency of alpha-delta sleep and subjective sleep depth and/or refreshing sleep [67,68].

Congestive heart failure

Other chronic medical conditions may have a significant impact on sleep continuity and on daytime function. Patients with severe congestive heart failure (CHF) have highly fragmented sleep, with frequent arousals and adverse sleep changes associated with the clinical manifestation of CHF [69]. More than half of patients with heart failure suffer from sleep-related breathing disorders [70]. A recent study showed that at least 21% of patients with congestive heart failure complained of EDS, and 48% complained of being awake more than 30 minutes during the course of the night [71]. Screening for sleep-related breathing complaints, referral, and treatment of any central or obstructive sleep apnea often improves alertness and well-being in these patients.

Cancer

Patients with cancer also have an elevated likelihood of EDS. Studies indicate prevalence rates of 54–68% for "feeling drowsy" and 21–40% for being "overly sleepy" in this population [72,73]. Causes of EDS in this population may be related to an increased risk of primary sleep disorders due to age alone (the average age at onset of cancer is 55 years) or a complex combination of etiologies. These include insufficient sleep due to insomnia, depression, or pain; disruption or erratic hormone secretion due to the malignancy or chemotherapy, with subsequent sleep disruption or shortened sleep periods; effects of cytokines and inflammatory mediators induced by cancer cells, biotherapy, or radiotherapy; and side-effects from chemotherapy or other adjunctive medications [74].

Endocrine disorders

Patients with chronic endocrine disorders may complain of EDS. Sleepiness is a well-recognized symptom of hypothyroidism. Additionally, hypothyroidism has been reported as a risk factor for the development of obstructive sleep apnea [75]. It is not clear in some patients with hypothyroidism whether the sleepiness they experience is due to a direct effect of the hypothyroid state or to a co-existing SRBD. Patients with acromegaly have also been shown to have an increased prevalence of sleep apnea, with reported rates from 39% to 58.8% [76,77]. On the other hand, patients with growth hormone deficiency consistently report low energy, fatigue, and impaired sleep quality [78].

Psychiatric disorders

Many psychiatric disorders and their treatments contribute to complaints of sleepiness and fatigue. The diagnostic criteria of many psychiatric disorders include fatigue, decreased vigilance, or sleepiness with the stipulation that these symptoms must not be due

---

Box 9.2 Symptom overlap between depression and sleep loss

Depression symptoms that may be associated with sleep loss
Decreased mood
Weight or appetite changes
Insomnia
Decreased activity
Fatigue/poor energy
Poor attention or concentration

Depression symptoms more specific to depression
Anhedonia
Worthlessness
Suicidal thoughts

---

to a primary sleep disorder; thus, attention to both psychiatric and potential sleep disorders provides the most comprehensive and appropriate care in the excessively sleepy patient (Box 9.2).

While it is true that tiredness, fatigue, and/or lack of energy are reported by a majority of patients with major depression, evaluation of EDS with subjective rating scales and objective measures suggests that frank sleepiness or a high sleep propensity may be less common than the complaint of fatigue or lack of energy [79]. Only a few studies have evaluated objective measures of sleepiness, such as the MSLT, in depression. These produce somewhat conflicting results, but overall suggest that most patients with depression maintain a normal level of daytime alertness and sleep propensity on MSLT [80]. Decreased sleep latency, shortened REM latency, and increased REM percentages are reported on overnight polysomnography in both sleep-deprived, non-depressed patients and suicidal patients [81,82]. Other studies suggest that insomnia, but not sleepiness or fatigue, correlates with thoughts of suicide, plans for suicide, or attempted suicide [83–85].

Medications and sleepiness

Side-effects from some psychiatric medications and non-prescription substances must be considered in the evaluation of a patient complaining of EDS. Special consideration should be given to sedating antidepressants, antipsychotics, antiepileptics, hypnotics, or sleep aids. Many psychotropic medications involve antidopaminergic, antiadrenergic, anticholinergic, or antihistaminic activity, all of which can contribute to sleepiness or fatigue. While side-effects are typically worse at drug initiation or during dose escalations, patients on stable dosing may continue to have sedation or fatigue related to their medication regimen. Many of the medications used in psychiatry have half-lives which lead to drug accumulation, and it is thus not surprising that even medications used at bedtime can produce EDS, as daytime serum levels of sedating medications can be many times higher than the maximum serum concentration immediately after drug initiation. For shorter-acting agents, one potential clue to the presence of medication-induced EDS is a maximum sleepiness in the morning, with improved alertness over the course of the day. A study evaluating side-effects of antidepressants found that 40% of 117 patients deemed to have a successful response to their antidepressant had symptoms of persistent fatigue or sleepiness [86]. It is difficult to determine the proportion of these symptoms due to the underlying disorder versus a medication side-effect; however, reductions in fatigue or sleepiness upon medication withdrawal suggest a significant component directly attributable to medications for some patients. Antihypertensives, specifically alpha 2 receptor agonists, beta-blockers, and alpha 1 receptor antagonists, should be considered as well, as these medications have been consistently reported to cause somnolence. Antiarrhythmic medications also may cause sedation. Stimulants or other medications causing insomnia, or upon withdrawal, may in turn contribute to EDS or fatigue complaints.

Counseling the patient with excessive sleepiness

Sleepiness while driving accounts for a significant proportion of traffic fatalities and injuries and is recognized as a legitimate public health concern. Sleepy drivers have reduced vigilance and response times regardless of the cause of their sleepiness. Remaining awake for a long day of 17–19 hours can result in neurocognitive impairment comparable to a blood alcohol level of 0.05% [87], which is considered hazardous and beyond the legal driving limit in many countries. One night of sleep deprivation combined with the normal circadian drive to sleep can result in neurocognitive impairment beyond that seen with a blood alcohol content of 0.08% or greater – considered the legal limit for driving while intoxicated in the USA [87]. The risks of driving while sleepy should be explained to all patients with EDS regardless

of cause or severity and they should be instructed to take appropriate measures to eliminate driving risks (e.g. avoid driving while sleepy; if driving and sleepy, pull over and take a nap, defer driving to another driver, or use appropriate alerting agents when indicated).

Conclusion

Excessive daytime sleepiness is a common problem in the general population that is frequently overlooked by clinicians of all specialties. In the psychiatric patient population, EDS can be a nebulous complaint that seems to cloud the overall clinical picture. It is important that the clinician evaluate a complaint of EDS distinct from the presenting psychiatric problem. There is obviously interplay between psychiatric disorders and EDS, which may make such a distinction difficult. However, appropriate workup, accurate diagnosis, and a suitable treatment plan often provides patients suffering from EDS with substantial improvement in quality of life. Timely referral to a sleep medicine specialist should be considered. While insufficient sleep is the most common cause of excessive daytime sleepiness in the general population, the other sources of hypersomnia of central origin outlined in this chapter are much less common, but must be considered nonetheless. Incorporating careful assessment that includes the broad differential diagnosis of EDS and provides effective treatment options for patients with excessive daytime sleepiness will result in the most comprehensive and appropriate care.

References

1. Sateia MJ, ed. *International Classification of Sleep Disorders: diagnostic and coding manual*, 2nd ed. Westchester, IL: American Academy of Sleep Medicine; 2005.

2. Ohayon MM, Priest RG, Zulley J, Smirne S, Paiva T. Prevalence of narcolepsy symptomatology and diagnosis in the European general population. *Neurology*. 2002;**58**(12):1826–1833.

3. National Sleep Foundation. Sleep in America Poll, 2002. http://www.sleepfoundation.org.

4. Johns MW. A new method of measuring sleepiness: the Epworth sleepiness scale. *Sleep*. 1991;**14**(6): 540–545.

5. Hoddes E, Zarcone V, Smythe H, Phillips R, Dement WC. Quantification of sleepiness: a new approach. *Psychophysiology*. 1973;**10**(4):431–436.

6. Rosenthal L, Roehr TA, Roth T. The sleep-wake activity inventory: a self-report measure of daytime sleepiness. *Biol Psychiatry*. 1993;**34**(11):810–820.

7. Richardson G, Carskadon M, Flagg W, et al. Excessive daytime sleepiness in man: multiple sleep latency measurements in narcoleptic and control subjects. *Electroencepholgr Clin Neurophysiol*. 1978;**45**(5):621–627.

8. Chua LWY, Yu NC, Golish JA, et al. Epworth sleepiness scale and the multiple sleep latency test: dilemma of the elusive link. *Sleep*. 1998;**21**(Suppl):184.

9. US Modafinil in Narcolepsy Multicenter Study Group. Randomized trial of modafinil for the treatment of pathological somnolence in narcolepsy. *Ann Neurol*. 1998;**43**(1):88–97.

10. Johns MW, Hocking B. Daytime sleepiness and sleep habits of Australian workers. *Sleep*. 1997;**20**(10):844–849.

11. Review by the MSLT and MWT Task Force of the Standards of Practice Committee of the American Academy of Sleep Medicine. *Sleep*. 2005;**28**(1):123–144.

12. Carskadon MA, Dement WC. Cumulative effects of sleep restriction on daytime sleepiness. *Psychophysiology*. 1981;**18**(2):107–113.

13. Sleep in America Poll, 2008. http://www.sleepfoundation.org

14. Rosenthal L, Roehrs TA, Rosen A, Roth T. Level of sleepiness and total sleep time following various time in bed conditions. *Sleep*. 1993;**16**(3):226–232.

15. Roehrs TA, Shore E, Papineau K, Rosenthal L, Roth T. A two-week sleep extension in sleepy normals. *Sleep*. 1996;**19**(7):576–582.

16. Beers T. Flexible schedules and shift work: replacing the '9-to-5' workday? *Monthly Labor Rev*. 2000:33–40.

17. Monk TH. Shift work. In: Kryger MH, Roth T, Dement WC, eds. *Priniciples and practices of sleep medicine*, 3rd ed. Philadelphia, PA: WB Saunders; 2000:602–603.

18. Akerstedt T. Sleepiness as a consequence of shift work. *Sleep*. 1988;**11**(1):17–34.

19. Budnick LD, Lerman SE, Baker TL, Jones H, Czeisler CA. Sleep and alertness in a 12-hour rotating shift work environment. *J Occup Med*. 1994;**36**(12):1295–1300.

20. Czeisler CA, Walsh JK, Roth T, et al. Modafinil for excessive sleepiness associated with shift-work sleep disorder. *New Engl J Med*. 2005;**353**(5):476–486.

21. Colton HR, Altevogt BM, eds. *Sleep disorders and sleep deprivation: an unmet public health problem. Committee on Sleep Medicine and Research*. The National Academies Press; 2006:55–172.

22. Van Dongen HP, Maislin G, Mullington JM, Dinges DF. The cumulative cost of additional wakefulness: dose-response effects on neurobehavioral functions and sleep physiology from chronic sleep restriction and total sleep deprivation. *Sleep*. 2003;**26**(2):117–126.

23. Chemelli RM, Willie JT, Sinton CM, et al. Narcolepsy in orexin knockout mice: Molecular genetics of sleep regulation. *Cell*. 1999;**98**(4):437–451.

24. Lin L, Faraco J, Li R, et al. The sleep disorder canine narcolepsy is caused by a mutation in the hypocretin (orexin) receptor 2 gene. *Cell*. 1999;**98**(3):365–376.

25. Mignot E, Nishino S. Emerging therapies in narcolepsy-cataplexy. *Sleep*. 2005;**28**(6):754–763.

26. Nishino S, Ripley B, Overeem S, Lammers GJ, Mignot E. Hypocretin (orexin) deficiency in human narcolepsy. *Lancet*. 2000;**355**(9197):39–40.

27. Black JE, Brooks SN, Nishino S. Narcolepsy and syndromes of primary excessive daytime somnolence. *Sem Neurol*. 2004;**24**(3):271–282.

28. Honda Y. Clinical features of narcolepsy: Japanese experiences. In: Honda Y, Juji T, eds. *HLA in narcolepsy*. Berlin: Springer-Verlag; 1988:24–57.

29. Ohayon MM, Priest RG, Caulet M, Guilleminault C. Hypnogogic and hypnopompic hallucinations: pathological phenomena? *Br J Psychiatry*. 1996; **169**(4):459–467.

30. Ohayon MM, Zulley J, Guilleminault C, Smirne S. Prevalence and pathologic associations of sleep paralysis in the general population. *Neurology*. 1999; **52**(6):1194–1200.

31. Mamelak M, Black J, Monplaisir J, Ristanovic R. A pilot study on the effects of sodium oxybate on sleep architecture and daytime alertness in narcolepsy. *Sleep*. 2004;**27**(7):1327–1334.

32. US Xyrem in Narcolepsy Multi-center Study Group. A randomized, double blind, placebo-controlled multicenter trial comparing the effects of three doses of orally administered sodium oxybate with placebo for the treatment of narcolepsy. *Sleep*. 2002;**25**(1):42–49.

33. Black J. Nightly administration of sodium oxybate is effective for the treatment of excessive daytime sleepiness in narcolepsy. *Sleep*. 2005;**28**:A218(abstract).

34. Mitler MM, Aldrich MS, Koob GF, Zarcone VP. Narcolepsy and its treatment with stimulants: ASDA standards of practice. *Sleep*. 1994;**17**(4):352–371.

35. Wisor JP, Ericksson KS. Dopaminergic-adrenergic interactions in the wake promoting mechanism of modafinil. *Neuroscience*. 2005;**132**(4):1027–1034.

36. US Modafinil in Narcolepsy Multicenter Study Group. Randomized trial of modafinil as a treatment for the excessive daytime somnolence of narcolepsy. *Neurology*. 2000;**54**(5):1166–1175.

37. Guilleminault C, Stoohs R, Clerk A, Cetel M, Maistros P. A cause of excessive daytime sleepiness:

The upper airway resistance syndrome. *Chest.* 1993;**104**(3):781–787.

38. Montplaisir J, Poirier G. HLA in disorders of excessive sleepiness without cataplexy in Canada. In: Honda Y, Juji T, eds. *HLA in narcolepsy.* Berlin: Springer-Verlag; 1988:186.

39. Montplaisir J, De Champlain J, Young SN, et al. Narcolepsy and idiopathic hypersomnia: biogenic amines and related compounds in CSF. *Neurology.* 1982;**32**(11):1299–1302.

40. Faull KF, Guilleminault C, Berger PA, Barchas JD. Cerebrospinal fluid monoamine metabolites in narcolepsy and hypersomnia. *Ann Neurol.* 1983; **13**(3):258–263.

41. Faull KF, Thiemann S, King RJ, Guilleminault C. Monoamine interactions in narcolepsy and hypersomnia: a preliminary report. *Sleep.* 1986; **9**(1 Pt 2):246–249.

42. Billiard M, Dauvillies Y. Idiopathic hypersomnia. *Sleep Med Rev.* 2001;**5**(5):351–360.

43. Roth B, Nevsimalova S, Rechtschaffen A. Hypersomnia with "sleep drunkenness." *Arch Gen Psychiatry.* 1972;**26**(5):456–462.

44. Critchley M. The syndrome of hypersomnia and periodical megaphagia in the adult male (Kleine-Levin): what is its natural course? *Rev Neurol.* 1967; **116**(6):647–650.

45. Arnulf I, Zeitzer JM, File J, Farber N, Mignot E. Kleine-Levin syndrome: a systematic review of 186 cases in the literature. *Brain.* **128**(12):2763–2776.

46. Rosenow F, Kotagal P, Cohen BH, Green C, Wyllie E. Multiple sleep latency test and polysomnography in diagnosing Kleine-Levin syndrome and periodic hypersomnia. *J Clin Neurophysiol* 2000; **17**(5):519–522.

47. Arias M, Crespo Iglesias JM, Perez J, et al. Klein-Levin syndrome: contribution of brain SPECT in diagnosis. *Rev Neurol.* 2003;**35**(6):531–533.

48. Billiard M, Guilleminault C, Dement WC. A menstruation-linked periodic hypersomnia. Kleine-Levin syndrome or a new clinical entity? *Neurology.* 1975;**25**(5):436–443.

49. Sachs C, Persson H, Hagenfeldt K. Menstruation-associated periodic hypersomnia: a case study with successful treatment. *Neurology.* 1982;**32** (12):1376–1379.

50. Bamford CR. Menstrual-associated sleep disorder: an unusual hypersomniac variant associated with both menstruation and amenorrhea with a possible link to prolactin and metoclopramide. *Sleep.* 1993;**16**(5):484–486.

51. Rothstein JD, Guidotti A, Tinuper P, et al. Endogenous benzodiazepine receptor ligands in idiopathic recurring stupor. *Lancet.* 1992;**340**(8826):1002–1004.

52. Lugaresi E, Montagna P, Tinuper P, et al. Endozepine stupor: recurring stupor linked to endozepine-4 accumulation. *Brain.* 1998;**121**(Pt 1):127–133.

53. Soriani S, Carrozzi M, De Carlo L, et al. Endozepine stupor in children. *Cephalalgia.* 1997;**17**(6):658–661.

54. Francisco GE, Ivanhoe CB. Successful treatment of post-traumatic narcolepsy with methylphenidate: a case report. *Am J Phys Med Rehabil.* 1996;**75**(1):63–65.

55. Manni R, Tantara A. Evaluation of sleepiness in epilepsy. *Clin Neurophysiol.* 2000;**111**(Suppl 2): S111–114.

56. Toth LA, Opp MR. Sleep and infection. In: Lee-Chiong TL, Sateia MJ, Carskadon MA, eds. *Sleep medicine.* Philadelphia, PA: Hanley & Belfus; 2002:77–83.

57. Guilleminault C, Mondini S. Mononucleosis and chronic daytime sleepiness: a long term follow-up study. *Arch Int Med.* 1986;**146**(7):1333–1335.

58. Askenasy JJM. Sleep in parkinson's disease. *Acta Neurol Scand.* 1993;**87**(3):167–170.

59. Chokroverty S. Sleep and degenerative neurologic disorders. *Neurol Clin.* 1996;**14**(4):807–826.

60. Trenkwalder C. Sleep dysfunction in Parkinson's disease. *Clin Neurosci.* 1998;**5**(2):107–114.

61. George CFP. Neuromuscular disorders. In: Kryger MH, Roth T, Dement WC, eds. *Principles and practice of sleep medicine,* 3rd ed. Philadelphia, PA: WB Saunders; 2000:1087–1092.

62. Gibbs JW, Ciafaloni E, Radtke RA. Excessive daytime somnolence and increased rapid eye movement pressure in myotonic dystrophy. *Sleep.* 2002;**25**(6): 662–665.

63. Campbell SM, Clark S, Tindall EA, Forehand ME, Bennett RM. Clinical characteristics of fibrositis, I: A "blinded" controlled study of symptoms and tender points. *Arthritis Rheum.* 1983;**26**(7):817–824.

64. Hyyppa MT, Kronhom E. Nocturnal motor activity in fibromyalgia patients with poor sleep quality. *J Psychosom Res.* 1995;**39**(1):85–91.

65. Moldofsky H, Saskin P, Lue FA. Sleep and symptoms in fibrositis syndrome after a febrile illness. *J Rheumatol.* 1988;**15**(11):1701–1704.

66. Moldofsky H, Lue FA, Smythe H. Alpha EEG sleep and morning symptoms of rheumatoid arthritis. *J Rheumatol.* 1983;**10**(3):373–379.

67. Perlis ML, Giles DE, Bootzin RR, et al. Alpha sleep and information processing, perception of sleep, pain,

and arousability in fibromyalgia. *Int J Neurosci.* 1997;**89**(3–4):265–280.

68. Moldolfsky H, Lue FA. The relationship of alpha delta EEG frequencies to pain and mood in "fibrositis" patients with chlorpromazine and L-tryptophan. *Electroencephalogr Clin Neurophysiol.* 1980;**50**(1–2):71–80.

69. Yamashiro Y, Kryger MH. Sleep in heart failure. *Sleep.* 1993;**16**(6):513–523.

70. Javaheri S, Parker TJ, Liming JD, et al. Sleep apnea in 81 ambulatory male patients with stable heart failure: types and their prevalences, consequences, and presentations. *Circulation.* 1998;**97**(21):2154–2159.

71. Brostrom A, Stromber A, Dahlsrom U, Fridland B. Sleep difficulties, daytime sleepiness, and health-related quality of life in patients with chronic heart failure. *J Cardiovasc Nurs.* 2004;**19**(4):234–242.

72. Davidson JR, MacLean AW, Brundage MD, Schulze K. Sleep disturbance in cancer patients. *Social Sci.* 2002; **54**(9):1309–1321.

73. Portenoy RK, Tahler HT, Kombilth AB, et al. Symptom prevalence, characteristics and distress in a cancer population. *Qual Life Res.* 1994;**3**(3):183–189.

74. Vena C, Parker K, Cunningham M, Clark J, McMillan S. Sleep-wake disturbances in people with cancer part I: an overview of sleep, sleep regulation, and effects of disease and treatment. *Oncol Nurs Forum.* 2004;**31**(4):735–746.

75. Resta O, Paanacciulli N, Di Gioia G, et al. High prevalence of previously unknown subclinical hypothyroidism in obese patients referred to a sleep clinic for sleep disordered breathing. *Nutr Metab Cardiovasc Dis.* 2004;**14**(5):248–253.

76. Blanco Perez JJ, Blanco-Ramos MA, Zamarron Sanz C, et al. Acromegaly and sleep apnea. *Arch Bronconeumol.* 2004;**40**(8):355–359.

77. Rosenow F, Reuter S, Deuss U, et al. Sleep apnoea in treated acromegaly: relative frequency and predisposing factors. *Clin Endocrinol (Oxf).* 1996; **45**(5):563–569.

78. Bjork S, Jonsson B, Westphal O, Levin JE. Quality of life of adults with growth hormone deficiency: a controlled study. *Acta Paediatr Scand Suppl.* 1989;**356**:55–59.

79. Tylee A, Gastpar M, Lepine JP, Mendlewicz J. DEPRES II (Depression Research in European Society II): a patient survey of the symptoms, disability and current management of depression in the community. DEPRES Steering Committee. *Int Clin Psychopharmacol.* 1999;**14**(3):139–151.

80. Reynolds CF 3rd, Coble PA, Kupfer DJ, Holzer BC. Application of the multiple sleep latency test in disorders of excessive sleepiness. *Electroencephalogr Clin Neurophysiol.* 1982;**53**(4):443–452.

81. Liu X, Buysse DJ. Sleep and youth suicidal behavior: A neglected field. *Curr Opin Psychiatry.* 2006;**19**: 288–293.

82. Fava M. Daytime sleepiness and insomnia as correlates of depression. *J Clin Psychiatry.* 2004; **65**:27–32.

83. Chellappa SL, Araujo JF. Sleep disorders and suicidal ideation in patients with depressive disorder. *Psychiatry Res.* 2007;**153**(2):131–136.

84. McCall WV, Harding D, O'Donovan C. Correlates of depressive symptoms in patients with obstructive sleep apnea. *J Clin Sleep Med.* 2006;**2**:424–426.

85. Sjostrom N, Waern M, Hetta J. Nightmares and sleep disturbances in relation to suicidality in suicide attempters. *Sleep.* 2007;**30**:91–95.

86. Fava M, Graves LM, Benazzi F, et al. A cross-sectional study of the prevalence of cognitive and physical symptoms during long-term antidepressant treatment. *J Clin Psychiatry.* 2006;**67**:1754–1759.

87. Williamson AM, Feyer AM. Moderate sleep deprivation produces impairments in cognitive and motor perfromance equivalent to legally prescribed levels of alcohol intoxication. *Occup Environ Med.* 2000;**57**:649–655.

Chapter 10

Parasomnias

Thomas D. Hurwitz and Carlos H. Schenck

Introduction

With the evolution of sleep medicine, the unwanted and mysterious physiological and behavioral events that have for centuries been associated with sleep and dreaming have been afforded their place within the currently utilized nosology of sleep disorders. The bizarre and often dangerous parasomnias such as sleepwalking and sleep terrors have been historically regarded as symptoms of psychiatric illness. Aristotle regarded dreaming as the sleep-related process that, when dissociated from the sleeping state into wakefulness, influenced the development of mental disease [1]. The incubus, in modern times described as sleep paralysis, was regarded as a demonic influence since the time of Plato, and over time came to be associated with states of psychopathology [2]. Caelius Aurelianus, a Roman physician of the late third century AD, likened the incubus to pavor nocturnes (now called night terrors) as "a fear of something obscure which the patient does not know ... which resides in the imagination ... there is also torpor of the body ... oppression ... sometimes inability to move ... and to speak ... often confusion." Though similar to epilepsy, it was thought to require little treatment other than peace and calm [3].

Later, during the nineteenth century, somnambulism was studied in fields as disparate as philosophy and literature. In medicine it was associated with mental disorders such as lethargy and catalepsy. Indeed, these three were known as "magnetic diseases" with some relationship to hysteria in the post-Mesmeric era when magnetic effects upon living tissue were thought to influence disease. Indeed, hypnosis had been considered an artificially induced form of somnambulism. Sleepwalking, then, was long considered to be a dissociative disorder [4]. Other psychiatric literature of the day addressed sleepwalking as "... a transient paroxysm of madness," [5] and as a manifestation of "some morbid condition in the ... cerebral organism" [6]. Freud, in *The Interpretation of Dreams*, did not address the issue of sleep "for that is essentially a problem of physiology," though he definitely associated cognitive dream experience with the core of unconscious life and a reflection of neurosis. He did not address motorically active dreaming in this work [7].

In our day, sleep-related behaviors may still be thought to be associated with psychopathological conditions, but frequently a presumed association may lead to erroneous diagnosis and inappropriate treatment. Because the symptomatic expression of parasomnias may be misinterpreted as a manifestation of a mental disorder, it behooves the modern psychiatric clinician to understand the differential diagnosis of these disorders so as to pursue timely and appropriate evaluation and treatment. This group of sleep disorders will be addressed from the perspective of clinical psychiatry.

Parasomnias are undesirable physical, experiential, or behavioral phenomena that occur exclusively during sleep or are exacerbated by the sleeping state. In the psychiatric nosology, DSM-IV-TR distinguishes nightmare disorder (formerly known as dream anxiety disorder), sleep terror disorder, sleepwalking disorder, and parasomnias not otherwise specified [8]. Unfortunately, this limited categorization understates the richness of the various disorders representing, as a group, the unusual and frequently bizarre manifestations of sleep–wake state misalignment. The International Classification of Sleep Disorders distinguishes them as disorders of arousal or partial arousal from non-REM sleep, disorders

Foundations of Psychiatric Sleep Medicine, ed. John W. Winkelman and David T. Plante. Published by Cambridge University Press.
© Cambridge University Press 2010.

Table 10.1 Parasomnia classification of DSM-IV and ICSD-2

	ICSD-2		
	Disorders of arousal (from NREM sleep)	**Parasomnias usually associated with REM sleep**	**Other parasomnias**
DSM-IV-TR	• Sleepwalking	• Nightmare disorder	• Parasomnia not otherwise specified/unspecified[†]
	• Sleep terrors		
	• Confusional arousals	• REM sleep behavior disorder*	• Sleep-related dissociative disorders
		• Recurrent isolated sleep paralysis	• Sleep enuresis
			• Sleep-related groaning (catathrenia)
			• Exploding head syndrome
			• Sleep-related hallucinations
			• Sleep-related eating disorder

Notes: This table indicates which disorders are included and excluded in each diagnostic schema. Note the ICSD-2 is more comprehensive with further delineation than the DSM-IV.
†Parasomnia not otherwise specified according to DSM-IV-TR would include those parasomnias shaded; while Parasomnia, unspecified according to ICSD-2 would include parasomnias not listed. Not listed are Parasomnias due to medical condition and Parasomnia due to drug or substance (ICSD-2) that would be classified as Sleep disorder due to a general medical condition, Parasomnia type and substance-induced sleep disorder, Parasomnia type respectively under DSM-IV-TR [8,9].
*Category includes parasomnia overlap disorder and status dissociatus.

usually associated with REM sleep, and other unusual parasomnias ranging from sleep-related groaning to eating and sexual behavior [9]. These categorizations are indicated in Table 10.1. They achieve clinical significance in proportion to their disruption of sleep, and risk of injury to patient as well as bed partner. As an indication of the prevalence of such disorders, a recent survey of 2078 adult men and 2894 women in the UK revealed a prevalence of 2.1% (N=106), occurring mostly in males, of self-reported sleep-related violent or injurious behavior [10].

The basic premise that underlies parasomnias is that rapid eye movement (REM) sleep, non-REM (NREM) sleep, and wakefulness are not always mutually exclusive states and that fundamental behavioral and electrophysiological components of each state may dissociate from the parent state and recombine in aberrant form. When components of NREM sleep and wakefulness occur in conjunction, there may be variable juxtapositions or oscillations of consciousness, memory, motor, and/or autonomic activation. When elements of wakefulness and REM phenomena intertwine, there may be intrusions of atonia and visual imagery into behavioral wakefulness such as in the cases of cataplexy, sleep paralysis, and hypnagogic hallucinations of narcolepsy, or dream enactment behavior during spells of REM sleep behavior disorder [11]. Such admixtures of sleep phenomena and wakefulness can easily be confused with primary psychiatric disorders such as when hypnagogic hallucinations are mistakenly interpreted as symptoms of waking psychosis.

NREM sleep parasomnias: disorders of arousal

The designation "disorders of arousal," first coined by Gastaut and Broughton [12], has reappeared as a category of NREM parasomnias and includes confusional arousals, sleepwalking, and sleep terrors. Confusional arousals are the mildest and the most common manifestation of this overlapping mixed state of wake and sleep, during which neither is completely established. Typically arising from deep NREM sleep (i.e. slow-wave sleep; SWS; stage N3), these arousals, or incomplete awakenings, have also been known as sleep drunkenness and sleep inertia [13,14]. The affected individuals demonstrate variable degrees of confusion, disorientation, retrograde and antero-grade amnesia, as well as disturbed and occasionally violent behavior during periods of variable duration. Mild, brief episodes often occur without recognition, as the individual may not even rise out of bed. Two variants in adolescents and adults, severe morning sleep inertia and sleep-related abnormal sexual behaviors, are also recognized [9]. Confusional arousals may affect individuals of all ages, and may be precipitated by sleep deprivation, circadian rhythm alteration (jet lag, shift work, etc.), alcohol, medications, and by conditions of excessive somnolence. Both sexes may be affected and there is a familial predisposition to deeper sleep. Epidemiological data suggest confusional arousals may occur in as many as 4.2% of the adult population, though due to the inherent difficulties in reporting these events, this may dramatically underestimate their prevalence [10].

Sleepwalking and sleep terrors: overview and clinical description

Sleepwalking (SW) represents motor activation during an abnormal arousal, usually from deep NREM sleep. Common during childhood (1–17%), SW tends to diminish in frequency following adolescence but can persist into or even begin during adult life (2.5%) [15,16]. Behaviors can vary from sitting up in the bed to full ambulation. Behaviors can be very complex and include walking, running, driving, eating, and violence. Mental activity is usually poorly recalled but may include dream-like visual imagery, which tends to be both less detailed and less bizarre than traditional REM dream reports. Individuals are variably amnestic for the episodes. Typically occurring during the early part of the sleep cycle and emerging from the "deeper" stage N3 of NREM sleep, they may technically derive from any NREM stage. Many individuals report that frequency and severity of sleepwalking increase with stressful life experiences. Cases have been associated with migraine and thyrotoxicosis [17,18]. There is often a familial predisposition and it occurs in both sexes. Spells can be precipitated in susceptible individuals by anything that stimulates arousals from sleep. These can include exogenous stimuli such as noises, or endogenous factors such as obstructive sleep apnea

(OSA), periodic limb movements of sleep (PLMS), gastroesophageal reflux disorder, other physical illness, or full bladder, without any specific psychological meaning [9,11,19,20–22]. Nathaniel Kleitman, father of American sleep research, wrote: "all the characteristics of somnambulism underline the difference between wakefulness and consciousness." [23] This idea is reinforced by a more recent report of SPECT imaging during a polygraphically documented SW episode, demonstrating increased cerebral blood flow (CBF) in the anterior cerebellum (vermis) and posterior cingulate cortex when compared to quiet slow-wave sleep. There were also large areas of frontal and parietal cortical decrements of CBF when compared with normal awake subjects. As anticipated by Kleitman, SW appears to represent a concurrence of increased motor activation and decreased executive function during incomplete, disordered arousals from sleep [24].

Sleep terrors (ST) are spells of abrupt arousals with profound autonomic activation including tachycardia, tachypnea, flushing, diaphoresis, and mydriasis that may include sitting up in bed and may progress to SW. The two disorders, often occurring in combination, represent a continuum of events with exclusively motor or autonomic activation as polar examples. Pure ST occur more frequently in young children, arising in approximately 3% of children and less than 1% of adults. Arising typically during the first third of the night, ST are followed by return to sleep and amnesia for the event. Precipitants are not necessarily present, but may include fever, prior sleep deprivation, or central nervous system depressant drugs including alcohol. Polysomnography (PSG) findings are essentially those described with SW below but with notable increases in cardiac and respiratory rates [9].

Though often unnecessary in typical, benign cases of SW and ST, PSG is indicated when they have an adult onset (as this may indicate another underlying precipitating sleep disorder), when there is risk of significant injury to oneself or another person, or when there is substantial disruption of one's sleep or the sleep of the bed partner. Such studies should include an expanded "seizure" montage of EEG channels, electromyographic (EMG) monitoring of four limbs to detect movement, and continuous audiovisual monitoring (that is time-synchronized to the PSG), in order to rule out seizure disorder, REM sleep behavior disorder (RBD), OSA, PLMS, or other primary sleep disorders [25,26]. Electrocardiogram

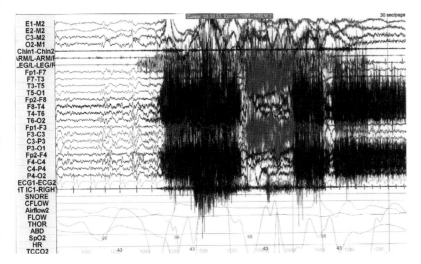

Figure 10.1 Nocturnal polysomnogram of 32-year-old man with history of SW/ST demonstrating an abrupt spontaneous arousal from non-REM stage N2 sleep as the record becomes suddenly obscured by muscular movement artifact. Tachycardia develops later during the arousal and the man subsequently left the bed and later reported dream recall of being in his son's house in a living room filled with red furniture and becoming convinced that "some disaster like a fire" was about to occur. He dreamed that he attempted to warn his wife when he, in fact, bolted from his bed and subsequently only slowly was convinced by the technologist that there was no real imminent danger. There is no epileptiform activity in the EEG. See plate section for color version.

provides constant observation of cardiac rhythm. Nasal pressure and nasal–oral airflow recording, full monitoring of chest and abdominal respiratory excursions, and audiovisual recording are essential during all such studies, with written notations by skilled technologists performing the studies. Sleep deprivation and forced arousals such as with an auditory stimulus may be used in an attempt to elicit a spell [27,28]. Urine toxicology screens should be utilized when indicated by history or clinical impression. Multiple sleep latency testing is carried out during the subsequent day in cases requiring quantification of patient-reported or clinically suspected excessive daytime sleepiness.

Periods of confusion may be observed during the study. When apparent, EEG activity often may not indicate clear wakefulness [29,30]. If the background EEG is not obscured by muscle artifact during the abnormal arousal, there may be persisting elements of sleep such as delta-wave activity, relatively low-voltage, mixed frequency activity, or diffuse, poorly reactive alpha frequency [29,31]. Movement often causes artifactually high amplitude and frequency deflections in the display, such that underlying EEG patterns may not be discernible. Epileptiform activity is typically not seen [32]. In the laboratory, behavioral events are frequently not recorded or are less severe than reported by history. Excessive abrupt spontaneous arousals from NREM sleep in the absence of behavioral events are supportive of the diagnosis. In a reported series of sleep-related injuries, PSG studies either established or supported the diagnosis of

SW/ST in 49/54 (90.7%) of cases [19]. In another report, actual behavioral spells were observed during PSG in 8/10 (80%) cases [33]. In children, an abnormal alternation of EEG amplitude during intermittent bursts of slow-wave activity has been reported to be a possible marker of neurophysiological predisposition to disorders of arousal [34]. Also, a study of cyclic alternating pattern, an EEG measure of NREM sleep instability, may reflect a physiological substrate for SW [35,36].

Historically, SW has been thought to be associated with psychopathology in adults. Two older reports from military medical sources describe a total of 48 cases of SW. Psychiatric diagnoses, based upon clinical interviews, were assigned to 42/48 (87.5%) of these cases. Eleven of the 48 (22.9%) were noted to have what might have been equivalent to modern axis I psychiatric disorders (7 schizophrenia, 1 obsessive-compulsive disorder, 3 probable adjustment disorders). Roughly two-thirds (31/48) had what may have been axis II personality disorders [37,38]. Another early report of young sleepwalkers aged 9–27 concluded that greater psychopathology was to be found in adults than in children with the disorder, even though only three subjects were older than 16 years, and no psychosis was reported in any of them [39]. A large group of 50 adult sleepwalkers recruited by advertisement and diagnosed without PSG has been studied with psychiatric interview, Minnesota multiphasic personality inventory (MMPI), and symptom checklist 90 (SCL90). Psychiatric diagnoses were assigned to 21/29 (72%) current, as opposed to 7/21 (33%) former, sleepwalkers.

Regrettably, diagnoses were not specified, but said to have been primarily personality disorders [40]. An accompanying report from the same center described 40 adults with current ST evaluated in the same way. Thirty-four of these (85%) were said to have psychiatric diagnoses, likewise not specified but roughly equally distributed between personality disorders and neuroses [41].

The previously cited report of 54 adults with SW/ST from a study of 100 patients with sleep-related injury is based upon PSG, psychiatric interview, MMPI, Beck depression inventory (BDI), and SCL90 [19]. Active DSM-III axis I diagnoses were found in only 19/54 (35.2%) cases, and included 14/19 (37.6%) with mood disorders, and 4/19 (21.1%) with alcohol and/or substance use disorders. These did not appear temporally associated with the presentation of parasomnias. An additional 7/54 (13%) had past histories of mood disorders (3/7) and alcohol/substance abuse (4/7). MMPI data available for 36/54 (66.7%) were available and personality disorder was suggested by the profiles in only 12/36 (33.3%). The overwhelming majority of these patients were enjoying good psychosocial adjustments [19].

More recent reports provide no basis for a psychiatric etiology of parasomnias. In a retrospective review of 11 cases of ST, though 7/11 patients reported an influence of stress on their disturbance, none had a diagnosis of panic disorder and the course of the sleep disorders did not overlap significantly with any lifetime mood or substance use disorders. The authors concluded that sleep terrors were "not simply symptoms of a psychiatric disorder" [42].

A larger series describes 41 patients, including 29 (19 male) who had demonstrated violent sleep-related behaviors, while 12 (7 male) were non-violent. Hamilton depression rating scores greater than 24 were seen in only 3 (10%) violent cases and 3 (25%) non-violent cases. Dysfunctional families were described in only 3 (10%) of violent and 3 (25%) of non-violent cases. Obsessive-compulsive personality disorder was noted in 6 (21%) violent and 6 (50%) non-violent cases. Though there was an interesting prevalence of this personality pattern, there was no clear psychiatric basis found to underlie these cases and even less apparent psychiatric disorder in the most severely affected. The authors also note that stress responsiveness can account for some increased frequency of parasomnia events [43].

Another large report documents the evaluation of 64 individuals with nocturnal behavioral spells categorized as non-violent (NV, N=26, 11 male), potentially harmful (PH, N=12, 6 male), and violent (V, N=26, 22 male). Histories of childhood abuse were found in 4 female cases (3 NV, 1 PH). Current DSM-III axis I diagnoses were described in 13/64 (20%) of cases. Alcohol abuse (as a stressor associated with sleep-related behavior, not necessarily an axis I disorder) was noted in 11/64 (17%) and some prior history of drug abuse in 24/64 (38%). There was no systematic association between the sleep disorders and any psychiatric diagnosis and, on the SCL 90, there was no difference between the three groups [44].

Of particular interest to psychiatrists are cases of parasomnias related to the use of psychotropic drugs. SW/ST, occasionally of severe and injurious intensity, have been reportedly associated with the use of neuroleptics including: olanzapine [45] and quetiapine [46]; antidepressants including paroxetine [47,48], reboxetine [49], and bupropion [50]; lithium [51,52]; sedative-hypnotics (zolpidem) [53]; anti-epileptics including topiramate [54], valproic acid combined with zolpidem [55]; stimulants; minor tranquilizers; and antihistamines, often in various combinations [20,21,56–62]. Other associated medications are metoprolol [63] and fluoroquinolone [64].

Treatment of SW/ST

The earliest pharmacological agents offered to individuals at serious risk of injury were diazepam [65] and imipramine [66]. Clonazepam has been reported to be effective in doses of 0.25–2.0 mg taken about 30–120 minutes before sleep. When given to 28/54 (51.9%) patients with SW/ST, it produced substantial benefit in over 80% [19]. Other agents anecdotally effective include other benzodiazepines, carbamazepine, paroxetine, doxepin, trazodone [57], and melatonin [67]. In cases with less imminent risk of injury, non-pharmacological therapy with clinical hypnosis may be preferred. This can also be offered initially in combination with medication, which can be gradually withdrawn. Patients are instructed in the induction of a relaxed, meditative state, with visual imagery of quiet, restful sleep associated with comfort, safety, and reinforcement of possible but minimally probable need for physical mobilization. With self-hypnosis utilized before retiring to bed, benefit has been reported in 20/27 (74%) patients who reported much or very much improvement

[68]. In another study with similar techniques, 3/6 (50%) SW patients were much improved or spell-free after 18 months and 2/3 (67%) were likewise after 5 years follow-up [69]. Progressive muscle relaxation training has also been utilized [70]. In children, use of anticipatory awakenings [71], clinical hypnosis [72,73], and a combination of acupuncture with medicinal herbs have been documented as helpful [74].

Although co-morbid psychiatric disorder must be treated if present, a straightforward symptomatic approach to the treatment of SW/ST remains very reasonable. Though psychotherapy has been reportedly helpful [75], it is not routinely indicated, and should only be considered for distinct psychiatric indications beyond SW/ST. Successful treatment of psychiatric illness, however, does not guarantee remission of the parasomnia.

Box 10.1 Case examples of sleepwalking/sleep terrors

Case 1:

A 24-year-old man, self-referred for evaluation of long-standing weekly "bad dreams," 1–3 hours after sleep onset, described sudden arousals with screaming, shortness of breath, fearfulness of panic proportions, and attempts to fight or flee from imagined threats resulting in injuries such as lacerations when putting his arms through glass windows. He was generally amnestic for the spells unless awakened by someone during their course. Dentists had commented to him about dental erosion suggestive of bruxism and bed partners had reported frequent somniloquy (sleep-talking). Past history included enuresis until age 11, childhood attention deficit disorder and learning disability, and alcohol and cannabis abuse in remission. PSG revealed unremarkable sleep architecture and three auditory stimulus-induced abrupt arousals, one with complex behavior of sitting up, screaming, and rapidly removing all firmly adherent electrodes while clearly not awake and misperceiving the environment. Diagnosis of SW/ST was made and the patient responded to therapy with self-hypnosis. Subsequently, he reported that arousals would still occur during some nights but without panic or problematic behaviors and were followed by rapid resumption of sleep.

Case 2:

A 71-year-old man complained of precipitous nocturnal arousals with sensations of air hunger and attendant inability to return easily to sleep, worsening after coronary artery bypass surgery 4 years prior to sleep disorder center evaluation. He also described a history of SW dating to childhood with awakenings "from a dream" and "with a hard time returning to reality." Commonly, he would dream that he had nails or toothpicks in his mouth. On one occasion, he arose from bed, walked to a neighbor's house and told her to "get some help." On another occasion, he dreamt that a dog was chasing him and he in fact jumped from the bed, tripped, hit his head on a dresser, and sustained a laceration requiring five sutures. More frequently, he will sit up in bed and call to his wife for help. As a youngster, he recalled arising

shortly after sleep onset, dressing, and going out to a barn to begin milking cows when he slowly awoke to realize that the hour was 9:00 p.m. and not early morning. Family history revealed a 38-year-old son with precipitous awakenings, believing there was an intruder in his home. The first night PSG revealed striking difficulty initiating and maintaining sleep with prolonged sleep-onset latency of 158 minutes. Non-apneic respiratory effort-related arousals (RERAs) occurred at a rate of 44 per hour of sleep. During the next night, PSG revealed frequent, prolonged awakenings and increased stages 3 and 4 sleep (54.8%) for age. Four non-breathing-related arousals occurred from SWS and were characterized by very complex motor behavior with confusion. During one of these, he left the bed rapidly and had to be restrained by the technologist who had difficulty convincing him that there was no imminent danger. Later, the patient recalled very detailed, complex, and prolonged dream-like mentation preceding the event. He has experienced improvement with the use of doxepin 25 mg at bedtime. This case reminds us that SW can occur well beyond childhood and of the precipitating effects of sleep deprivation.

Case 3:

A 38-year-old woman was referred because of childhood onset SW with pronounced worsening during the 18 months prior to evaluation. During a period of intense stress, she had gained 70 pounds to a weight of 295 pounds. She had become depressed with complaints of diminished memory and concentration. SW spells had been occurring once or more nightly and included injuries to ankles, knees, hips, and shoulders from falling. When awakening outside of her bedroom, she had found herself lighting cigarettes, and occasionally eating food. She admitted to snoring and also suffered significant excessive daytime sleepiness with embarrassing sleep onsets and at least one instance of missing her stop when sleeping on a bus. Past history included some difficulty with bladder control and alleged childhood physical, emotional, and sexual

Box 10.1 (*cont.*)

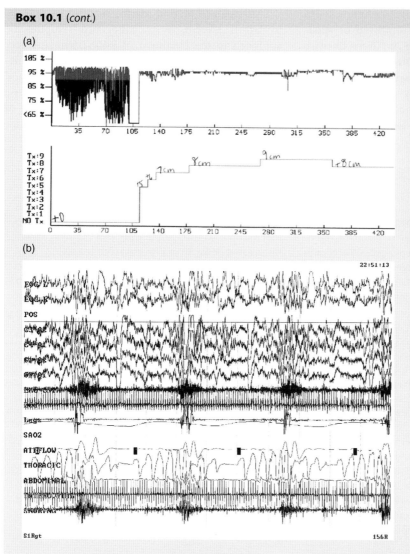

Figure 10.2 (a) Oximetry tracing from an obese 38-year-old woman showing frequent desaturations of oxyhemoglobin, reaching a nadir of <60% during polysomnographically documented non-REM sleep, secondary to obstructive sleep apnea. Apnea and hypopnea events occurred at a rate of 80 per hour of sleep. Each desaturation is accompanied by evidence of arousal from sleep on the corresponding polysomnogram. She had complained of frequent spells of SW, which included eating foods from her cupboards and refrigerator. She responded well to CPAP at 8–9 cmH$_2$O pressure, with resolution of obstructive sleep apnea and SW. See plate section for color version. (b) Polysomnogram corresponding to 2 minutes of sleep during baseline recording of sleep in the case of a 38-year-old obese woman with obstructive sleep apnea, demonstrated by reduction of oral–nasal airflow in the presence of respiratory effort noted by deflections representing chest and abdominal movements. The ensuing arousals from sleep represent events that had historically been likely to have precipitated confusional arousals and sleepwalking.

abuse at the hands of a violent, alcoholic father. PSG revealed profound sleep fragmentation with OSA at a rate of 72 apneas or hypopneas per hour of sleep and additional respiratory effort-related arousals at a rate of 73 per hour. Oxyhemoglobin saturation reached a low of 60% during the night (Figure 10.2a). She responded well to nasal continuous positive airway pressure (CPAP) therapy at a pressure of 12 cm of water with 28% supplemental oxygen (Figure 10.2b). Her worsening SW, obviously in response to sleep disordered breathing-induced arousals, was eliminated entirely by effective CPAP in spite of continued severe financial stress.

Parasomnias usually associated with REM sleep

REM sleep behavior disorder: overview

First predicted by animal experimentation in 1965 and certainly having existed for centuries in humans,

REM sleep behavior disorder (RBD) was first reported in 1985 after systematic evaluation of an elderly gentleman complaining of injurious dream-enactment behavior. He would fly out of bed during dreams of playing football, and then collide with furniture or a wall. Countless cases have now been contributed to the world literature. The disorder is based upon persistent or intermittent loss of normal atonia of skeletal muscles during REM sleep along with complex motor activity associated with dream mentation [76,77,78].

RBD typically involves a prolonged, chronic course and is identified most frequently in elderly males. There tends to be a lengthy prodrome in about 25% of patients with increased action-packed dream content along with somniloquy and limb jerking. As the disorder becomes established, there is a tendency for abrupt, often violent movement concordant with dream content. Dream reports tend to be much more vivid than those reported when dream mentation is recalled during SW/ST. Patients typically dream of themselves as defenders, rarely as aggressors. The bed partner may receive blows believed by the dreamer to be defensive. RBD spells are likely to occur during the latter part of the night when REM sleep tends to be more prolonged and intense, in contrast to SW/ST, which may occur earlier in the course of the night when stage N3 is more likely.

RBD may be misconstrued from history alone to represent conditions such as seizure disorders, other parasomnias, OSA, post-traumatic stress disorder, and various psychiatric illnesses. Patients have carried mistaken diagnoses of "repressed aggression," "familial alcoholic personality disorder," and post-traumatic stress disorder. PSG is diagnostic of the disorder with fluctuating levels of skeletal motor (rarely autonomic) activation during REM sleep. Normally, alpha motor neurons are hyperpolarized during REM sleep with resulting atonia of voluntary muscles. This is disrupted in RBD, and manifested by varying degrees of muscle tone on EMG monitoring of submental (chin) and limb muscles. Increased muscular twitching is also seen, even when complex behavior is not recorded, but documented by history. There is often an increase in the percentage of sleep time spent in stage REM (>25%), a reduction of the REM sleep latency <75 minutes, and an increase in the actual number of rapid eye movements. There tends to be an increase of stage N3 beyond that expected for age [77,79]. A technique for quantitative scoring of motor activation during REM sleep has been described [80].

This disorder may produce severe sleep-related injury that has included lacerations, fractures, and joint injuries that afflict patients as well as bed partners. Patients have attempted to protect themselves with restraints, padded waterbeds, pillow barricades, plastic screens, and sleeping on a floor mattress in an empty room. Injuries are often the presenting complaints and patients rarely complain of sleep disruption or daytime sleepiness.

During the decade following the initial description of RBD, approximately half of cases appeared to be associated with central nervous system disorders, ranging from degenerative processes to narcolepsy, vascular disorders, cerebral astrocytoma, multiple sclerosis, and Guillain-Barré syndrome. Conversely, of the initial 166 published cases, 47% were designated as idiopathic, without apparent neurological explanation [78]. Neuropsychological evaluations suggested short- and long-term verbal and visual memory impairment not due to global dementia. With time, gradual development of Parkinson's disease was reported in 38% of 29 previously idiopathic cases, suggesting a pathophysiological relationship [81]. After another 7 years, the same cohort revealed an increased prevalence of delayed emergence of parkinsonism and/or dementia of 65% [82]. Indeed, RBD is now recognized as "cryptogenic" rather than idiopathic, and appears to be an early component of neurodegenerative disease. More specifically, these are disorders marked by deposits of alpha synuclein such as Parkinson's Disease, Lewy Body disease, and multisystem atrophy [83,84]. Pathophysiology of REM sleep motor control seems to be localized in the subcoeruleus region of the pons, which is involved in the generation of REM sleep components such as atonia [85]. In cases of various synucleinopathies, RBD prevalence appears to be 19–77%. Conversely, in tauopathies such as Alzheimer's disease, corticobasal degeneration, progressive supranuclear palsy, and frontotemporal dementia, RBD is quite rare at 0–27% [86]. Neuropsychological testing, though not indicated for diagnosis, has revealed dysfunctional visuospatial constructional ability and altered visuospatial learning in early, apparently idiopathic RBD. This may be consistent with the possibility of underlying neurodegenerative disorder [87]. Long-term prospective follow-up studies will eventually clarify if there is any predictive value of this relationship between neuropsychological findings and idiopathic RBD. If there is, it will present a clear opportunity for prophylaxis when neuroprotective therapies become known and available.

Acute, transient cases may occur in the context of intoxication or withdrawal, such as with alcohol.

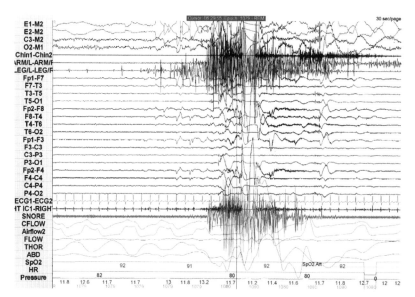

Figure 10.3 Polysomnogram of a 72-year-old man with REM sleep behavior disorder. Although the rapid eye movements are typical of REM sleep and the EEG is characteristically desynchronized, chin muscle atonia is incomplete during this burst of phasic eye movements, and there is prominent electromyographic activation of muscles of upper and lower extremities movements with corresponding movement. Patient yelled out during this event and, retrospectively, recalled dreaming of fighting. See plate section for color version.

Many psychotropic drugs can be associated with REM sleep without atonia or frank RBD. These include selective and non-selective serotonergic antidepressants, monoamine oxidase inhibitors (MAOI), and withdrawal from TCA and MAOI. This drug-related RBD may be self-limiting, affect young persons, and include both sexes [56,58,60,77,86,88]. It is not yet known if there is any particular predisposition to drug-induced REM without atonia or RBD, or if these cases present similar probability of developing subsequent neurodegenerative disorders.

About 20% of RBD cases include an active axis I psychiatric disorder while about 13% have a history of past axis I illness. Diagnoses have been confined to mood disorders (generally recurrent major depression) and alcohol/substance use disorders (largely in remission). In a report of 96 patients with RBD, 9 (9.4%) appeared to have had onset of the sleep disorder temporally linked with a psychiatric illness. Five (4 male) of these 9 had RBD related to drug abuse including cessation of alcohol, cocaine, and amphetamine. Mean age ± SD was 44.0 (range 31–60), and RBD had been occurring for months to 17 years (unpublished data). A principal mechanism in these cases may be the effect of pathological REM rebound after withdrawal of REM suppressant drugs as was likely the case in a 67-year-old woman with acute, transient RBD following rapid withdrawal of imipramine for treatment of major depression [89].

However, RBD may also arise as the result of antidepressant treatment, as was the case for a 34-year-old man who developed RBD with typical dream enactment during fluoxetine treatment of obsessive-compulsive disorder. [90] A psychiatric disorder rarely associated with RBD is adjustment disorder in response to severe psychosocial stress. A 69-year-old man presented after the stress of divorce and a 61-year-old man had a similar course following an automobile accident with a major risk of death but no actual injury. In both cases, RBD persisted long after the stresses had subsided. Pathological dreaming in these cases was typical of RBD, rather than involving obvious post-traumatic imagery, and may represent a manifestation of central nervous system (CNS) reorganization in response to psychological stress. It is possible that CNS plasticity in response to stress may influence the possibility of a post-traumatic form of RBD, which has also been reported in two cases by other authors [19,89,91,92,93,94].

It must be underscored that parasomnias including RBD have been misconstrued as psychiatric disorders. Such patients may even find their way to psychiatric intensive care units as was the case for a 62-year-old man hospitalized for recurrent major depression with suicidality. Other patients and staff in spite of no wakeful manifestations of psychosis or threatening behavior misattributed his dream enactment violence as a manifestation of a psychiatric disorder [95].

Treatment of RBD

Treatment of RBD with clonazepam has been gratifying. The highly activated dream and behavioral manifestations of the disorder generally respond to modest doses of 0.5–2.0 mg taken about 30 minutes before retiring. Inappropriate escalation of dosage or tachyphylaxis is rare, side-effects modest, and there has been minimal risk of abuse or addiction with this agent in these patients [96]. The mechanism of action is apparently suppression of phasic motor activity and behavioral release rather than restoration of normal REM atonia.

Melatonin is now considered to be a second-line, or at times a first-line therapy of RBD, with the mechanism of action apparently involving substantial restoration of REM atonia [97,98,99]. Pramipexole may be the preferred third-line therapy based on two published series [100,101]. There is anecdotal support for other medications being beneficial in patients who do not respond to clonazepam. These include carbidopa/levodopa, donepezil, quetiapine, clozapine, clonidine, L-tryptophan, carbamazepine, and gabapentin. Though REM-suppressing drugs such as antidepressants usually cause or worsen RBD, there are also some reports of benefit with desipramine and imipramine [77,79,86,97–99,100–102].

Box 10.2   Case examples of REM sleep behavior disorder

Case 1:

A 72-year-old man complained of being "very active during the first half of my sleep period … I have fallen out of bed from my dreams and once walked in my sleep for 10 feet before awakening." He had demonstrated jerking and twitching in his sleep beginning at least 42 years prior to evaluation and, 37 years later, began shouting profanity during sleep. Three years before evaluation, he found himself falling from bed when dreaming of kicking an unfamiliar attacking animal or unfamiliar human assailant. His wife had avoided awakening him from such dreams because she "then become[s] incorporated in his dream which could be dangerous." He began sleeping tethered into the bed by a belt or rope several months before presenting for sleep disorder center consultation in order to confine himself to the bed during the night. He had no history of any psychiatric or neurological disorder and was medically healthy and led a vigorous life.

Case 2:

A 72-year-old woman was referred for evaluation of a complaint of excessive sleepiness with chronic depression. There was no history of cataplexy or sleep paralysis. She complained of longstanding restless legs when lying still which interfered with sleep onset and vigorous kicking movements during sleep. There was no history of SW/ST but she had demonstrated occasional loud yelling during sleep. There was increasing action-filled dreaming described during the past year, and some recall of frightening dreams concordant with her kicking movements during sleep. These seemed to worsen when imipramine 125 mg nightly had been prescribed for over 1 month before being discontinued 4 days prior to PSG study. Alprazolam had been tapered and discontinued over a period of time as well. The first night PSG revealed very brief REM latency of 11 minutes, markedly increased REM sleep (52.2% of total sleep time) with loss of atonia during REM sleep. There were very prominent extremity movements and frequent random extremity twitching during REM and non-REM sleep. On one occasion during REM sleep, there was an episode of dream enactment behavior with waving of arms concordant with recall of gesturing to her daughter in a dream. The second night PSG, 1 month later, was similar, with REM latency of 8 minutes and 39.6% of total sleep time in stage REM, with active upper and lower extremity movements and vocalizations. Submental EMG showed persisting periods of elevated tone during REM sleep. She also demonstrated periodic limb movements of sleep at a rate of 19 per hour. There was no evidence of excessive sleepiness on the multiple sleep latency test. She subsequently did well on a regimen of clonazepam 0.5 mg and pramipexole 0.5 mg nightly.

Nightmare disorder

Formerly termed dream anxiety attacks, nightmare disorder is now recognized as a REM sleep phenomenon, distinct from NREM ST. Nightmares are frightening dreams, frequently associated with moderate to intense autonomic activation and full awakening from sleep, usually with full recollection of dream content. Emotional manifestations of fear, anger, and sadness may predominate. Nightmares occur in 5–8% of adults, more commonly women, and individuals with "type A" personality characteristics [103–105]. They can be induced by a number of drugs including some antidepressants and neuroleptics, antiparkinsonian drugs such as L-DOPA, amantadine, lisuride, clonidine, methyldopa, prazosin, reserpine, lipophilic beta blockers, ciprofloxacin, donepezil, and amiodarone. Withdrawal from REM-suppressing agents such as tricyclic antidepressants, monoamine oxidase inhibitors, clonidine, alcohol, and amphetamines may cause nightmares as a result of REM sleep rebound. Nightmares not uncommonly occur following traumatic experiences, and occasional psychotic episodes may be heralded by their occurrence [106]. Non-psychotic individuals suffering frequent lifelong nightmares tend to be open, trusting, defenseless, vulnerable, creative people described as having "thin" interpersonal, ego, and sleep–wake boundaries [107–109]. Schizotypal personality characteristics have been associated with nightmare distress in one report but individuals with those traits also reported enjoyable dreaming. This implicates a more general notion of imaginativeness influencing dream experience [110].

Reported treatments include a cognitive strategy known as imagery rehearsal, which treats the disorder as a sleep disturbance rather than a manifestation of specific psychopathology. Patients are taught to restructure the dream scenario into a more acceptable experience by rewriting the script as an exercise during wakefulness [111]. Instruction in lucid dreaming has also been cited in a case report [112]. Pharmacotherapy, based largely on experience with post-traumatic stress disorder, includes reported benefit with cyproheptadine and prazosin [113,114] (see Chapter 17: Sleep in anxiety disorders).

Recurrent isolated sleep paralysis

Sleep paralysis is essentially the atonia of REM sleep that has become dissociated and occurs at times other than the typical periods of REM sleep during the night. It can either intrude into light NREM sleep at sleep onset or persist into awakening at the offset of sleep. In either case, its occurrence during sleep–wake transitions is often experienced as discomforting or frightening. It is classically found in association with the quintessential dissociation of REM sleep components in narcolepsy, but it is not specific for this disorder (see Chapter 9: Hypersomnias of central origin). In this case, it is similar to cataplexy, or the intrusion of atonia during a period of full wakefulness. Isolated sleep paralysis may occur with a lifetime prevalence of 2.3–40%, depending on the country and study population. Unless the history includes hypersomnia or cataplexy, there is no need for PSG.

Treatment is usually unnecessary unless there is significant sleep disruption or subjective distress. In that case, REM-suppressing agents such as fluoxetine or imipramine may be indicated [115].

The term *nachtmahr* originally referred to the perception of an oppressive presence of a spirit (*mare*), causing a feeling of suffocation and an awakening. As in the incubus or succubus attacks of ancient times and middle ages, the experience was attributed to demonic influence. The conjunction of vivid visual imagery and muscular paralysis suggests that this has always been associated with the REM sleep state, and when occurring closer to the time of sleep onset, is a manifestation of abnormally timed, sleep-onset REM periods and can be described as hypnagogic hallucination with sleep paralysis. This experience has been explained in various ways in different cultures. In Newfoundland, tradition has held that these experiences represented supernatural attacks of "the Old Hag," that could result in feeling tired or "haggard" (hag-ridden) the next day [116,117].

Other parasomnias
Sleep-related dissociative disorders

Dissociative disorders may also occur during the sleep period, typically in individuals suffering daytime syndromes such as dissociative identity disorder (DID), psychogenic amnesia, and dissociative disorder not otherwise specified (NOS). In a report of polysomnographic studies of 21 patients with dissociative disorders, 6/21 (27.5%) demonstrated nocturnal dissociative episodes, with two of them showing a clear transition to an alter personality [118]. The original published report includes only one case of exclusively sleep-related DID without daytime dissociation in a 19-year-old male. This unusual case presented with nocturnal arousals and subsequent behavior consistent with vague dream recall of being a large cat following a female zookeeper in anticipation of feeding on raw meat. During events, he would demonstrate great strength such as grasping furniture in his jaws and moving a mattress gripped between his teeth. He had walked about with raw bacon in his mouth. Other patients with diurnal dissociative disorders have demonstrated nocturnal behaviors resembling SW/ST that can be quite prolonged, often with amnesia. If observed in the sleep laboratory during PSG, these complex, lengthy, and repetitive behaviors are seen to

Box 10.3 Case example of sleep-related dissociative disorder

A 30-year-old woman with dissociative disorder, primarily psychogenic amnesia, had a history of severe and recurrent self-mutilation. She had allegedly endured severe childhood physical and sexual abuse and had longstanding diurnal flashbacks and nocturnal disturbed dreaming experiences wherein she would re-experience sexually traumatic events. During night-time spells, she would inflict cuts and bruises upon herself, often including lacerations of her genitalia for which she would be typically amnestic. PSG was diagnostic by virtue of absent epileptiform features and multiple episodes of restlessness, apparent distress, crying out, and unresponsiveness to technicians. These spells clearly began during periods of EEG-defined wakefulness. Treatment with doxepin was associated with a modest sense of subjectively improved sleep and she was referred to a psychotherapist skilled in treatment of dissociative disorders.

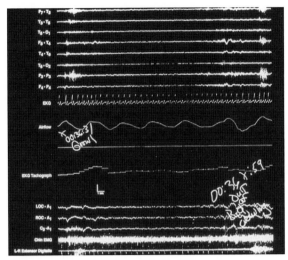

Figure 10.4 Polysomnogram showing an episode of dissociative disorder emerging during a period of clear electroencephalographic nocturnal wakefulness in a 19-year-old man, 53 minutes after sleep onset when he suddenly begins to growl, and then 28 seconds later he leaves his bed and crawls away in the manner of a large jungle cat, as noted by the sleep technologist. A 9-channel EEG indicates a corresponding wakeful state. Reprinted from Schenck CH, et. al. Dissociation 1989;2:194–204, with permission from the Ridgeview Institute.

follow after the development of EEG wakefulness in spite of no obvious behavioral awakening. In the published report noted above, 4/8 (50%) cases demonstrated these electrographically wakeful behaviors, while another 4/8 (50%) had histories of nocturnal and diurnal dissociative disorders though PSG studies recorded no behavioral spells. In the latter cases, the diagnosis was supported by absence of EEG seizure activity, REM or NREM motor abnormality, or any sleep-related respiratory disorder [119]. Therapy is typically that which is provided for the wakeful dissociative disorder.

Sleep-related enuresis

Sleep enuresis was originally included as one of the disorders of arousal. It is no longer linked with arousal disorders from slow-wave or any other sleep stage. When bladder activity and EEG are monitored, sudden, single-event bladder contractions occur independent of any sleep stage. It is very frequent in childhood and may occur in 4–15% of school age children and as many as 2% of 18-year-olds. Prevalence in boys is twice that of girls until it equalizes following puberty. No etiology has yet been clearly implicated but there is a strong genetic predisposition for primary enuresis (no prior dry period for 6 or more months). For secondary enuresis, with such a prior dry period, there is more likely to be a relationship with an underlying disorder such as sleep disordered breathing, diabetes mellitus or insipidus, or epilepsy. Urological explanations may be found in 2–4% of pediatric cases. Pathophysiology may include small bladder capacity, insufficient inhibition of spontaneous bladder contractions, and decreased nocturnal secretion of vasopressin. There is no known specific psychopathology known to cause this disorder, though social and familial consequences may impact negatively on self-image [120].

Treatment is generally unnecessary before age 5–6 years. After that age, depending on the extent of the symptom, therapy could include behavioral conditioning with a bell-and-pad device and a wet-ness-induced auditory stimulus leading to wakening and normal voiding. If behavior therapy is ineffective, imipramine, desipramine, oxybutynin, and desmopressin have been used. Hypnosis, or exercises utilizing relaxation and mental imagery, have been reported to be helpful [21,91,120,121,122].

Sleep-related groaning (catathrenia)

Catathrenia (nocturnal groaning) is typically a longstanding, nightly disorder characterized by expiratory groaning during sleep, especially during the second half of the night. Polysomnography documents recurrent bradypneic episodes that occur mainly during REM sleep and often appear in clusters, in which a deep inspiration is followed by prolonged expiration that is accompanied by a monotonous vocalization closely resembling groaning. There is no observed respiratory distress or anguished facial expression despite the presence of moaning.

The affected person is usually unaware of the groaning and it is the bed partner or roommate who is disturbed by it, especially since the groaning is often loud and may resemble cracking, humming, or roaring sounds. The groaning is not associated with any body movements, sleepwalking, or dreaming. The affected person, who could be a young adult or older adult, usually has no sleep-related complaint. No association with respiratory disorders or with psychological problems or psychiatric disorders has been found. General physical examinations and routine laboratory testing, along with neurological and otorhinolaryngological examinations, are unremarkable. The prevalence is unknown. However, it appears to be quite rare. No predisposing factors have been identified and few of the reported patients have a history of any other parasomnia. The main complication is interpersonal, as the bed partner or others in the same household have their sleep disrupted, or become distressed from the groaning. Therapy can be problematic, with nasal CPAP being effective in some patients [123,124].

Exploding head syndrome

Exploding head syndrome is characterized by the sudden sensation of a loud noise or sense of a violent explosion in the head occurring as the affected person is falling asleep or waking during the night. Descriptions of these events also include a painless loud bang, an explosion, or a clash of cymbals, but less alarming sounds can be experienced. This can be very frightening, and many patients believe they are having a stroke. The number of attacks can vary widely. It is important to emphasize that this is not a headache disorder. The prevalence is unknown. The median age of onset is 58 years, but onsets at all ages have been reported. Most patients cannot identify precipitating factors. The course is benign with no reported neurological sequelae. Symptoms often appear to remit spontaneously. The condition appears to be a sensory variant of the better-known transient (and benign) motor phenomenon of

"sleep starts" or hypnic jerks occurring at wake–sleep transitions [125,126].

Sleep-related hallucinations

The most common hallucinations emerging in relation to sleep involve the hypnagogic (occurring in the twilight of sleep onset) and hypnopompic (occurring on awakening in the morning) hallucinations that are often associated with narcolepsy, although they can occur as isolated phenomena. In addition, "complex nocturnal visual hallucinations" are another recently recognized form of sleep-related hallucinations [127]. Most patients with this condition are women (without history of daytime hallucinations), who wake up suddenly from sleep, usually without prior dream recall, and see vivid, realistic images of relatively immobile, usually silent, and sometimes distorted people or animals that vanish when a light is turned on. The patient is clearly awake and sometimes responds by jumping out of bed in terror. Unlike hypnagogic and hypnopompic hallucinations, which are usually less vivid, these hallucinations are often difficult to distinguish from waking phenomena. They may be auditory, tactile, or kinetic and are often associated with sleep paralysis. In contrast, the visual hallucinations of sleep-related complex partial epileptic seizures are usually brief, stereotyped, and fragmentary, although occasionally more vivid visual imagery may be present. Sleep-related migraine with aura at times can be associated with complex visual hallucinations, but a headache should follow. Complex nocturnal visual hallucinations can represent a benign, idiopathic condition, or it can be associated with the use of beta-adrenergic receptor blocking medications, dementia with Lewy bodies, visual loss (Charles Bonnet hallucinations), and other brain pathology (peduncular hallucinosis) [127].

Sleep-related eating disorder

Among the interesting behavioral manifestations of disorders of arousal is sleep-related eating disorder (SRED), often a relentless, chronic condition. It is characterized by consumption of high caloric foods and sometimes bizarre substances. Foods high in carbohydrates and fats are typically eaten, and binging is common. The majority of patients report that breads, pies, and dairy products such as ice cream, and also chocolate, other sweets, and peanut butter are most commonly consumed. Interestingly, hunger is typically absent in SRED and the food choices are often not consumed during the daytime.

Of 38 adults with complaints of sleep-related involuntary nocturnal eating in an early study, the problematic behaviors appeared to be related to SW in 26 (68.4%), restless legs syndrome/periodic limb movement disorder (RLS/PLMD) in 5 (13.2%), triazolam abuse in 1 (2.6%), and obstructive sleep apnea syndrome in 4 (10.5%). Over half (57.9%) described nocturnal eating frequency as nightly, but sometimes more than once in a night. Eighteen of the patients (47.4%) had evidence of DSM-III axis I psychiatric disorders and only 2 (5.3%) had daytime eating disorders, which were in remission for 3–7 years prior to sleep evaluation. Eating behaviors included sloppy preparation or consumption, injuries from cooking or eating, and weight gain. A similar earlier series of 23 consecutive cases included 11/23 (48%) based upon SW. The majority of patients described a long history of involuntary nocturnal eating (mean duration 15.8 years) and nearly all reported eating on a nightly basis (1–6 times per night). A lifetime diagnosis of daytime eating disorder was noted in 8/23 (35%) of these individuals [128]. In a prior study, Winkelman noted that sleep-related eating disorder was found in 8.7% of outpatient eating disorders, 16.7% of inpatient eating disorders, 1.0% of obese patients, 3.4% of depressed outpatients, and 4.6% of student controls. There was an association with depressed mood in those outpatients with both daytime and sleep-related eating disorders [129]. In a more recent study reporting 35 patients with nocturnal eating, 25 ate more than once a night and 8 ate more than 5 times a night [130].

Food preparation and consumption has resulted in safety concerns and adverse health consequences. Hazardous activity has included: drinking excessively hot liquids, choking on thick foods, and lacerations from careless food preparation. Furthermore, inedible and toxic substances have been consumed such as frozen food, uncooked spaghetti, cat food, egg shells, coffee grounds, sunflower shells, buttered cigarettes, glue, and cleaning solutions. It is important for psychiatrists to query patients receiving monoamine oxidase inhibitor antidepressants and their families regarding nocturnal eating or SW/ST because of the risk of possible hypertensive crisis in a patient unwittingly vulnerable to ingestion of proscribed foods.

Various medical and dental consequences can occur from repeated nocturnal eating. Weight gain is commonly reported, and the increased BMI may then precipitate, or aggravate, pre-existing diabetes mellitus (type I or II), hyperlipidemia, hypercholesterolemia, hypertension, and OSA. Furthermore, patients with SRED are at risk of ingesting poisonous substances or food to which they are allergic. Patients with SRED are at risk for poor dentition as the feeding behavior, usually high in carbohydrates, is not typically followed by dental hygiene practices. Furthermore, many patients will sleep with an oral bolus of food which combined with the circadian decline in salivary flow promotes the development of caries. Finally, failure to exhibit control over nocturnal eating can lead to secondary depressive disorders related to excessive weight gain.

SRED has been associated with psychotropic medications, in particular sedative-hypnotics. Sporadic cases of SRED have been reported with agents, such as tricyclic antidepressants, anticholinergics, lithium, triazolam, olanzapine, and risperidone. More recently SRED has been implicated with use of the benzodiazepine receptor agonist zolpidem [62,131,132]. Because of its association with sometimes complex automatic behavior, the drug should be discontinued.

Various forms of psychotherapy, hypnotherapy, and behavior therapy have proven ineffective. Generally, therapy for these disorders includes various combinations of dopaminergics (carbidopa/levodopa, bromocriptine), codeine (usually combined in an acetaminophen preparation), and clonazepam which were found associated with sustained pharmacological control in 23/27 (85.2%) of patients for whom outcome data were available [133,134]. More recently, the anticonvulsant topiramate has been shown to be efficacious in two open-label series in suppressing nocturnal eating in roughly two-thirds of patients with either the sleepwalking or the idiopathic variant of SRED [135,136].

The major differential diagnosis is night eating syndrome (NES), in which there is overeating in the evening, and often also during full nocturnal awakenings with subsequent recall the next day. NES is considered to be a sleep maintenance insomnia disorder with eating (usually not binging) helping induce the resumption of sleep, whereas SRED is a parasomnia (often with binging) with reduced awareness and compromised subsequent recall. SRED is not associated with overeating in the evening. There

Box 10.4 Case example of sleep-related eating disorder

A 19-year-old female presented 2 months before she was due to leave home to attend university. Her chief complaint was a 3-year history of increasingly frequent episodes of sleepwalking with eating. These episodes usually began 1–2 hours after she fell asleep, and she could have up to 3 episodes on a single night for 3–6 nights each week. She usually had some vague recall of her eating during the night. The patient was concerned about what her new roommates at university would think about her on account of her peculiar and disruptive sleep behaviors, and she was also concerned about her safety in wandering around a college dormitory or going outside searching for food during the night. Also, she had gained almost 15 pounds from the nocturnal eating, and was worried about further weight gain at university from her sleep-eating. She no longer had a desire to eat breakfast, and many mornings she awakened with food in her mouth and with her stomach feeling full. She worried about the possibility of choking in her sleep from unswallowed food. She felt thoroughly disgusted about her loss of control during sleep. She never, however, considered purging herself in any manner, day or night. She had an accurate appraisal of her body size and shape.

Treatment with topiramate, with an initial dose of 25 mg gradually increased to 100 mg qhs, controlled nearly all episodes of sleep-eating throughout the first half of the school year.

Box 10.5 Case example of sexsomnia

A 32-year-old married man, with a chief complaint of "fondling my wife during sleep," presented with his wife of 10 years who had urged him to seek help for his sleep problem that had begun 4 years earlier, when he commenced to snore and also grope and fondle his wife sexually while being sound asleep. His snoring became progressively louder over time and his wife reported that "he would keep trying to hump me while he was asleep." She was "shocked" to observe her husband engage in a full repertoire of sexual behavior with her while he was clearly asleep, 4 nights weekly over a period of years. His wife reported that he was somewhat insistent with his sleep sex initiatives with her, but never aggressive or violent, and he always responded promptly to her setting of limits. There had been no underlying marital problems at the time of referral or in the past. The sleep sex eventually did influence a growing strain on their marriage. They endorsed having a normal sexual relationship and could not identify any psychosocial triggering factor for the emergence of sleep sex 4 years previously, such as disordered sexual function, sexual deprivation, or other stress. There was no history of prior sleep disorder, and specifically no childhood or subsequent history of parasomnia. There was no history of medical, neurological, or psychiatric disorder, nor any loss of consciousness or seizure-like spells. There was no history of paraphilia, or criminal sexual misconduct, and he denied having problems with compulsive masturbation, or excessive/inappropriate sexual fantasies or preoccupations. He denied any history of having been sexually molested during childhood or subsequently. There was no history of alcohol or substance abuse, or excessive caffeine use; he smoked a pack of cigarettes daily.

PSG evaluation revealed moderately severe obstructive apnea, with an apnea-hypopnea index of 19/hour, oxygen desaturation nadir of 78%, and average duration of apnea, 22.7 seconds. Administration of CPAP 10 cmH$_2$O pressure completely eliminated the sleep disordered breathing. At 3-month follow-up, the patient's wife reported that nightly CPAP therapy had controlled his snoring and also completely eliminated his sexsomnia, which presumably had emerged during ongoing OSA-induced confusional arousals.

are a number of overlapping and divergent features between NES and SRED, as recently reviewed [134].

Additional varieties

Sexsomnia

Sexsomnia has been classified in the ICSD-2 within the group of parasomnias named "disorders of arousal (from NREM sleep)," with the designation of "sleep-related abnormal sexual behaviors" being a variant of confusional arousals (and SW). There is an established and growing literature on the latter phenomenon that has also been named "sleepsex," "sexsomnia," and "atypical sexual behaviors in sleep." A recent review has provided the first classification of all reported abnormal sexual behaviors associated with sleep disorders, including the sexual parasomnias. The majority of published cases involve young adult males with

rich histories of NREM sleep parasomnias, such as sleepwalking and sleep terrors. Most patients responded to standard therapy for disorders of arousal (e.g. clonazepam at hs), or CPAP therapy of OSA [137]. This parasomnia can present serious forensic implications by virtue of the variety of reported behaviors including masturbation, fondling, intercourse, and sexual vocalizations, all of which can include aggressive and even assaultive degrees of sexual behavior. These can afflict adults and minors. It is important to note that there has not been any reported case of sexsomnia in a person with either daytime paraphilia or sexual assault history, or with any suggestion of sexual deprivation playing a contributing role for the sexsomnia. This is strictly a sleep-related sexual disorder, with release of unrestrained appetitive and aggressive behaviors released during sleep.

Sleep-related epilepsy

Approximately 10% of epileptic disorders will present with exclusively or predominantly sleep-related seizures. Diagnosis is often not aided by a history of classical generalized tonic-clonic convulsions and conventional EEG studies may be inconclusive. All night PSG studies utilizing a full montage of EEG leads, and continuous audiovisual recording with

technologist observation and written commentary are essential. In spite of careful recording, some unusual ictal events may be unaccompanied by EEG dysrrhythmias, but are frequently responsive to anticonvulsant therapy. Diagnostic confusion is compounded by atypical, unconventional seizures that can present as recurrent dreams, nightmares, sleepwalking, sleep terrors, or psychiatric illness. Orbitofrontal seizures particularly may cause bizarre behavior, peculiar clustering, and a tendency to be nocturnal. Any sleep-related behavior, even such events as apnea, stridor, coughing, laryngospasm, chest pain, arrhythmias, paroxysmal flushing, and localized hyperhydrosis, may be caused by unconventional

---

Box 10.6 Case example of sleep-related epilepsy

An 11½-year-old girl was referred for evaluation of unusual arousals from sleep. These tended to occur during the latter part of the night and were noted to begin with mouthing movements leading to a generalized arousal wherein she would stand on her bed, scream, and appear very frightened. There would frequently be loss of bladder control during these episodes. There would be no tonic-clonic movement or eye deviation. She would either return promptly to sleep or arise to void, return to bed, and then fall back asleep. She would typically be amnestic for these spells on the following morning. She did have a history of earlier nocturnal generalized tonic-clonic seizures treated successfully with carbamazepine. The more recent spells were thought to represent sleep terrors possibly precipitated by epileptic discharges. In the sleep laboratory, she was found to have very frequent polyspike and slow-wave complexes in the EEG and brief runs of "epileptiform fast activity" confined to the left anterior quadrant. Clinical events occurred with characteristic repetitive screaming and axial tonic-clonic movements accompanied by focal left anterior epileptiform activity. After a difficult course, she responded to the addition of diphenylhydantoin to her regimen of carbamazepine.

Box 10.7 Case example of nocturnal frontal lobe seizures

A 27-year-old pregnant woman complained of repeated, sudden, violent, spontaneous arousals occurring shortly after falling asleep nightly. She awakens with violent movements that have even caused her to fall from the bed. She awakens instantly with awareness of tremulousness and shaking of her limbs and racing pulse. This may occur 2 or more times each night and is also observed by her husband. PSG revealed sudden, spontaneous arousals accompanied by forceful dystonic posturing of the legs for which she retained full recall. Extensive EEG monitoring revealed no epileptiform activity. Because of pregnancy, pharmacotherapy was avoided and the patient did not return for further follow-up.

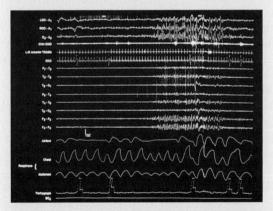

Figure 10.5 Polysomnogram showing widely distributed EEG epileptiform activity, apparently following an obstructive apnea event. The patient had a history of abrupt stereotypical arousals from sleep with loud vocalizations and thrashing arm and leg movements. There had been no apparent history of any spells during wakefulness.

seizures. They should be considered in the differential diagnosis of any sleep-related behavior that is recurrent, stereotyped, and/or inappropriate [11,138].

Nocturnal frontal lobe seizure disorder, originally described as nocturnal paroxysmal dystonia, is a condition characterized by stereotypic, repetitive spells of dystonic musculature or dyskinesia such as ballistic or choreo-athetoid movements. Frequently, the individual will demonstrate EEG and behavioral wakefulness and will recall the event, which may be accompanied by vocalization. Fearfulness during the spells can achieve the intensity of a panic attack. Though epileptiform EEG changes are typically not found during spells, response to carbamazepine is often gratifying. These conditions must be distinguished from sleep terrors and sleep-related panic attacks [139,140].

Psychiatric disorders presenting as parasomnias

Panic disorder

Some primary psychiatric disorders may include symptoms that occur prominently or exclusively in association with the sleep period. Though favored or precipitated by the sleep state physiology, they must be distinguished from primary sleep parasomnias. Panic disorder is well known in its diurnal form. Up to 69% of individuals with this disorder have had a sleep-related panic attack and 33% report recurrent sleep-related spells. Patients with panic disorder also complain of more middle and terminal insomnia than do controls [141,142]. Published PSG studies have documented increased sleep-onset latency, decreased sleep efficiency (decreased time asleep during monitored time in bed), and increased duration between sleep onset and the occurrence of the first REM period (increased REM latency), contrary to what has been reported for major depression. Sleep-related panic, when observed in the laboratory, tends to occur during transitions from lighter (stage N2) to deeper (stage N3) non-REM sleep. Clinical features of these nocturnal spells resemble those of diurnal attacks, and they arouse the patient who rapidly achieves full wakefulness with anxiety and subsequent difficulty returning to sleep. Patients retain full recall of these events [141–146]. Diagnostic caution must be emphasized because of the myriad other disorders which can masquerade as nocturnal panic, such as SW/ST, RBD, seizures, gastroesophageal reflux, OSA, bruxism, nocturnal asthma, and nocturnal cardiac arrhythmias.

Post-traumatic stress disorder

Post-traumatic stress disorder (PTSD), known for centuries as war neurosis, shell shock, combat fatigue, etc. has been studied extensively since 1980 following reports of its occurrence in combat veterans of the Vietnam war. Sleep disturbances have figured prominently in descriptions of the disorder and have been designated as "hallmark[s]" [147]. Sleep complaints include initial insomnia, sleep discontinuity with increased arousal, limb movements, night terrors, nightmares and even purposeful behavior, sometimes dream enactment that can result in injury to a bed partner who is misperceived as a threat. Earlier PSG studies describe poor sleep continuity, with increased percentages of "lighter" non-REM stages 1 and 2 and decreased deeper stages 3 and 4 [148–150]. Nightmares tend to occur less frequently in the laboratory than in the naturalistic environment [149]. Conflicting claims have appeared concerning the timing of rapid eye movement (REM) sleep, with reports of diminished REM latency [151,152] and a lengthening of this interval [153,154,155,156]. Nightmares, occurring during REM and NREM sleep, tend to be recurrent with repetitive imagery of the traumatic event [150]. No study characterizes a definitive, descriptive, polysomnographic pattern that would ultimately have therapeutic implications. In two reports, motor activation during REM sleep suggests the possibility of RBD [89,93,149]. Repetitive body movements seen in other stages may resemble those seen in non-PTSD patients with SW/ST, and rhythmic movement disorder [157]. Kardiner, in his original descriptions of war neurosis, presents a case that may represent nocturnal dissociative disorder [158].

Some studies of Vietnam combat veterans with PTSD have noted a paucity of any specific findings. As in patients with conditioned, psychophysiological insomnia, sleep laboratory findings can be substantially milder than would be predicted by the history of sleep in the usual home environment [159,160]. Indeed, careful review of sleep-related symptoms of PTSD in Vietnam theater veterans in the National Vietnam Veterans Readjustment Study has confirmed that frequent nightmares are hallmark symptoms in those with current

PTSD and correlate more with level of combat exposure than insomnia symptoms [161]. It is very possible that objective studies of sleep in PTSD may underreport nightmare frequency and severity because more severely affected subjects may avoid participation [162].

A striking finding in the PTSD sleep literature is the elevation of auditory arousal thresholds in affected subjects during NREM as well as REM sleep [163–165]. Kramer interprets these findings as evidence that in chronic PTSD there is a heightened responsiveness to internal events while individuals are less arousable by external stimuli [166]. Increased depth of sleep may represent a chronic adaptation to trauma. Kaminer and Lavie describe the diminished dream recall of their better-adjusted Holocaust survivors compared with those less well adjusted [167]. The common subjective sleep complaints of patients may reflect a breakdown of this adaptation but with enough resilience to allow intact sleep in a safe, neutral environment such as a sleep laboratory.

Treatment of PTSD has progressed in recent years. There are a number of reports of improvement in PTSD nightmares with pharmacotherapy and some studies suggest benefit from 5-HT$_2$ receptor antagonists such as nefazodone. Effectiveness of clonidine, GABAergic drugs such as tiagabine, atypical neuroleptics such as quetiapine, and anticonvulsants such as topiramate have also been reported [168–173]. Few placebo-controlled studies have been reported, and there is some evidence for utility of olanzapine as well as prazosin [174,175]. Prazosin is an alpha 1 adrenoreceptor antagonist, which has been effective in reducing frequency and intensity of nightmares as well as non-nightmare distressed awakenings [114,176,177]. Non-pharmacological therapies have included clinical hypnosis for relief of insomnia and dream rehearsal therapy for nightmares [111, 178–180]. There is accumulating evidence of efficacy for the technique known as eye movement desensitization and reprocessing therapy (EMDR), which has been theorized to modulate the intensity of PTSD by shifting the memory processing of the brain into a mode resembling REM sleep [181].

Box 10.8   Case example of PTSD

A 44-year-old veteran of combat during the Vietnam War suffered post-traumatic stress disorder (PTSD) beginning about 2 years after his tour of duty. He had symptoms satisfying DSM-IIIR criteria for it and also described cycles of waxing and waning sleep disturbance with a periodicity of around 2 weeks. Following 2 or 3 nights of terribly disturbed sleep with traumatic nightmares, he has calmer, improved sleep but with a crescendo once again to a new peak of disturbed sleep. Alcohol abuse had long been in remission. He had PSG study at a time when he expected to be at a peak level of sleep disruption. During 3 nights, PSG revealed no significant abnormality in spite of increasing subjective distress that he felt to be usually predictive of impaired sleep. He subsequently attributed his improvement in the laboratory to sleeping in the supine position and found that this position continued to be associated with improved sleep in his home until he began returning to the lateral position and again experienced poor sleep.

Factitious parasomnia

Rarely, an individual may present for evaluation with a factitious parasomnia. There is no reason to assume that such a disorder could not be chosen for this purpose. The forensic literature includes numerous examples of sleep-related violence, some of which result in exculpation because of the presence of a sleep disorder [182–184]. A particular form of factitious disorder is the Munchausen syndrome, which can even occur by proxy, such as the bizarre case of a mother who described obstructive sleep apnea in her child. When studied in the sleep laboratory, the child was observed on video recording to be suffocated by the mother who then summoned the technologist for assistance [185].

Malingering might be expected in situations involving litigation, correctional institutions, military settings, and many others. This must be very carefully considered as a diagnosis by exclusion, supported by observations, reliable reports, or other factors that would support the likelihood of malingering. Likewise, even though diagnostic findings may emerge during PSG, they do not necessarily prove that alleged acts are attributable to the disorder. The ideal role of the sleep specialist in these cases is to educate the court about the complexity of these disorders and the likelihood of the diagnoses, rather than to adopt an adversarial position [186,187].

Table 10.2 Characteristics of parasomnias

Parasomnia	Non-REM parasomnias			REM parasomnias			Other parasomnias		
	Confusional arousals	Sleepwalking	Sleep terrors	RBD	Sleep paralysis	Nightmare disorder	SRED	SRH*	SRDD
Stage of arousal	II, III, IV	III, IV	III, IV	REM	REM	REM	II, III, IV	REM	NREM or REM
Typical time of night	Anytime	First 2 hours	First 2 hours	Anytime	Anytime (first 2 hours)	Anytime	Anytime	Onset/offset of sleep	Anytime
EEG during event	NA	Mixed	Mixed	REM pattern	Wake pattern	NA	Mixed	Wake pattern	Wake pattern
EMG activity during event	↑	↑	↑	↑	↓	NA	↑	NA	↑
Decreased responsiveness during event	+	+	+	+	-	+	+	-	+
Autonomic hyperactivity	-	-	+	+	+/-	+	-	+/-	+/-
Amnesia	+	+	+	- (dream recall)	- (experience recall)	- (dream recall)	+/- (partial)	-	+
Confusion post episode	+	+	+	-	-	-	+	-	+
Family history	+	+	+	-	+/-	-	+	+/-	Unknown

EEG, electroencephalogram; EMG, electromyogram; NREM, non-rapid eye movement; RBD, REM behavior disorder; REM, rapid eye movement; SRED, sleep-related eating disorder; SRH, sleep-related hallucinations; SRDD, sleep-related dissociative disorder.

Note: *SRH for this table includes hypnagogic/pompic hallucinations. The few EEG studies of complex nocturnal hallucinations suggest they can occur from NREM. Reproduced from Plante DT, Winkelman JW. Parasomnias: Psychiatric Considerations. *Sleep Med Clin.* 2008; **3**(2):217–229, with permission from Elsevier.

Evaluation and treatment

Although the most typical and benign parasomnias require no treatment, the anxiety and concern they arouse can be calmed through education and reassurance. Any parasomnia that is significantly disruptive to individual or family life warrants careful evaluation and may require consultation with an experienced sleep medicine specialist. Any parasomnia that is potentially or actually injurious to self or others must be evaluated thoroughly at an accredited sleep disorders center with staff skilled in such evaluation. Description of clinical history must be based upon as many sources of information as possible in view of difficulties with subjective self-reports from individuals whose symptoms include varying degrees of amnesia. Initial history must include age of onset, estimations of frequency of spells at various periods in the course of the disorder, any changes over time, medical and psychiatric history, family history, general sleep history with reference to sleep hygiene and observations of respiration, sleep disruption and body movements during sleep, apparent precipitating factors including drug/alcohol abuse or dependence, and prior responses to treatment. Description of the spells must include reference to typical time of onset in the sleep period, recent frequency, specific behaviors with special regard for dangers posed to self or others, dream recall, and degree of amnesia for either dream content or actual behavior. Psychiatric assessment should focus especially on the presence or absence of mood disorders as well as drug and/or alcohol abuse or dependence. Psychiatric interview as well as screening instruments such as the MMPI, Beck depression inventory, SCL90, dissociative experiences scale, and Zung or Beck self-rating anxiety inventories may indicate areas deserving of further psychiatric assessment or therapy. A recent publication includes Table 10.2, which summarizes the clinical and polysomnographic features that distinguish various parasomnias.

When behavioral spells are observed during PSG study, the diagnosis can be confirmed. In a report of 100 consecutive adult patients with sleep-related injury, diagnoses were established by PSG in 65% of cases (42.6% of SW/ST, 100% of RBD, 42.9% of dissociative disorders, 100% of nocturnal seizures, and 100% of PLMS). Diagnoses were strongly supported in another 26% (48.1% of SW/ST), accounting for an overall positive yield of PSG studies of 91%. Confirmatory findings include behaviors such as moaning, somniloquy, yelling, limb movements, gesturing including violent movements, finger pointing, sitting up abruptly, looking around in a confused manner, apparently hallucinated behavior, and leaving the bed during particular stages of sleep or arousals. Supportive findings include excessive abrupt, spontaneous arousals from stages of NREM sleep in cases of SW/ST [19,34].

While behavioral manifestations of many disorders can lead to diagnostic confusion, proper evaluation can lead to gratifying therapeutic results with reduction of the risk of sleep-related injury for sufferers and their bed partners. Seemingly obvious SW/ST can occasionally be found to arise from a seizure disorder. Many parasomnias with bizarre, complex behaviors can be misrepresented as psychiatric illness. Treatment of nocturnal dissociative disorder with clonazepam as if it were SW/ST could be unsuccessful or even worsen the spells [119]. Treatment of RBD with neuroleptic medication as if it represented nocturnal agitation in a geriatric patient could allow the untreated parasomnia to pose continued risk of serious injury to the patient and/or bed partner and antidepressant therapy could precipitate or worsen RBD. Furthermore, the presence of RBD signals the need for careful neurological assessment and follow-up for detection of emergent neurodegenerative disorders. Only careful clinical and polysomnographic evaluations can definitively clarify the nature of the most difficult and dangerous of these disorders.

References

1. Roccatagliata G. In: *A history of ancient psychiatry.* Westport, Connecticut: Greenwood Press; 1986:107–108.

2. Roccatagliata G. In: *A history of ancient psychiatry.* Westport, Connecticutt: Greenwood Press; 1986:216.

3. Roccatagliata G. In: *A history of ancient psychiatry.* Westport, Connecticut: Greenwood Press; 1986:241.

4. Ellenberger H. *The discovery of the unconscious: the history and evolution of dynamic psychiatry.* New York: Basic Books; 1970.

5. Rush B. Of dreaming, incubus, or night mare, and somnambulism. In: *Medical inquiries and observations upon the diseases of the mind.* Philadelphia: Kimber and Richardson; 1812:300–305.

6. Ray I. Somnambulism (Chapter 19), Legal consequences of somnambulism (Chapter 20), and Simulated somnambulism (Chapter 21). In: *Treatise*

on the medical jurisprudence of insanity. Boston: Charles C. Little and James Brown; 1838:386–400.

7. Freud S. *The Interpretation of dreams.* New York: Basic Books; 1953.

8. American Psychiatric Association. *Diagnostic and statistical manual of mental disorders*, 4th ed, text revision. Washington, DC: American Psychiatric Association; 2000.

9. American Academy of Sleep Medicine. *International classification of sleep disorders, 2nd ed: Diagnostic and coding manual.* Westchester, IL: American Academy of Sleep Medicine; 2005.

10. Ohayon M, Guilleminault C, Priest R. Night terrors, sleepwalking, and confusional arousals in the general population: Their frequency and relationship to other sleep; and mental disorders. *J Clin Psychiatry.* 1999; **60**(4):268–276.

11. Mahowald M, Ettinger M. Things that go bump in the night: the parasomnias revisited. *J Clin Neurophysiol.* 1990;**7**(1):119–143.

12. Gastaut H, Broughton R. A clinical and polygraphic study of episodic phenomena during sleep. In: Wortis J, ed. *Recent advances in biological psychiatry.* New York: Plenum Press; 1965:197–223.

13. Roth B, Nevsimalova S, Rechtschaffen A. Hypersomnia with sleep drunkenness. *Arch Gen Psychiatry.* 1972;**26**:456–462.

14. Tassi P, Muzet A. Sleep inertia. *Sleep Med Rev.* 2000;**4**:341–353.

15. Klackenberg G. Somnambulism in childhood: prevalence, course and behavioral correlations. *Acta Paediatr Scand.* 1982;**71**:494–499.

16. Bixler E, Kales A, Soldatos C, et al. Prevalence of sleep disorders in the Los Angeles metropolitan area. *Am J Psychiatry.* 1979;**136**:1257–1262.

17. Casez O, Dananchet Y, Besson G. Migraine and somnambulism. *Neurology* 2005;**65**(8):1334–1335.

18. Ajlouni K, Ahmad A, El-Zahiri M, et al. Sleepwalking associated with hyperthyroidism. *Endocr Pract.* 2005;**11**(4):294.

19. Schenck C, Milner D, Hurwitz T, Bundlie S, Mahowald M. A polysomnographic and clinical report on sleep-related injury in 100 adult patients. *Am J Psychiatry.* 1989;**146**(9):1166–1173.

20. Guilleminault C, Sylvestri R. Disorders of arousal and epilepsy during sleep. In: Sterman M, Shouse M, Passouant P, eds. *Sleep and epilepsy.* New York: Academic Press; 1982:513–531.

21. Millman R, Kipp G, Carskadon M. Sleepwalking precipitated by treatment of sleep apnea with nasal CPAP. *Chest.* 1991;**99**:750–751.

22. Espa F, Dauvilliers Y, Ondze B, Billiard M, Besset A. Arousal reactions in sleepwalking and night terrors in adults: the role of respiratory events. *Sleep.* 2002; **25**(8):871–875.

23. Kleitman N. *Sleep and wakefulness,* revised and enlarged edition. Chicago: University of Chicago Press; 1963.

24. Bassetti C, Vella S, Donati F, Wielepp P, Weder B. SPECT during sleepwalking. *Lancet.* 2000;**356**:484–485.

25. Chesson A, Ferber F, Fry J, et al. The indications for polysomnography and related procedures. *Sleep.* 1997;**20**(6):423–487.

26. Kushida C, Littner M, Morgenthaler T, et al. Practice parameters for the indications for polysomnography and related procedures: an update for 2005. *Sleep.* 2005;**28**(4):499–521.

27. Pilon M, Montplaisir J, Zadra A. Precipitating factors of somnambulism: impact of sleep deprivation and forced arousals. *Neurology.* 2008;**70**(24):2284–2290.

28. Zadra A, Pilon M, Montplaisir J. Polysomnographic diagnosis of sleepwalking: effects of sleep deprivation. *Ann Neurol.* 2008;**63**(4):513–519.

29. Schenck C, Pareja J, Patterson A, Mahowald M. Analysis of polysomnographic events surrounding 252 slow-wave sleep arousals in thirty-eight adults with injurious sleepwalking and sleep terrors. *J Clin Neurophysiol.* 1998;**15**(2):159–166.

30. Zadra A, Pilon M, Joncas S, Rompre S, Montplaisir J. Analysis of postarousal EEG activity during somnambulistic episodes. *J Sleep Res.* 2004;**13** (3):279–284.

31. Diagnostic Classification Steering Committee TM, Chairman. *International classification of sleep disorders: Diagnostic and coding manual.* Rochester, Minnesota: American Sleep Disorders Association; 1990.

32. Denesle R, Gosselin A, Zadra A, Nicolas A, Montplaisir J. Arousals from REM and non-REM sleep in sleepwalkers and normal controls. *Sleep.* 1998;**21**(3 Suppl):254.

33. Kavey N, Whyte J, Resor S, Gidro-Frank S. Somnambulism in adults. *Neurology.* 1990;**40**: 749–752.

34. Bruni O, Ferri R, Novelli L, et al. NREM sleep instability in children with sleep terrors: the role of slow wave activity interruptions. *Clin Neurophysiol.* 2008;**119**(5):985–992.

35. Guilleminault C, Kirisoglu C, da Rosa A, Lopes C, Chan A. Sleepwalking, a disorder of NREM sleep instability. *Sleep Med.* 2006;**7**(2):163–170.

36. Guilleminault C, Lee J, Chan A, et al. Non-REM sleep instability in recurrent sleepwalking in pre-pubertal children. *Sleep Med.* 2005;**6**(6):515–521.

37. Pierce C, Lipcon H. Somnambulism: Psychiatric interview studies. *US Armed Forces Med J.* 1956; 7(8):1143–1153.

38. Sours J, Frumkin P, Indermill R. Somnambulism, its clinical significance and dynamic meaning in late adolescence and adulthood. *Arch Gen Psychiatry.* 1963;9:400–413.

39. Kales A, Jacobson A, Paulson M, Kales J. Somnambulism: psychophysiological correlates, II. Psychiatric interviews, psychological testing, and discussion. *Arch Gen Psychiatry.* 1966;14:595–604.

40. Kales A, Soldatos C, Caldwell A, et al. Somnambulism, clinical characteristics and personality patterns. *Arch Gen Psychiatry.* 1980;37:1406–1410.

41. Kales J, Kales A, Soldatos C, et al. Night terrors, clinical characteristics and personality patterns. *Arch Gen Psychiatry.* 1980;37:1413–1417.

42. Llorente M, Currier M, Norman S, Mellman T. Night terrors in adults: phenomenology and relationship to psychopathology. *J Clin Psychiatry.* 1992; 53(11):392–394.

43. Guilleminault C, Moscovitch A, Leger D. Forensic sleep medicine: nocturnal wandering and violence. *Sleep.* 1995;18(9):740–748.

44. Moldofsky H, Gilbert R, Lue F, MacLean A. Sleep-related violence. *Sleep.* 1995;18(9):731–739.

45. Chiu Y, Chen C, Shen W. Somnambulism secondary to olanzapine treatment in one patient with bipolar disorder. *Prog Neuropsychopharmacol Biol Psychiatry.* 2008;15(2):581–582.

46. Hafeez A, Kalinowski C. Two cases of somnambulism induced by quetiapine. *Prim Care Companion J Clin Psychiatry.* 2007;9(4):313.

47. Khawaja I, Hurwitz T, Schenck C. Violent parasomnia associated with a serotonin reuptake inhibitor (SSRI): A case report. *J Clin Psychiatry.* 2008;69:1982–1983.

48. Kawashima T, Yamada S. Paroxtine-induced somnambulism. *J Clin Psychiatry.* 2003;64(4):483.

49. Kunzel H, Schuld A, Pollmacher T. Sleepwalking associated with reboxetine in a young female patient with major depression: a case report. *Pharmacopsychiatry.* 2004;37(6):307–308.

50. Khazaal Y, Krenz S, Zullino D. Bupropion-induced somnambulism. *Addict Biol.* 2003;8:359–362.

51. Landry P, Warnes H, Nielsen T, Montplaisir J. Somnambulistic-like behaviour in patients attending a lithium clinic. *Int Clin Psychopharmacol.* 1999; 14(3):173–175.

52. Landry P, Montplaisir J. Lithium-induced somnambulism. *Can J Psychiatry.* 1998; 43(9):957–958.

53. Tsai J, Yang P, Chung W, et al. Zolpidem-induced amnesia and somnambulism: Rare occurrences? *Eur Neuropsychopharmacol.* 24 Sept 2008; Epub ahead of print.

54. Varkey B, Varkey L. Topiramate induced somnambulism and automatic behavior. *Indian J Med Sci.* 2003;57(11):508–510.

55. Sattar S, Ramaswamy S, Bhatia S, Petty F. Somnambulism due to probable interaction of valproic acid and zolpidem. *Ann Pharmacother.* 2003; 37(10):1429–1433.

56. Mahowald M, Schenck C. REM-sleep behavior disorder. In: Thorpy M, ed. *Handbook of sleep disorders.* New York: Marcel Dekker; 1990:567–593.

57. Mahowald M, Schenck C. NREM sleep parasomnias. *Neurol Clin.* 1996;14(4):675–696.

58. Charney D, Kales A, Soldatos C, Nelson J. Somnambulistic-like episodes secondary to combined lithium-neuroleptic treatment. *Br J Psychiatry.* 1979;135:418–424.

59. Hartmann E. Two case reports: night terrors with sleepwalking: a potentially lethal disorder. *J Nerv Ment Dis.* 1983;171:503–505.

60. Landry P, Warnes H, Osivka S, Montplaisir J. Somnambulistic-like behaviors induced by lithium taken with or without other pharmacological agents. *Sleep Res.* 1997;26:407.

61. Mendelson W. Sleepwalking associated with zolpidem. *J Clin Psychopharmacol.* 1994;14(2):150.

62. Morgenthaler T, Silber M. Amnestic sleep-related eating disorder associated with zolpidem. *Sleep Med.* 2002;3(4):323–327.

63. Hensel J, Pillman F. Late-life somnambulism after therapy with metoprolol. *Clin Neuropsychopharmacol.* 2008;31(4):248–250.

64. von Vigier R, Vella S, Bianchetti M. Agitated sleepwalking with fluoroquinolone therapy. *Pediatr Infect Dis J.* 1999;18(5):484–485.

65. Glick B, Schulman D, Turecki S. Diazepam (Valium) treatment in childhood sleep disorders: A preliminary investigation. *Dis Nerv Syst.* 1971;32(8):565–566.

66. Cooper A. Treatment of coexistent night-terrors and somnambulism in adults with imipramine and diazepam. *J Clin Psychiatry.* 1987;48(5):209–210.

67. Jan J, Freeman R, Wasdell M, Bomben M. A child with severe night terrors and sleep-walking responds to melatonin therapy. *Dev Med Child Neurol.* 2004;46(11):789.

68. Hurwitz T, Mahowald M, Schenck C, Schluter J, Bundlie S. A retrospective outcome study and review of hypnosis as treatment of adults with sleepwalking

and sleep terror. *J Nerv Ment Dis*. 1991;
179(4):228–233.

69. Hauri P. The treatment of parasomnias with hypnosis: a 5-year follow-up study. *J Clin Sleep Med*. 2007; **3**(4):369–373.

70. Kellerman J. Behavioral treatment of night terrors in a child with acute leukemia. *J Nerv Ment Dis*. 1979;**167**:182–185.

71. Tobin J. Treatment of somnambulism with anticipatory awakening. *J Pediatr*. 1993;**122**: 426–427.

72. Koe G. Hypnotic treatment of sleep terror disorder: a case report. *Am J Clin Hypn*. 1989;**32**(1):36–40.

73. Kohen D, Mahowald M, Rosen G. Sleep-terror disorder in children: the role of self-hypnosis in management. *Am J Clin Hypn*. 1992;**34**(4):233–244.

74. Jiarong L. 10 cases of somnambulism treated with combined acupuncture and medicinal herbs. *J Tradit Chin Med*. 1989;**9**:174–175.

75. Kales J, Cadieux R, Soldatos C, Kales A. Psychotherapy with night-terror patients. *Am J Psychother*. 1982;**36**:399–407.

76. Schenck C, Bundlie S, Ettinger M, Mahowald M. Chronic behavioral disorders of human REM sleep: a new category of parasomnia. *Sleep*. 1986;**9**:293–308.

77. Schenck C, Mahowald M. Polysomnographic, neurologic, psychiatric, and clinical outcome report on 70 consecutive cases with REM sleep behavior disorder (RBD): sustained clonazepam efficacy in 89.5% of 57 treated patients. *Cleveland Clin J Med*. 1990;**57** (Suppl):9–23.

78. Schenck C, Hurwitz T, Mahowald M. REM sleep behaviour disorder: an update on a series of 96 patients and a review of the world literature. *J Sleep Res*. 1993;**2**:224–231.

79. Mahowald M, Schenck C. REM sleep behavior disorder. In: Kryger M, Roth T, Dement W, eds. *Principles and practice of sleep medicine*. Philadelphia: WB Saunders; 1989:389–401.

80. Consens F, Chervin R, Koeppe R, et al. Validation of a polysomnographic score for REM sleep behavior disorder. *Sleep*. 2005;**28**(8):993–997.

81. Schenck C, Bundlie S, Mahowald M. Delayed emergence of a parkinsonian disorder in 38% of 29 older men initially diagnosed with idiopathic rapid eye movement sleep behavior disorder. *Neurology*. 1996;**46**:388–393.

82. Schenck C, Bundlie S, Mahowald M. REM behavior disorder (RBD): delayed emergence of parkinsonism and/or dementia in 65% of older men initially diagnosed with idiopathic RBD, and analysis of the minimum and maximum tonic and/or phasic electromyographic abnormalities found during REM sleep. *Sleep*. 2003;**26**(Abstract Suppl):A316.

83. Fantini M, Ferini-Strambi L, Montplaisir J. Idiopathic REM sleep behavior disorder: toward a better nosologic definition. *Neurology*. 2005;**64**:780–786.

84. Iranzo A, Molinuevo J, Santamaria J, et al. Rapid-eye-movement sleep behaviour disorder as an early marker for a neurodegenerative disorder: a descriptive study. *Lancet Neurol*. 2006;**5**(7):552–553.

85. Boeve B, Silber M, Saper C, et al. Pathophysiology of REM sleep behaviour disorder and relevance to neurodegenerative disease. *Brain*. 2007;**130** (Pt 11):2770–2788.

86. Thomas A, Bonanni L, Onofrj M. Symptomatic REM sleep behavior disorder. *Neurol Sci*. 2007;**28**: S21–S36.

87. Ferini-Strambi L, Di Gioia M, Castronovo V, et al. Neuropsychological assessment in idiopathic REM sleep behavior disorder (RBD): does the idiopathic form of RBD really exist? *Neurology*. 2004; **62**:41–45.

88. Winkelman J, James L. Serotonergic antidepressants are associated with REM sleep without atonia. *Sleep*. 2004;**27**:317–321.

89. Schenck C, Milner D, Hurwitz T, et al. Sleep-related injury in 85 adult patients: a polysomnographic study. *Sleep Res*. 1988;**17**:247.

90. Schenck C, Mahowald M, Kim S, O'Connor K, Hurwitz T. Prominent eye movements during NREM sleep and REM sleep behavior disorder associated with fluoxetine treatment of depression and obsessive-compulsive disorder. *Sleep*. 1992; **15**(3):226–235.

91. Schenck C, Hurwitz T, Mahowald M. REM sleep behavior disorder. *Am J Psychiatry*. 1988; **145**:652.

92. Kandel E. Cellular mechanisms of learning and the biological basis of individuality. In: Kandel E, Schwartz J, Jessell T, eds. *Principles of neural science*, 3rd ed. New York: Elsevier; 1991:1009–1031.

93. Hefez A, Metz L, Lavie P. Long-term effects of extreme situational stress on sleep and dreaming. *Am J Psychiatry*. 1987;**144**(3):344–347.

94. Sugita Y, Taniguchi M, Terashima K, et al. A young case of idiopathic REM sleep behavior disorder (RBD) specifically induced by socially stressful conditions. *Sleep Res*. 1991;**20A**:394.

95. Schenck C, Mahowald M. Injurious sleep behavior disorders (parasomnias) affecting patients on intensive care units. *Intensive Care Med*. 1991;**17**: 219–224.

96. Schenck C, Mahowald M. Long-term, nightly benzodiazepine treatment of injurious parasomnias and other disorders of disrupted nocturnal sleep in 170 adults. *Am J Med.* 1996;**100**:333–337.

97. Kunz D, Bes F. Melatonin as a therapy in REM sleep behavior disorder patients: an open-labeled pilot study on the possible influence of melatonin on REM-sleep regulation. *Mov Disord.* 1999;**14**(3): 507–511.

98. Takeuchi N, Uchimura N, Hashizume Y, et al. Melatonin therapy for REM sleep behavior disorder. *Psychiatry Clin Neurosci.* 2001;**55**(3):267–269.

99. Boeve B, Silber M, Ferman T. Melatonin therapy for treatment of REM sleep behavior disorder in neurologic disorders: results in 14 patients. *Sleep Med.* 2003;**4**:281–284.

100. Fantini M, Gagnon J, Filipini D, Montplaisir J. The effects of pramipexole in REM sleep behavior disorder. *Neurology.* 2003;**61**(10):1418–1420.

101. Schmidt M, Koshal V, Schmidt H. Use of pramipexole in REM sleep behavior disorder: results from a case series. *Sleep Med.* 2006;**7**(5):418–423.

102. Schenck C, Mahowald M. REM sleep parasomnias. *Neurol Clin.* 1996;**14**(4):697–720.

103. Zadra A, Donderi D. Nightmares and bad dreams: their prevalence and relationship to well-being. *J Abn Psychol.* 2000;**109**:273–281.

104. Ohayon M, Morselli P, Guilleminault C. Prevalence of nightmares and their relationship to psychopathology and daytime functioning in insomnia subjects. *Sleep.* 1997;**20**:340–348.

105. Tan V, Hicks R. Type A-B behavior and nightmare types among college students. *Percept Mot Skills.* 1995;**81**(1):15–19.

106. Kitabayashi Y, Ueda H, Tsuchida H, et al. Doepezil-induced nightmares in mild cognitive impairment. *Psychiatry Clin Neurosci.* 2006;**60**(1):123–124.

107. Hartmann E. *The nightmare: the psychology and biology of terrifying dreams.* New York: Basic Books; 1984.

108. Hartmann E. Normal and abnormal dreams. In: Kryger M, Roth T, Dement W, eds. *Principles and practice of sleep medicine.* Philadelphia: WB Saunders; 1989:191–195.

109. Dey S. Nightmare due to ciprofloxacin. *Indian Ped.* 1995;**32**(8):918–920.

110. Claridge G, Clark K, Davis C. Nightmares, dreams, and schizotypy. *Br J Clin Psychology.* 1997;**36**(Pt 3):377–86.

111. Krakow B, Zadra A. Clinical management of chronic nightmares: imagery rehearsal therapy. *Behav Sleep Med.* 2006;**4**(1):45–70.

112. Abramovitch H. The nightmare of returning home: a case of acute onset nightmare disorder treated by lucid dreaming. *Israel J Psychiatry Rel Sci.* 1995; **32**(2):140–145.

113. Kinzie J, Fredrickson R, Ben R, Fleck J, Karls W. Posttraumatic stress disorder among survivors of Cambodian concentration camps. *Am J Psychiatry.* 1984;**141**(5):645–650.

114. Raskind M, Peskind E, Hoff D, et al. A parallel group placebo controlled study of prazosin for trauma nightmares and sleep disturbance in combat veterans with posttraumatic stress disorder. *Biol Psychiatry.* 2007;**61**(8):928–934.

115. Koran L, Raghavan S. Fluoxetine for isolated sleep paralysis. *Psychosomatics.* 1993;**34**:184–187.

116. Hufford D. *The terror that comes in the night.* Philadelphia: University of Pennsylvania Press; 1982.

117. Hinton D, Hufford D, Kirmayer L. Culture and sleep paralysis. *Transcult Psychiatry.* 2005;**42**:5–10.

118. Agargun M, Kara Y, Ozer O, et al. Characteristics of patients with nocturnal dissociative disorders. *Sleep and Hypnosis.* 2001;**3**(4):131–134.

119. Schenck C, Milner D, Hurwitz T, Bundlie S, Mahowald M. Dissociative disorders presenting as somnambulism: polysomnographic, video and clinical documentation (8 cases). *Dissociation* 1989; **2**(4):194–204.

120. Kotagal S. Parasomnias of childhood. *Curr Opin Pediatr.* 2008;**20**(6):659–665.

121. Ferber R. Sleep-associated enuresis in the child. In: Kryger M, Roth T, Dement W, eds. *Principles and practice of sleep medicine.* Philadelphia: WB Saunders; 1989:643–647.

122. Gardner G, Olness K. *Hypnosis and hypnotherapy with children.* New York: Grune and Stratton; 1981:130–135.

123. Pevernagie D, Boon P, Mariman A, Verhaeghen D, Pauwels R. Vocalization during episodes of prolonged expiration: a parasomnia related to REM sleep. *Sleep Med.* 2001;**2**:19–30.

124. Vertrugno R, Provini F, Plazzi G, et al. Catathrenia (nocturnal groaning): a new type of parasomnia. *Neurology.* 2001;**56**:681–683.

125. Pearce J. Clinical features of the exploding head syndrome. *J Neurol Neurosurg Psychiatr.* 1989;**52**:907–910.

126. Sachs C, Svanborg E. The exploding head syndrome: polysomnographic recordings and therapeutic suggestions. *Sleep.* 1991;**14**:263–266.

127. Silber M, Hansen M, Girish M. Complex nocturnal visual hallucinations. *Sleep Med.* 2005;**6**:363–366.

128. Winkelman J W. Clinical and polysomnographic features of sleep-related eating disorder. *J Clin Psychiatry*. 1998;**59**(1):14–19.

129. Winkelman JW, Herzog DB, Fava M. The prevalence of sleep-related eating disorder in psychiatric and non-psychiatric populations. *Psychol Med*. 1999; **29**:1461–1466.

130. Vetrugno R, Manconi M, Ferini-Strambi L, et al. Nocturnal eating: sleep-related eating disorder or night eating syndrome? A videopolysomnographic study. *Sleep*. 2006;**29**:949–954.

131. Schenck C, Connoy D, Castellanos M, et al. Zolpidem-induced sleep-related eating disorder (SRED) in 19 patients. *Sleep*. 2005;**28**:A259.

132. Howell M, Schenck C, Crow S. A review of night-time eating disorders. *Sleep Med Rev*. 2008; doi:10.1016/j.smrv.2008.07.005.

133. Schenck C, Hurwitz T, Bundlie S, Mahowald M. Sleep-related eating disorders: polysomnographic correlates of a heterogeneous syndrome distinct from daytime eating disorders. *Sleep*. 1991;**14**(5):419–431.

134. Schenck C, Hurwitz T, O'Connor K, Mahowald M. Additional categories of sleep-related eating disorders and the current status of treatment. *Sleep*. 1993; **16**(5):457–466.

135. Schenck C. A study of circadian eating and sleeping patterns in night eating syndrome (NES) points the way to future studies on NES and sleep-related eating disorder. *Sleep Med*. 2006;**7**(8):653–656.

136. Winkelman J. Efficacy and tolerability of open-label topiramate in the treatment of sleep-related eating disorder: a retrospective case series. *J Clin Psychiatry*. 2006;**67**:1729–1734.

137. Schenck C, Arnulf I, Mahowald M. Sleep and sex: what can go wrong? A review of the literature on sleep related disorders and abnormal sexual behaviors and experiences. *Sleep*. 2007;**30**:683–702.

138. Pedley T, Guilleminault C. Episodic nocturnal wanderings responsive to anti-convulsant drug therapy. *Ann Neurol*. 1977;**2**:30–35.

139. Lugaresi E, Cirignotta F, Montagna P. Nocturnal paroxysmal dystonia. *J Neurol Neurosurg Psychiatry*. 1986;**49**:375–380.

140. Tinuper P, Cerullo A, Cirignotta F, et al. Nocturnal paroxysmal dystonia with short-lasting attacks: three cases with evidence for an epileptic frontal lobe origin of seizures. *Epilepsia*. 1990;**31**:549.

141. Mellman T, Uhde T. Electroencephalographic sleep in panic disorder, a focus on sleep-related panic attacks. *Arch Gen Psychiatry*. 1989;**46**:178–184.

142. Mellman T, Uhde T. Sleep panic attacks: New clinical findings and theoretical implications. *Am J Psychiatry*. 1989;**146**(9):1204–1207.

143. Lesser I, Poland R, Holcomb C, Rose D. Electroencephalographic study of nighttime panic attacks. *J Nerv Ment Dis*. 1985;**173**(12):744–746.

144. Lydiard R, Zealberg J, Laraia M, et al. Electroencephalography during sleep of patients with panic disorder. *J Neuropsychiatry Clin Neurosci*. 1989;**1** (Fall):372–376.

145. Hauri P, Friedman M, Ravaris C. Sleep in patients with spontaneous panic attacks. *Sleep*. 1989;**12**(4):323–337.

146. Mellman T, Uhde T. Sleep in panic and generalized anxiety disorders. In: Ballenger J, ed. *Neurobiology of panic disorder*. New York: Wiley-Liss; 1990:365–376.

147. Ross R, Ball W, Sullivan K, Caroff S. Sleep disturbance as the hallmark of posttraumatic stress disorder. *Am J Psychiatry*. 1989;**146**(6):697–707.

148. Friedman M. Post-Vietnam syndrome: recognition and management. *Psychosomatics*. 1981;**22**(11):931–943.

149. van der Kolk B, Blitz R, Burr W, Sherry S, Hartmann E. Nightmares and trauma: A comparison of nightmares after combat with lifelong nightmares in veterans. *Am J Psychiatry*. 1984;**14**(2):187–190.

150. Friedman M. Toward a rational pharmacotherapy for posttraumatic stress disorder: an interim report. *Am J Psychiatry*. 1988;**145**(3):281–285.

151. Kauffman C, Reist C, Djenderedjian A, Nelson J, Haier R. Biological markers of affective disorders and posttraumatic stress disorder: a pilot study with desipramine. *J Clin Psychiatry*. 1987;**48**(9):366–367.

152. Greenberg R, Pearlman C, Gampel D. War neuroses and the adaptive function of REM sleep. *Br J Med Psychol*. 1972;**45**:27–33.

153. Kramer M, Kinney L, Scharf M. Sleep in delayed-stress victims. *Sleep Res*. 1982;**11**:113.

154. Kramer M, Schoen L, Kinney L. The dream experience in dream-disturbed Vietnam veterans. In: Kolk BAVD, ed. *Post-traumatic stress disorder: psychological and biological sequelae*. Washington, DC: American Psychiatric Press; 1984:82–95.

155. Schlossberg A, Benjamin M. Sleep patterns in three acute combat fatigue cases. *J Clin Psychiatry*. 1978;**39**:546–548.

156. Lavie P, Hefez A, Halperin G, Enoch D. Long-term effects of traumatic war-related events on sleep. *Am J Psychiatry*. 1979;**136**(2):175–178.

157. Lavie P, Hertz G. Increased sleep motility and respiration rates in combat neurotic patients. *Biol Psychiatry*. 1979;**14**(6):983–987.

158. Kardiner A. *The traumatic neuroses of war*. Washington, DC: Hoeber; 1941.

159. Hurwitz T, Mahowald M, Kuskowski M, Engdahl B. Polysomnographic sleep is not clinically impaired in Vietnam combat veterans with chronic posttraumatic

stress disorder. *Biol Psychiatry*. 1998; **44**(10):1066–1073.

160. Breslau N, Roth T, Rosenthal L, Andreski P. Sleep disturbance and psychiatric disorders: A longitudinal epidemiological study of young adults. *Biol Psychiatry*. 1996;**39**:411–418.

161. Neylan T, Marmar C, Metzler T, et al. Sleep disturbances in the Vietnam generation: findings from a nationally representative sample of male Vietnam veterans. *Am J Psychiatry*. 1998; **155**(7):929–933.

162. Woodward S, Stegman W, Pavao J, et al. Self-selection bias in sleep and psychophysiological studies of posttraumatic stress disorder. *J Trauma Stress*. 2007; **20**(4):619–623.

163. Dagan Y, Lavie P. Subjective and objective characteristics of sleep and dreaming in war-related PTSD patients: lack of relationships. *Sleep Res*. 1991;**20**A:270.

164. Schoen L, Kramer M, Kinney L. Auditory thresholds in the dream disturbed. *Sleep Res*. 1984;**13**:102.

165. Lavie P, Katz N, Pillar G, Zinger Y. Elevated awaking thresholds during sleep: characteristics of chronic war-related posttraumatic stress disorder patients. *Biol Psychiatry*. 1998;**44**:1060–1065.

166. Kramer M. Developing delayed, chronic PTSD: the contribution of disturbances in sleep, dreams and responsivity. In: *International Society for Traumatic Stress Studies*. San Antonio; 1993.

167. Kaminer H, Lavie P. Sleep and dreaming in holocaust survivors, dramatic decrease in dream recall in well adjusted survivors. *J Nerv Ment Dis*. 1991; **179**(11):664–669.

168. Boehnlein J, Kinzie J. Pharmacologic reduction of CNS noradrenergic activity in PTSD: the case for clonidine and prazosin. *J Psychiatr Pract*. 2007;**13**(2):72–78.

169. Kinzie J, Sack R, Riley C. The polysomnographic effects of clonidine on sleep disorders in posttraumatic stress disorder: a pilot study with Cambodian patients. *J Nerv Ment Dis*. 1994;**182**(10):585–587.

170. Connor K, Davidson J, Meisler R, Zhang W, Abraham L. Tiagabine for posttraumatic stress disorder: effects of open-label and double-blind discontinuation treatment. *Psychopharmacology*. 2006;**184**(1):21–25.

171. Robert S, Hamner M, Kose S, et al. Quetiapine improves sleep disturbances in combat veterans with PTSD: sleep data from a prospective, open-label study. *J Clin Psychopharm*. 2005;**25**(4):387–388.

172. Neylan T, Lenoci M, Maglione M, et al. The effect of nefazodone on subjective and objective sleep quality in posttraumatic stress disorder. *J Clin Psychiatry*. 2003;**64**(4):445–450.

173. Berlant J. Topiramate in posttraumatic stress disorder: preliminary clinical observations. *J Clin Psychiatry*. 2001;**62**(Suppl 17):60–63.

174. van Liempt S, Vermetten E, Geuze E, Westenberg H. Pharmacotherapy for disordered sleep in post-traumatic stress disorder: a systematic review. *Int Clin Psychopharmacol*. 2006;**21**(4):193–202.

175. Stein M, Kline N, Matloff J. Adjunctive olanzapine for SSRI-resistant combat-related PTSD: a double-blind placebo-controlled study. *Am J Psychiatry*. 2002; **159**(10):1777–1779.

176. Thompson C, Taylor F, McFall M, Barnes R, Raskind E. Non-nightmare distressed awakenings in veterans with posttraumatic stress disorder: response to prazosin. *J Trauma Stress*. 2008;**21**(4):417–420.

177. Miller L. Prazosin for the treatment of posttraumatic stress disorder sleep disturbances. *Pharmacotherapy*. 2008;**28**(5):656–666.

178. Abramowitz E, Barak Y, Ben-Avi I, Knobler H. Hypnotherapy in the treatment of chronic combat-related PTSD patients suffering from insomnia: a randomized, zolpidem-controlled clinical trial. *Int J Clin Exp Hypn*. 2008;**56**(3):270–280.

179. Moore B, Krakow B. Imagery rehearsal therapy for acute posttraumatic nightmares among combat soldiers in Iraq. *Am J Psychiatry*. 2007;**164**(4):683–684.

180. Germain A, Shear M, Hall M, Buysse D. Effects of a brief behavioral treatment for PTSD-related sleep disturbances: a pilot study. *Behav Res Ther*. 2007;**45**:3.

181. Stickgold R. EMDR: a putative neurobiological mechanism of action. *J Clin Psychol*. 2002;**58**(1):61–75.

182. Mahowald M, Bundlie S, Hurwitz T, Schenck C. Sleep violence – forensic science implications: polysomnographic and video documentation. *J Forensic Sci*. 1990;**35**(2):413–432.

183. Broughton R, Billings R, Cartwright R, et al. Homicidal somnambulism: a case report. *Sleep*. 1994;**17**(3):253–264.

184. Broughton R, Shimizu T. Sleep-related violence: A medical and forensic challenge. *Sleep*. 1995; **18**(9):727–730.

185. Mahowald MW, Schenck CH, Rosen GM, Hurwitz T D. The role of a sleep disorder center in evaluating sleep violence. *Arch Neurol*. 1992;**49**:604–607.

186. Bornemann M, Mahowald M, Schenck C. Parasomnias: clinical and forensic implications. *Chest*. 2006;**130**(2):605–610.

187. Pressman M, Schenck C, Mahowald M, Bornemann M. Sleep science in the courtroom. *J Forensic Leg Med*. 2007;**14**(2):108–111.

Circadian rhythm disorders

Katy Borodkin and Yaron Dagan

Overview

Humans, like many other mammals, are awake through the daytime hours and sleep during the night. Sometimes, sleep and wake episodes are chronically misaligned with the 24-hour social and physical environment. When this mismatch involves (1) complaints of insomnia or excessive daytime sleepiness or both, and (2) impaired academic, occupational, social, or family functioning, a circadian rhythm sleep disorder (CRSD) is established [1].

CRSDs can be classified as primary, secondary, or behavioral according to their etiology. Primary CRSDs arise from an abnormality of the intrinsic biological clock and include four types. *Delayed sleep phase type* (or delayed sleep phase disorder, DSPD) occurs when habitual sleep–wake times are delayed usually more than 2 hours relative to conventional or socially acceptable times (see Figure 11.1). When forced to follow an environmentally imposed schedule, these patients complain of difficulties falling asleep and waking up in the morning, and feel sleepy during the day. *Advanced sleep phase type* (or advanced sleep phase disorder, ASPD) is characterized by habitual sleep onset and wake-up times that are several hours earlier than desired or socially accepted (see Figure 11.2). This pattern results in symptoms of compelling evening sleepiness, early sleep onset, and awakening that is earlier than desired.

The third type of primary CRSD is the *non-entrained type* (or non-24-hour sleep–wake syndrome), in which the sleep–wake cycle is usually longer than a 24-hour period (see Figure 11.3). Sleep and wake episodes are progressively delayed each day to later times, thus alternating between synchrony and complete asynchrony with the environmental schedule. Lastly, the *irregular sleep–wake type* (or irregular sleep–wake rhythm) is characterized by sleep and wake episodes that are temporally disorganized and variable throughout the 24-hour period (see Figure 11.4). These patients are likely to manifest inability to initiate and maintain sleep at night, frequent daytime napping, and excessive daytime sleepiness [1].

Secondary CRSDs are diagnosed if the CRSD is due to an underlying medical or neurological condition, among which are brain tumor [2,3], head trauma [4,5], dementia [6], and Parkinson's disease [7]. The CRSD is presumed to result from the effects of the underlying condition on the circadian timing system. The sleep–wake disruption can be similar to any of the four primary types of CRSD (DSPD, ASPD, non-24-hour sleep–wake syndrome, and irregular sleep–wake rhythm). Secondary CRSDs can also arise as a side-effect of a drug or substance, as will be described later in this chapter.

Behavioral CRSDs are disorders that emerge when the activity of the normal intrinsic biological clock is disrupted by external factors. One such CRSD is shift work sleep disorder, which occurs as a result of working hours scheduled during the habitual sleep hours. The disorder is most commonly reported in night and early morning shift workers and might involve complaints of daytime sleepiness, difficulty initiating sleep and awakening, and insufficient sleep. The condition may last as long as the person continues working shifts. In some cases, it may persist beyond the duration of shift work.

Another type of behavioral CRSD is jet leg syndrome, in which there is a temporary incompatibility between the intrinsic sleep–wake cycle and the environmental 24-hour cycle following a change in time zone. The disorder can arise following a

Foundations of Psychiatric Sleep Medicine, ed. John W. Winkelman and David T. Plante. Published by Cambridge University Press.
© Cambridge University Press 2010.

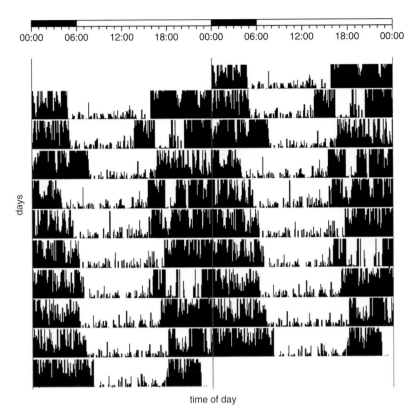

Figure 11.1 Sleep–wake schedule of a patient with delayed sleep phase disorder, represented by an actogram. Sleep episodes (represented by white areas) start at 4 a.m. to 6 a.m. and end at 3 p.m. to 5 p.m. Thus, the sleep–wake cycle is delayed, but relatively stable throughout the monitoring period.

transmeridian flight across at least two time zones and begins within 1-2 days following the air travel. Jet lag syndrome is associated with complaints of sleep disturbances, insomnia, daytime sleepiness, decreased alertness, difficulties in daytime functioning, general malaise, and sometimes, gastrointestinal disturbance. The severity and duration of the symptoms usually depend on the number of time zones crossed and the direction of the flight. This chapter will mainly focus on primary and secondary CRSDs; the reader is referred to recent reviews on behavioral CRSDs for further information [8,9].

Limited data are available regarding the prevalence of CRSDs (both primary and secondary) in the general population. DSPD is more common (7.3%) [10] among adolescents living in Western countries than among adults, where the estimated prevalence ranges from 0.13% [11] to 0.17% [12]. ASPD is estimated to occur in 1% of middle-aged and older adults [13]. Non-24-hour sleep–wake syndrome and irregular sleep–wake rhythm are assumed to be rare conditions in the general population. Non-24-hour sleep–wake syndrome is common among totally blind individuals. Irregular sleep–wake rhythm is usually

secondary to a neuropsychiatric condition, particularly those requiring institutionalization. Among patients with CRSDs referred to sleep clinics, the vast majority receive the diagnosis of DSPD (83.5%), 12.3% have non-24-hour sleep–wake syndrome, while only a handful of patients suffer from an irregular sleep–wake rhythm (1.9%) and ASPD (1.3%) [14].

The majority of patients with CRSD (89.6%) report that the disorder typically began in early childhood or adolescence [14]. Secondary CRSDs can occur at any age. All primary and secondary CRSDs are chronic conditions, which can last throughout life, unless treated. There are no known gender differences.

Pathophysiology

Diurnal rhythms are regulated by the circadian timing system. The core component of this system is the suprachiasmatic nucleus of the hypothalamus. This internal biological clock has self-generated, endogenous near-circadian rhythmicity, which it conveys through direct and indirect pathways to a widespread network of subcortical and cortical sites. Regulation of the circadian rhythm of the sleep–wake

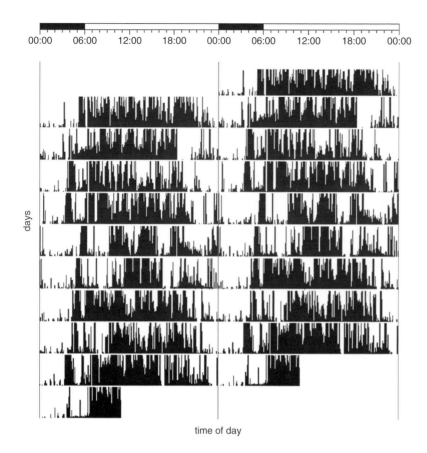

Figure 11.2 Sleep–wake schedule of a patient with advanced sleep phase disorder, represented by an actogram. Sleep episodes (represented by white areas) start at 8 p.m. to 10 p.m. and end at 4 a.m. to 5 a.m. Thus, the sleep–wake cycle is advanced, but relatively stable throughout the monitoring period.

cycle involves secretion of the hormone melatonin by the pineal gland, one of the central target sites of the suprachiasmatic nucleus [15].

Several findings indicate that CRSDs can arise as a result of an altered circadian timing system. DSPD is associated with delayed circadian rhythms of melatonin [16–18], cortisol, thyroid-stimulating hormone [17], and body temperature [19], indicating that a phase delay in the internal circadian clock might underlie DSPD. In addition, the coupling between the sleep–wake cycle and melatonin rhythms is also altered in DSPD [18,20] as well as non-24-hour sleep–wake syndrome [21]. Similarly, altered phase relationships between the sleep–wake cycle and body temperature rhythms exist in DSPD [19,22–24] and in non-24-hour sleep–wake syndrome [24]. Thus, in some patients, CRSD may reflect not a simple alteration in the phase of the internal clock, but an inability of the clock to coordinate among endogenous physiological systems, and to keep these systems properly entrained to the 24-hour day [22].

The endogenous biological pacemaker is synchronized or entrained with the environment through time cues, such as light [25]. Exposure to bright light at night acutely reduces melatonin concentration in subjects with a typical sleep–wake rhythm [26]. Interestingly, patients with DSPD show even greater melatonin suppression in response to light than controls [27], whereas patients with non-24-hour sleep–wake syndrome seem to be less sensitive than controls to this manipulation [28]. Thus, altered sensitivity of the circadian timing system to external cues might also be a factor precipitating and maintaining abnormalities in the timing and coupling of circadian rhythms noted in CRSDs.

Some findings suggest that the pathophysiology of CRSDs, particularly DSPD, might also involve deficiencies of the sleep homeostatic process, which regulates the balance between sleep and wakefulness periods. One manifestation of this process is growing sleep pressure with prolonged wakefulness. Thus, after total sleep deprivation sleep pressure increases, and recovery sleep can occur regardless of the time of the day in healthy subjects. In contrast, patients with DSPD are able to compensate for previous sleep loss

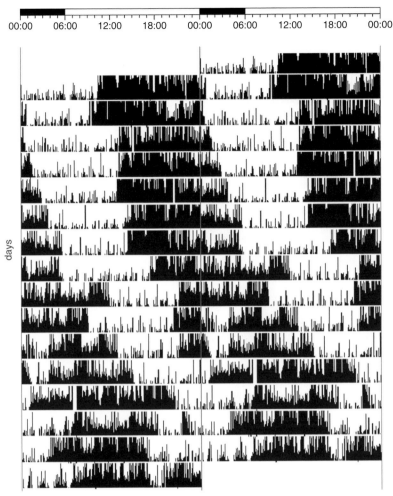

Figure 11.3 Sleep–wake schedule of a patient with non-24-hour sleep–wake syndrome, represented by an actogram. On the first 2 days of monitoring, sleep episodes (represented by white areas) begin at around 1 a.m. During the following 5 days, sleep onset is delayed each day by an hour, thus by the end of the first week the patient falls asleep at approximately 6 a.m. During the second week, sleep episodes are further and further delayed and so, by the end of the monitoring period, sleep episodes occur during the day and early evening hours. Due to his longer than 24-hour sleep–wake cycle, the patient sometimes sleeps at night and sometimes during the day.

time of day

only during their circadian night [20,29]. Patients with DSPD also show different temporal distribution of slow-wave sleep [22,24]. These alterations in sleep propensity and sleep architecture, along with differences in phase relationships of the sleep–wake cycle and physiological markers of the endogenous clock, can be interpreted as evidence of an imbalance between circadian and sleep homeostatic systems in the pathophysiology of DSPD. However, it is unclear if these physiological abnormalities described above are caused by the CRSDs, or an effect of the abnormal exposure to light which is characteristic of the syndromes.

Lastly, a genetic origin was demonstrated in some CRSDs. As many as 44% of patients with a CRSD have other family members with similar sleep–wake patterns as the patient [14]. In a pedigree of one family with DSPD, the trait was found to segregate with either an autosomal dominant mode of heritance with incomplete penetrance or a multifactorial mode of inheritance [30]. Structural polymorphisms on one of the haplotypes of the human period3 gene (*hper3*) were implicated as contributors to increased susceptibility to DSPD [31]. Several pedigrees of familial ASPD were also reported, in which the ASPD trait segregated as an autosomal dominant mode of inheritance [32,33]. Although a mutation of human period2 (*hper2*) gene was identified in a large family with ASPD [34], other findings indicate genetic heterogeneity in this disorder [35].

Diagnosis

The diagnosis of CRSDs can be established through three procedures: clinical interview, longitudinal

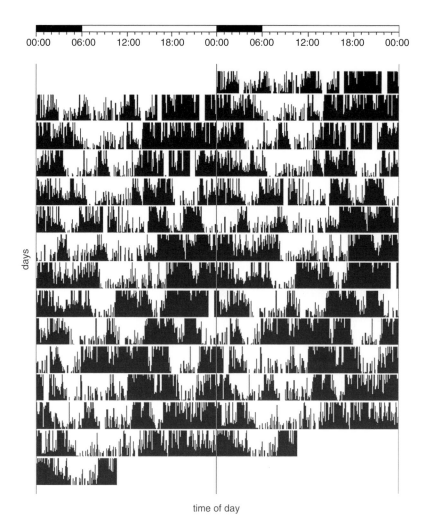

00:00 06:00 12:00 18:00 00:00 06:00 12:00 18:00 00:00

days

time of day

Figure 11.4 Sleep–wake schedule of a patient with irregular sleep–wake rhythm, represented by an actogram. During the monitoring days, sleep (represented by white areas) alternates chaotically with wakefulness (represented by black areas). Most of the 24-hour periods contain more than a single sleep episode. Thus, the sleep–wake cycle is unstable and sleep is frequently fragmented into several episodes.

monitoring of the sleep–wake cycle, and assessment of biological markers of the internal circadian rhythmicity. During the clinical interview, the patient is asked about sleep onset and offset times, sleep-related symptoms, timing of hunger and preferred cognitive activity, hereditary trends, presence of other diseases, and use of medications. In most types of these disorders, clinical interview is helpful in establishing the general diagnosis of CRSD, but the particular type is usually defined by longitudinal monitoring of sleep–wake patterns.

Sleep–wake patterns should be studied for several days (at least 7–10 days are recommended) using actigraphy or a sleep log. An actigraph is a watch-sized device worn on the non-dominant wrist, which samples hand motion. The output of this device is an actogram, in which periods of inactivity (presumed to

be sleep episodes) are represented by white areas and periods of activity (presumed to be wake episodes) by black areas. The 24-hour period can be double-plotted in a raster format (see Figures 11.1–4 for examples). Visual screening of an actogram is usually sufficient to recognize the sleep–wake pattern. Actigraphy also produces quantitative data for more precise evaluation of such sleep variables as sleep onset and offset, sleep duration, number of awakenings, number of limb movements, and sleep efficiency.

It is important to note that periods of inactivity as measured by actigraphy are not always sleep (e.g. the patient may be meditating, reading, or may remove the actigraph temporarily), and thus actigraphy is often combined with sleep diaries/logs and patient report to more accurately determine sleep–wake periods. Sleep logs are records of bedtime and awakening time made by the patient. If actigraphic devices are unavailable, sleep logs alone can be a reliable substitution for clinical purposes. In the evaluation of a potential CRSD, actigraphic/sleep log monitoring should be carried out in unconstrained conditions, such that the patient is free to choose bedtime and wake-up hours. This feature is highly important in CRSD diagnosis, since a sleep–wake schedule obtained under forced conditions can mask the true pattern of the schedule, thus obscuring the diagnosis.

The third diagnostic procedure is assessment of biological markers of the internal biological clock, as captured by melatonin and body temperature circadian rhythms. This procedure is not mandatory, but can be helpful in complicated cases, especially when non-24-hour sleep–wake syndrome or irregular sleep–wake rhythm is suspected. In clinical practice, salivary melatonin and oral temperature samplings can be made simultaneously every 2 hours for 36 hours during wakefulness. The acrophase (time of the rhythm's maximal values) of melatonin rhythm and the nadir of temperature rhythm (time of the rhythm's minimal values) are the most straightforward chronobiological markers to establish the phase of the rhythm. The period of each rhythm and phase relationships between the rhythms are also useful in defining the abnormality of the intrinsic biological clock.

Differential diagnosis

Primary CRSDs, especially DSPD and ASPD, should be distinguished from "normal" sleep patterns. Some individuals without sleep disorders might demonstrate a DSPD-like sleep–wake cycle. This might occur when sleep onset is delayed voluntarily, as a consequence of occupational, academic, and social activities in the late evening hours. These individuals differ from patients with DSPD mainly in the flexibility of their biological clock. Thus, an individual with an intact biological clock who is used to falling asleep later than accepted is able to adjust his or her sleep–wake schedule to environmental changes (such as transition from weekend to weekday, vacations, new working hours, etc.). Patients with DSPD seem to be unable to readily phase shift sleep episodes by motivation or education alone. Similarly, early sleep onset and awakening in the elderly should not be confused with ASPD. Whereas normal advancement in the phase of the sleep–wake cycle tends to occur in the elderly, ASPD is a chronic condition that can appear as early as childhood, but typically begins in middle age.

CRSDs should also be differentiated from other primary sleep disorders, especially those presenting with excessive daytime sleepiness (such as idiopathic hypersomnia, sleep apnea, and narcolepsy). Patients with CRSDs are not sleepy if allowed to follow their intrinsic preferred sleep–wake cycle. Insomnia disorders can also be confused with DSPD, due to complaints of difficulties falling asleep that are present in both disorders. Patients suffering from sleep-onset insomnia may feel sleepy at the desired bedtime, but have difficulty initiating sleep. By comparison, patients with DSPD who attempt to move their bedtime earlier (i.e. advance their sleep–wake cycle) will not be sleepy and thus will be unable to fall asleep. Further, sleep-onset difficulties endure for as long as the patient keeps his bedtime out of phase with his endogenous sleep–wake rhythm. When allowed to maintain the preferred schedule, sleep initiation is normal, unlike insomnia patients who often have difficulties initiating or maintaining sleep regardless of the timing of sleep.

Primary CRSDs should be distinguished from behavioral and secondary CRSDs. A thorough patient interview and physical examination (when an underlying medical condition is suspected) may help to establish the etiology of the CRSD in such cases.

Lastly, the various types of primary CRSDs should be differentiated from each other. Some individuals with non-24-hour sleep–wake syndrome might show DSPD-like symptoms, such as difficulty falling asleep, daytime sleepiness, and delayed sleep onset. To establish the diagnosis, actigraphic/sleep log monitoring is often required. In unconstrained conditions, rest–activity patterns of a patient with DSPD show relative stability in sleep onset and offset, whereas sleep episodes of a patient with a non-24-hour sleep–wake syndrome are progressively delayed to later hours from day to day. If the actogram/sleep log is inconclusive, as might occur in atypical cases, assessment of melatonin/temperature circadian rhythm is helpful. In DSPD, both rhythms have a clear 24-hour periodicity, whereas in non-24-hour sleep–wake syndrome the period is usually longer than 24 hours. Further, if both melatonin and temperature rhythms are measured simultaneously, their phases will be desynchronized with each other only in the case of non-24-hour sleep–wake syndrome.

Treatment

Bright light therapy and melatonin treatment, or a combination of these two, have proved to be the most effective treatment modalities for patients with CRSDs. These techniques aim to reset the sleep–wake cycle of patients to match the external 24-hour schedule.

Bright light is the most powerful time cue to the internal circadian timing system. Light exposure at specific times of the 24-hour period can result in a phase shift of the endogenous circadian rhythms of various functions, such as melatonin secretion, body temperature, and sleep propensity [36–38]. In general, exposure to bright light in the morning induces a phase advance, whereas evening bright light exposure induces phase delay. Bright light exposure as a therapy can be provided by means of artificial light devices. The patient is required to sit in front of a light-box at a prespecified time. In patients with DSPD, exposure to 2000–2500 lux from 6 a.m. to 9 a.m. helps to advance the sleep–wake rhythm, and avoidance of bright light in the evening may be necessary to prevent the circadian rhythm from being further delayed [39]. In patients with ASPD, 2500 lux for 4 hours from 8 p.m. to midnight, or 4000 lux for 2 or 3 hours from 8 or 9 p.m. to 11 p.m. [40] is recommended to induce phase delay. Some evidence supports the effectiveness of light therapy in the treatment of non-24-hour sleep–wake syndrome [41], jet lag [42], and shift work [43]. Further recommendations on intensities and time limits for bright light therapy in the treatment of CRSDs have been provided by the American Academy of Sleep Medicine [44].

Endogenous melatonin secreted by the pineal gland is another potent regulator of the sleep–wake cycle. It is thought that the night-time increase in melatonin concentration reduces body temperature, which promotes the onset of sleep [45]. Pharmacological preparations of melatonin can mimic the effects of endogenous melatonin. These effects are time dependent: phase advance is produced by melatonin administered in the evening, whereas melatonin administration in the morning induces phase delays [46]. These effects are the opposite of those produced by light. For example, melatonin may be administered in the evening (roughly 2 hours before the desired sleep onset, rather than at bedtime) in DSPD to help advance the circadian rhythm. Of note, the use of morning melatonin to delay the circadian rhythm, which would be theoretically useful in ASPD, can be problematic as melatonin can also be sedating, thus decreasing daytime alertness in some instances. Administration of melatonin might be a preferable therapeutic strategy for many patients who find bright light therapy too demanding, leading to decreased compliance. The beneficial effects of melatonin 0.5–5 mg/day were demonstrated in several types of CRSD [47–51], and in some instances, higher doses may have no added effect (or even be less effective) in shifting the circadian rhythm compared to lower doses. Importantly, treatment with melatonin not only synchronizes the sleep–wake cycle of patients with CRSD, but may also significantly improve several dimensions of their daytime functioning [52]. Although the long-term effects of melatonin administration remain to be fully researched, the treatment appears to be promising. Recent well-designed studies indicate that even relatively large doses of melatonin (10 mg/day for a month) have no toxic effects [53]. Further, a prolonged-release 2 mg melatonin preparation (Circadin™) was approved by the European Medicines Agency for the short-term treatment of primary insomnia in patients who are aged 55 or above.

Patients not responding to bright light or melatonin therapies may adopt a rehabilitative approach, according to which the patients would accept that their condition is permanent and consider changes in lifestyle that will be congruent with their sleep–wake cycle (e.g. working evening shifts in the case of DSPD) [54].

Circadian rhythm sleep disorders in psychiatry

Generally, otherwise healthy patients with CRSDs seem to suffer from more emotional and cognitive disturbances than healthy controls [55]. Psychiatric disorders are also very common in these patients. For example, in a sample of 126 patients with CRSDs attending sleep clinics, 29% had a psychiatric diagnosis [56]. In another study, 62% of sighted patients with non-24-hour sleep–wake syndrome had a psychiatric co-morbidity [57]. While CRSDs can co-occur with a wide variety of mental disorders, the present chapter will review the disorders that have been systematically examined with regard to CRSDs, specifically mood disorders, attention-deficit/hyperactivity disorder (ADHD), personality disorders, and obsessive-compulsive disorder (OCD).

The etiology of the relationship between CRSDs and psychiatric disorders is a matter of debate. It has been suggested that in patients who developed a CRSD after the onset of a psychiatric disorder, the sleep–wake alteration is an epiphenomenon that arises due to changes in behavioral patterns [57,58]. In other cases, the incompatibility of the sleep–wake cycle and the social environment might be the primary factor predisposing patients with CRSDs to psychiatric illness [59]. Another intriguing possibility is that the sleep–wake abnormality and the psychiatric disorder share a common pathology [60], possibly in the circadian timing system.

Mood disorders

Diurnal variation in mood, a common feature of depressive illness, has led many researchers to look for irregularities in circadian rhythms in these patients. Altered amplitude and phase of melatonin, cortisol, prolactin, and body temperature were found in patients with major depressive disorder (MDD) [61,62], bipolar depression (BD) [63], and seasonal affective disorder (SAD) [64,65]. Recent studies have also demonstrated polymorphisms of several clock genes (such as Period3, CLOCK, BMAL1, TIMELESS) in MDD [66], BD [67–70], and SAD [71] that may be associated with the development of the mood disorder and/or specific sleep–wake patterns during the course of the illness.

Sleep disturbance is one of the hallmarks of depression. Complaints of insomnia (difficulty initiating sleep, nocturnal arousals, and early morning wakening) are very common in MDD. Subjective reports of hypersomnia tend to occur in BD during depressive episodes [72] and in SAD [73]. Sleep in MDD, as measured by polysomnography, is characterized by longer sleep onset, more fragmented sleep, shorter total sleep time, reduced time spent in SWS, and several abnormalities in REM sleep (reviewed in [74]). Interestingly, nocturnal sleep patterns in BD seem to be similar to those in MD, despite differences in the clinical manifestations of these disorders [75]. SAD is also characterized by sleep abnormalities, but these are different from those seen in MDD and BD. For example, some studies reported longer (rather than shorter) total sleep time [73], increased (rather than reduced) SWS duration [76], and normal (rather than shortened) REM latency [73] in SAD patients compared to healthy controls.

Based on the aforementioned findings, several researchers hypothesized that depression is a chronobiological disorder that arises as a result of a mismatch between circadian rhythms [77–79]. According to these approaches, insomnia symptoms are a manifestation of this mismatch. The pathology of CRSDs is also linked to alterations in the circadian timing system, and thus it is not surprising that these disorders are also highly co-morbid with mood disorders. In a study of clinical profiles of DSPD in 22 adolescents, 36% showed features of depression and 27% received prior treatment for depression [80]. In 33 adult patients with DSPD, as many as 76% were treated with antidepressants in the past or at the time of research, although such a high prevalence was possibly a result of self-referral bias [81]. When a large sample of DSPD patients was compared to healthy controls, the results showed the same trends: DSPD was associated with greater current depression ratings, lifetime history of unipolar depression, depression treatment, antidepressant use, and family history of depression [60].

Depression also seems to be a frequent co-morbidity in non-24-hour sleep–wake syndrome. Among 57 sighted individuals with non-24-hour sleep–wake syndrome, major depression preceded the CRSD onset in 5.3% of the sample. Interestingly, 34% developed major depression following the onset of non-24-hour sleep–wake syndrome. One-third of these reported that depression severity varied according to changes in sleep phase: it was aggravated when sleep episodes occurred during the daytime and slightly ameliorated when sleep episodes occurred during the night-time [57].

Several mechanisms have been proposed to explain the association between CRSDs and depression. Since patients with DSPD often have a family history of depression, the disorders might share genetic susceptibility factors [60]. Alternatively, a sleep–wake cycle that is discrepant with the environment might lead to social isolation and reduced light exposure. Since both factors are considered synchronizers of the internal biological clock, inappropriate exposure (both to light and social cues) might also predispose to depression. Conversely, depression itself can cause social withdrawal and decrease in outdoor activities, exacerbating or leading to a CRSD [57,60].

While these suggestions are plausible, they cannot fully account for CRSDs without depression. Future research should further explore the conditions that lead to co-occurrence of the disorders. Depressive disorders are commonly recognized as heterogeneous.

It is therefore possible that different subtypes can also be characterized by sleep disturbances with distinct etiologies, some of which may be related to circadian mechanisms. Such differentiation between subtypes might be clinically important, since previous findings indicate that the type of sleep disturbance can be predictive of depression recurrence. For example, residual insomnia in patients with depression treated with antidepressants and psychotherapy confers greater risk for subsequent depression [82]. On the other hand, melatonin administration in patients with DSPD may successfully treat the sleep disorder and significantly reduce depressive symptoms [52,83]. Thus, careful examination of the sleep disturbance associated with depression might improve our understanding of the underlying pathology as well as the treatment outcome.

Attention-deficit/hyperactivity disorder

ADHD is frequently associated with sleep disturbances. The characteristics and the implications of sleep disorders such as sleep apnea and restless legs syndrome in ADHD received broad attention in the literature (reviewed in [84,85]). Recently, a few studies also provided a description of the characteristics of CRSDs in ADHD patients. Van der Heijden and colleagues examined a group of children with ADHD and sleep disturbance, which was defined by the authors as idiopathic sleep-onset insomnia [86]. Compared to ADHD without insomnia, the ADHD with insomnia group had later sleep onset and wake-up time, and delayed melatonin rhythm. Importantly, no differences between the groups were found in measures of sleep maintenance. This profile of sleep disturbance has led the authors to suggest that insomnia in children with ADHD is, in fact, pediatric DSPD.

The prevalence of ADHD in pediatric patients with DSPD seems to be high. In one study [87], as many as 28 out of 62 (45%) children with suspected DSPD were previously diagnosed with ADHD. We found a similar prevalence in our sample of children and adolescents diagnosed with DSPD: among 33 patients, 15 (45%) had been previously diagnosed with ADHD [88]. When adults with ADHD were studied, 40.7% described themselves as evening types, as assessed by the morningness–eveningness questionnaire [89]. Greater evening preference was associated in this study with more subjective and objective deficits in functioning.

Treatment with melatonin generally improves sleep disturbances in children with ADHD and DSPD. Compared to placebo, a 1-month treatment with 3-6 mg melatonin administered at 7 p.m. advanced sleep onset and melatonin rhythm, reduced sleep latency, and increased total sleep time [87,90]. Long-term treatment with 3–5 mg melatonin taken 2 hours before bedtime advanced sleep onset and total sleep time in children and adolescents with DSPD and co-morbid ADHD [88]. It also reduced the frequency of sleep-related complaints typical of DSPD: difficulty falling asleep and waking up, as well as daytime sleepiness.

Some of the findings indicate that chronobiological treatments might prove helpful not only for sleep disturbances, but also for ADHD-related symptomatology. Treatment with 5 mg melatonin at 7 p.m. improved health and functional status of children with ADHD and suspected DSPD [87]. We also found that long-term treatment with 3–5 mg melatonin taken 2 hours before sleep reduced the frequency of self-reported behavioral/social difficulties and of absences/late arrivals at school in children and adolescents with DSPD and ADHD [88]. However, in another study, no effect of melatonin was found on problem behavior, cognitive performance, or quality of life [90]. Adults with ADHD treated with light (10 000 lux) administered for half an hour before 8 a.m. for 3 weeks showed advance in circadian preference, which also was the best predictor of improvement in the severity of ADHD symptoms [91].

The frequent co-occurrence of ADHD and DSPD in clinical samples could be related to selection bias, i.e. patients with ADHD exhibit more behavioral problems and are more likely to receive professional guidance. Other possibilities are that DSPD is secondary to primary abnormalities in the central nervous system associated with ADHD or to treatment with stimulants. However, there is no evidence at present to support such an etiology. Alternatively, DSPD might be the underlying condition that contributes to hyperactive and inattentive behaviors. DSPD in school-aged students involves chronic and substantial sleep loss [88]. Insufficient sleep and ADHD are both associated with impairment of executive functions regulated by the prefrontal cortex [92]. Thus, chronic sleep loss during the school years might lead to and/or exacerbate ADHD symptomatology.

It was recently reported that one of the alleles of the CLOCK polymorphism is associated with adult ADHD [93]. Thus, it is possible that co-occurrence of ADHD and DSPD arises as a result of a genetic alteration of the circadian clock system. Lastly, the overlap between ADHD and DSPD might be attributed to frequent underrecognition and misinterpretation of symptoms of DSPD on the part of health professionals. The incompatibility of sleep–wake habits with school schedule is frequently associated with dysfunctional school behaviors and underachievement, which in some cases might be severe enough to be mistakenly interpreted as symptoms of ADHD. Interestingly, many of the patients with DSPD in our sample were able to reduce or discontinue psychotherapy and/or stimulant medication during melatonin therapy [88]. This finding indicates that at least in some cases, CRSD-related dysfunctional behaviors might be erroneously interpreted as symptoms of ADHD.

Personality disorders

Personality disorders are also a frequent psychiatric co-morbidity in CRSDs. For example, as many as 22% of patients with CRSDs attending sleep clinics were diagnosed with personality disorders based on clinical interview [14]. In another study, a higher prevalence of personality disorders was found in patients with DSPD or non-24-hour sleep–wake syndrome than in healthy controls [94]. In both of these studies, no specific profile of personality disorders could be clearly detected over and above the existence of general personality pathology. To explore this association further, the sleep–wake habits of 63 adolescents with a variety of mental disorders hospitalized in psychiatric wards were examined [59]. Sixteen percent were diagnosed as having DSPD. The probability of co-morbid DSPD among patients with personality disorders was significantly higher than among patients with any other psychiatric disorder. Further, all of the patients with DSPD suffered from disorders characterized by affective lability, namely bipolar disorder, schizoaffective disorder classified as mainly affective, and borderline personality disorder [59].

These findings have led some to suggest that there may be an interrelationship between CRSD and personality disorders. It is noticeable that both disorders are defined [95] as primarily involving a mismatch between the expectations of the society in which the individual lives and his or her own behavioral pattern. Thus, it might be that personality disorders are characterized by a deviant sleep–wake pattern as one expression of the general deviation from the expectations of society.

On the other hand, it could be speculated that peculiarities of the biological clock might lead to emotional, social, and functional difficulties that subsequently give rise to a personality disorder. According to this latter hypothesis, a deviant sleep–wake schedule frequently emerges early in life, possibly harming the mother and the child's mutual ability to adapt to each other. The mother, required to adjust to a biological clock of her infant that differs markedly from her own, becomes tired, frustrated, and angry, causing the infant to respond accordingly. The resulting emotional burden, carried by both parties, might jeopardize the attachment processes, thus affecting future prospects of personal and social relationships of the child. At later stages of life, such a child has difficulties following the school timetable of activities, fails to obtain sufficient amount of sleep at night, loses concentration during the morning and early afternoon hours, and, eventually, falls behind other children in school.

Frequently, the abnormal sleep–wake cycle of individuals with CRSD and the accompanying dysfunction at school or work are misattributed by parents, educators, psychologists, and other healthcare professionals to psychological rather than biological factors, such as laziness and low motivation. This attitude toward individuals with CRSD, to which they are subjected since early childhood or adolescence, adds psychological distress to the practical difficulties of coping with life and may theoretically contribute to the development of personality disorders [14,59,94].

Obsessive-compulsive disorder

The occurrence of OCD was occasionally reported in studies of clinical features of CRSDs. In a sample of 126 patients with CRSDs, approximately 5.5% had co-morbid OCD [56]. In another sample of 57 patients with non-24-hour sleep–wake syndrome, 3.5% suffered from OCD that preceded the onset of the sleep disorder [57]. Recently, the possible association between OCD and CRSDs has received more focused attention. In a retrospective study of 187 OCD inpatients [96], 17.6% showed symptoms of DSPD, which is considerably higher than the prevalence reported in the general population [12,13]. In a prospective study of OCD inpatients, even higher prevalence of DSPD was found: among

36 patients, 42% fulfilled criteria for DSPD [58]. In both studies, patients with DSPD had more severe OCD and experienced higher levels of functional disability than patients with OCD and a normal sleep phase.

The authors found that the OCD groups with and without DSPD did not differ in the severity of depressive symptoms, the extent of rituals around bedtime, or in prescribed medications. Having alternative explanations ruled out, they suggested that a direct link between DSPD and OCD might exist. Further, the authors raised the possibility that DSPD was secondary to OCD in their sample, since all patients in the DSPD group reported that the delay in sleep phase occurred after the onset of OCD. Accordingly, the alteration of the sleep–wake cycle in OCD might have occurred as a result of common daily routines (such as lengthy in-house rituals in the morning), social isolation, and lack of regularity in meal times, all of which can diminish the impact of external time cues on the internal biological clock. Other findings suggest that some of the physiological circadian rhythms are altered in OCD [97,98], suggesting that sleep–wake schedule disorders in OCD might result from an interaction of an abnormal intrinsic biological clock and lack of appropriate external time signals. Clearly, more research is required to further explore the nature of the association between OCD and CRSDs.

Psychoactive medication

Several cases of disrupted sleep–wake schedule as iatrogenic effects of psychoactive drugs are documented in the literature. Treatment with the typical neuroleptic haloperidol in a patient with chronic schizophrenia was associated with an irregular sleep–wake cycle. Switching treatment to the atypical neuroleptic clozapine established a more organized and stable sleep–wake pattern and improved the clinical state of the patient [99]. In another study [100], patients receiving typical neuroleptics (flupentixol or haloperidol) showed a variety of abnormalities in the daily rest–activity rhythm (e.g. delayed circadian phase syndrome, free-running sleep–wake syndrome, and irregular sleep–wake rhythm). In contrast, rest–activity cycles of those patients treated with the atypical neuroleptic clozapine were highly organized and synchronized with the environmental schedule.

Similar effects were observed in a patient with early-onset Alzheimer's disease: when treated with haloperidol, her rest–activity patterns became completely arrhythmic, which was accompanied by marked worsening of cognitive state. When haloperidol was replaced by clozapine, rapid normalization of her sleep–wake cycle occurred and cognitive functioning improved [101]. Similar effects of haloperidol were described in a patient with Gilles de la Tourette syndrome [102]. Prior to haloperidol treatment, the patient reported having a normal sleep–wake schedule. Two years after commencing the treatment, his sleep–wake cycle became irregular. When therapy with haloperidol was changed to the atypical neuroleptic risperidone, the timing and duration of sleep episodes became more organized, although his sleep–wake schedule still remained somewhat disturbed. The patient's sleep–wake circadian rhythm was fully recovered after addition of melatonin as a secondary therapy. This was accompanied by improvement in quality of life, social interactions, and employment status.

These findings suggest that typical neuroleptics like haloperidol and flupentixol might alter the circadian sleep–wake rhythm, whereas atypical neuroleptics like clozapine and risperidone tend to enhance the congruity of the individual's sleep–wake cycle with the environment. Since this effect was evident in several medical disorders, e.g. schizophrenia, Alzheimer's disease, and Tourette syndrome, it was argued that CRSDs might be a side-effect of typical neuroleptics, rather than illness-related phenomena [99–102]. The exact mechanisms through which typical and atypical neuroleptics exert their differential effects on the sleep–wake cycle remain to be elucidated.

Other psychoactive drugs, such as selective serotonin reuptake inhibitors (SSRIs), can also trigger the emergence of CRSD as a side-effect. Treatment with fluvoxamine in patients with OCD was associated with DSPD [103]. It was postulated that DSPD in these patients was secondary to fluvoxamine since: (1) all patients received no other medications except fluvoxamine prior to the onset of DSPD, (2) in all patients, DSPD first occurred following fluvoxamine initiation, (3) when fluvoxamine was withdrawn or the dose considerably reduced, the sleep–wake cycle returned to normal, and (4) with re-exposure to fluvoxamine, DSPD recurred. Interestingly, emergence of DSPD may be specific to fluvoxamine; treatment with two other serotonin reuptake inhibitors (clomipramine and fluoxetine) was not associated with any adverse effects on the sleep–wake cycle of these patients [103]. The authors hypothesized that the alteration of the sleep–wake schedule or the lack of it by different antidepressant agents might depend on the differential effects of these drugs on serum melatonin levels.

To summarize, the above described cases indicate that certain psychoactive medications might have adverse effects on the circadian rhythm of the sleep–wake cycle. To date, there is clinical evidence of such effects for haloperidol, flupentixol, and fluvoxamine. Further research exploring whether additional psychotropics are associated with disruptions of the sleep–wake schedule, whether the response is dose- and time-dependent, and what patient characteristics contribute to development of CRSDs while on these drugs is needed. At this stage, however, sleep-related complaints of patients treated with psychoactive drugs, especially haloperidol, flupentixol and fluvoxamine, should not always be regarded as drug-induced insomnia or daytime somnolence. In some cases, CRSDs should be considered as a possible side-effect. When iatrogenic CRSD is suspected, changing therapy and/or adding melatonin and/or light therapy might be indicated.

Conclusion

There is an intimate relationship between CRSDs and psychiatric disorders, such as mood disorders, ADHD, personality disorders, and OCD. It is plausible that in some cases the CRSD is secondary to the psychiatric disorder, whereas in others the sleep pathology may lead to the development of psychiatric symptoms. Another possibility is that common pathology underlies both sleep and mental abnormalities. Conventional treatment of CRSDs (i.e. by means of melatonin or bright light therapies) can sometimes improve not only sleep–wake disturbances, but also psychiatric symptomatology. Thus, research into the nature of the association between CRSDs and mental disorders might be extremely helpful in developing appropriate treatment options for such patients.

It should be emphasized that CRSDs in otherwise healthy individuals are associated with significant emotional distress and multilevel disturbances in daily functioning. In extreme cases, these characteristics of CRSDs might be severe enough to be mistakenly interpreted as symptoms of psychiatric disorders. As was previously described [54,104], many cases of CRSDs are under-recognized and misdiagnosed as psychiatric disorders or psychophysiological insomnia. Consequently, these patients receive inappropriate treatment, which can enhance the psychological distress and add to the adjustment difficulties that accompany CRSDs. Thus, it is clearly of great importance to raise awareness of these disorders among pediatricians, physicians, neurologists, psychiatrists, and psychologists.

References

1. American Academy of Sleep Medicine. *International classification of sleep disorders: diagnostic and coding manual*, 2nd ed. Westchester, IL: American Academy of Sleep Medicine; 2005.

2. Borodkin K, Ayalon L, Kanety H, Dagan Y. Dysregulation of circadian rhythms following prolactin-secreting pituitary microadenoma. *Chronobiol Int.* 2005;**22**(1):145–156.

3. Cohen RA, Albers HE. Disruption of human circadian and cognitive regulation following a discrete hypothalamic lesion: a case study. *Neurology.* 1991;**41**(5):726–729.

4. Ayalon L, Borodkin K, Dishon L, Kanety H, Dagan Y. Circadian rhythm sleep disorders following mild traumatic brain injury. *Neurology.* 2007;**68**(14):1136–1140.

5. Boivin DB, James FO, Santo JB, Caliyurt O, Chalk C. Non-24-hour sleep–wake syndrome following a car accident. *Neurology.* 2003;**60**(11):1841–1843.

6. Witting W, Kwa IH, Eikelenboom P, Mirmiran M, Swaab DF. Alterations in the circadian rest-activity rhythm in aging and Alzheimer's disease. *Biol Psychiatry.* 1990;**27**(6):563–572.

7. Bliwise DL, Watts RL, Watts N, et al. Disruptive nocturnal behavior in Parkinson's disease and Alzheimer's disease. *J Geriatr Psychiatry Neurol.* 1995;**8**(2):107–110.

8. Sack RL, Auckley D, Auger RR, et al. Circadian rhythm sleep disorders: part I, basic principles, shift work and jet lag disorders. An American Academy of Sleep Medicine review. *Sleep.* 2007;**30**(11):1460–1483.

9. Waterhouse J, Reilly T, Atkinson G, Edwards B. Jet lag: trends and coping strategies. *Lancet.* 2007;**369**(9567):1117–1129.

10. Paleo RP, Thorpy MJ, Glovinsky P. Prevalence of delayed sleep phase syndrome among adolescents. *Sleep Res.* 1998;**17**:391.

11. Yazaki M, Shirakawa S, Okawa M, Takahashi K. Demography of sleep disturbances associated with circadian rhythm disorders in Japan. *Psychiatry Clin Neurosci.* 1999;**53**(2):267–268.

12. Schrader H, Bovim G, Sand T. The prevalence of delayed and advanced sleep phase syndromes. *J Sleep Res.* 1993;**2**(1):51–55.

13. Ando K, Kripke DF, Ancoli-Israel S. Estimated prevalence of delayed and advanced sleep phase syndromes. *Sleep Res.* 1995;**24**:509.

14. Dagan Y, Eisenstein M. Circadian rhythm sleep disorders: toward a more precise definition and diagnosis. *Chronobiol Int.* 1999;**16**(2):213–222.

15. Klein DC, Moore RY. Pineal N-acetyltransferase and hydroxyindole-O-methyltransferase: control by the retinohypothalamic tract and the suprachiasmatic nucleus. *Brain Res.* 1979;**174**(2):245–262.

16. Rahman SA, Kayumov L, Tchmoutina EA, Shapiro CM. Clinical efficacy of dim light melatonin onset testing in diagnosing delayed sleep phase syndrome. *Sleep Med.* 2009;**10**(5):549–555.

17. Shibui K, Uchiyama M, Kim K, et al. Melatonin, cortisol and thyroid-stimulating hormone rhythms are delayed in patients with delayed sleep phase syndrome. *Sleep and Biological Rhythms.* 2003;**1**(3):209–214.

18. Shibui K, Uchiyama M, Okawa M. Melatonin rhythms in delayed sleep phase syndrome. *J Biol Rhythms.* 1999;**14**(1):72–76.

19. Ozaki S, Uchiyama M, Shirakawa S, Okawa M. Prolonged interval from body temperature nadir to sleep offset in patients with delayed sleep phase syndrome. *Sleep.* 1996;**19**(1):36–40.

20. Uchiyama M, Okawa M, Shibui K, et al. Poor compensatory function for sleep loss as a pathogenic factor in patients with delayed sleep phase syndrome. *Sleep.* 2000;**23**(4):553–558.

21. Uchiyama M, Shibui K, Hayakawa T, et al. Larger phase angle between sleep propensity and melatonin rhythms in sighted humans with non-24-hour sleep–wake syndrome. *Sleep.* 2002;**25**(1):83–88.

22. Campbell SS, Murphy PJ. Delayed sleep phase disorder in temporal isolation. *Sleep.* 2007;**30**(9):1225–1228.

23. Uchiyama M, Okawa M, Shibui K, et al. Altered phase relation between sleep timing and core body temperature rhythm in delayed sleep phase syndrome and non-24-hour sleep–wake syndrome in humans. *Neurosci Lett.* 2000;**294**(2):101–104.

24. Watanabe T, Kajimura N, Kato M, et al. Sleep and circadian rhythm disturbances in patients with delayed sleep phase syndrome. *Sleep.* 2003;**26**(6):657–661.

25. Czeisler CA, Kronauer RE, Allan JS, et al. Bright light induction of strong (type 0) resetting of the human circadian pacemaker. *Science.* 1989;**244**(4910):1328–1333.

26. Lewy AJ, Wehr TA, Goodwin FK, Newsome DA, Markey SP. Light suppresses melatonin secretion in humans. *Science.* 1980;**210**(4475):1267–1269.

27. Aoki H, Ozeki Y, Yamada N. Hypersensitivity of melatonin suppression in response to light in patients with delayed sleep phase syndrome. *Chronobiol Int.* 2001;**18**(2):263–271.

28. McArthur AJ, Lewy AJ, Sack RL. Non-24-hour sleep–wake syndrome in a sighted man: circadian rhythm studies and efficacy of melatonin treatment. *Sleep.* 1996;**19**(7):544–553.

29. Uchiyama M, Okawa M, Shibui K, et al. Poor recovery sleep after sleep deprivation in delayed sleep phase syndrome. *Psychiatry Clin Neurosci.* 1999;**53**(2):195–197.

30. Ancoli-Israel S, Schnierow B, Kelsoe J, Fink R. A pedigree of one family with delayed sleep phase syndrome. *Chronobiol Int.* 2001;**18**(5):831–840.

31. Ebisawa T, Uchiyama M, Kajimura N, et al. Association of structural polymorphisms in the human period3 gene with delayed sleep phase syndrome. *EMBO Rep.* 2001;**2**(4):342–346.

32. Jones CR, Campbell SS, Zone SE, et al. Familial advanced sleep-phase syndrome: A short-period circadian rhythm variant in humans. *Nat Med.* 1999;**5**(9):1062–1065.

33. Reid KJ, Chang AM, Dubocovich ML, et al. Familial advanced sleep phase syndrome. *Arch Neurol.* 2001;**58**(7):1089–1094.

34. Toh KL, Jones CR, He Y, et al. An hPer2 phosphorylation site mutation in familial advanced sleep phase syndrome. *Science.* 2001;**291**(5506):1040–1043.

35. Satoh K, Mishima K, Inoue Y, Ebisawa T, Shimizu T. Two pedigrees of familial advanced sleep phase syndrome in Japan. *Sleep.* 2003;**26**(4):416–417.

36. Drennan M, Kripke DF, Gillin JC. Bright light can delay human temperature rhythm independent of sleep. *Am J Physiol.* 1989;**257**(1 Pt 2):R136–141.

37. Honma K, Honma S, Nakamura K, et al. Differential effects of bright light and social cues on reentrainment of human circadian rhythms. *Am J Physiol.* 1995;**268**(2 Pt 2):R528–535.

38. Tzischinsky O, Lavie P. The effects of evening bright light on next-day sleep propensity. *J Biol Rhythms.* 1997;**12**(3):259–265.

39. Rosenthal NE, Joseph-Vanderpool JR, Levendosky AA, et al. Phase-shifting effects of bright morning light as treatment for delayed sleep phase syndrome. *Sleep.* 1990;**13**(4):354–361.

40. Campbell SS, Dawson D, Anderson MW. Alleviation of sleep maintenance insomnia with timed exposure to bright light. *J Am Geriatr Soc.* 1993;**41**(8):829–836.

41. Partonen T, Vakkuri O, Lamberg-Allardt C. Effects of exposure to morning bright light in the blind and sighted controls. *Clin Physiol.* 1995;**15**(6):637–646.

42. Honma K, Honma S, Sasaki M, Endo T. Bright lights accelerate the re-entrainment of circadian clock

to 8-hour phase-advance shift of sleep–wake schedule: 1 Circadian rhythms in rectal temperature and plasma melatonin level. *Jpn J Psychiatry Neurol.* 1991;**45**(1):153–154.

43. Czeisler CA, Johnson MP, Duffy JF, et al. Exposure to bright light and darkness to treat physiologic maladaptation to night work. *N Engl J Med.* 1990;**322**(18):1253–1259.

44. Chesson AL Jr, Anderson WM, Littner M, et al. Practice parameters for the nonpharmacologic treatment of chronic insomnia. An American Academy of Sleep Medicine report. Standards of Practice Committee of the American Academy of Sleep Medicine. *Sleep.* 1999;**22**(8):1128–1133.

45. Cagnacci A, Elliott JA, Yen SS. Melatonin: a major regulator of the circadian rhythm of core temperature in humans. *J Clin Endocrinol Metab.* 1992;**75**(2): 447–452.

46. Lewy AJ, Ahmed S, Jackson JM, Sack RL. Melatonin shifts human circadian rhythms according to a phase-response curve. *Chronobiol Int.* 1992;**9**(5):380–392.

47. Dagan Y, Yovel I, Hallis D, Eisenstein M, Raichik I. Evaluating the role of melatonin in the long-term treatment of delayed sleep phase syndrome (DSPS). *Chronobiol Int.* 1998;**15**(2):181–190.

48. Dahlitz M, Alvarez B, Vignau J, et al. Delayed sleep phase syndrome response to melatonin. *Lancet.* 1991;**337**(8750):1121–1124.

49. Nagtegaal JE, Kerkhof GA, Smits MG, Swart AC, Van Der Meer YG. Delayed sleep phase syndrome: A placebo-controlled cross-over study on the effects of melatonin administered five hours before the individual dim light melatonin onset. *J Sleep Res.* 1998;**7**(2):135–143.

50. Oldani A, Ferini-Strambi L, Zucconi M, et al. Melatonin and delayed sleep phase syndrome: ambulatory polygraphic evaluation. *Neuroreport.* 1994;**6**(1):132–134.

51. Sack RL, Brandes RW, Kendall AR, Lewy AJ. Entrainment of free-running circadian rhythms by melatonin in blind people. *N Engl J Med.* 2000;**343** (15):1070–1077.

52. Nagtegaal JE, Laurant MW, Kerkhof GA, et al. Effects of melatonin on the quality of life in patients with delayed sleep phase syndrome. *J Psychosom Res.* 2000;**48**(1):45–50.

53. Seabra ML, Bignotto M, Pinto LR Jr, Tufik S. Randomized, double-blind clinical trial, controlled with placebo, of the toxicology of chronic melatonin treatment. *J Pineal Res.* 2000;**29**(4):193–200.

54. Dagan Y, Abadi J. Sleep-wake schedule disorder disability: a lifelong untreatable pathology of the

circadian time structure. *Chronobiol Int.* 2001;**18** (6):1019–1027.

55. Shirayama M, Shirayama Y, Iida H, et al. The psychological aspects of patients with delayed sleep phase syndrome (DSPS). *Sleep Med.* 2003;**4**(5):427–433.

56. Yamadera W, Sasaki M, Itoh H, Ozone M, Ushijima S. Clinical features of circadian rhythm sleep disorders in outpatients. *Psychiatry Clin Neurosci.* 1998;**52**(3):311–316.

57. Hayakawa T, Uchiyama M, Kamei Y, et al. Clinical analyses of sighted patients with non-24-hour sleep–wake syndrome: a study of 57 consecutively diagnosed cases. *Sleep.* 2005;**28**(8):945–952.

58. Turner J, Drummond LM, Mukhopadhyay S, et al. A prospective study of delayed sleep phase syndrome in patients with severe resistant obsessive-compulsive disorder. *World Psychiatry.* 2007; **6**(2):108–111.

59. Dagan Y, Stein D, Steinbock M, Yovel I, Hallis D. Frequency of delayed sleep phase syndrome among hospitalized adolescent psychiatric patients. *J Psychosom Res.* 1998;**45**(1 Spec No):15–20.

60. Kripke DF, Rex KM, Ancoli-Israel S, et al. Delayed sleep phase cases and controls. *J Circadian Rhythms.* 2008;**6**:6.

61. Koenigsberg HW, Teicher MH, Mitropoulou V, et al. 24-h monitoring of plasma norepinephrine, MHPG, cortisol, growth hormone and prolactin in depression. *J Psychiatr Res.* 2004;**38**(5):503–511.

62. Szymanska A, Rabe-Jablonska J, Karasek M. Diurnal profile of melatonin concentrations in patients with major depression: relationship to the clinical manifestation and antidepressant treatment. *Neuro Endocrinol Lett.* 2001;**22**(3):192–198.

63. Nurnberger JI Jr, Adkins S, Lahiri DK, et al. Melatonin suppression by light in euthymic bipolar and unipolar patients. *Arch Gen Psychiatry.* 2000;**57** (6):572–579.

64. Avery DH, Dahl K, Savage MV, et al. Circadian temperature and cortisol rhythms during a constant routine are phase-delayed in hypersomnic winter depression. *Biol Psychiatry.* 1997;**41**(11):1109–1123.

65. Wehr TA, Duncan WC Jr, Sher L, et al. A circadian signal of change of season in patients with seasonal affective disorder. *Arch Gen Psychiatry.* 2001;**58** (12):1108–1114.

66. Pirovano A, Lorenzi C, Serretti A, et al. Two new rare variants in the circadian "clock" gene may influence sleep pattern. *Genet Med.* 2005;**7**(6):455–457.

67. Benedetti F, Dallaspezia S, Colombo C, et al. A length polymorphism in the circadian clock gene Per3

influences age at onset of bipolar disorder. *Neurosci Lett.* 2008;**445**(2):184–187.

68. Benedetti F, Dallaspezia S, Fulgosi MC, et al. Actimetric evidence that CLOCK 3111 T/C SNP influences sleep and activity patterns in patients affected by bipolar depression. *Am J Med Genet B Neuropsychiatr Genet.* 2007;**144B**(5):631–635.

69. Mansour HA, Wood J, Logue T, et al. Association study of eight circadian genes with bipolar I disorder, schizoaffective disorder and schizophrenia. *Genes Brain Behav.* 2006;**5**(2):150–157.

70. Nievergelt CM, Kripke DF, Barrett TB, et al. Suggestive evidence for association of the circadian genes PERIOD3 and ARNTL with bipolar disorder. *Am J Med Genet B Neuropsychiatr Genet.* 2006;**141B**(3):234–241.

71. Johansson C, Willeit M, Smedh C, et al. Circadian clock-related polymorphisms in seasonal affective disorder and their relevance to diurnal preference. *Neuropsychopharmacology.* 2003;**28**(4):734–739.

72. Detre T, Himmelhoch J, Swartzburg M, et al. Hypersomnia and manic-depressive disease. *Am J Psychiatry.* 1972;**128**(10):1303–1305.

73. Anderson JL, Rosen LN, Mendelson WB, et al. Sleep in fall/winter seasonal affective disorder: effects of light and changing seasons. *J Psychosom Res.* 1994;**38**(4): 323–337.

74. Benca RM, Obermeyer WH, Thisted RA, Gillin JC. Sleep and psychiatric disorders: A meta-analysis. *Arch Gen Psychiatry.* 1992;**49**(8):651–668.

75. Duncan WC Jr, Pettigrew KD, Gillin JC. REM architecture changes in bipolar and unipolar depression. *Am J Psychiatry.* 1979;**136**(11): 1424–1427.

76. Schwartz PJ, Rosenthal NE, Kajimura N, et al. Ultradian oscillations in cranial thermoregulation and electroencephalographic slow-wave activity during sleep are abnormal in humans with annual winter depression. *Brain Res.* 2000;**866**(1–2):152–167.

77. Borbely AA, Wirz-Justice A. Sleep, sleep deprivation and depression: A hypothesis derived from a model of sleep regulation. *Hum Neurobiol.* 1982;**1**(3):205–210.

78. Ehlers CL, Frank E, Kupfer DJ. Social zeitgebers and biological rhythms: A unified approach to understanding the etiology of depression. *Arch Gen Psychiatry.* 1988;**45**(10):948–952.

79. Lewy AJ, Sack RL, Miller LS, Hoban TM. Antidepressant and circadian phase-shifting effects of light. *Science.* 1987;**235**(4786):352–354.

80. Thorpy MJ, Korman E, Spielman AJ, Glovinsky PB. Delayed sleep phase syndrome in adolescents. *J Adolesc Health Care.* 1988;**9**(1):22–27.

81. Regestein QR, Monk TH. Delayed sleep phase syndrome: a review of its clinical aspects. *Am J Psychiatry.* 1995;**152**(4):602–608.

82. Dombrovski AY, Mulsant BH, Houck PR, et al. Residual symptoms and recurrence during maintenance treatment of late-life depression. *J Affect Disord.* 2007;**103**(1–3):77–82.

83. Srinivasan V, Smits M, Spence W, et al. Melatonin in mood disorders. *World J Biol Psychiatry.* 2006;**7**(3): 138–151.

84. Owens JA. The ADHD and sleep conundrum: a review. *J Dev Behav Pediatr.* 2005;**26**(4):312–322.

85. Philipsen A, Hornyak M, Riemann D. Sleep and sleep disorders in adults with attention deficit/hyperactivity disorder. *Sleep Med Rev.* 2006;**10**(6):399–405.

86. Van der Heijden KB, Smits MG, Van Someren EJ, Gunning WB. Idiopathic chronic sleep onset insomnia in attention-deficit/hyperactivity disorder: a circadian rhythm sleep disorder. *Chronobiol Int.* 2005;**22**(3):559–570.

87. Smits MG, van Stel HF, van der Heijden K, et al. Melatonin improves health status and sleep in children with idiopathic chronic sleep-onset insomnia: a randomized placebo-controlled trial. *J Am Acad Child Adolesc Psychiatry.* 2003;**42**(11):1286–1293.

88. Szeinberg A, Borodkin K, Dagan Y. Melatonin treatment in adolescents with delayed sleep phase syndrome. *Clin Pediatr (Phila).* 2006;**45**(9):809–818.

89. Rybak YE, McNeely HE, Mackenzie BE, Jain UR, Levitan RD. Seasonality and circadian preference in adult attention-deficit/hyperactivity disorder: clinical and neuropsychological correlates. *Compr Psychiatry.* 2007;**48**(6):562–571.

90. Van der Heijden KB, Smits MG, Van Someren EJ, Ridderinkhof KR, Gunning WB. Effect of melatonin on sleep, behavior, and cognition in ADHD and chronic sleep-onset insomnia. *J Am Acad Child Adolesc Psychiatry.* 2007;**46**(2):233–241.

91. Rybak YE, McNeely HE, Mackenzie BE, Jain UR, Levitan RD. An open trial of light therapy in adult attention-deficit/hyperactivity disorder. *J Clin Psychiatry.* 2006;**67**(10):1527–1535.

92. Dahl RE. The regulation of sleep and arousal: development and psychopathology. *Dev Psychopathol.* 1996;**8**:3–27.

93. Kissling C, Retz W, Wiemann S, et al. A polymorphism at the 3′-untranslated region of the CLOCK gene is associated with adult attention-deficit hyperactivity disorder. *Am J Med Genet B Neuropsychiatr Genet.* 2008;**147**(3):333–338.

94. Dagan Y, Sela H, Omer H, Hallis D, Dar R. High prevalence of personality disorders among circadian

rhythm sleep disorders (CRSD) patients. *J Psychosom Res.* 1996;**41**(4):357–363.

95. American Psychiatric Association. *Diagnostic and statistical manual of mental disorders*, 4th ed. Washington, DC: American Psychiatric Association; 1994.

96. Mukhopadhyay S, Fineberg NA, Drummond LM, et al. Delayed sleep phase in severe obsessive-compulsive disorder: a systematic case-report survey. *CNS Spectr.* 2008;**13**(5):406–413.

97. Millet B, Touitou Y, Poirier MF, et al. Plasma melatonin and cortisol in patients with obsessive-compulsive disorder: relationship with axillary temperature, physical activity, and clinical symptoms. *Biol Psychiatry.* 1998;**44**(9):874–881.

98. Monteleone P, Catapano F, Del Buono G, Maj M. Circadian rhythms of melatonin, cortisol and prolactin in patients with obsessive-compulsive disorder. *Acta Psychiatr Scand.* 1994;**89**(6):411–415.

99. Wirz-Justice A, Cajochen C, Nussbaum P. A schizophrenic patient with an arrhythmic circadian rest-activity cycle. *Psychiatry Res.* 1997;**73**(1–2):83–90.

100. Wirz-Justice A, Haug HJ, Cajochen C. Disturbed circadian rest-activity cycles in schizophrenia patients: an effect of drugs? *Schizophr Bull.* 2001;**27**(3):497–502.

101. Wirz-Justice A, Werth E, Savaskan E, et al. Haloperidol disrupts, clozapine reinstates the circadian rest-activity cycle in a patient with early-onset Alzheimer disease. *Alzheimer Dis Assoc Disord.* 2000;**14**(4):212–215.

102. Ayalon L, Hermesh H, Dagan Y. Case study of circadian rhythm sleep disorder following haloperidol treatment: reversal by risperidone and melatonin. *Chronobiol Int.* 2002;**19**(5):947–959.

103. Hermesh H, Lemberg H, Abadi J, Dagan Y. Circadian rhythm sleep disorders as a possible side effect of fluvoxamine. *CNS Spectr.* 2001;**6**(6):511–513.

104. Dagan Y, Ayalon L. Case study: psychiatric misdiagnosis of non-24-hours sleep–wake schedule disorder resolved by melatonin. *J Am Acad Child Adolesc Psychiatry.* 2005;**44**(12):1271–1275.

Principles of insomnia

Wendy M. Troxel and Daniel J. Buysse

Overview

Insomnia is the most common sleep disorder, with prevalence estimates ranging from 10% to 20% of the population [1]. The term "insomnia" is used in the vernacular to refer to various complaints about poor sleep quality or an inability to fall asleep or stay asleep. The 1-year prevalence of insomnia *symptoms* in the general population ranges from 30% to 40%, and up to 66% in primary care and psychiatric settings [2]. Clinically, the insomnia *disorder* refers to complaints of an inability to fall asleep, stay asleep, or non-restorative sleep, despite an adequate opportunity for sleep, combined with some form of daytime impairment (e.g. fatigue, occupational problems, relational problems, etc.). One of the inherent challenges in diagnosing and treating insomnia is that there are no known physiological markers to indicate the presence or absence of the phenotype. Rather, it is a disorder defined solely by the subjective complaints of poor sleep and daytime impairment. As with all subjective symptoms, these complaints may reflect a general negative affect bias [3] or a bias common to other psychiatric disorders (most notably, depression and anxiety), rather than a distinct disorder, *per se*. Moreover, given the high prevalence of insomnia symptoms in the general population, the assessment and diagnosis of the clinical disorder of insomnia poses a number of clinical challenges. Primarily for these reasons, the field of insomnia research and treatment has historically struggled to establish the disorder's legitimacy as a distinct clinical entity associated with significant morbidity, rather than being merely a symptom of another disorder or secondary diagnosis. Over the past several decades, however, accumulating evidence has documented the high prevalence of insomnia in the population at large,

and in specific subpopulations, the significant psychiatric and medical morbidity associated with insomnia, and the efficacy of insomnia treatments for improving sleep as well as overall well-being, and other psychiatric co-morbidities. Indeed, based on consistencies in clinical features, course, and response to treatment, a 2005 National Institutes of Health Conference suggested that the term "co-morbid" insomnia may be more appropriate terminology for insomnia co-occurring with other psychiatric or medical diagnoses, rather than "secondary." Such a change in terminology reflects the growing recognition that insomnia is a significant public health concern in its own right. To provide an overview of the current state-of-the-science in insomnia research and clinical applications, the current chapter will review topics pertaining to the assessment and diagnosis, prevalence and course, epidemiology and risk factors, and consequences of insomnia.

Assessment and diagnosis

An insomnia disorder is a syndrome consisting of at least one insomnia complaint (difficulty falling asleep, staying asleep, or non-restorative sleep) in an individual with adequate opportunity/circumstances for sleep, combined with significant daytime impairment or distress. Common daytime impairments in insomnia patients include mood disturbances (irritability, mild dysphoria, low stress/frustration tolerance), impaired cognitive function (problems with memory, concentration, or difficulty completing complex, abstract, or creative tasks), daytime fatigue, or role impairments (difficulty at work or in family roles) [4]. Interestingly, while *fatigue* is a very common daytime impairment in insomnia, physiological "*sleepiness*" is not [5], although patients may

Foundations of Psychiatric Sleep Medicine, ed. John W. Winkelman and David T. Plante. Published by Cambridge University Press.
© Cambridge University Press 2010.

initially believe the terms are synonymous. To clarify with patients, it is often helpful to describe "sleepiness" as the actual likelihood of falling asleep, which can be asked directly or subjectively measured with scales such as the Epworth sleepiness scale [6]. In contrast, fatigue is the feeling of mental or physical weariness or exhaustion. Indeed, once this terminology is clarified, patients will commonly make statements such as, "Yes, I feel fatigued all the time, but I could never fall asleep. That's the problem."

A key clinical feature of insomnia is that sleep complaints are present despite the fact that the individual has an adequate opportunity for sleep. Establishing whether one has opportunity for sleep is particularly relevant in today's 24–7 society where it is common for people to regularly get less than 6 hours of sleep, due to the demands of work, family life, social roles, etc [7]. Moreover, in certain populations such as the military, irregular sleep schedules and sleep deprivation are common during deployment [8]. Insomnia disorders are also highly prevalent in returning military veterans [9]. However, it is important to distinguish the development of insomnia, which is distinct from, though likely related to, the irregular sleep schedules and prolonged work hours, as well as other characteristics of deployment.

Current classification systems

The importance of a consistent diagnosis and classification system cannot be overstated. For clinical purposes, such consistency facilitates effective communication across care providers and may also be critical for reimbursement for services provided. For research purposes, such consistency guides recruitment and treatment response criteria, which will ultimately inform our understanding of the pathophysiology and treatment of insomnia. The three primary classification schemes used to describe insomnia are included within the *International Classification of Sleep Disorders*, 2nd Edition (ICSD-2 [10]), the *Diagnostic and Statistical Manual of Mental Disorders*, 4th Edition (DSM-IV [11]) and the World Health Organization's (WHO) *International Classification of Diseases* (ICD-9CM and ICD-10 [12]). In addition, in 2004, the American Academy of Sleep Medicine (AASM) published research diagnostic criteria for insomnia, to operationally define the disorder for insomnia research [13]; however, the current chapter will focus on the primary classification systems for clinical practice.

Broadly speaking, the ICSD-2 provides the most complete and specific system for defining the various insomnia disorders (i.e. specific subtypes); however, it is less widely used as compared to the DSM-IV or ICD. The ICSD-2 insomnia disorders are included as one of six major categories of sleep disorders. Both the DSM-IV and ICD have fewer subclassifications and include more global diagnostic categories for insomnia than the ICSD-2. The DSM-IV has a specific category for primary insomnia, defined as a disorder which does not occur "exclusively during the course of Narcolepsy, Breathing-Related Sleep Disorder, Circadian Rhythm Disorder, or a parasomnia" or "another mental disorder" (e.g. major depressive disorder, generalized anxiety disorder, a delirium) or is due to a substance or medication. In DSM-IV secondary diagnoses include co-morbid insomnia disorders, such as insomnia related to another mental disorder or substance-induced insomnia. The ICD system classifies sleep disorders according to presumptive etiology, organic versus non-organic.

Despite their differences, in general, each of the classification systems describes three major categories of insomnia:

1. *Insomnia secondary to or co-morbid with other conditions.* Consistent with the previously described DSM-IV criteria for secondary diagnoses, this category refers to insomnias related to other medical or psychiatric disorders, or due to the direct physiological effects of substance use or withdrawal. By far, this category is the single most common type of insomnia diagnosis seen in epidemiological studies and in clinical samples [14,15].

2. *Insomnia as a symptom of other sleep-specific disorders.* This category includes insomnia symptoms that occur within restless legs syndrome, some cases of obstructive sleep apnea, and some cases of parasomnias.

3. *Primary insomnias.* This category refers to disorders in which insomnia complaints are the primary symptoms, with no other disorder as a putative cause.

Differential diagnosis

Given that the underlying causes of insomnia are often complex and multifactorial and that co-morbid insomnias are the most prevalent type of insomnia disorder [15], carefully differentiating between insomnia symptoms and other co-morbid conditions that may contribute to or be exacerbated by the insomnia symptoms, is critical for optimizing treatment efforts.

Psychiatric disorders

Roughly half of individuals presenting with chronic insomnia have a current or past psychiatric diagnosis [14,15]. In addition, complaints of poor sleep or sleep disturbances are included within the clinical profiles of many psychiatric disorders, including mood disorders, anxiety disorders, post-traumatic stress disorder, and substance use disorders. Given evidence that insomnia symptoms often appear as prodromal symptoms preceding the onset of "full-blown" psychiatric disorders [2,16] and that insomnia symptoms often do not remit even with successful treatment of the psychiatric disorder [17], a thorough psychiatric history is necessary for the adequate assessment and treatment of insomnia.

Other sleep disorders

Occult or untreated sleep disorders, such as periodic leg movement disorder, restless legs syndrome, and sleep-related breathing disorders can cause insomnia symptoms, including difficulty falling asleep, sleep fragmentation, and daytime impairments, such as fatigue. Polysomnography may be necessary for some insomnia patients who have another suspected sleep disorder. Insomnia complaints are also often present within *circadian rhythm disorders*. Inclusion of sleep diaries within the insomnia evaluation is particularly useful for evaluating the presence of a circadian rhythm disorder. Although they are significantly less commonly reported in conjunction with insomnia complaints, *parasomnias*, which are characterized by a complaint of unusual behavior or events during sleep that may lead to nocturnal arousals, should also be considered as part of the insomnia differential diagnosis.

Medical and neurological conditions

Another critical element of the differential diagnosis is the evaluation of medical disorders (e.g. hyperthyroidism, stroke, neuropathy) and use of medications which may underlie insomnia complaints [18]. Such a determination should be based on the patient's medical history, available laboratory findings, and/or physical examination.

The insomnia evaluation and assessment tools

Polysomnography, which is typically considered the "gold standard" in the measurement of sleep and critical for the diagnosis of other sleep disorders, such as periodic leg movement disorder or obstructive sleep apnea, is generally "not recommended for the routine evaluation of insomnia" [5] (except as a rule-out for other sleep disorders). Rather, the assessment of insomnia depends on a thorough clinical history focusing on specific sleep symptoms and associated daytime impairments, chronology of symptoms, including any identifiable or suspected precipitating events, exacerbating and alleviating factors (e.g. seasonal effects, how insomnia symptoms are affected by changes in usual bedroom environment), and response to previous treatments. Patient's usual sleep and wake periods and the degree of variability in these patterns, as well as behaviors (including napping), cognitions, and environmental factors related to bedtime routines are also critical elements of the insomnia history. Symptoms of restless legs syndrome (RLS; e.g. restlessness or need to move legs during or prior to falling asleep), symptoms of obstructive sleep apnea (snoring, gasping, or breathing problems, morning dry mouth), nightmares, and pain or limitations to mobility or comfort during sleep should also be assessed as a part of the differential diagnosis. Regularity of daytime routines, including work, social interactions, exercise routines, and mealtimes should also be considered in the history.

Given that insomnia is often co-morbid with other psychiatric, sleep, and medical conditions, a thorough insomnia assessment should include a comprehensive sleep history, including common sleep disturbances and sleep habits, and a review of the patient's psychiatric, medical, and social history.

Assessment tools

In our laboratory and clinic, we routinely use a number of self-report instruments, including a self-reported sleep history, the Epworth sleepiness scale [6], the Pittsburgh sleep quality index (PSQI [19]), and self-report measures of depression or anxiety symptoms, to facilitate the assessment process. Moreover, in efforts to make the assessment as efficient as possible, new patients are sent a package of these screening measures and a sleep diary at least 2 weeks prior to the initial evaluation.

Sleep–wake diaries

Sleep-wake diaries covering 1–2 weeks of the patient's usual sleep times and behaviors related to sleep are critical tools in the assessment and treatment of insomnia (Figure 12.1). Ask a patient to verbally report their "usual" sleep and wake time and you are likely to get a report of how he/she slept last night or his/her worst night of sleep. Thus, a sleep diary is essential to avoid such primacy and recency biases, in order to receive a more valid representation of the patient's typical sleep patterns, as well as day-to-day variability in sleep hours, and the specific sleep problems experienced by the patient. Such an accurate representation is necessary not only for diagnosis, but also for treatment purposes, whether treatment is behavioral or pharmacological. For instance, a central feature of virtually all behavioral treatments is restricting time in bed to coincide with actual time spent asleep. Thus, a careful assessment of the patient's *usual* sleep times is essential. Similarly, knowledge of the patient's usual bedtime routines and sleep problems is also important for appropriate choice of pharmacological treatment and dosing instructions.

Actigraphy

Actigraphy is useful as an objective measure of assessing rest–activity patterns. The actigraph itself is a non-invasive wrist-watch style device, typically worn on the individual's non-dominant wrist for several days to weeks. Used in conjunction with a sleep diary, actigraphy can provide useful information regarding temporal patterns, variability in rest–activity, and responses to treatment. A number of studies have shown moderate to strong correlations between actigraphy patterns and sleep as monitored by polysomnography (PSG) [20].

Epidemiology

The experience of transient insomnia symptoms at some point during the life course is a nearly universal experience. The commonality of these symptoms within the normative population has made the epidemiology of insomnia complicated and prevalence rates have varied widely across sources. Epidemiological studies which generally rely on single or few-item measures of sleep complaints, and rarely include measures of associated daytime impairments, yield information about insomnia symptomatology.

These studies have led to somewhat alarming prevalence rates, in the range of 30–40% in the general population and up to 66% in the primary care and psychiatric settings [1,21]. Symptom-based definitions, however, are only modestly associated with more stringently defined criteria for the insomnia disorder [22]. Prevalence rates for insomnia as a specific disorder have ranged from 4.4% to 11.7% [1]. The disparity between prevalence rates for insomnia symptoms and those meeting DSM-IV diagnostic criteria for insomnia, highlights the fact that a significant proportion of the population is affected by sleep complaints, though the majority of those complaints do not meet clinically significant criteria.

Risk factors

A number of demographic, psychosocial, and behavioral risk factors have been identified as important risk factors for chronic insomnia (persisting for 1 month or longer). Moreover, among the risk factors identified, they can be broadly categorized into those that *predispose* an individual to developing insomnia, those that *precipitate* the onset of the disorder, and those that *perpetuate* the disorder. Among the predisposing or vulnerability factors, female sex has consistently been shown to be a risk factor for insomnia [2,23]. The sex disparity in insomnia rates may reflect women's greater tendency to report symptoms, more generally, or may reflect sex differences in traditional gender roles which are associated with sleep disturbances, such as parenting responsibilities and caregiving [24].

Older adults also have higher rates of insomnia than younger adults [25–27]; however, more recent studies that carefully control for other co-morbidities show weaker correlations between advancing age and insomnia risk [28,29]. Thus, age, *per se*, is not a risk factor for insomnia, but age-related deteriorations in mental and physical health status are associated with increased risk of insomnia [28].

Marital status has also been identified as an important risk factor for insomnia. Divorced/separated or widowed individuals are at increased risk for insomnia as compared to their married counterparts [30]; however, the magnitude of this effect is generally greater in women than in men [31]. A number of studies have shown that low socioeconomic status and unemployment are also risk factors for insomnia [32,33]. Finally, research on race/ethnicity and insomnia risk presents a more complicated picture, suggesting that the effects

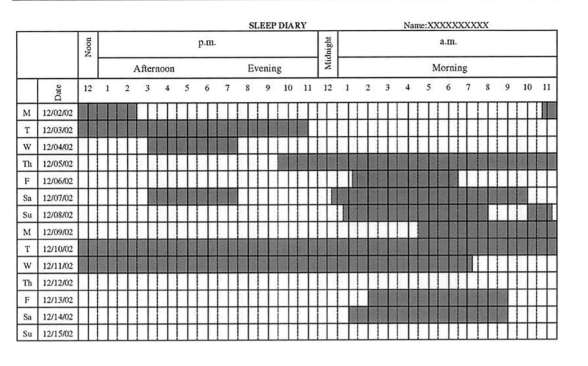

Figure 12.1 Example sleep diaries. Adapted from Buysse DJ. Introduction. In: *Sleep disorders and psychiatry*. Arlington, VA: American Psychiatric Publishing, Inc: American Psychiatric Publishing Review of Psychiatry; 2005.

Table 12.1 Medical and neurological diseases associated with insomnia

Disorder	Possible cause(s) for insomnia
Cardiovascular diseases:	
Congestive heart failure	Central sleep apnea, orthopnea
Coronary artery disease	Angina (may occur during sleep)
Pulmonary diseases:	
Chronic obstructive pulmonary disease	Breathing difficulty; sleep apnea
Asthma	Asthma attacks commonly occur during sleep
Neurological diseases:	
Stroke	Damage to sleep-regulating brain structures; mobility limitations
Parkinson's disease	Mobility limitation; direct effects of impaired dopamine neurotransmission; periodic limb movement disorder
Neuropathy	Pain
Traumatic brain injury	Damage to sleep-regulating brain structures
Gastrointestinal diseases:	
Gastroesophageal reflux	Pain; initiation of apneas
Renal diseases:	
Chronic renal failure	Restless legs syndrome; obstructive sleep apnea
Endocrine disorders:	
Diabetes	Associated obesity; sleep apnea; neuropathy
Hyperthyroidism	Hyperarousal
Rheumatological diseases:	
Rheumatoid arthritis, osteoarthritis	Pain; microarousals; high-frequency EEG activity during NREM sleep
Fibromyalgia	Pain; microarousals; high-frequency EEG activity during NREM sleep

Source: Adapted from Buysse DJ. Insomnia. In: *Sleep disorders and psychiatry*. Arlington, VA: American Psychiatric Publishing, Inc: American Psychiatric Publishing Review of Psychiatry; 2005.

of race/ethnicity on insomnia depend on (i.e. are moderated by) other demographic and sociocultural characteristics. For instance, older African Americans report fewer insomnia symptoms than age-matched Caucasians [34,35]; however, among younger samples, African Americans have higher rates of symptoms as compared to their Caucasian counterparts [36]. Older African American women appear to be a particularly vulnerable group, with prevalence rates of 19% versus 12% in African American males, and 14% in Caucasian males and females [37]. Recent research speculates that these complex relationships between race/ethnicity and insomnia suggest that race itself may not be a vulnerability factor; however, racial differences in the experience of other precipitating factors for insomnia, such as chronic stress, low socioeconomic status, and increased medical and psychiatric morbidities, may contribute to racial disparities in insomnia risk [38].

Co-morbid psychiatric or medical conditions are also associated with increased risk for insomnia [14,39]. Notably, clinical depression and depressive symptoms are among the largest and most consistent risk factors for insomnia [15] (see Table 12.1). Finally, emerging evidence suggests strong familial aggregation of insomnia risk [40,41], with limited data from twin studies further suggesting that such aggregation is largely due to genetic rather than shared factors [42].

Psychosocial stressors, including major life transitions, such as job changes, residential moves, occupational or interpersonal problems, or caregiving responsibilities, are common events that may precipitate the onset of insomnia symptoms or maintain them [43]. Another important perpetuating factor that plays an important role in many behavioral interventions for insomnia is the adoption of counterproductive sleep habits [44] (discussed in greater detail in Chapter 14: Cognitive behavioral therapy for insomnia).

Natural history of insomnia

Population-based data on the natural history of insomnia are limited. However, follow-up studies of clinical and population-based samples have generally shown that insomnia follows a persistent course, often lasting for several years, and tends to worsen over time [45,46]. A recent 20-year prospective study from the Zurich Study cohort confirmed the persistent nature of insomnia, with prevalence rates for more chronic forms of insomnia (lasting 1 month or longer) increasing gradually over time [47]. Similarly, results from a population-based study in Sweden confirmed the high prevalence of insomnia and persistent course of the illness over a 1-year follow-up period [48].

Pathophysiology of insomnia

The physiological model of insomnia is based on the central assumption that insomnia represents a disorder of increased physiological arousal. Arousal is believed to be a centrally mediated phenomenon related to the function of wake-promoting regions in the ascending reticular activating system, hypothalamus, and basal forebrain, which interact with sleep-promoting brain centers in the anterior hypothalamus and hypothalamus. Insomnia, according to this model, represents a disorder of increased arousal or "hyperarousal," which may be present tonically or in response to specific cues, such as the sleep environment. Importantly, emerging evidence suggests that arousal and sleep are not mutually exclusive neurobehavioral states, as was originally predicted by this model [49,50]. Rather, both states may co-occur in insomnia and it is precisely this simultaneous activation of sleep and arousal states that may contribute to certain paradoxical findings in the insomnia literature (e.g. reports of daytime sleepiness and fatigue with an inability to nap). Indeed, a number of studies using a variety of techniques, including psychophysiological and metabolic, electrophysiological, neuroendocrine, and functional neuroanatomic methods, support the basic contention that hyperarousal plays a role in the pathophysiology of insomnia.

Psychophysiological, metabolic, and electrophysiological measures of arousal

Findings from studies utilizing measures of heart rate, respiration, galvanic skin response, respiration rate, peripheral blood flow or vasoconstriction, and whole body metabolic rate generally support the notion of increased physiological arousal in poor sleepers as compared to good sleepers, with some evidence suggesting that such arousal is particularly evident at sleep onset [51–56]. For instance, Bonnet and Arand [57,58] showed that whole body metabolic rate, measured by volume of oxygen consumption per unit of time (VO_2) is higher during sleep in patients with insomnia compared to good sleepers. Although there are important limitations in several of these earlier studies, including the use of symptom-based definitions of insomnia rather than clinically defined criteria, and inclusion of a heterogeneous group of insomnia participants, including those with secondary diagnoses, the consistency of the results suggests that individuals with insomnia do exhibit heightened physiological arousal.

Neuroendocrine measures of arousal

Activation of the hypothalamic-pituitary-adrenal (HPA) axis is a critical component of the stress response system and is thought to play a role in the purported hyperarousal in insomnia. Consistent with this notion, several studies have shown that insomnia patients have elevated cortisol and adrenocorticotropic hormone levels prior to and during sleep, with the largest differences present in the first half of the night as compared to good sleepers [59,60].

Functional neuroanatomic measures of arousal

Single photon emission computed tomography (SPECT) and positron emission tomography (PET) are methods used to identify regional blood flow or metabolic activity associated with specific tasks or states. Only a handful of studies have utilized these techniques thus far in the context of insomnia. In the first PET study of primary insomnia, Nofzinger and colleagues [50] found that patients had increased global metabolic rates during both wakefulness and NREM sleep compared with good sleepers. Moreover, in insomnia patients, the usual sleep-related declines in wake-promoting brain regions, including the ascending reticular activating system, hypothalamus, and thalamus, were attenuated. However, during wakefulness insomnia participants showed reduced dorsolateral prefrontal cortical activity. Together, these findings suggesting hyperarousal during NREM sleep and hypoarousal during wakefulness may correspond to insomnia patients' sleep and daytime impairments. In patients with co-morbid insomnia with major depression, EEG beta activity was positively associated with metabolic activity in the orbitofrontal cortex, and with complaints of poor sleep quality [61], further supporting the hyperarousal hypothesis. In contrast to these findings, a study using

Tc-HMPAO SPECT found that patients with insomnia showed a consistent pattern of hypoperfusion (i.e. decreased blood flow) across eight a priori defined brain regions, with the most prominent effect observed in the basal ganglia [62]. Taken together, this limited literature suggests that there are indeed functional neuroanatomic changes during NREM sleep associated with insomnia; however, the precise nature of these changes and how they relate to insomnia complaints requires further investigation [63,64].

Cognitive behavioral models

All cognitive behavioral models of insomnia share a basic framework outlining the relationships between sleep-related thoughts, behaviors, and perceived arousal, their antecedents, and consequences. However, the core dysfunction purported to underlie the clinical disorder of insomnia differs across these models.

Behavioral models

Spielman and colleagues articulated a behavioral model in which insomnia develops as a result of the interaction between *predisposing* or vulnerability factors (e.g. heightened physiological or cognitive arousal) and external *precipitating* factors (e.g. life stressors) [44]. Importantly, the factors that predispose or precipitate the development of insomnia are distinct from the factors that *perpetuate* or maintain the disorder. In particular, maladaptive, compensatory sleep habits, such as spending more time in bed by going to bed earlier or having weekend "catch-up" sleep serve as perpetuating factors which maintain and reinforce the insomnia even after the original precipitants recede. Thus, an individual may be prone to insomnia due to enduring, trait-level characteristics, and may experience acute episodes of insomnia as a result of exposure to precipitating factors, such as life events. However, it is behavioral factors which are believed to underlie the chronic manifestations of the disorder.

Cognitive models

In contrast to Spielman's focus on maladaptive behaviors as the critical factor underlying chronic insomnia, cognitive models highlight the role of cognitive factors, in particular, ruminative thoughts and worries, particularly around bedtime, as the central components underlying insomnia [65]. Repeated pairings between these cognitions and temporal (e.g. bedtime routines) and environmental (e.g. bed, bedroom) cues are purported to result in a conditioned arousal response particularly around bedtime. Consistent with the physiological models, the cognitive models contend that conditions of hyperarousal are antithetical to the sleep state. Thus, such conditioned cognitive arousal begets sleeplessness. The resulting sleep disturbance and ruminations about one's ability to sleep ultimately leads to daytime consequences such as mood disturbances and fatigue. Over time, these experiences can lead to dysfunctional beliefs and attitudes about one's ability to sleep and the consequences of sleep difficulties [66]. Ultimately, these dysfunctional beliefs lead to the development of strategies aimed at maximizing sleep (e.g. going to bed earlier, sleeping later) which further reinforce sleep disturbances and cognitive hyperarousal.

Harvey [67] reconceptualized the cognitive model to emphasize the specific role of attentional biases and monitoring of threat-related cues in the maintenance of insomnia. According to this model, excessive negative cognitive activity (e.g. worries, ruminative thoughts) leads to increased physiological hyperarousal and distress, which in turn, leads to selective attention and monitoring towards internal and external cues indicative of sleeplessness. Such selective attention operates 24 hours a day, leading to both cognitive distortions regarding sleep deficits and daytime consequences. These distorted beliefs regarding the consequences of sleep loss and threats to sleep, in turn, lead to the development of "safety behaviors" during the daytime, such as avoidance of work or social activities, and at night-time, such as going to bed early or "catching up" on sleep after a poor night's sleep. These safety behaviors are adopted in order to avoid some feared outcome – in this case, sleeplessness. However, in actuality, these behaviors further reinforce rumination and worry, physiological arousal, and perpetuate erroneous beliefs regarding sleep and daytime deficits seen in insomnia. In support of Harvey's model, evidence suggests that patients with insomnia do, in fact, selectively attend to sleep-related stimuli (e.g. a pillow), have exaggerated ("catastrophic") thoughts about sleep loss, and engage in daytime safety behaviors [68–70].

Neurocognitive model

Perlis and colleagues [71] proposed a neurocognitive model of insomnia which focuses on the central role of cortical arousal in the pathophysiology of insomnia. Specifically, this model suggests that both physiological and cognitive arousal arise from increased cortical arousal at or around the sleep-onset period and during NREM sleep, as measured by high-frequency (beta) EEG activity (14–45 Hz). They further posit that this arousal can be conditioned, and is critical to the insomnia experience, and in particular, the phenomenon of sleep-state misperception. Specifically, cortical arousal is hypothesized to lead to enhanced sensory processing around sleep onset and during NREM sleep, which may obscure the insomnia patient's ability to distinguish between sleep and wakefulness[71,72]. Such a blurring of the distinction between sleep and wakefulness may account for the tendency for insomniacs to perceive themselves to be awake when polysomnography indicates sleep [73]. In support of the role of cortical arousal in sleep-state misperception and for the neurocognitive model in general, patients with sleep-state misperception disorder have higher levels of beta EEG activity than good sleepers or patients with primary insomnia without sleep-state misperception [74], and patients with primary insomnia have higher EEG activity as compared to good sleepers or patients with insomnia secondary to major depression [72].

Consequences of insomnia

The consequences of insomnia are substantial and represent a significant public health concern. A preponderance of evidence suggests that insomnia is both a cause and a consequence of psychiatric disorders. Several studies have shown that insomnia presages the development of psychiatric disorders, most notably, depressive, anxiety, and substance use disorders [75–80]. In patients with major depressive disorder (MDD), insomnia is associated with worse initial treatment response [81], symptom persistence [82], and increased likelihood of recurrence [83,84]. Moreover, a number of studies have shown that insomnia in the context of MDD is associated with increased risk of suicidal ideation or completed suicide, and in most cases this association persisted even after adjusting for depression severity [85]. Insomnia is also associated with persistence and relapse in alcohol dependence [86].

Insomnia may be associated with increased motor vehicle and other accidents [87,88] and has been linked with increased incidence of falls in the elderly

[89,90]. Recent research has suggested that insomnia may also be associated with increased risk for cardio-vascular diseases [91,92] and mortality [93]; however, the evidence is equivocal with regard to whether insomnia represents an independent risk [94–96].

In contrast, the results are unequivocal with regard to the association between insomnia and reduced quality of life. Indeed, a number of studies have shown reduced quality of life (QoL) in individuals with insomnia [97,98] – a reduction similar in magnitude to that seen with chronic conditions such as congestive heart failure and MDD [99]. As compared to individuals without sleep/wake problems, individuals with insomnia report greater daytime fatigue, poorer mood, more anxiety or stress, less vigor, difficulty coping with life demands, less ability to complete tasks, and role impairments across a broad set of domains such as job performance, social life, and family life [2,100].

In addition to the compromised quality of life and increased medical and physical burden experienced by insomnia sufferers themselves, the burden of insomnia also exacts a significant toll on the health-care system and employers, particularly given the prevalence of insomnia [101]. In particular, insomnia is associated with increased medical care utilization, more absenteeism from work [87,102], and increased direct and indirect medical costs [100,101,103,104]. Indeed, direct costs associated with insomnia have been estimated to be $13.9 billon annually, with the vast percentage of those costs attributable to nursing home care [104]. Striking as these estimates are, they are likely to be a conservative estimate of the actual public health toll of insomnia given that a substantial number of insomnia sufferers do not actively seek treatment for their disorder [105,106]. Thus, adequately diagnosing and treating insomnia represents a significant public health concern.

Summary and conclusions

Insomnia is a prevalent health complaint that is often co-morbid with psychiatric and medical disorders. Recent studies on the pathophysiology of insomnia have implicated increased CNS arousal as well as cognitive and behavioral factors as critical factors in the development and course of insomnia. Given that insomnia complaints are ubiquitous phenomena, diagnosis of the insomnia disorder rests on a detailed and accurate clinical history, supplemented by sleep diaries and other assessment tools. The consequences of insomnia are substantial and affect virtually all aspects of the patient's life, including decreased quality of life, impaired daytime functioning, increased risk for the development of psychiatric disorders, and poorer prognosis in psychiatric and medically ill populations. Despite the high prevalence of insomnia symptoms reported in population-based studies, insomnia continues to be an underdiagnosed and undertreated condition, and thus remains a significant public health concern.

References

1. Ohayon MM. Epidemiology of insomnia: what we know and what we still need to learn. *Sleep Med Rev.* 2002;**6**:97–111.

2. Buysse DJ, Germain A, Moul DE. Diagnosis, epidemiology, and consequences of insomnia. *Prim Psychiatry.* 2005;**12**(8):37–44.

3. Watson D, Pennebaker JW. Health complaints, stress, and distress: exploring the central role of negative affectivity. *Psychol Rev.* 1989;**96**:234–254.

4. Moul DE, Nofzinger EA, Pilkonis PA, et al. Symptom reports in severe chronic insomnia. *Sleep.* 2002;**25**(5):548–558.

5. Buysse DJ, Ancoli-Israel S, Edinger JD, Lichstein KL, Morin CM. Recommendations for a standard research assessment of insomnia. *Sleep.* 2006;**29**(9):1155–1173.

6. Johns MW. Sleepiness in different situations measured by the Epworth Sleepiness Scale. *Sleep.* 1994;**17**(8):703–710.

7. Kryger MH, Roth T, Dement WC. *Principles and practice in sleep medicine.* Philadelphia: Elsevier; 2005.

8. Peterson AL, Goodie JL, Satterfield WA, Brim WL. Sleep disturbance during military deployment. *Mil Med.* 2008;**173**(3):230–235.

9. Hoge CW, Terhakopian A, Castro CA, Messer SC, Engel CC. Association of posttraumatic stress disorder with somatic symptoms, health care visits, and absenteeism among Iraq war veterans. *Am J Psychiatry.* 2007;**164**(1):150–153.

10. American Academy of Sleep Medicine. *The international classification of sleep disorders, 2nd edition (ICSD-2): Diagnostic and statistical coding manual.* Westchester, Illinois: American Academy of Sleep Medicine; 2005.

11. American Psychiatric Association. *Diagnostic and statistical manual of mental disorders (DSM-IV-TR),* 4th ed, Text Revision. Washington, DC: American Psychiatric Association; 2000.

12. World Health Organization (WHO). *International statistical classification of diseases and related health problems,* 10th Revision. Geneva: WHO; 1992.

13. Edinger JD, Bonnet MH, Bootzin RR, et al. Derivation of research diagnostic criteria for insomnia: Report of an American Academy of Sleep Medicine Work Group. *Sleep.* 2004;**27**:1567–1596.

14. Buysse DJ, Reynolds CF, Kupfer DJ, et al. Clinical diagnoses in 216 insomnia patients using the International Classification of Sleep Disorders (ICSD), DSM-IV and ICD-10 categories: A report from the APA/NIMH DSM-IV field trial. *Sleep.* 1994;**17**(7):630–637.

15. Ohayon MM. Prevalence of DSM-IV diagnostic criteria of insomnia: distinguishing insomnia related to mental disorders from sleep disorders. *J Psychiatr Res.* 1997;**31**:333–346.

16. Perlis ML, Giles DE, Buysse DJ, et al. Self-reported sleep disturbance as a prodromal symptom in recurrent depression. *J Affect Disord.* 1997;**42**(2–3):209–212.

17. Nierenberg A, Keefe BR, Leslie VC, et al. Residual symptoms in depressed patients who respond acutely to fluoxetine. *J Clin Psychiatry.* 1999;**60**:221–225.

18. Taylor DJ, Mallory LJ, Lichstein KL, et al. Comorbidity of chronic insomnia with medical problems. *Sleep.* 2007;**30**:213–218.

19. Buysse DJ, Reynolds CF, Monk TH, Berman SR, Kupfer DJ. The Pittsburgh Sleep Quality Index: A new instrument for psychiatric practice and research. *Psychiatry Res.* 1989;**28**(2):193–213.

20. Lichstein KL, Stone KC, Donaldson J, et al. Actigraphy validation with insomnia. *Sleep.* 2006;**29**:232–239.

21. Ford DE, Kamerow D. Epidemiologic study of sleep disturbances and psychiatric disorders: an opportunity for intervention? *JAMA.* 1989;**262**:1479–1484.

22. Ohayon MM, Roth T. What are the contributing factors for insomnia in the general population? *J Psychosom Res.* 2001;**51**(6):745–755.

23. Soares CN, Murray BJ. Sleep disorders in women: clinical evidence and treatment strategies. *Psychiatr Clin North Am.* 2006;**29**(4):1095–1113.

24. Hislop J, Arber S. Sleepers Wake! The gendered nature of sleep disruption among mid-life women. *Sociology.* 2003;**37**:695–711.

25. Foley DJ, Monjan AA, Brown SL, et al. Sleep complaints among elderly persons: an epidemiologic study of three communities. *Sleep.* 1995;**18**(6):425–432.

26. Roth T, Roehrs T. Insomnia: epidemiology, characteristics, and consequences. *Clinical Cornerstone*. 2003;**5**(3):5–15.

27. Morphy H, Dunn KM, Lewis M, Boardman HF, Croft PR. Epidemiology of insomnia: a longitudinal study in a UK population. *Sleep*. 2007; **30**(3):274–280.

28. Ohayon MM, Zulley J, Guilleminault C, Smirne S, Priest RG. How age and daytime activities are related to insomnia in the general population: consequences for older people.[see comment]. *J Am Geriatr Soc*. 2001;**49**(4):360–366.

29. Reynolds CF III, Buysse DJ, Nofzinger EA, et al. Age wise: Aging well by sleeping well. *J Am Geriatr Soc*. 2001;**49**(4):491.

30. Hajak G, Group SS. Epidemiology of severe insomnia and its consequences in Germany. *Eur Arch Psychiatry Clin Neurosci*. 2001;**251**(2):49–56.

31. Hale L. Who has time to sleep? *J Pub Health*. 2005;**27** (2):205–211.

32. Doi Y, Minowa M, Okawa M, Uchiyama M. Prevalence of sleep disturbance and hypnotic medication use in relation to sociodemographic factors in the general Japanese adult population. *J Epidemiol*. 2000;**10** (2):79–86.

33. Gellis LA, Lichstein KL, Scarinci IC, et al. Socioeconomic status and insomnia. *J Abnorm Psychol*. 2005;**114**(1):111–118.

34. Jean-Louis G, Magai CM, Cohen CI, et al. Ethnic differences in self-reported sleep problems in older adults. *Sleep*. 2001;**24**(8):926–933.

35. Whitney CW, Enright PL, Newman AB, et al. Correlates of daytime sleepiness in 4578 elderly persons: the Cardiovascular Health Study. *Sleep*. 1998;**21**(1):27–36.

36. Hicks RA, Lucero-Gorman K, Bautista J, Hicks GJ. Ethnicity, sleep duration, and sleep satisfaction. *Percept Mot Skills*. 1999;**88**(1):234–235.

37. Blazer DG, Hays JC, Foley DJ. Sleep complaints in older adults: a racial comparison. *Journals of Gerontology Series A, Biological Sciences & Medical Sciences*. 1995;**50**(5):M280–284.

38. Hall M, Matthews KA, Kravitz HM, et al. Race and financial strain are independent correlates of sleep in mid-life women: The SWAN Sleep Study. *Sleep*. 2009; **32**(1):73–82.

39. Okuji Y, Matsuura M, Kawasaki N, et al. Prevalence of insomnia in various psychiatric diagnostic categories. *Psychiatry Clin Neurosci*. 2002;**56**(3):239–240.

40. Dauvilliers Y, Morin C, Cervena K, et al. Family studies in insomnia. *J Psychosom Res*. 2005;**58**(3): 271–278.

41. Drake CL, Scofield H, Roth T. Vulnerability to insomnia: the role of familial aggregation. *Sleep Med*. 2008;**9**(3):297–302.

42. Watson NF, Goldberg J, Arguelles L, Buchwald D. Genetic and environmental influences on insomnia, daytime sleepiness, and obesity in twins. *Sleep*. 2006;**29**(5):645–649.

43. Bastien CH, Vallieres A, Morin CM. Precipitating factors of insomnia. *Behav Sleep Med*. 2004; **2**(1):50–62.

44. Spielman A, Caruso L, Glovinsky P. A behavioral perspective on insomnia treatment. *Psychiatr Clin North Am*. 1987;**10**:541–553.

45. Mendelson WB. Long-term follow-up of chronic insomnia. *Sleep*. 1995;**18**:698–701.

46. Vollrath M, Wicki W, Angst J. The Zurich Study, VIII. Insomnia: association with depression, anxiety, somatic syndromes, and course of insomnia. *Eur Arch Psychiatry Neurol Sci*. 1989;**239**:113–124.

47. Buysse DJ, Angst J, Gamma A, et al. Prevalence, course, and comorbidity of insomnia and depression in young adults.[see comment]. *Sleep*. 2008;**31** (4):473–480.

48. Jansson-Frojmark M, Linton SJ. The course of insomnia over one year: a longitudinal study in the general population in Sweden. *Sleep*. 2008;**31** (6):881–886.

49. Cano G, Mochizuki T, Saper CB. Neural circuitry of stress-induced insomnia in rats. *J Neurosci*. 2008;**28** (40):10167–10184.

50. Nofzinger EA, Buysse DJ, Germain A, et al. Functional neuroimaging evidence for hyperarousal in insomnia. *Am J Psychiatry*. 2004;**161**(11): 2126–2129.

51. Bastien CH, St-Jean G, Morin CM, Turcotte I, Carrier J. Chronic psychophysiological insomnia: hyperarousal and/or inhibition deficits? An ERPs investigation. *Sleep*. 2008;**31**(6):887–898.

52. Drake CL, Roth T. Predisposition in the evolution of insomnia: Evidence, potential mechanisms, and future directions. *Sleep Med Clin*. 2006; **1**(3):333–349.

53. Roth T, Roehrs T, Pies R. Insomnia: Pathophysiology and implications for treatment. *Sleep Med Rev*. 2007;**11**:71–79.

54. Vgontzas AN, Tsigos C, Bixler EO, et al. Chronic insomnia and activity of the stress system: a preliminary study. *J Psychosom Res*. 1998;**45** (1 Spec No):21–31.

55. Bonnet MH, Arand DL. Heart rate variability in insomniacs and matched normal sleepers. *Psychosom Med*. 2003;**60**(5):610–615.

56. Hall M, Thayer JF, Germain A, et al. Psychological stress is associated with heightened physiological arousal during NREM sleep in primary insomnia. *Behav Sleep Med.* 2007;**5**(3):178–193.

57. Bonnet MH, Arand DL. Physiological activation in patients with Sleep State Misperception. *Psychosom Med.* 1997;**59**(5):533–540.

58. Bonnet MH, Arand DL. 24-hour metabolic rate in insomniacs and matched normal sleepers. *Sleep.* 1995;**18**(7):581–588.

59. Rodenbeck A, Hajak G. Neuroendocrine dysregulation in primary insomnia. *Rev Neurol (Paris).* 2001;**157** (11 Pt 2):S57–61.

60. Vgontzas AN, Bixler EO, Lin HM, et al. Chronic insomnia is associated with nyctohemeral activation of the hypothalamic-pituitary-adrenal axis: clinical implications. *J Clin Endocrinol Metab.* 2001;**86** (8):3787–3794.

61. Nofzinger EA, Price JC, Meltzer CC, et al. Towards a neurobiology of dysfunctional arousal in depression: The relationship between beta EEG power and regional cerebral glucose metabolism during NREM sleep. *Psychiatry Res: Neuroimaging.* 2000;**98** (2):71–91.

62. Smith MT, Perlis ML, Chengazi VU, et al. Neuroimaging of NREM sleep in primary insomnia: a Tc-99_HMPAO single photon emission computed tomography study. *Sleep.* 2002;**25**:325–335.

63. Nofzinger EA. Neuroimaging of sleep and sleep disorders. *Curr Neurol Neurosci Rep.* 2006;**6** (2):149–155.

64. Winkelman J, Buxton O, Jensen J, et al. Reduced brain GABA in primary insomnia: preliminary data from 4T proton magnetic resonance spectroscopy (1H-MRS). *Sleep.* 2008;**31**(11):1499–1506.

65. Morin CM. *Insomnia: psychological assessment and management.* New York: Guilford; 1993.

66. Morin CM, Blaise F, Savard J. Are changes in beliefs and attitudes about sleep related to sleep improvements in the treatment of insomnia? *Behav Res Ther.* 2002;**40**:741–752.

67. Harvey AG. A cognitive model of insomnia. *Behav Res Ther.* 2002;**40**:869–893.

68. Harvey AG. Pre-sleep cognitive activity: a comparison of sleep-onset insomniacs and good sleepers. *Br J Clin Psychol.* 2000;**39**(Pt 3):275–286.

69. Harvey AG. Identifying safety behaviors in insomnia. *J Nerv Ment Dis.* 2002;**190**(1):16–21.

70. Harvey AG, Greenall E. Catastrophic worry in primary insomnia. *J Behav Ther Exp Psychiatry.* 2003;**34** (1):11–23.

71. Perlis ML, Giles DE, Mendelson WB, Bootzin RR, Wyatt JK. Psychophysiological insomnia: the behavioural model and a neurocognitive perspective. [see comment]. *J Sleep Res.* 1997;**6**(3):179–188.

72. Perlis ML, Smith MT, Andrews PJ, Orff H, Giles DE. Beta/Gamma EEG activity in patients with primary and secondary insomnia and good sleeper controls. *Sleep.* 2001;**24**(1):110–117.

73. Mercer JD, Bootzin RR, Lack LC. Insomniacs' perception of wake instead of sleep. *Sleep.* 2002;**25**:564–571.

74. Krystal AD, Edinger JD, Wohlgemuth WK, Marsh GR. NREM sleep EEG frequency spectral correlates of sleep complaints in primary insomnia subtypes. *Sleep.* 2002;**25**(6):630–640.

75. Perlis ML, Smith LJ, Lyness JM, et al. Insomnia as a risk factor for onset of depression in the elderly. *Behav Sleep Med.* 2006;**4**(2):104–113.

76. Neckelmann D, Mykletun A, Dahl AA. Chronic insomnia as a risk factor for developing anxiety and depression. *Sleep.* 2007;**30**(7):873–880.

77. Riemann D, Voderholzer U. Primary insomnia: a risk factor to develop depression? *J Affect Disord.* 2003;**76** (1–3):255–259.

78. Taylor DJ, Lichstein KL, Durrence HH, Bush AJ, Riedel BW. Epidemiology of insomnia, depression, and anxiety. *Sleep Med.* 2005;**28**:1299–1306.

79. Weissman MM, Greenwald S, Nino-Murcia G, et al. The morbidity of insomnia uncomplicated by psychiatric disorders. *Gen Hosp Psychiatry.* 1997;**19**:245–250.

80. Johnson EO, Roth T, Breslau N. The association of insomnia with anxiety disorders and depression: exploration of the direction of risk. *J Psychiatr Res.* 2006;**40**(8):700–708.

81. Buysse DJ, Tu XM, Cherry CR, et al. Pretreatment REM sleep and subjective sleep quality distinguish depressed psychotherapy remitters and nonremitters. *Biol Psychiatry.* 1999;**45**(2):205–213.

82. Pigeon WR, Hegel M, Unutzer J, et al. Is insomnia a perpetuating factor for late-life depression in the IMPACT cohort?[see comment]. *Sleep.* 2008;**31** (4):481–488.

83. Cho HJ, Lavretsky H, Olmstead R, et al. Sleep disturbance and depression recurrence in community-dwelling older adults: a prospective study.[see comment]. *Am J Psychiatry.* 2008; **165**(12):1543–1550.

84. Reynolds CF 3rd, Frank E, Houck P, et al. Which elderly patients treated with remitted depression remain well with continued interpersonal

psychotherapy after discontinuation of antidepressant medication? *Am J Psychiatry.* 1997;**154**:958–962.

85. Liu X, Buysse DJ. Sleep and youth suicidal behavior: A neglected field. *Curr Opin Psychiatry.* 2006;**19**(3):288–293.

86. Brower KJ, Aldrich MS, Robinson EA, et al. Insomnia, self-medication, and relapse to alcoholism. *Am J Psychiatry.* 2001;**158**:399–404.

87. Leger D, Massuel MA, Metlaine A, Group SS. Professional correlates of insomnia.[see comment]. *Sleep.* 2006;**29**(2):171–178.

88. Powell NB, Schectman KB, Riley RW, et al. Sleepy driving: accidents and injury. *Otolaryngol Head Neck Surg.* 2002;**126**(3):217–227.

89. Fitzpatrick P, Kirke PN, Daly L, et al. Predictors of first hip fracture and mortality post fracture in older women. *Ir J Med Sci.* 2001;**170**(1):49–53.

90. Brassington GS, King AC, Bliwise DL. Sleep problems as a risk factor for falls in a sample of community-dwelling adults aged 64–99 years. *J Am Geriatr Soc.* 2000;**48**(10):1234–1240.

91. Schwartz S, McDowell AW, Cole SR, et al. Insomnia and heart disease: a review of epidemiologic studies. *J Psychosom Res.* 1999;**47**(4):313–333.

92. Schwartz SW, Cornoni-Huntley J, Cole SR, et al. Are sleep complaints an independent risk factor for myocardial infarction? *Ann Epidemiol.* 1998;**8**(6):384–392.

93. Pollak CP, Perlick D, Linsner JP, et al. Sleep problems in the elderly as predictors of death and nursing home placement. *J Comm Health.* 1990;**15**:123–135.

94. Phillips B, Mannino DM. Do insomnia complaints cause hypertension or cardiovascular disease? *J Clin Sleep Med.* 2007;**3**(5):489–494.

95. Althuis MD, Fredman L, Langenberg PW, Magaziner J. The relationship between insomnia and mortality among community-dwelling older women. *J Am Geriatr Soc.* 1998;**46**(10):1270–1273.

96. Kripke DF, Garfinkel L, Wingard DL, et al. Mortality associated with sleep duration and insomnia. *Arch Gen Psychiatry.* 2002;**59**:131–136.

97. Byles JE, Mishra GD, Harris MA. The experience of insomnia among older women. *Sleep.* 2005;**28**(8):972–979.

98. Philip P, Leger D, Taillard J, et al. Insomniac complaints interfere with quality of life but not with absenteeism: respective role of depressive and organic comorbidity. *Sleep Med.* 2006;**7**(7):585–591.

99. Katz DA, McHorney CA. The relationship between insomnia and health-related quality of life in patients with chronic illness. *J Fam Pract.* 2002;**51**(3):229–235.

100. Leger D, Guilleminault C, Bader G, Levy E, Paillard M. Medical and socio-professional impact of insomnia. *Sleep.* 2002;**25**(6):625–629.

101. Ozminkowski RJ, Wang S, Walsh JK. The direct and indirect costs of untreated insomnia in adults in the United States. *Sleep.* 2007;**30**(3):263–273.

102. Godet-Cayre V, Pelletier-Fleury N, Le Vaillant M, et al. Insomnia and absenteeism at work. Who pays the cost? [see comment]. *Sleep.* 2006;**29**(2):179–184.

103. Metlaine A, Leger D, Choudat D. Socioeconomic impact of insomnia in working populations. *Ind Health.* 2005;**43**(1):11–19.

104. Walsh JK. Clinical and socioeconomic correlates of insomnia. *J Clin Psychiatry.* 2004;**65**(Suppl 8):13–19.

105. Stinson K, Tang NK, Harvey AG. Barriers to treatment seeking in primary insomnia in the United Kingdom: a cross-sectional perspective. *Sleep.* 2006;**29**(12):1643–1646.

106. Leger D. Public health and insomnia: economic impact. *Sleep.* 2000;**23**(Suppl 3):S69–76.

Chapter 3

Treatment of insomnia: pharmacotherapy

Andrew D. Krystal

Introduction

A large number of different types of medications are used to treat insomnia. This includes benzodiazepines, non-benzodiazepines, melatonin receptor agonists, antidepressants, antipsychotics, anticonvulsants, and antihistamines [1]. These agents exert therapeutic effects on insomnia through a number of different pharmacological mechanisms. Some enhance the sleep-promoting effects of GABA and melatonin systems (benzodiazepines, non-benzodiazepines, melatonin agonists) while others have therapeutic effects on sleep disturbance by blocking the wake-promoting effects of serotonin, norepinephrine, acetylcholine, and histamine (antidepressants, antipsychotics, and antihistamines). The particular mechanism by which these agents act affects the properties of their therapeutic effects on insomnia. This mechanism, along with the other pharmacological effects, determines the side-effect profile of a given insomnia medication. This chapter reviews the pharmacology of the therapeutic and adverse effects of these medications and identifies their distinguishing characteristics when used to treat insomnia in clinical practice. The available data on the treatment of insomnia in key patient subgroups is also discussed. For each agent the available placebo-controlled trials are reviewed. These trials serve as the basis for weighing the risks and benefits of each of these agents when making treatment decisions [1].

Optimally, the decision of whether to administer a therapy for insomnia, which therapy to administer, and whether to continue a therapy should be based on an empirically based weighing of the risks and benefits of the treatment options [1]. This should include the risks of not treating insomnia, which is reflected in the degree of impairment in function and quality of life associated with the insomnia. There is evidence that insomnia

treatment decisions in clinical practice are not being made based on empirical evidence. Some of the most frequently administered insomnia agents have not been established to have efficacy in the treatment of insomnia and their side-effect profile in insomnia therapy remains uncharacterized [2]. It is hoped that by reviewing the placebo-controlled trials that can serve as an empirical basis for clinical decision-making, this chapter will facilitate optimizing the treatment of insomnia among psychiatric practitioners.

Medications used to treat insomnia

Benzodiazepines

The benzodiazepines are a group of chemically related agents that have a therapeutic effect on insomnia through enhancing the inhibitory effects of gamma-amino-butyric acid (GABA), the predominant inhibitory neurotransmitter in the brain and the most important sleep-promoting system [1,3]. Benzodiazepines have a binding site on one of the types of GABA receptors, the GABA-A receptor, which is a channel comprised of five protein subunits that controls the flow of chloride ions across neuronal membranes [3]. When benzodiazepines bind to this allosteric binding site, they cause a conformational change in the subunits which facilitates the inward flow of chloride ions that occurs when GABA binds to the receptor complex. This enhances GABA's inhibitory effect because the extra inward negative ion flux results in added membrane hyperpolarization, which further biases the neuron away from exceeding the threshold of depolarization needed to fire an action potential. This inhibition promotes sleep through GABAergic projections to key wake-promoting regions of the brain. These regions include the histaminergic

Foundations of Psychiatric Sleep Medicine, ed. John W. Winkelman and David T. Plante. Published by Cambridge University Press.
© Cambridge University Press 2010.

tuberomammillary nucleus, the orexinergic/hypocretinergic perifornical area, the serotonergic raphe nuclei, the cholinergic laterodorsal tegmentum/pedunculopontine tegmentum, the dopaminergic ventral periaqueductal grey and the noradrenergic locus coeruleus (see Chapter 2: Neuroanatomy and neurobiology of sleep and wakefulness) [4].

GABA-A receptors are located in many regions of the brain other than those that affect sleep/wake function. As a result, benzodiazepines have clinical effects in addition to sleep enhancement. These may include anxiolysis, anticonvulsant effects, myorelaxation, memory impairment, motor impairment, and reinforcement. This accounts for the adverse effects of these agents which include sedation, cognitive impairment, motor impairment, and the potential for abuse (see Table 13.1). The associated anxiolytic and myorelaxant effects may be important assets when treating insomnia patients because insomnia frequently occurs in conjunction with anxiety and/or pain [5].

Benzodiazepines most commonly used in the treatment of insomnia include triazolam, flurazepam, temazepam, estazolam, quazepam, clonazepam, lorazepam, and alprazolam. The properties of these agents appear in Table 13.1. The primary feature which distinguishes these agents from each other is their half life. Half life and dosage determine the duration of clinical effects. Longer half life and higher dosage both tend to lead to longer lasting effects. The shortest half-life benzodiazepine commonly used in the treatment of insomnia is triazolam. As a result, it is least likely to be associated with next-day effects when used in the recommended range of dosing. In contrast, flurazepam, quazepam, and clonazepam have half lives which exceed 24 hours and, as a result, are relatively likely to lead to next-day effects.

A number of the benzodiazepines have well-established efficacy in the treatment of insomnia. Placebo-controlled trials in insomnia patients aged 18–65 have identified a therapeutic effect on sleep onset and maintenance for triazolam, temazepam, flurazepam, quazepam, and estazolam (see Table 13.1) [1]. Efficacy in the treatment of insomnia in older adults has been reported for triazolam and flurazepam in terms of both sleep onset and maintenance, and a therapeutic effect on sleep maintenance has been reported for temazepam [1]. A few placebo-controlled studies have evaluated the use of benzodiazepines in the treatment of insomnia occurring with medical and psychiatric conditions (co-morbid insomnia). One study compared the combination of clonazepam plus fluoxetine versus placebo plus fluoxetine for the treatment of insomnia occurring co-morbid with major depressive disorder [6]. Adjunctive clonazepam significantly improved sleep compared with placebo and also led to a greater antidepressant response. Another study compared the use of triazolam versus placebo in treating insomnia associated with rheumatoid arthritis [7]. Triazolam was associated with significantly greater improvement in sleep and also led to less morning stiffness than placebo. These placebo-controlled trials in primary and co-morbid insomnia represent the empirical basis for making clinical treatment decisions with regard to the benzodiazepines. The established efficacy of a number of these agents in primary insomnia and the two studies in co-morbid insomnias represent the expected benefit that must be weighed against the known risks. The most common risks are sedation, dizziness, memory side-effects, abuse, and ataxia [1]. All of these risks increase in likelihood as the dosage is increased. Adverse effects associated with impairment in daytime function are also more likely to occur with longer half-life agents [1].

Of the agents used to treat insomnia, benzodiazepines are most suited for use in the treatment of individuals with insomnia occurring with anxiety and/or pain given their profile of therapeutic effects. However, as is evident from the above review of placebo-controlled trials, there has been minimal systematic research on the use of these agents for the treatment of insomnia occurring in association with pain or anxiety. As a result, the actual risk–benefit profile of their use in this setting remains unknown. The abuse potential of these agents suggests that they should be used with caution in those with a predisposition to substance abuse. In this regard it should be noted that, among insomnia patients without a history of substance abuse, benzodiazepines are used for therapeutic purposes (in order to address their sleep disturbance) and the risk of non-therapeutic use appears to be very low [8].

Non-benzodiazepines

The term "non-benzodiazepines" has been used to refer to a group of medications, zolpidem, zaleplon, and eszopiclone, which have a sleep-promoting effect through binding to the same site on the GABA-A receptor complex as the benzodiazepines; however, they are chemically unrelated to the benzodiazepines.

Table 13.1 Attributes of medications used in the treatment of insomnia

Medication	Type	Insomnia dosage (mg)	Tmax (hours)	T1/2 (hours)	Mechanisms of sleep effect	Positive placebo-controlled primary insomnia trials	Possible non-insomnia therapeutic effects	Most important side-effects
Agents that enhance effects of sleep-promoting systems:								
Triazolam	Benzodiazepine	0.25	1–3	2–4	Enhancement of GABA inhibition	8/8	Anxiety, myorelaxation	Sedation, cognitive impairment, motor impairment, abuse potential
Temazepam	Benzodiazepine	15–30	1–3	8–20	Enhancement of GABA inhibition	2/2	Anxiety, myorelaxation	Sedation, cognitive impairment, motor impairment, abuse potential
Estazolam	Benzodiazepine	1–2	1.5–2	10–24	Enhancement of GABA inhibition	3/3	Anxiety, myorelaxation	Sedation, cognitive impairment, motor impairment, abuse potential
Quazepam	Benzodiazepine	15	2	25–41	Enhancement of GABA inhibition	2/2	Anxiety, myorelaxation	Sedation, cognitive impairment, motor impairment, abuse potential
Flurazepam	Benzodiazepine	15–30	0.5–1.5	24–100	Enhancement of GABA inhibition	4/4	Anxiety, myorelaxation	Sedation, cognitive impairment, motor impairment, abuse potential
Clonazepam	Benzodiazepine	0.25–2	1–2	35–40	Enhancement of GABA inhibition	–	Anxiety, myorelaxation	Sedation, cognitive impairment, motor impairment, abuse potential
Lorazepam	Benzodiazepine	0.125–1	1–3	12–15	Enhancement of GABA inhibition	–	Anxiety, myorelaxation	Sedation, cognitive impairment, motor impairment, abuse potential
Alprazolam	Benzodiazepine	0.125–1	1–3	12–14	Enhancement of GABA inhibition	–	Anxiety, myorelaxation	Sedation, cognitive impairment, motor impairment, abuse potential
Zaleplon	Non-benzodiazepine	10	1.1	1	Enhancement of GABA inhibition	5/5	–	Sedation, cognitive impairment, motor impairment, abuse potential

Drug	Class				Mechanism		Other uses	Side effects
Zolpidem	Non-benzodiazepine	5–10	1.7–2.5	1.5–2.5	Enhancement of GABA inhibition	8/8	–	Sedation, cognitive impairment, motor impairment, abuse potential
Zolpidem CR	Non-benzodiazepine	6.25–12.5	1.7–2.5	1.5–2.5	Enhancement of GABA inhibition	3/3	–	Sedation, cognitive impairment, motor impairment, abuse potential
Eszopiclone	Non-benzodiazepine	1–3	1.3–1.6	5–7	Enhancement of GABA inhibition	8/8	Anxiety, depression, pain	Sedation, cognitive impairment, motor impairment, abuse potential
Melatonin	Hormone	0.3–10	0.3–1	0.6–1	Melatonin receptor agonism	13/14		Headache, sedation
Ramelteon	Melatonin receptor agonist	8	0.7–0.95	0.8–2	Melatonin receptor agonism	4/4		Drowsiness, fatigue, dizziness
Tiagabine	Antiepileptic agent	2–16	1–1.5	8	GABA reuptake inhibition	2/4	Seizures	Sedation, nausea, dizziness, seizures
Agents that block the effects of wake-promoting systems:								
Amitriptyline	Antidepressant	10–100	2–5	10–100	Antagonism of NE, HA, Ach	–	Anxiety, depression, chronic pain	Sedation, dizziness, weight gain, OH, dry mouth, blurred vision, constipation, urinary retention
Doxepin	Antidepressant	1–25	1.5–4	10–50	Antagonism of NE, HA, Ach; in low doses HA only	5/5	Anxiety, depression, chronic pain	Sedation, dizziness, weight gain, OH, dry mouth, blurred vision, constipation, urinary retention
Trimipramine	Antidepressant	25–100	2–8	15–40	Antagonism of NE, HA, Ach	2/2	Anxiety, depression, chronic pain	Sedation, dizziness, weight gain, OH, dry mouth, blurred vision, constipation, urinary retention
Trazodone	Antidepressant	25–150	1–2	7–15	Antagonism of $5HT_2$, NE, HA	0/1	Anxiety, depression	Sedation, dizziness, headache, dry mouth, blurred vision, OH, priapism

Table 13.1 (cont.)

Medication	Type	Insomnia dosage (mg)	Tmax (hours)	T1/2 (hours)	Mechanisms of sleep effect	Positive placebo-controlled primary insomnia trials	Possible non-insomnia therapeutic effects	Most important side-effects
Mirtazapine	Antidepressant	7.5–30	0.25–2	20–40	Antagonism of $5HT_2$, HA	–	Anxiety, depression	Sedation, dry mouth, increased appetite, weight gain, constipation
Olanzapine	Antipsychotic	2.5–20	4–6	20–54	Antagonism of HA, NE, Ach, $5HT_2$, DA	–	Psychosis, mania, anxiety	Sedation, agitation, dizziness, constipation, OH, akathisia, weight gain, increased incidence of cerebrovascular events in dementia patients
Quetiapine	Antipsychotic	25–200	1–2	7	Antagonism of HA, NE, Ach, $5HT_2$, DA	–	Psychosis, depression, mania, anxiety	Sedation, OH, dry mouth, tachycardia, weight gain
Gabapentin	Antiepileptic agent	100–900	3–3.5	5–9	Decreasing release of GLU and NE	0/1	Pain, anxiety, seizures	Sedation, dizziness, ataxia, diplopia
Pregabalin	Antiepileptic agent	50–300	1	4.5–7	Decreasing release of GLU and NE	1/1	Pain, anxiety, seizures	Sedation, dizziness, dry mouth, cognitive impairment, increased appetite, discontinuation effects
Diphen-hydramine	Antihistamine	25–50	2–2.5	5–11	Antagonism of HA and Ach	2/2	Allergy	Sedation, dizziness, dry mouth, blurred vision, constipation, urinary retention
Doxylamine	Antihistamine	25–50	1.5–2.5	10–12	Antagonism of HA and Ach	–	Allergy	Sedation, dizziness, dry mouth, blurred vision, constipation, urinary retention

HA=histamine; DA=dopamine; OH=orthostatic hypotension; NE=norepinephrine; Ach=acetylcholine; GLU=glutamate; GABA=gamma-amino-butyric acid; $5HT_2$=serotonin type 2 receptor.

They also differ from the benzodiazepines in that they bind more specifically to subtypes of GABA-A receptors [9]. The 5-protein subunits of the GABA-A receptor are comprised of two identical α type subunits, two identical β type subunits, and a γ subunit [3]. These subunits occur in a variety of forms which tend to be localized in different brain regions, and, as a result, inhibit different aspects of brain function. GABA-A receptor complexes include one of six different α subunits. While benzodiazepines generally have effects at GABA-A receptors containing α_1, α_2, α_3, and α_5 subunits, the non-benzodiazepines appear to have effects that are more specific [10]. Zolpidem and zaleplon have relative selectivity for α_1 subunit-containing GABA-A receptors [9]. The alpha subunit effect profile of eszopiclone is less well established but there is some evidence that it may have effects predominantly on α_2 and/or α_3 subunit-containing GABA-A receptors [11].

The relative specificity of the effects of the non-benzodiazepines on GABA-A receptor subtypes would be expected to manifest in more specific clinical effects than the benzodiazepines. As a result of their preferential impact on α_1 subunit-containing GABA-A receptors, zolpidem and zaleplon would be expected to have effects that are limited to anticonvulsant, amnestic, and motor-impairing effects in addition to sleep enhancement [12]. In contrast, eszopiclone would be expected to have predominantly anxiolytic and myorelaxant effects in addition to sleep promotion to the extent that it is α_2 and α_3 subunit specific [3].

The available placebo-controlled trials do not allow a meaningful determination of whether these pharmacological considerations translate into actual differences in the profile of clinical effects of the non-benzodiazepines and benzodiazepines. Limited head-to-head data exist comparing these two types of agents. Studies of the non-benzodiazepines suggest a profile of adverse effects that are similar to those of the benzodiazepines with the most important being sedation, dizziness, and psychomotor impairment. There is some evidence that the abuse potential of the non-benzodiazepines may be less than that of the benzodiazepines when used at the recommended dosages, though a dose-dependent increase in abuse liability should be considered [13].

As was the case with the benzodiazepines, the half lives of the non-benzodiazepines are an important differentiating feature (see Table 13.1). All of the non-benzodiazepines have relatively short half lives compared with all of the benzodiazepines except triazolam and, as a result, relatively less next-day effects would be expected with these agents. Commensurate with the relatively short half lives of zaleplon and zolpidem, their therapeutic effects in insomnia are largely limited to difficulties with sleep onset [1]. On the other hand, eszopiclone and a controlled-release version of zolpidem have effects both on difficulties initiating and maintaining sleep.

The non-benzodiazepines have well-established efficacy in the treatment of insomnia. Placebo-controlled trials indicate the sleep-onset efficacy of zolpidem and zaleplon in younger and older adults with primary insomnia [1]. Zolpidem CR has been found to have onset and maintenance efficacy in adults ages 18–65, while eszopiclone has been noted to have onset and maintenance efficacy both in this population and in older adults [1]. Of note, far better data exist establishing the long-term efficacy and safety profile of the non-benzodiazepines compared with the benzodiazepines. Eszopiclone has sustained efficacy in two 6-month placebo-controlled trials, one of which included a 6-month open-label extension phase [14,15]. Efficacy was also maintained over 6 months in a placebo-controlled study of zolpidem CR dosed 3–7 nights per week [16]. The safety of zaleplon in long-term treatment has also been established in an open-label study of nightly dosing for 6–12 months in older adults [17]. The empirical basis for making clinical decisions regarding the non-benzodiazepines also includes a number of studies of the treatment of co-morbid insomnia. In a trial comparing fluoxetine plus eszopiclone versus fluoxetine plus placebo in the treatment of insomnia occurring with major depressive disorder, eszopiclone-treated subjects not only experienced greater improvement in sleep but also had a greater and more rapid improvement in depression (Hamilton depression score with sleep items removed) [18]. A study of the same design was carried out in patients with insomnia occurring with generalized anxiety disorder where eszopiclone was evaluated as adjunctive therapy to escitalopram [19]. As in the major depression study, eszopiclone not only improved sleep but was also associated with greater improvement in anxiety. Lastly, both eszopiclone and zolpidem were found to improve sleep in menopausal insomnia [20,21].

Among the options for medication therapy of insomnia, the non-benzodiazepines are relatively well suited for use in a number of conditions. These agents have a strong empirical base establishing their efficacy in insomnia therapy. Zaleplon and zolpidem are among the shorter half-life agents available which make them well suited for the treatment of sleep-onset difficulties. Eszopiclone and zolpidem CR are the only agents other than benzodiazepines that are approved by the US Food and Drug Adminstration (FDA) for the treatment of difficulties with both sleep onset and maintenance. Because of their relatively longer half lives, most of the benzodiazepines that can be used to treat sleep maintenance difficulties are likely to be associated with more next-day effects. The non-benzodiazepines may be associated with less abuse liability than the benzodiazepines; however, these agents should also be used with caution in abuse-prone individuals. Eszopiclone has better established long-term efficacy and safety with nightly dosing than any other agent, while the utility of zolpidem CR for long-term intermittent dosing has also been demonstrated. Lastly, controlled trials support the use of eszopiclone as adjunctive therapy for insomnia occurring with major depressive disorder and generalized anxiety disorder while studies indicate the utility of eszopiclone and zolpidem in the treatment of menopausal insomnia.

Melatonin receptor agonists

Available melatonin receptor agonists include melatonin and ramelteon. These agents are believed to exert their therapeutic effects on insomnia primarily through binding to MT1 and MT2 melatonin receptors. Melatonin is a hormone produced by the pineal gland that is obtainable as an "over-the-counter" medication. Ramelteon is an agent that is approved by the US FDA for the treatment of insomnia.

Melatonin has circadian rhythm modifying effects as well as a small but consistent effect on sleep-onset latency. The effect on sleep latency has been demonstrated in a wide range of patient populations including normal sleepers, children and adults with insomnia, patients with Alzheimer's disease, those with insomnia co-morbid with medical disorders, those with mood disorders, patients with schizophrenia, children with attention-deficit disorder, and children with neurodevelopmental disorders [22–36]. The great variation in the methods employed in these studies limits their application to clinical practice [37,38]. Most problematic in this regard is that they evaluated dosages of melatonin varying from 0.1 to 75 mg

(2–6 mg in most studies) which were administered from 30 minutes to 3 hours before bedtime.

A factor complicating the determination of the time of optimal dose and timing of dosing of melatonin is that, unlike benzodiazepines and non-benzodiazepines, the sleep-enhancing effects of melatonin agonists are not tightly linked to the serum blood level. A dose–response relationship does not exist for melatonin or ramelteon and a number of studies suggest that the time lag from dosing of melatonin to when its effects on sleep become evident depends on the time of day of administration [39–41]. Despite the fact that the peak blood level of melatonin occurs around 30 minutes after ingestion, some studies have identified that the sleep effects may not occur until up to 3 hours after dosing.

Ramelteon also has a therapeutic effect on sleep-onset latency. Despite the lack of a clear relationship between serum level and effects on sleep, the available studies have focused on a dosage of 8 mg administered 30 minutes prior to lights out [1]. Studies in both adults 18–65 years of age and older adults with insomnia indicate a consistent therapeutic effect on sleep-onset latency which is more consistent when assessed with measures derived from the overnight sleep study (polysomnogram) than with self-report measures.

Both melatonin and ramelteon have relatively favorable profiles of adverse effects. Headache is the most frequent side-effect of melatonin, and sedation and slowing of reaction time have been observed when melatonin has been taken during the day [39,42,43]. There is some evidence that melatonin may affect fertility in both men and women [44–47]. As a result, it has been suggested that melatonin should not be used by individuals attempting to conceive. The most common side-effects associated with ramelteon are somnolence, dizziness, nausea, and fatigue [48,49]. There is evidence that ramelteon can be safely used in those with sleep apnea and mild to moderate chronic obstructive pulmonary disease [50,51]. Neither melatonin nor ramelteon appear to have significant abuse potential and would therefore be well suited for use in individuals with insomnia who have a history of substance abuse; however, neither agent has been studied in a substance-abuse prone population.

Antidepressants

Antidepressants are frequently used to treat insomnia in clinical practice, though relatively little data exist on the treatment of insomnia patients with these agents [1,2]. As a result, it is not possible to carry out a meaningful risk–benefit analysis. This should be a consideration in the use of antidepressants in the clinical treatment of insomnia.

When used to treat insomnia, antidepressants are typically dosed well below the range generally used for the treatment of depression. These agents enhance sleep by antagonism of receptors of wake-promoting systems including: serotonin, norepinephrine, acetylcholine, and histamine (compendium). The antidepressants most commonly used to treat insomnia are the tricyclic antidepressants doxepin, amitriptyline, and trimipramine, as well as trazodone and mirtazapine.

Tricyclic antidepressants

These agents promote sleep by antagonism of the wake-promoting systems norepinephrine, histamine, and acetylcholine. Effects on sleep onset and mainten- ance have been noted with a number of these agents in depression trials [52]. However, studies in insom- nia patients have only been carried out with two tricyclic antidepressants: trimipramine and doxepin. Two studies in primary insomnia patients have been carried out with trimipramine at dosages from 50 to 200 mg [53,54]. These studies reported improvement in sleep quality and sleep efficiency (total sleep time divided by time in bed), but did not find a significant effect on sleep-onset latency. Three studies carried out with doxepin at dosages from 25 to 50 mg reported that this agent had efficacy in terms of sleep quality, sleep onset, and sleep maintenance [53,55–57]. Dox- epin has also been studied at dosages of 1–6 mg where it becomes a relatively selective blocker of the hista- mine H1 receptor [58,59]. At these lower dosages doxepin has been found to have therapeutic effects on both onset and maintenance of sleep with the greatest and most consistent effects on sleep difficul- ties occurring in the last third of the night [58,59].

This effect that doxepin appears to have on sleep difficulties occurring towards the end of the night is another example of how the pharmacological mechan- isms of insomnia agents can affect their clinical effects. Intuition gained from experience with benzodiazep- ine-related agents cannot explain how an agent with a peak blood level occurring 1.5–4 hours after dosing can have its predominant effect 7–8 hours after dosing [60–62]. Further evidence for a dissociation of serum level and clinical effects with doxepin is the lack of significant sedation or impairment 1 hour after waking

or evidence of greater daytime somnolence than pla- cebo, despite the 10–50-hour half life of this agent [58]. Only limited data exist that might explain these novel clinical effects of doxepin 1–6 mg. However, it is evi- dent that the clinical effects depend on the time of day and perhaps activity level (whether one is awake or asleep) and that low-dose doxepin may be well suited for the treatment of individuals with sleep difficulty occurring towards the end of the night.

The primary side-effects of the tricyclic anti- depressants include sedation, weight gain, orthostatic hypotension, and anticholinergic side-effects (dry mouth, blurred vision, constipation, urinary reten- tion, exacerbation of narrow-angle glaucoma, and risk of delirium) [61,63]. Less common but more severe side-effects include impairment of cardiac electrical conduction which can lead to heart block in some instances, and seizures. These side-effects derive from the antihistaminergic, anticholinergic, antisero- tonergic, and antiadrenergic effects of the tricyclic antidepressants. The dose-dependence of these side- effects is illustrated by the evidence that doxepin dosed from 1 to 6 mg has substantially less side-effects (sedation, weight gain, and anticholinergic effects) than have been reported with this agent dosed at 25 mg and above [58,59].

The tricyclic antidepressants may be considered for use in abuse-prone insomnia patients because they appear to lack abuse potential. These agents may also be useful in the treatment of insomnia patients with significant anxiety or chronic pain as they have often been used to treat these conditions [64]. They could also be considered for use in patients with insomnia occurring with major depression, however, it remains unclear whether they have antidepressant effects in the dosages typically used to treat insomnia and the efficacy and safety of combining these agents with non-sedating antidepressants is not established [65]. Low-dose doxepin may also be particularly useful for the treatment of those with difficulty with sleep in the last third of the night, including early morning awak- enings. Caution should be exercised when adminis- tering tricyclic antidepressants to patients with significant heart disease and those at risk for compli- cations from the anticholinergic effects of these medications [61,63].

Trazodone

Trazodone, dosed at 200–600 mg when used to treat major depression, is used at a dosage of 25–150 mg "off-label" for treating insomnia [1]. In fact, it has been among the most frequently administered treatments for insomnia over the last 20 years [2]. Trazodone's sleep-enhancing effects are believed to derive from antagonism of several wake-promoting systems including serotonin ($5HT_2$ receptors), norepinephrine (α_1 receptors), and histamine (H1 receptors). A factor which complicates the use of trazodone is that it is metabolized into methyl-chlorophenylpiperazine (mCPP) which has a wake-promoting effect and somewhat unpredictably (because of the highly variable metabolism of trazodone and mCPP in the population) may undermine the therapeutic effects of trazodone [66,67].

Despite the frequency with which trazodone is used in the treatment of insomnia, there is remarkably scant evidence that it is safe and effective when used for this purpose. Only one placebo-controlled study of the treatment of insomnia patients has been carried out with trazodone [68]. In this 2-week study, patients treated with 50 mg had significantly better self-reported sleep than placebo-treated subjects in the first but not second week of treatment. Evidence of the sleep-promoting effect of trazodone has been noted in two small placebo-controlled studies, one carried out in abstinent alcoholics and another in patients with depression treated with either fluoxetine or bupropion [69,70].

The most common adverse effects seen with trazodone treatment are sedation, dizziness, headache, dry mouth, blurred vision, and orthostatic hypotension [1,68]. A rare side-effect of trazodone in men is priapism, a prolonged erection associated with pain, which may result in irreversible impotence [71].

Like the tricyclic antidepressants, trazodone appears to be without significant abuse potential and, as a result, can be considered for use in abuse-prone insomnia patients. The small placebo-controlled trial carried out in abstinent alcoholics provides some support for this use [69]. While trazodone probably lacks antidepressant efficacy in the dose range generally used to treat insomnia, this has not been systematically evaluated. Preliminary evidence suggests that it can be safely used to treat insomnia in patients taking fluoxetine and bupropion but its use with other antidepressants remains unknown [70].

Mirtazapine

The effects of mirtazapine are believed to derive from antagonism of serotonergic ($5HT_2$ and $5HT_3$),

adrenergic (α_1 and α_2), and histaminergic (H1) receptors [72]. All of these pharmacological effects enhance sleep except for the antagonism of the α_2 receptor, which is a presynaptic receptor that inhibits the release of norepinephrine [73]. It is believed that, as a result of this α_2 antagonism, the sleep-enhancing effects of mirtazapine may diminish with increasing dosage. For this reason, dosages of 30 mg and less are generally used to treat insomnia, while the range of antidepressant dosing is 7.5–45 mg. No placebo-controlled trials of the use of mirtazapine for the treatment of insomnia patients have been carried out. Data indicating that mirtazapine has sleep-enhancing effects derive from a double-blind study evaluating mirtazapine versus fluoxetine carried out in depressed patients and open-label studies in a group of healthy volunteers without sleep complaints and a group of depressed patients [74–76]. The most common side-effects associated with mirtazapine are sedation, increased appetite, weight gain, dry mouth, and constipation [73]. Like the other antidepressants discussed, mirtazapine does not appear to be associated with abuse potential and, therefore, could be considered for use in substance abuse-prone patients with insomnia. Because the dosages used to treat insomnia and depression with mirtazapine overlap, this agent can be considered for single-agent therapy in depressed patients with insomnia. Future studies will be needed to determine the effectiveness of this approach compared to combining a non-sedating antidepressant with an established insomnia therapy.

Antipsychotics

Like the antidepressants, antipsychotic agents are sometimes used "off-label" for the treatment of insomnia [2]. These agents enhance sleep through antagonism of the following wake-promoting systems: dopamine, histamine (H1 receptors), serotonin ($5HT_2$ receptors), acetylcholine (muscarinic receptors), and norepinephrine (α_1 receptors) [1]. When used to treat insomnia, antipsychotic agents are typically administered at a lower dosage than used for the treatment of thought disorders and mood disorders. The agents most commonly used to treat insomnia, quetiapine and olanzapine, are dosed at 25–250 mg and 2.5–20 mg, respectively [2,77].

No placebo-controlled trials of the treatment of insomnia patients have been carried out with any of the antipsychotic medications. This is a factor which limits the ability to make risk–benefit assessments with these agents. Quetiapine dosed at from 25 to 75 mg has been found to have a sleep-enhancing effect in a population of primary insomnia patients and in healthy volunteers in open-label studies [78]. Olanzapine has been noted to enhance sleep in an open-label study of healthy volunteers [77]. Both of these agents have also been reported to enhance sleep in a number of studies in patients with thought disorders and mood disorders [77,79,80]. The pharmacokinetics of olanzapine (tmax of 4–6 hours) make it better suited for the treatment of sleep maintenance problems than sleep-onset problems, while quetiapine's pharmacokinetics suggest that it has the potential to be helpful for both problems, staying asleep and falling asleep (tmax of 1–2 hours; half life of 7 hours) [1].

The most common side-effects of the antipsychotic agents used to treat insomnia are: sedation, dizziness, anticholinergic side-effects (dry mouth, blurred vision, constipation, urinary retention), and increased appetite [77]. The frequency of these side-effects varies among the antipsychotic agents. Antipsychotic agents also have other potential side-effects. Among these are extrapyramidal side-effects that occur as a result of dopamine antagonism (parkinsonism, acute dystonic reactions, akathisia, and tardive dyskinesia) [78]. These extrapyramidal side-effects appear to occur rarely with the atypical antipsychotics as compared to typical antipsychotics. Olanzapine has been associated with an increased risk of insulin resistance, impaired cognition, and mortality in dementia patients, and all antipsychotics should be used with caution in older adults because of a potential increased risk of cardiac-related mortality [81].

Antipsychotic agents are most appropriate for the treatment of patients who have insomnia occurring in the setting of psychosis or a mood disorder. In addition to having FDA indications for the treatment of psychosis, a number of these agents are approved for the treatment of mania and quetiapine is approved for the treatment of bipolar depression. Antipsychotic agents can also be considered for use in substance abuse-prone patients with insomnia as these agents do not have significant abuse potential.

Antihistamines

Many agents are significant antagonists of H1 histamine receptors and could therefore be referred to as antihistamines. This includes the antidepressants doxepin and mirtazapine, which are among the more potent and selective H1 antagonists, and the antipsychotics quetiapine and olanzapine [1]. However, the term "antihistamine" is generally reserved for agents that were developed primarily for the treatment of allergies. Among these agents, diphenhydramine and doxylamine are used the most commonly for the treatment of insomnia and are important constituents of many insomnia treatments available "over-the-counter." These two medications have similar properties. The usual dosage of both agents for the treatment of insomnia is 25–50 mg and both have significant muscarinic cholinergic antagonist effects.

Several placebo-controlled trials in insomnia patients have been carried out with diphenhydramine, though no such studies have evaluated the efficacy and safety of doxylamine. Diphenhydramine has been observed to improve sleep in trials in the following populations: primary insomnia, psychiatric patients, primary care patients, and nursing home residents [82–86]. In these studies diphenhydramine appeared to have a stronger effect on maintenance than sleep onset. This is consistent with the findings observed with low-dose doxepin, another potent H1 antagonist, suggesting that a greater effect on sleep maintenance may be a characteristic of agents acting via blocking the wake-promoting effects of histamine. One study where diphenhydramine was administered during the day found that the therapeutic effect was lost by the 4th day of treatment [87]. Further studies will be needed to determine if tolerance occurs to night-time dosing of this medication. The only study of doxylamine was a large double-blind trial carried out in post-operative patients where a significant effect on subjective measures of sleep was observed [88].

The predominant adverse effects associated with both diphenhydramine and doxylamine are: anticholinergic effects (dry mouth, blurred vision, constipation, urinary retention, risk of delirium), sedation, dizziness, and weight gain. Infrequent side-effects of diphenhydramine are agitation and insomnia while doxylamine has been associated with coma and rhabdomyolysis in case reports [89].

Neither of these medications has significant abuse potential and, therefore, may be considered for use in abuse-prone insomnia patients. Both of these agents are particularly well suited for use in the treatment of insomnia occurring with allergies or significant nasal/sinus congestion. These agents should be avoided in those at risk for complications due to anticholinergic effects, such as those with dementia, urinary retention, and narrow-angle glaucoma.

Anticonvulsants

Anticonvulsants sometimes used in the treatment of insomnia include gabapentin, pregabalin, and tiagabine. Gabapentin and pregabalin enhance sleep by decreasing the activity of the wake-promoting systems glutamate and norepinephrine (by binding to the alpha-2-delta subunit of N-type voltage-gated calcium channels) while tiagabine enhances the sleep-promoting effects of GABA by inhibiting the reuptake of GABA [90,91]. While all three agents have FDA indications for the treatment of seizures, gabapentin and pregabalin also have indications for the treatment of pain and pregabalin is indicated for the treatment of fibromyalgia.

Sleep-enhancing effects of gabapentin and pregabalin have been reported in trials carried out with healthy volunteers, patients with restless legs syndrome, chronic pain patients, and patients being treated for partial epilepsy [92–95]. A therapeutic effect on sleep was observed with gabapentin compared with placebo in a small study of the treatment of insomnia in patients with alcohol dependence [96]. Given the relatively high tmax of gabapentin (3–3.5 hours), it is relatively less likely to be effective for sleep-onset difficulties than sleep-maintenance problems. In placebo-controlled trials in primary insomnia patients, tiagabine has been found to consistently increase slow-wave sleep; however, it did not improve sleep onset and inconsistently affected sleep maintenance [97–100].

For all three of these agents the most common adverse effects are sedation and dizziness. Other common side-effects are: gabapentin – ataxia, diplopia; pregabalin – dry mouth, cognitive impairment, peripheral edema, and increased appetite; tiagabine – nausea.

Gabapentin and tiagabine do not have significant abuse potential and could be considered for use in abuse-prone patients with insomnia. However, pregabalin may have abuse potential and should be used with caution in this population [101]. In this regard, preliminary evidence supports the use of gabapentin in patients with alcohol dependence. Gabapentin and pregabalin could also be considered for use in patients with insomnia occurring in conjunction with pain. Pregabalin could also be considered for treating insomnia in fibromyalgia patients as it is indicated

for the treatment of this syndrome. Preliminary evidence also supports the use of gabapentin in patients with restless legs syndrome and periodic limb movements of sleep.

The pharmacological treatment of insomnia in psychiatric patients

The majority of insomnia cases occur with medical and psychiatric conditions [5]. Longstanding clinical guidelines published in 1983 discouraged targeting treatment to insomnia in those with medical and psychiatric disorders [102]. This view was based on a model in which chronic insomnia was assumed to be a symptom of an underlying medical or psychiatric disorder. As such, treatment of the underlying disorder was indicated and this was assumed to result in resolution of the insomnia along with all of the other symptoms of the underlying condition. Thus, insomnia-specific treatment was superfluous. Over time, research suggests that the symptom model of insomnia is too limited and indicates the need to consider implementing therapy directed to insomnia along with treatment of the associated medical or psychiatric condition [103]. In this regard, a number of pharmacological treatment studies of insomnia have been carried out in those with psychiatric disorders. While most such studies were discussed above, they are reviewed again here to focus attention on the treatment of insomnia specifically in patients with psychiatric disorders. These studies provide further support for the need to directly target insomnia when it occurs with psychiatric conditions to improve sleep and potentially the outcome of the associated psychiatric conditions. However, these studies also highlight the relatively limited body of research carried out in this area and the great need for more trials in these populations.

Major depression

Several studies have been carried out in which patients with insomnia occurring with major depression were treated with insomnia pharmacotherapy along with antidepressant medication. In one such study, 53 subjects were randomized to receive the benzodiazepines flunitrazepam, lormetazepam, or placebo along with one of several tricyclic antidepressant medications [104]. Of the two agents, only lormetazepam led to improved sleep versus placebo in this study. The addition of clonazepam or placebo to fluoxetine antidepressant treatment has been evaluated in three trials carried out by the same group [6,105,106]. Clonazepam improved sleep compared with placebo but also was noted to improve non-sleep depressive symptoms in two of the studies; however, in a longer-duration study it was found that the benefit on depressive symptoms versus placebo was not sustained. In the largest study of insomnia co-therapy of antidepressant treatment, subjects treated with fluoxetine were randomized to receive insomnia treatment with either eszopiclone or placebo [18]. In this study, eszopiclone not only improved sleep but led to greater and more rapid improvement in non-sleep depression symptoms versus placebo.

An option for treating patients with insomnia and depression other than combining a non-sedating anti-depressant with an insomnia agent is to administer a sedating antidepressant. There are relatively few placebo-controlled studies of the effects on sleep of these agents, however, controlled trials indicate the efficacy of mirtazapine and several tricyclic antidepressants on sleep in depressed patients treated with these agents [52,74]. No studies have been carried out evaluating the relative utility of using a sedating antidepressant versus combining a sleep agent with a non-sedating antidepressant. As a result, while the available data suggest the need to treat insomnia in patients with insomnia occurring with major depression and point to a number of agents that appear to be effective in this setting, these data do not allow a determination of whether there is an optimal therapeutic approach. However, whereas the sleep agent can be discontinued after 4–6 weeks, the antidepressant will most probably be maintained for a minimum of 6–9 months after resolution of depressive symptoms. Therefore, clinicians should be comfortable with the other properties (e.g. weight gain, anticholinergic effects) of a sedating antidepressant which are initially used for both anti-depressant and hypnotic effects.

Insomnia associated with successful antidepressant therapy

Two placebo-controlled studies have been carried out of the treatment of insomnia in those otherwise successfully treated with antidepressant medication. In one study of 15 patients randomized to "add-on" therapy with trazodone or placebo, trazodone led to greater improvement in sleep compared to placebo

[70]. In a trial of 110 patients with persistent insomnia who had otherwise remitted to treatment with either fluoxetine, sertraline, or paroxetine, the addition of zolpidem was associated with significantly greater improvement in sleep than placebo [107]. Some ambiguity exists related to these studies because it is not clear if the insomnia represents a side-effect of the antidepressant medication, incomplete anti-depressant response, or a pre-existing and perhaps somewhat independent condition. Further, only a very few combinations of antidepressants and insomnia agents have been evaluated. Until additional work is completed the risk–benefit profile of combining many insomnia agents with antidepressants will remain unknown.

Generalized anxiety disorder

Given the very high prevalence of insomnia in those with anxiety disorders, surprisingly little research has been carried out on the treatment of insomnia in patients with anxiety disorders [5]. Only one placebo-controlled trial of the treatment of insomnia has been carried out in those with anxiety disorders. In this study, 595 patients with insomnia and generalized anxiety disorder treated with escitalopram were randomized to receive adjunctive treatment with either eszopiclone or placebo [19]. Eszopiclone was associated with significantly greater improvement in sleep than placebo as well as a significantly greater benefit in non-sleep features of generalized anxiety disorder. Studies of the treatment of generalized anxiety disorder with other agents are needed. Further treatment studies of insomnia in other anxiety disorders such as post-traumatic stress disorder where sleep difficulty is frequently reported, and from clinical experience, can be challenging to treat, are also needed.

Insomnia in abstinent alcoholics

Like anxiety disorders, alcoholism is a condition where insomnia is frequent and also the subject of little research. Only one study of the pharmacotherapy of insomnia in those with alcohol difficulties has been carried out. This study was undertaken in 16 recently alcohol-abstinent subjects who were randomized to treatment with trazodone or placebo. Sleep was improved to a significantly greater extent in those subjects treated with trazodone compared with placebo-treated subjects [69]. Trazodone and other agents that do not act via the benzodiazepine binding site may be preferred in this population because of a lack of abuse potential. However, these agents are relatively unstudied for use in the treatment of insomnia. Because of the large number of individuals with alcohol-related sleep difficulties there is motivation to study these agents specifically in the population of abuse-prone individuals.

Schizophrenia

Sleep disturbance is commonly reported by patients with schizophrenia and is evident when polysomnographic assessment of sleep is carried out in this population [103]. However, there have been no placebo-controlled trials of the treatment of insomnia in patients with schizophrenia. Because many of the antipsychotic agents used to treat schizophrenia have a sleep-promoting effect, it may be possible to address sleep disturbance in this population by choosing an antipsychotic agent that is likely to enhance sleep, based on the considerations discussed above [77]. However, in some patients this might not be desirable due to the associated side-effect profile of the sleep-enhancing antipsychotic medications, in which case the combination of a non-sedating antipsychotic and a sleep aid should be considered.

Bipolar disorder

A decrease in sleep is a core symptom of mania [77]. However, it is not clear if this represents insomnia, which is defined by an inability to sleep enough to feel restored given the adequate opportunity to do so, or a decrease in sleep need. It has been hypothesized that sleep loss is part of a positive feedback cycle that triggers mania, based in part on evidence that patients with bipolar disorder may develop mania in response to sleep deprivation [77]. As a result, it is natural to consider pharmacological interventions aimed at increasing sleep in this population, though it has never been demonstrated that improving sleep either prevents the development of mania or is integral to resolving mania once it occurs. Despite the absence of data on this issue, it has become standard practice to administer sedating agents for preventing or addressing mania. Indeed, it is difficult to do otherwise because all of the primary agents used to treat mania may enhance sleep (lithium, valproate, and antipsychotic medications). Whether the addition of agents other than mood stabilizers targeted at further

enhancing sleep might improve the ability to prevent or treat mania remains unknown.

Insomnia in chronic pain patients

Two placebo-controlled trials have been carried out of the treatment of insomnia in patients with chronic pain. Both were carried out in patients with rheumatoid arthritis. In one study, 15 patients with rheumatoid arthritis were randomized to triazolam or placebo [7]. In this study triazolam was associated with significantly greater improvement in sleep than placebo, as well as less daytime sleepiness, and less morning stiffness. In the other controlled trial of insomnia therapy in this population, subjects were randomized to receive either eszopiclone or placebo [108]. Eszopiclone led to greater improvement in both sleep and pain than placebo. While limited data exist these studies suggest that the treatment of insomnia in those with pain, at least rheumatoid arthritis, may lead not only to improvement in sleep but also to better pain management.

Summary

A large number of different types of medications are used to treat insomnia. The clinical effects of these agents derive from the pharmacological mechanism by which they enhance sleep, their other pharmacological effects, and their pharmacokinetics. The risk–benefit profile of a number of medications used to treat insomnia are well established. However, for a number of agents frequently prescribed for the treatment of insomnia little or no placebo-controlled research has been carried out. This presents a significant challenge to their use as data from placebo-controlled studies are needed to make the risk–benefit decisions needed to optimize the treatment of insomnia in clinical practice. Limited research has also been carried out on the pharmacological treatment of insomnia in those with psychiatric disorders. The studies that have been completed suggest that some agents are effective in the treatment of insomnia in disorders such as major depression, generalized anxiety disorder, alcohol dependence, and chronic pain. Further, these studies suggest that in some cases the treatment of insomnia may not only improve sleep but may improve the treatment outcome of the associated psychiatric condition. Further studies are needed to determine if this benefit occurs due to improvement in insomnia or is a direct pharmacological effect of the agents studied.

References

1. Krystal A. A compendium of placebo-controlled trials of the risks/benefits of pharmacologic treatments for insomnia: The empirical basis for clinical practice. *Sleep Med Rev.* 2009;**13**(4):265–274.

2. Walsh J K. Drugs used to treat insomnia in 2002: regulatory-based rather than evidence-based medicine. *Sleep.* 2004;**27**(8):14441–14442.

3. Sieghart W, Sperk G. Subunit composition, distribution and function of GABA(A) receptor subtypes. *Curr Top Med Chem.* 2002;**2**:795–816.

4. Saper C, Scammell TE, Lu J. Hypothalamic regulation of sleep and circadian rhythms. *Nature.* 2005;**437** (7063):1257–1263.

5. Ford D, Kamerow D. Epidemiologic study of sleep disturbances in psychiatric disorders. *JAMA.* 1989;**262**:1479–1484.

6. Londborg P, Smith WT, Glaudin V, Painter J R. Short-term cotherapy with clonazepam and fluoxetine: anxiety, sleep disturbance and core symptoms of depression. *J Affect Disord.* 2000;**61**:73–79.

7. Walsh J, Muehlbach MJ, Lauter SA, Hilliker NA, Schweitzer P K. Effects of triazolam on sleep, daytime sleepiness, and morning stiffness in patients with rheumatoid arthritis. *J Rheumatol.* 1996;**23**(2): 245–252.

8. Roehrs T, Pedrosi B, Rosenthal L, et al. Hypnotic self administration and dose escalation. *Psychopharmacology (Berl).* 1996;**127**:150–154.

9. Sanna E, Busonero F, Talani G, et al. Comparison of the effects of zaleplon, zolpidem, and triazolam at various GABA(A) receptor subtypes. *Eur J Pharmacol.* 2002;**451**(2):103–110.

10. Mohler H, Fritschy JM, Rudolph U. A new benzodiazepine pharmacology. *J Pharmacol Exp Ther.* 2002;**300**:2–8.

11. Jia F, Goldstein PA, Harrison N L. The modulation of synaptic GABA(A) receptors in the thalamus by eszopiclone and zolpidem. *J Pharmacol Exp Ther.* 2009;**328**(3):1000–1006.

12. Crestani F, Assandri R, Tauber M, et al. Contribution of the alpha1-GABA(A) receptor subtype to the pharmacological actions of benzodiazepine site inverse agonists. *Neuropharmacology.* 2002;**43**:679–684.

13. Griffiths RR, Johnson MW. Relative abuse liability of hypnotic drugs: a conceptual framework and algorithm for differentiating among compounds. *J Clin Psychol.* 2005;**66**(Suppl 9):31–41.

14. Krystal AD, Walsh JK, Laska E, et al. Sustained efficacy of eszopiclone over six months of nightly treatment: Results of a randomized, double-blind, placebo controlled study in adults with chronic insomnia. *Sleep.* 2003;**26**:793–799.

15. Walsh J, Krystal AD, Amato DA. Nightly treatment of primary insomnia with eszopiclone for six months: Effect on sleep, quality of life and work limitations. *Sleep.* 2007;**30**(8):959–968.

16. Krystal AD, Erman M, Zammit GK, et al. Long-term efficacy and safety of zolpidem extended-release 12.5 mg, administered 3 to 7 nights per week for 24 weeks, in patients with chronic primary insomnia: a 6-month, randomized, double-blind, placebo-controlled, parallel-group, multicenter study. *Sleep.* 2008;**31**(1):79–90.

17. Ancoli-Israel S, Richardson GS, Mangano RM, et al. Long-term use of sedative hypnotics in older patients with insomnia. *Sleep Med.* 2005;**6**(2):107–113.

18. Fava M, McCall WV, Krystal A, et al. Eszopiclone co-administered with fluoxetine in patients with insomnia co-existing with major depressive disorder. *Biol Psychiatry.* 2006;**59**:1052–1060.

19. Pollack M, Kinrys G, Krystal A, et al. Eszopiclone co-administered with escitalopram in patients with insomnia and comorbid generalized anxiety disorder. *Arch Gen Psychiatry.* 2008;**65**(5):551–562.

20. Soares C, Rubens R, Caron J, et al. Eszopiclone treatment during menopausal transition: Sleep effects, impact on menopausal symptoms, and mood. *Sleep.* 2006;**29**:A239.

21. Dorsey C, Lee KA, Scharf MB. Effect of zolpidem on sleep in women with perimenopausal and postmenopausal insomnia: a 4-week, randomized, multicenter, double-blind, placebo-controlled study. *Clin Ther.* 2004;**26**(10):1578–1586.

22. Hughes R, Sack RL, Lewy AJ. The role of melatonin and circadian phase in age-related sleep-maintenance insomnia: assessment in a clinical trial of melatonin replacement. *Sleep.* 1998;**21**:52–68.

23. Singer C, Tractenberg RE, Kaye J, et al. A multicenter, placebo-controlled trial of melatonin for sleep disturbance in Alzheimer's disease. *Sleep.* 2003;**26** (7):893–901.

24. Smits M, Nagtegaal EE, van der Heijden J, Coenen AM, Kerkhof GA. Melatonin for chronic sleep onset insomnia in children: a randomized placebo-controlled trial. *J Child Neurol.* 2001;**16**(2):86–92.

25. Zhdanova I, Wurtman RJ, Morabito C, Piotrovska VR, Lynch HJ. Effects of low oral doses of melatonin, given 2–4 hours before habitual bedtime, on sleep in normal young humans. *Sleep.* 1996;**19**(5):423–431.

26. Zhdanova I, Wurtman RJ, Wagstaff J. Effects of a low dose of melatonin on sleep in children with Angelman syndrome. *J Pediatr Endocrinol.* 1999;**12**(1):57–67.

27. Zhdanova IV, Wurtman RJ, Regan MM, et al. Melatonin treatment for age-related insomnia. *J Clin Endocrinol Metab*. 2001;**86**:4727–4730.

28. Waldhauser F, Saletu B, Trinchard-Lugan I. Sleep laboratory investigations on hypnotic properties of melatonin. *Psychopharmacology*. 1990;**100**(2):222–226.

29. Dalton E, Rotondi D, Levitan RD, Kennedy SH, Brown GM. Use of slow-release melatonin in treatment-resistant depression. *J Psychiatr Neurosci*. 2000;**25**(1):48–52.

30. Andrade C, Srihari BS, Reddy KP, Chandramma L. Melatonin in medically ill patients with insomnia: a double-blind, placebo-controlled study. *J Clin Psychol*. 2001;**62**(1):41–45.

31. Serfaty M, Kennell-Webb S, Warner J, Blizard R, Raven P. Double blind randomised placebo controlled trial of low dose melatonin for sleep disorders in dementia. *Int J Geriatr Psychiatry*. 2002;**17**(12):1120–1127.

32. Suresh Kumar P, Andrade C, Bhakta SG, Singh NM. Melatonin in schizophrenic outpatients with insomnia: a double-blind, placebo-controlled study. *J Clin Psychol*. 2007;**68**(2):237–241.

33. Van der Heijden K, Smits MG, Van Someren EJ, Ridderinkhof KR, Gunning WB. Effect of melatonin on sleep, behavior, and cognition in ADHD and chronic sleep-onset insomnia. *J Am Acad Child Adolesc Psychiatry*. 2007;**46**(2):233–241.

34. Wasdell M, Jan JE, Bomben MM, et al. A randomized, placebo-controlled trial of controlled release melatonin treatment of delayed sleep phase syndrome and impaired sleep maintenance in children with neurodevelopmental disabilities. *J Pineal Res*. 2008;**44**(1):57–64.

35. Braam W, Didden R, Smits M, Curfs L. Melatonin treatment in individuals with intellectual disability and chronic insomnia: a randomized placebo-controlled study. *J Intellect Disabil Res*. 2008;**52**(3):256–264.

36. Haimov I, Lavie P, Laudon M, et al. Melatonin replacement therapy of elderly insomniacs. *Sleep*. 1995;**18**(7):598–603.

37. Mendelson WB. Efficacy of melatonin as a hypnotic agent. *J Biol Rhythms*. 1997;**12**(6):651–656.

38. Sack R, Hughes RJ, Edgar DM, Lewy AJ. Sleep-promoting effects of melatonin: at what dose, in whom, under what conditions, and by what mechanisms? *Sleep*. 1997;**20**(10):908–915.

39. Krystal A. The possibility of preventing functional imapairment due to sleep loss by pharmacologically enhancing sleep. *Sleep*. 2005;**28**:16–17.

40. Slotten H, Krekling S. Does melatonin have an effect on cognitive performance. *Psychoneuroendocrinol*. 1996;**21**:673–680.

41. Hughes R, Badia P. Sleep-promoting and hypothermic effects of daytime melatonin administration in humans. *Sleep*. 1997;**20**:124–131.

42. Graw P, Werth E, Krauchi K, et al. Early morning melatonin administration impairs psychomotor vigilance. *Behav Brain Res*. 2001;**121**:167–172.

43. Dollins A, Zhdanova IV, Wurtman RJ, Lynch HJ, Deng MH. Effect of inducing nocturnal serum melatonin concentrations in daytime on sleep, mood, body temperature and performance. *Proc Natl Acad Sci USA*. 1994;**91**:1824–1828.

44. Lerchl A. Melatonin administration alters semen quality in normal men. *J Androl*. 2004;**25**(2):185–186.

45. Ianas O, Manda D, Câmpean D, Ionescu M, Soare G. Effects of melatonin and its relation to the hypothalamic-hypophyseal-gonadal axis. *Adv Exp Med Biol*. 1999;**460**:321–328.

46. Partonen T. Melatonin-dependent infertility. *Med Hypotheses*. 1999;**52**(3):269–270.

47. Pang SF, Li L, Ayre EA, et al. Neuroendocrinology of melatonin in reproduction: recent developments. *J Chem Neuroanat*. 1998;**14**(3–4):157–166.

48. Roth T, Seiden D, Sainati S, et al. Effects of ramelteon on patient-reported sleep latency in older adults with chronic insomnia. *Sleep Med*. 2006;**7**(4):312–318.

49. Zammit G, Erman M, Wang-Weigand S, et al. Evaluation of the efficacy and safety of ramelteon in subjects with chronic insomnia. *J Clin Sleep Med*. 2007;**3**(5):495–504.

50. Kryger M, Roth T, Wang-Weigand S, Zhang J. The effects of ramelteon on respiration during sleep in subjects with moderate to severe chronic obstructive pulmonary disease. *Sleep Breath*. 2009;**13**(1):79–84.

51. Kryger M, Wang-Weigand S, Roth T. Safety of ramelteon in individuals with mild to moderate obstructive sleep apnea. *Sleep Breath*. 2007;**11**(3):159–164.

52. Dunleavy D, Brezinova V, Oswald I, MacLean AW, Tinker M. Changes during weeks in effects of tricyclic drugs on the human sleep brain. *Br J Psychiatry*. 1972;**120**:663–672.

53. Riemann D, Voderholzer U, Cohrs S, et al. Trimipramine in primary insomnia: results of a polysomnographic double-blind controlled study. *Pharmacopsychiatry*. 2002;**35**(5):165–174.

54. Hohagen F, Montero RF, Weiss E. Treatment of primary insomnia with trimipramine: an alternative to benzodiazepine hypnotics? *Eur Arch Psychiatry Clin Neurosci*. 1994;**244**(2):65–72.

55. Rodenbeck A, Cohrs S, Jordan W, Huether G, Ruther E, Hajak G. The sleep-improving effects of doxepin are paralleled by a normalized plasma cortisol secretion in

primary insomnia. *Psychopharmacology (Berl)*. 2003;**170**:423–428.

56. Hajak G, Rodenbeck A, Adler L, et al. Nocturnal melatonin secretion and sleep after doxepin administration in chronic primary insomnia. *Pharmacopsychiatry*. 1996;**29**(5):187–192.

57. Hajak G, Rodenbeck A, Voderholzer U, et al. Doxepin in the treatment of primary insomnia: a placebo-controlled, double-blind, polysomnographic study. *J Clin Psychol*. 2001;**62**(6):453–463.

58. Roth T, Rogowski R, Hull S, et al. Efficacy and safety of doxepin 1 mg, 3 mg, and 6 mg in adults with primary insomnia. *Sleep*. 2007;**30**(11):1555–1561.

59. Scharf M, Rogowski R, Hull S, et al. Efficacy and safety of doxepin 1 mg, 3 mg, and 6 mg in elderly patients with primary insomnia: a randomized, double-blind, placebo-controlled crossover study. *J Clin Psychol*.; in press.

60. Virtanen R, Scheinin M, Iisalo E. Single dose pharmacokinetics of doxepin in healthy volunteers. *Acta Pharmacol Toxicol (Copenh)*. 1980;**47**(5):371–376.

61. Ziegler V, Biggs JT, Ardekani AB, Rosen SH. Contribution to the pharmacokinetics of amitriptyline. *J Clin Pharmacol*. 1978;**18**(10):462–467.

62. Rudorfer M, Potter W Z. Metabolism of tricyclic antidepressants. *Cell Mol Neurobiol*. 1999;**19**(3):373–409.

63. Richelson E, Nelson A. Antagonism by antidepressants of neurotransmitter receptors of normal human brain in vitro. *J Pharmacol Exp Ther*. 1984;**230**(1):94–102.

64. Murphy D, Siever LJ, Insel TR. Therapeutic responses to tricyclic antidepressants and related drugs in non-affective disorder patient populations. *Prog in Neuropsychopharm Biol Psychiatry*. 1985;**9**(1):3–13.

65. Schweitzer I, Tuckwell V. Risk of adverse events with the use of augmentation therapy for the treatment of resistant depression. *Drug Saf*. 1998;**19**(6):455–464.

66. Caccia S, Ballabio M, Fanelli R, Guiso G, Zanini MG. Determination of plasma and brain concentrations of trazodone and its metabolite, 1-m-chlorophenylpiperazine, by gas-liquid chromatography. *J Chromatogr*. 1981;**5**(210):311–318.

67. Greenblatt DJ, Friedman H, Burstein ES, et al. Trazodone kinetics: Effects of age, gender and obesity. *Clin Pharmacol Ther*. 1987;**42**:193–200.

68. Walsh JK, Erman M, Erwin CW, et al. Subjective hypnotic efficacy of trazodone and zolpidem in DSM-III-R primary insomnia. *Hum Psychopharm*. 1998;**13**:191–198.

69. Le Bon O, Murphy JR, Staner L, et al. Double-blind, placebo-controlled study of the efficacy of trazodone in alcohol post-withdrawal syndrome: polysomnographic and clinical evaluations. *J Clin Psychopharmacol*. 2003;**23**(4):377–383.

70. Nierenberg AA, Adler LA, Peselow E, et al. Trazodone for antidepressant-associated insomnia. *Am J Psychiatry*. 1994;**151**:1069–1072.

71. Warner M, Peabody CA, Whiteford HA, Hollister LE. Trazodone and priapism. *J Clin Psychiatry*. 1987;**48**(6):244–245.

72. De Boer T. The pharmacologic profile of mirtazapine. *J Clin Psychol*. 1996;**57**(Suppl 4):19–25.

73. Fawcett J, Barkin RL. Review of the results from clinical studies on the efficacy, safety and tolerability of mirtazapine for the treatment of patients with major depression. *J Affect Disord*. 1998;**51**(3):267–285.

74. Winokur A, Sateia MJ, Hayes JB, et al. Acute effects of mirtazapine on sleep continuity and sleep architecture in depressed patients: a pilot study. *Biol Psychiatry*. 2000;**48**(1):75–78.

75. Winokur A DeMartinis NA, McNally DP, Gary EM, Cormier JL, Gary KA. Comparative effects of mirtazapine and fluoxetine on sleep physiology measures in patients with major depression and insomnia. *J Clin Psychol*. 2003;**64**(10):1224–1229.

76. Sørensen MJJ, Viby-Mogensen J, Bettum V, Dunbar GC, Steffensen K. A double-blind group comparative study using the new anti-depressant Org 3770, placebo and diazepam in patients with expected insomnia and anxiety before elective gynaecological surgery. *Acta Psychiatr Scand*. 1985;**71**(4):331–346.

77. Krystal A, Goforth HW, Roth T. Effects of antipsychotic medications on sleep in schizophrenia. *Int Clin Psychopharmacol*. 2008;**23**(3):150–160.

78. Wiegand MH Landry F, Brückner T, Pohl C, Veselý Z, Jahn T. Quetiapine in primary insomnia: a pilot study. *Psychopharmacology (Berl)*. 2008;**196**(2):337–338.

79. Moreno R, Hanna MM, Tavares SM, Wang YP. A double-blind comparison of the effect of the antipsychotics haloperidol and olanzapine on sleep in mania. *Braz J Med Biol Res*. 2007;**40**(3):357–366.

80. Todder D, Caliskan S, Baune BT. Night locomotor activity and quality of sleep in quetiapine-treated patients with depression. *J Clin Psychopharmacol*. 2006;**26**(6):638–642.

81. Kirshner H. Controversies in behavioral neurology: the use of atypical antipsychotic drugs to treat neurobehavioral symptoms in dementia. *Curr Neurol Neurosci Rep*. 2008;**8**(6):471–474.

82. Kudo Y, Kurihara MC. Clinical evaluation of diphenhydramine hydrochloride for the treatment of insomnia in psychiatric patients: a double-blind study. *J Clin Pharmacol*. 1990;**30**(11):1041–1048.

83. Rickels K, Morris RJ, Newman H, et al. Diphenhydramine in insomniac family practice

patients: a double-blind study. *J Clin Pharmacol.* 1983;**23**(5–6):234–242.

84. Morin C, Koetter U, Bastien C, Ware JC, Wooten V. Valerian-hops combination and diphenhydramine for treating insomnia: a randomized placebo-controlled clinical trial. *Sleep.* 2005;**28**(11):1465–1471.

85. Meuleman J, Nelson RC, Clark RL. Evaluation of temazepam and diphenhydramine as hypnotics in a nursing-home population. *Drug Intell Clin Pharm.* 1987;**21**(9):716–720.

86. Glass JR SB, Herrmann N, Busto UE. Effects of 2-week treatment with temazepam and diphenhydramine in elderly insomniacs: a randomized, placebo-controlled trial. *J Clin Psychopharmacol.* 2008;**28**(2):182–188.

87. Richardson G, Roehrs TA, Rosenthal L, Koshorek G, Roth T. Tolerance to daytime sedative effects of H1 antihistamines. *J Clin Psychopharmacol.* 2002;**22**(5):511–515.

88. Smith G, Smith, PH. Effects of doxylamine and acetaminophen on postoperative sleep. *Clin Pharmacol Ther.* 1985;**5**:549–557.

89. Koppel C, Tenczer J, Ibe K. Poisoning with over-the-counter doxylamine preparations: an evaluation of 109 cases. *Hum Toxicol.* 1987;**6**(5):355–359.

90. Rose M, Kam C A. Gabapentin: pharmacology and its use in pain management. *Anaesthesia.* 2002;**57**:451–462.

91. Gajraj N. Pregabalin: its pharmacology and use in pain management. *Anesth Analg.* 2007;**105**(6):1805–1815.

92. Gilron I. Gabapentin and pregabalin for chronic neuropathic and early postsurgical pain: current evidence and future directions. *Curr Opin Anaesthesiol.* 2007;**20**(5):456–472.

93. Hindmarch I, Dawson J, Stanley N. A double-blind study in healthy volunteers to assess the effects on sleep of pregabalin compared with alprazolam and placebo. *Sleep.* 2005;**28**(2):187–193.

94. de Has S, Otte A, de Weerd A, et al. Exploratory polysomnographic evaluation of pregabalin on sleep disturbance in patients with epilepsy. *J Clin Sleep Med.* 2007;**3**(5):473–478.

95. Garcia-Borreguero D, Larrosa O, de la Llave Y, et al. Treatment of restless legs syndrome with gabapentin: a double-blind, cross-over study. *Neurology.* 2002;**59**(10):1573–1579.

96. Brower K, Myra Kim, H, Strobbe S, et al. A randomized double-blind pilot trial of gabapentin versus placebo to treat alcohol dependence and comorbid insomnia. *Alcohol Clin Exp Res.* 2008;**32**(8):1429–1438.

97. Walsh J, Zammit G, Schweitzer PK, Ondrasik J, Roth T. Tiagabine enhances slow wave sleep and sleep maintenance in primary insomnia. *Sleep Med.* 2006;**7**(2):155–161.

98. Roth T, Wright KP Jr, Walsh J. Effect of tiagabine on sleep in elderly subjects with primary insomnia: a randomized, double-blind, placebo-controlled study. *Sleep.* 2006;**29**(3):335–341.

99. Walsh J, Perlis M, Rosenthal M, et al. Tiagabine increases slow-wave sleep in a dose-dependent fashion without affecting traditional efficacy measures in adults with primary insomnia. *J Clin Sleep Med.* 2006;**2**(1):35–41.

100. Walsh J, Randazzo AC, Frankowski S, et al. Dose-response effects of tiagabine on the sleep of older adults. *Sleep.* 2005;**28**(6):673–676.

101. Guay D. Pregabalin in neuropathic pain: a more "pharmaceutically elegant" gabapentin? *Am J Geriatr Pharmacother.* 2005;**3**(4):274–287.

102. NIH. Consensus conference – Drugs and insomnia: The use of medications to promote sleep. *JAMA.* 1984;**11**(251):2410–2414.

103. Krystal A, Thakur M, Roth T. Sleep disturbance in psychiatric disorders: effects on function and quality of life in mood disorders, alcoholism, and schizophrenia. *Ann Clin Psychol.* 2008;**20**(1):39–46.

104. Nolen W, Haffmans PM, Bouvy PF, Duivenvoorden H J. Hypnotics as concurrent medication in depression: A placebo-controlled, double-blind comparison of flunitrazepam and lormetazepam in patients with major depression, treated with a (tri) cyclic antidepressant. *J Affect Disord.* 1993;**28**(3):179–188.

105. Smith W, Londborg PD, Glaudin V, et al. Short-term augmentation of fluoxetine with clonazepam in the treatment of depression: a double-blind study. *Am J Psychiatry.* 1998;**155**(10):1339–1345.

106. Smith WT, Londborg PD, Glaudin V, Painter JR. Is extended clonazepam cotherapy of fluoxetine effective for outpatients with major depression? *J Affect Disord.* 2002;**70**(3):251–259.

107. Asnis GM, Chakraburtty A, DuBoff EA, et al. Zolpidem for persistent insomnia in SSRI-treated depressed patients. *J Clin Psychiatry.* 1999;**60**:668–676.

108. Schnitzer T, Rubens R, Wessel T, et al. The effect of eszopiclone 3 mg compared with placebo in patients with rheumatoid arthritis and co-existing insomnia. *Prim Care Comp J Clin Psychiatry* 2009;**11**(6):292–301.

Cognitive behavioral therapy for insomnia

Philip R. Gehrman, Dieter Riemann, Donn Posner, and Michael Perlis

Introduction

The present chapter is divided into three sections. The first section addresses the question "why treat insomnia?" The second section provides a review of the various definitions of insomnia, with special reference to not only type but the issue of severity as defined in terms of symptom frequency, intensity, and chronicity. This section also contains a review of the behavioral model of insomnia. The third section contains a brief review of "how" cognitive behavioral therapy for insomnia (CBT-I) is conducted.

Why treat insomnia?

Insomnia, when chronic, tends to be unremitting, disabling, costly, pervasive, and pernicious. These factors, in combination with the existence of effective treatments, provide more than sufficient justification for the perspective that *insomnia should be a primary focus for treatment, even when it occurs in the context of psychiatric and/or medical disorders.*

Insomnia is unremitting

To our knowledge, there are only a handful of investigations on the natural history of insomnia [1–4]. In general, these studies find that chronic insomnia usually does not spontaneously resolve [2,4] and the presenting form of insomnia (i.e. initial, middle, or late) tends to be unstable or variable over time. Mendelson [2] reported that subjects with difficulty sleeping at their initial assessment continued to report insomnia at two follow-up intervals (70% at 40 months and 88% at 64 months).

Insomnia is disabling

To date there are a number of investigations that suggest that individuals with chronic insomnia, compared to those with no or occasional insomnia, have more difficulty with intellectual, social, and/or vocational functioning.

In terms of intellectual functioning, there are a number of studies (cf. [5–7]) documenting that patients with chronic insomnia report impaired cognitive performance. In fact, this type of complaint constitutes one of the defining attributes of insomnia as it is delineated in the International Classification of Sleep Disorders, 2nd edition (ICSD-2). This said, neuropsychological evaluations of patients with chronic insomnia have often failed to find evidence of specific cognitive deficits [8]. This discrepancy between perceived and measured impairment may be reflective of several things. First, individuals with insomnia may have an attentional bias towards perceiving negative performance in the absence of actual deficits [9,10]. Second, there may be a preoccupation with poor performance irrespective of whether or not it occurs. Third, and finally, the perception of performance deficits may not be related to actual poor performance, or altered self-monitoring, but rather to the patient's real appreciation of the fact that extra effort is required to maintain normal or near normal performance [8].

Patients with chronic insomnia reliably report difficulties with social functioning, including decreased interest in, facility with, and satisfaction from interpersonal relationships and social interactions. For example, in patients being seen in a primary care practice, chronic insomnia was associated with decreased ability to handle minor irritations, decreased ability to enjoy family/social life, and poorer interpersonal relationships with spouses [7].

With respect to vocational performance, several studies have found that sleep disturbance and/or

Foundations of Psychiatric Sleep Medicine, ed. John W. Winkelman and David T. Plante. Published by Cambridge University Press.
© Cambridge University Press 2010.

chronic insomnia is associated with less job satisfaction, lower performance scores, less productivity, and higher rates of absenteeism [11,12]. A more recent study by Leger and colleagues found higher rates of absenteeism compared to good sleepers (31% vs. 19%), more errors at work in the previous month (15% vs. 6%), and more frequent self-reported poor work efficiency in the past month (18% vs. 8%) [13].

Insomnia is costly

In the USA alone, the direct and indirect costs attributable to insomnia exceed $100 billion annually [14]. Direct costs, including physician visits, prescriptions, and procedures, equal or exceed $13 billion per annum [15]. These costs are, in part, related to the increased tendency of patients with insomnia to use healthcare resources [13]. The estimated cost of physician visits is over $600 million per year and the cost of prescription medications is estimated at over $800 million per year [15]. Indirect costs associated with motor vehicle and workplace accidents, reduced productivity, and absenteeism are thought to account for the majority of the economic consequences of insomnia with cost estimates between 77 and 92 billion dollars per annum. Viewed at the individual as opposed to the societal level, work by Ozminkowski suggests that the per person cost per annum direct healthcare costs are $1253 in younger adults and $1143 in older adults [16].

Insomnia is pervasive

As stated in the National Institutes of Health (NIH) State of the Science Statement on Manifestations and Management of Chronic Insomnia in Adults "…chronic insomnia is known to be common… Population-based studies suggest that about 30 percent of the general population complains of sleep disruption, while approximately 10 percent have associated symptoms of daytime functional impairment consistent with the diagnosis of insomnia" [17]. Thus, chronic insomnia affects a substantial proportion of the population.

Insomnia is pernicious

While it may seem an overstatement to say "insomnia is pernicious" there are a variety of studies suggesting that chronic insomnia is a significant risk factor for both new-onset and recurrent medical and psychiatric illness.

With respect to medical disease, preliminary data suggest that insomnia confers risk. Only a few epidemiological studies have been conducted and even fewer studies have assessed the association prospectively. This said, the data that exist suggest that patients with insomnia are more likely to suffer from pain conditions and gastrointestinal distress [12] and that untreated insomnia puts sufferers at risk for hypertension [18,19] and heart disease [18,20]. It has also been suggested that insomnia may be a risk factor for the development of diabetes in that patients with type 2 diabetes have shown that poor sleep quality is associated with poor glycemic regulation [21]. Whether these associations are causal remains to be determined as does what factors specifically related to insomnia confer and moderate/mediate risk.

With respect to psychiatric disease, there is a preponderance of data to suggest that insomnia confers increased risk for new-onset and recurrent illness, and that this is particularly true for depression/major depressive disorder (MDD) [22]. There are now at least 14 longitudinal studies showing that subjects with chronic insomnia are between 2 and 6 times more likely to have a new-onset or recurrent episodes of depression (within 6 months to 3 years) as compared to subjects without chronic insomnia [23–36]. In addition to the risk for new-onset and recurrent illness, there are two studies which suggest that insomnia is associated with the clinical course of MDD such that insomnia acts as a prodromal symptom and risk factor for relapse [37,38].

Taken together, these data suggest that insomnia may serve as a predisposing, precipitating, and/or perpetuating factor for depression. This said, as with medical disorders, it remains to be (1) shown that these associations are causal and (2) determined as to what factors related to insomnia confer and mediate risk. For additional information on the association between insomnia and depression, the reader is referred to the chapter dedicated to this topic (Chapter 15: Depressive disorders).

Insomnia treatment is safe and effective

There are a number of meta-analyses that summarize the literatures for both benzodiazepines (BZs) and benzodiazepine receptor agonists (BzRAs, i.e. zolpidem, eszopiclone, and zaleplon) and for cognitive behavioral therapy for insomnia (CBT-I) (e.g. [39–42]). There is also one comparative meta-analysis which evaluates the relative efficacy of benzodiazepines and BzRAs as compared to CBT-I [43]. The data from this last meta-analysis suggests, consistent with the conclusions of the NIH State of the Science Conference [17], that: (1) BzRAs and CBT-I are effective to treat insomnia in the short term, and CBT-I has more durable effects when active treatment is discontinued; and (2) there is limited evidence that BzRAs retain their efficacy during long-term treatment. As for safety, most agree that the first-line treatment modalities have very benign safety profiles. To date, only a few studies have been conducted on the relative safety of BZs and BzRAs and no studies have been conducted comparing the efficacy and safety of medications with an indication for insomnia to either CBT-I or medications that are used off-label. Figure 14.1 (below) presents the data from the comparative meta-analysis conducted by Smith and colleagues. In this figure, CBT-I appears to be superior to pharmacotherapy for its effects on sleep latency, with the remaining effects being approximately comparable. The authors suggest that sleep latency effect is an artifact of how the trials were conducted (prescribing the medications at time of bed as opposed to 30–60 minutes in advance of bed time) and conservatively conclude that the acute effects of CBT-I and pharmacotherapy are likely to be equivalent.

EFFECT SIZE DIFFERENCES WITH ACUTE TX

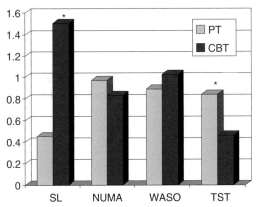

Figure 14.1 Effect sizes of pharmacotherapy (PT) and cognitive behavioral therapy for insomnia (CBT) in the acute treatment of insomnia on sleep latency (SL), number of awakenings (NUMA), wake after sleep onset (WASO), and total sleep time (TST). Based on data presented in Smith MT, Perlis ML, Park A, et al. Comparative meta-analysis of pharmacotherapy and behavior therapy for persistent insomnia. *Am J Psychiatry.* 2002; 159(1):5–11.

Are these reasons enough to justify treatment?

The central proposition for this introduction is: *Because chronic insomnia tends to be unremitting, disabling, costly, pervasive, and pernicious, and because there are effective treatments, this is more than sufficient justification for the perspective that insomnia should be a primary focus for treatment.* While reasonable, this proposition doesn't address the issue that would eliminate any and all doubt about the appropriateness of aggressive treatment for insomnia; the possibility that insomnia is a modifiable risk factor for medical and psychiatric illness. To date, all that can be definitively said is that insomnia treatment diminishes the severity of insomnia and/or the psychological distress that accompanies this disorder. While a laudable end, there is very little information available regarding the effects of treatment on daytime functioning. This is the case because treatment outcome has almost exclusively focused on the sleep continuity variables [44,45] and there is not yet a consensus regarding the criteria to determine what constitutes successful outcomes [46]. What is needed are clear demonstrations that insomnia treatment not only reduces the incidence and severity of insomnia, but that such outcomes serve to improve daytime function/quality of life and/or reduce the incidence and severity of other forms of medical and psychiatric symptomatology and/or morbidity. To date there are only a handful of such studies.

Within the daytime function arena there are three studies which show that treatment positively impacts this domain. Leger and colleagues have shown that medical treatment for insomnia results in significant improvements with respect to quality of life [47]. Krystal and colleagues have shown that pharmacological treatment results in improved self-reported health, mood, concentration/alertness, daytime functioning, and quality of life [45]. Walsh and colleagues show similar gains with pharmacotherapy on quality of life measures and extend these findings to include positive outcomes with respect to work limitations [48].

Within the medical and psychiatric domain there are two studies with medical outcomes and three investigations with psychiatric outcomes. With respect to medical outcomes, Edinger and colleagues found that CBT-I leads to improvements in medical and psychological functioning in patients with fibromyalgia [49]. Preliminary data from Pigeon et al. [50] show that CBT-I in chronic pain patients with co-morbid insomnia leads to significant reductions in insomnia, depression, and perceived pain (as measured by the pain disability index and the multidimensional pain inventory) as compared to patients who received non-directive-supportive therapy or were randomized to a wait list condition.

With respect to psychiatric outcomes, Fava and colleagues [51] have shown that concomitant treatment for insomnia in the context of acute depression (fluoxetine $+/-$ eszopiclone) yields: (1) effects on insomnia that are comparable with those seen in primary insomnia; and (2) effects on the clinical course of the co-morbid disorder. That is, a larger proportion of patients treated with dual therapy experienced treatment response and/or remission and did so at an accelerated rate. Similar preliminary data with CBT-I were recently reported by Manber et al [52]. Finally, there is a study by Taylor and colleagues [53] suggesting that CBT-I, when administered as a monotherapy, is associated with a significant decrease in depression severity in acutely ill patients with mild depression. Taken together these data provide the first examples that insomnia treatment may improve quality of life and have larger effects on medical and mental health.

Why treat insomnia? At present the answer is simply: because insomnia can be effectively treated and treatment can be expected to reduce insomnia-related distress and suffering in the tens of millions of patients who live with this disorder. In the future, the answer to this query is likely to be more compelling. If it can be shown that insomnia is a modifiable risk factor for medical and/or psychiatric illness and/or that targeted treatment for co-morbid insomnia reliably reduces illness severity, promotes remission, and/or reduces relapse then the answer to the question will be: *because treatment for insomnia promotes better medical and/or psychiatric health*. In fact the question "why treat insomnia?" will, at that time, be moot and the new question to answer will be "when isn't insomnia treatment indicated?"

What is insomnia?

The DSM-IV differentiates between primary insomnia, in which the sleep disorder occurs as an isolated condition, and secondary insomnia, in which it occurs in the context of another disorder. It is noteworthy that primary insomnia accounts for only 10–20% of cases [54,55]. Most insomnias, therefore, are related to medical conditions (e.g. chronic pain, cancer), psychiatric conditions (e.g. depression, post-traumatic stress disorder), substance abuse, and medication side-effects. As behavioral and cognitive models of insomnia predict, the precipitating agents or factors leading to insomnia (be they a life stressor like a divorce or a condition like depression), do not generally change the developmental course of insomnia [56].

It is important to distinguish primary insomnia from secondary insomnia in the clinical evaluation of the patient. First, clinical experience suggests that while medical and psychiatric disorders may precipitate insomnia, the sleep initiation and maintenance problems may often persist long after the parent conditions are stable or resolved. This is often the case in psychiatric illness where insomnia persists despite improvement in the "primary" disorder. The common strategy of treating what might be considered primary (e.g. depression) and forgoing insomnia interventions rests in the belief that the latter is only a symptom. While this is certainly true for some individuals, such a strategy may not serve a sizable number of patients. In this reality, it may be more accurate to consider the insomnia to be "co-morbid" rather than secondary.

A careful clinical history may indeed determine that the inability to fall asleep, stay asleep, or the tendency to awaken early in the morning may be related to a variety of factors including primary medical or psychiatric conditions, drug use or abuse, or other extrinsic or intrinsic sleep disorders. Typical medical exclusions for beginning with insomnia treatment include untreated or unstable gastrointestinal disorders (e.g. gastroesophageal reflux disease), cardiopulmonary disorders (e.g. heart disease), and neuroendocrine disorders (e.g. estrogen deficiency). Typical psychiatric exclusions include untreated or unstable affective and/or anxiety disorders. Typical drug use or abuse exclusions include the use of medications and/or "recreational" drugs that have insomnia as a direct effect or as a withdrawal effect. Typical sleep disorder exclusions include other intrinsic sleep disorders (e.g. sleep apnea), circadian rhythm disorders (e.g. shift work sleep disorder), and extrinsic sleep disorders (e.g. inadequate sleep hygiene).

This said, it is important to understand that if the insomnia has become co-morbid then treatment of the primary disorder alone may in fact not yield the desired improvements in sleep even as the primary disorder ameliorates. In this condition rather than increasing the treatment for the primary disorder to improve the residual "symptom of insomnia," what may be required is that the insomnia be treated in conjunction with the treatment of a "primary" disorder or even as a front-line intervention. This has been demonstrated in several populations including in patients with depression, post-traumatic stress disorder, and chronic pain. How insomnia evolves into a co-morbid disorder worthy of treatment in its own right will now be described.

The behavioral model of insomnia

The behavioral model, as originally set forth by Spielman and colleagues [57], posits that insomnia occurs acutely in relation to both trait and precipitating factors. Thus, an individual may be prone to insomnia due to trait characteristics, but experiences acute episodes because of precipitating factors. The acute insomnia becomes subchronic when it is reinforced by maladaptive coping strategies. These strategies, in turn, result in conditioned arousal and chronic insomnia. A graphic representation of this model is presented in Figure 14.2.

When an insomnia episode is initiated there are a variety of maladaptive strategies that individuals adopt in the attempt to get more sleep. Research and treatment have focused on two in particular: excessive time in bed and the practice of staying in bed while awake. Excessive time in bed refers to the tendency of

patients with insomnia to go to bed earlier, get out of bed later, and/or nap. Such changes are enacted in order to increase the opportunity to get more sleep. These behaviors, however, lead to decreased sleep efficiency. That is, when the opportunity to sleep exceeds basal ability to generate sleep, the consequence is more frequent and longer awakenings. The practice of staying in bed while awake, as with the prior strategy, is enacted to increase the opportunity to get more sleep. In addition, the practice is often adopted under the rationale that staying in bed is at least "restful." While a seemingly reasonable behavior, staying in bed while awake leads to an association of the bed and bedroom with arousal, not sleepiness and sleep. In addition, as the insomnia fails to remit, while staying in bed the individual is likely to become more frustrated and anxious about the lack of sleep and its possible consequences. Over time when confronted with stimuli that are typically associated with sleep (bed and bedroom), they elicit considerable arousal responses via classical conditioning. The two maladaptive behaviors are likely to occur concurrently and promote one another. Excessive time in bed increases the likelihood that the individual will be awake while in bed. Being awake while in bed increases the likelihood that the individual will attempt to get more sleep by increasing sleep opportunity. The end result is conditioned arousal during the traditional sleep period and chronic insomnia.

The Spielman model of insomnia offers the theoretical foundation for CBT-I. There are, however, other models that contribute to our understanding of the etiology of insomnia [58] by drawing our

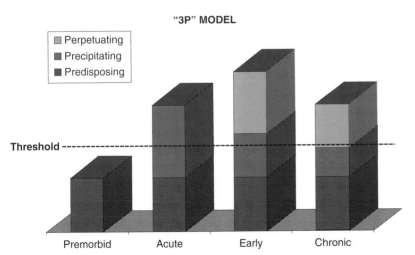

"3P" MODEL

- Perpetuating
- Precipitating
- Predisposing

Threshold

Premorbid   Acute   Early   Chronic

Figure 14.2 The "3P" model is one of several names for the Spielman model. The 3P refers to three etiological factors posited by the model. The y-axis represents insomnia intensity where below threshold is presumed to be normal sleep and above threshold significant sleep continuity disturbance. The figure is based on the original graphic presented in Spielman AJ, Caruso LS, Glovinsky PB. A behavioral perspective on insomnia treatment. *Psychiatr Clin North Am.* 1987;10(4):541–553.

attention to how patients may engage in maladaptive safety behaviors, harbor dysfunctional beliefs about sleep, engage in excessive rumination and catastrophizing, as well as being cortically primed for presleep arousal and overt attention to stimuli that good sleepers easily ignore [9,10,59,60]. All of these are antithetical to initiating and maintaining sleep and can be the focus of treatment.

Cognitive behavioral treatment of insomnia (CBT-I)

In general there are three main types of therapy that can be employed, from a behavioral standpoint, to deal with chronic insomnia (in order of priority): stimulus control, sleep restriction, and sleep hygiene therapies. These therapies comprise the standard behavioral therapy of insomnia. The session to session clinical regimen is described below. A description of other therapies follows in the next section.

Stimulus control therapy

Stimulus control therapy is considered to be the first-line behavioral treatment for chronic primary insomnia and therefore should be prioritized accordingly [61]. Stimulus control instructions limit the amount of time patients spend awake in bed or the bedroom and are designed to decondition presleep arousal. Typical instructions include: (1) keep a fixed wake-time 7 days per week, irrespective of how much sleep you get during the night; (2) avoid any behavior in the bed or bedroom other than sleep or sexual activity; (3) sleep only in the bedroom; (4) leave the bedroom if not asleep after approximately 15 to 20 minutes; (5) return only when sleepy; and (6) if still unable to fall asleep repeat steps 4 and 5 as often as is necessary. The combination of these instructions re-establishes the bed and bedroom as strong cues for sleep and entrains the circadian sleep–wake cycle to the desired phase. It is important to note that such reconditioning will only take place over several days and, as such, overall sleep continuity is likely to be unchanged or worse in the early phase of the treatment.

Sleep restriction

Sleep restriction therapy requires patients to limit the amount of time they spend in bed to an amount equal to their average total sleep time. In order to accomplish this, the clinician works with the patient to

(1) establish a fixed wake-time and (2) decrease sleep opportunity by prescribing a later bedtime. Initially, the therapy results in a reduction in total sleep time, but over the course of several days, results in decreased sleep latency, and decreased wake-time after sleep onset. As sleep efficiency increases, patients are instructed to gradually increase the amount of time they spend in bed. In practice, patients "roll back" their bedtime in 15-minute increments, given sleep diary data which shows that on the prior week the patient's sleep was efficient (85% or more of the time spent in bed was spent asleep). This therapy is thought to be effective for two reasons. First, it reverses the patients' strategy of coping with their insomnia by extending sleep opportunity. The strategy of extending time in bed, while increasing the opportunity to get more sleep, produces a form of sleep that is shallow and fragmented. Second, the initial sleep loss that occurs with sleep restriction therapy is thought to increase the "pressure for sleep" which in turn produces quicker sleep latencies, less wake after sleep onset, and more efficient sleep. It should be noted that the treatment has a paradoxical aspect to it. Patients who report being unable to sleep are in essence being told: "sleep less." Such a prescription needs to be delivered with care and compliance must be monitored. Sleep restriction is contraindicated in patients with histories of mania or seizure disorder, because it may aggravate these conditions. Patients also need to be made aware of the increased sleepiness that results from sleep restriction and the need to take extra precautions when driving or engaging in other behaviors which may be unsafe due to sleepiness.

Sleep hygiene

This requires that the clinician and patient review a set of instructions which are geared toward helping the patient maintain good sleep habits (see Table 14.1). It should be noted that sleep hygiene instructions are not helpful when provided as a monotherapy [62] and might be even less helpful when provided as written instructions which are not tailored to the individual or are cast in absolute terms. With respect to the former, providing patients with a "handout" (especially without an explanation of the clinical science behind the issues) undermines patient compliance. With respect to the latter, sleep hygiene instructions have within them several absolute

Table 14.1 Sleep hygiene instructions

1. **Sleep only as much as you need to feel refreshed during the following day**. Restricting your time in bed helps to consolidate and deepen your sleep. Excessively long times in bed lead to fragmented and shallow sleep. Get up at your regular time the next day, no matter how little you slept.

2. **Get up at the same time each day, 7 days a week**. A regular wake-time in the morning leads to regular times of sleep onset, and helps to set your "biological clock."

3. **Exercise regularly**. Schedule exercise times so that they do not occur within 3 hours of when you intend to go to bed. Exercise makes it easier to initiate sleep and deepen sleep.

4. **Make sure your bedroom is comfortable and free from light and noise**. A comfortable, noise-free sleep environment will reduce the likelihood that you will wake up during the night. Noise that does not awaken you may also disturb the quality of your sleep. Carpeting, insulated curtains, and closing the door may help.

5. **Make sure that your bedroom is at a comfortable temperature during the night**. Excessively warm or cold sleep environments may disturb sleep.

6. **Eat regular meals and do not go to bed hungry**. Hunger may disturb sleep. A light snack at bedtime (especially carbohydrates) may help sleep, but avoid greasy or "heavy" foods.

7. **Avoid excessive liquids in the evening**. Reducing liquid intake will minimize the need for night-time trips to the bathroom.

8. **Cut down on all caffeine products**. Caffeinated beverages and foods (coffee, tea, cola, chocolate) can cause difficulty falling asleep, awakenings during the night, and shallow sleep. Even caffeine early in the day can disrupt night-time sleep.

9. **Avoid alcohol, especially in the evening**. Although alcohol helps tense people fall asleep more easily, it causes awakenings later in the night.

10. **Smoking may disturb sleep**. Nicotine is a stimulant. Try not to smoke during the night when you have trouble sleeping.

11. **Don't take your problems to bed**. Plan some time earlier in the evening for working on your problems or planning the next day's activities. Worrying may interfere with initiating sleep and produce shallow sleep.

12. **Train yourself to use the bedroom only for sleeping and sexual activity**. This will help condition your brain to see bed as the place for sleeping. Do *not* read, watch TV, or eat in bed.

13. **Do not *try* to fall asleep**. This only makes the problem worse. Instead, turn on the light, leave the bedroom, and do something different like reading a book. Don't engage in stimulating activity. Return to bed only when you are sleepy.

14. **Put the clock under the bed or turn it so that you can't see it**. Clock watching may lead to frustration, anger, and worry, which interfere with sleep.

15. **Avoid naps**. Staying awake during the day helps you to fall asleep at night.

Author's note: The above list includes the usual practices described as "good sleep hygiene," but it also includes some principles subsumed under "stimulus control therapy" (#2,12,13), "sleep restriction therapy" (#1,2,15), and "relaxation" (#11,13).

dictums, e.g. "Avoid caffeinated products" and "Do Not Nap." Both of these instructions are too simple. For example, caffeine may be used to combat some of the daytime sequelae of insomnia and withdrawal from the substance, if timed appropriately, may actually enhance subjects' ability to fall asleep more quickly. Napping may be useful to sustain high levels of daytime function and performance. Such a compensatory strategy, however, should only be allowed provided that time to bed is delayed.

Step-by-step procedures
Session 1

Clinical evaluation and 2-week baseline. During this session, the patient's sleep complaints are reviewed with the clinician responsible for treatment and, if deemed to be appropriate for CBT-I, the patient is instructed to keep a sleep diary for a baseline period of 2 weeks. All subjects are carefully instructed on how to complete this measure. Diaries can be commenced simultaneously with treatment for other existing conditions; however, some time must be taken to decide whether or not the patient will continue on sleep medication during this baseline data gathering. Consideration should be given to the fact that if the patient remains on any sleeping medication the baseline data will misrepresent what their true sleep pattern might look like without the medication. In addition, the patient should be alerted to the possibility that at the end of treatment if they are sleeping well and wish to discontinue their medication at that time that this could result in some relapse of the problem. If the patient chooses to come off medication before treatment this should be done in such a way that the 2-week baseline sleep diary is started when the patient is already off or nearly off the medication. This is done so that the diary data will reflect the patient's pattern of sleep without medication and not a pattern of withdrawal from medication. Any reduction in medication must be done in collaboration with a qualified physician. Note that Session 2 is scheduled 2 weeks after Session 1 (or more depending on medication taper); all other sessions are scheduled at 1-week intervals.

Session 2

Sleep restriction and stimulus control therapy. Baseline sleep diary data are reviewed. This information sets the parameters for sleep restriction therapy and guides the patient toward the treatment to be prescribed. The standard approach is interactive/didactic. The patient and the clinician evaluate the data together. After reviewing the data and identifying basic assumptions, most patients easily deduce what might represent a good "counter strategy." The primary assumption most patients identify is what we call "the positive correlation fallacy": the more time in bed, the more sleep one will get. When the patient has identified one or more components of therapy, the clinician explains in detail the rationale and procedures for sleep restriction and stimulus control therapy (see above).

Session 3

Sleep hygiene and sleep restriction therapy adjustments. As with all sessions, sleep diary data are reviewed and charted. If sufficient progress has been made (diaries reflect higher than 85% sleep efficiency) then an upward titration process can be started. If progress has not yet reached the desired goals, this

may be an opportunity to assess for non-adherence, and much of the rest of the session may be spent problem solving and reviewing rationales. With the remaining time, sleep hygiene instructions can be reviewed by having the patient read aloud the various imperatives and the corresponding rationales. After the patient and the clinician have identified the relevance of a particular issue, the clinician reviews in more detail the basic concepts and related clinical research. The amount of, and manner in which, information is presented varies according to specific patient need.

Session 4

Sleep hygiene and sleep restriction therapy adjustments. Sleep diary data are reviewed and charted. Upward titration can either continue after being started in the last session or will be initiated here, provided that the patient has been compliant and the proper gains have been made. Any information from sleep hygiene that was not already covered can now be reviewed.

Sessions 5–7

Sleep restriction therapy adjustments. Sleep diary data are reviewed and charted. Upward titration can proceed. During these sessions work can be done to reinforce what the patient has learned and problem solve any issues that arise. Patients should be cautioned that expansion of sleep opportunity does not usually proceed in a consistent manner. There may be times when the requisite cut-offs will not be reached and upward titration may not be possible. Given that the patient is compliant it may just be that there are other transient factors that influenced sleep efficiency (e.g. having a cold, an argument with ones spouse, etc.). Setting the expectation that expansion will probably not be perfect can help to prevent panic when sleep efficiency is not exactly where one expects it to be. In these cases the patient should be encouraged to exercise patience and follow the titration formula. Often, after a short time, upward titration can proceed.

Session 8

Relapse prevention. This last session is largely psychoeducational. The clinician reviews (1) "how insomnia gets started" and the strategies that maintain poor sleep and (2) the strategies that are likely to abort an extended episode of insomnia. These strategies should include maintaining good sleep hygiene, always engaging in proper stimulus control, and using sleep restriction as necessary when problems arise.

Adjunctive therapies

In addition to these principal behavioral techniques, there are also several adjunctive therapies which may prove helpful to the patient and can be included in the treatment plan. These include cognitive therapy, relaxation training, and phototherapy. It may also be useful to combine pharmacotherapy with CBT-I.

Cognitive therapy

Interestingly, while therapy for insomnia is ubiquitously referred to as cognitive behavioral therapy for insomnia (CBT-I) the "C" is often not a core component [41,42]. This said, it is by far the most common adjuvant treatment. Several forms of cognitive therapy for insomnia have been developed and often overlap. The forms of cognitive therapy utilize techniques including psychoeducation [63], paradoxical intention [64], cognitive restructuring [63], and treatments that focus on safety behaviors [65] and attention bias [10]. While the approaches differ in procedure, all are based on the observation that patients with insomnia have negative thoughts and beliefs about their condition and its consequences. Helping patients to challenge the veracity and usefulness of these beliefs is thought to decrease the anxiety and arousal associated with insomnia.

Relaxation training

Different relaxation techniques target different physiological systems. Progressive muscle relaxation is used to diminish skeletal muscle tension. Diaphragmatic breathing is used to make breathing slower and shallower and resembles the form of breathing, interestingly, that naturally occurs at sleep onset. Autogenic training focuses on increasing peripheral blood flow. Biofeedback may similarly target specific systems with a common goal of achieving a "relaxed state." To the list of relaxation techniques can be added hypnosis and mindfulness-based stress reduction. While the latter involves more than learning a relaxation technique, this is nonetheless its core practice. Most practitioners select the optimal relaxation method based upon which technique is easiest for the patient to learn, which is most consistent with how the patient manifests arousal, and which technique is

not contraindicated by medical conditions (e.g. progressive muscle relaxation might not be an ideal choice for patients with certain neuromuscular disorders).

Phototherapy

The sleep-promoting effects of bright light may occur via several mechanisms including shifting the circadian system; enhancement of the amplitude of the circadian pacemaker, promoting wakefulness during the day and sleep at night; or indirectly via its antidepressant effects. In practice, bright light is used to shorten or lengthen the diurnal phase of the patient's day. In the case where the patient's insomnia has a phase delay component (i.e. the patient prefers to go to bed late and wake up late) waking early by alarm and being exposed to bright light in the morning for a period of time may enable them to "feel sleepy" at an earlier time in the evening. In the case where the patient's insomnia has a phase advance component (i.e. the patient prefers to go to bed early and wake up early) bright light exposure in the evening may enable them to stay awake later and wake up later. It is generally assumed that phototherapy has no significant side-effects, but this is not always the case. Mania may be triggered by bright light in patients with bipolar mood disorder. Other side-effects include insomnia, hypomania, agitation, visual blurring, eye strain, and headaches. Individuals with eye-related problems or who are at risk for such conditions such as diabetes should consult an eye care specialist prior to initiating light therapy.

Combining CBT-I with pharmacotherapy

One of the disadvantages of CBT-I, compared to pharmacotherapy, is that the impact on sleep is gradual. Patients often may not experience any improvement until after 2–4 weeks of treatment. Although this length of time is short relative to the typical duration of insomnia experienced by most patients prior to treatment, it can be a barrier to treatment adherence. Faced with the daytime effects of sleep restriction therapy, some patients abandon treatment before experiencing benefits. An alternate strategy is to combine CBT-I with hypnotic medication in order to capitalize on the rapid effects of pharmacotherapy while waiting for CBT-I to "kick in." Medications are then gradually tapered in the second half of treatment.

In perhaps the most experimentally rigorous test of this approach, Morin and colleagues randomly assigned older adults to receive CBT-I alone, temazepam alone, combined CBT-I and temazepam, or placebo [66]. At the post-treatment time point all three treatment groups had improved sleep relative to placebo, with a trend towards superior outcomes in the combined group. By the last assessment at 24 months post-treatment, the temazepam only group had returned to baseline severity, whereas both CBT-I groups maintained the treatment gains. Interestingly, the CBT-I only group had better outcomes than the combined group. Other studies with different medications have yielded similar outcomes, although some found better outcomes in the combined treatment group. It has been hypothesized that individuals who receive combined treatment may ascribe their treatment gains to the results of the medication and failed to develop self-efficacy, or confidence in their ability to sleep without medication. Once the medication was withdrawn, they no longer felt capable of sleeping unaided, which likely would lead to feelings of anxiety about sleep and subsequent difficulty sleeping [66]. Despite mixed findings thus far, there is still considerable potential to develop treatment strategies that combine CBT-I and pharmacotherapy in an effective manner.

An alternate approach is to combine CBT-I with wake-promoting medication using a daytime dosing schedule. While seemingly counterintuitive, there is a solid rationale for this strategy which spans three related possibilities. First, since sleep restriction therapy is associated with increased daytime sleepiness that can lead to treatment drop-out, counteracting this side-effect may enhance treatment adherence. Second, insomnia is often associated with anxiety about the negative consequences of poor sleep. This anxiety, in turn, likely exacerbates patients' difficulties by augmenting existing arousal (somatic, cognitive, and/or cortical). Thus, if the daytime consequences of insomnia could be attenuated or eliminated, it stands to reason that this factor (or related factors like attention bias or the engagement of safety behaviors) would cease to be contributive. Third, and lastly, the use of wake-promoting agents such as modafinil may enhance the patient's ability to extend wakefulness. This will enable the patient to reverse the tendency to "extend sleep opportunity," reduce the mismatch between sleep ability and sleep opportunity, and will prime the homeostatic drive for sleep via the prolongation of wakefulness and/or increased activation during wakefulness.

The first effort to evaluate the proposition that wakefulness promotion may be useful for the management of insomnia was conducted by Perlis and colleagues [67]. In this study, the effects of modafinil were assessed alone and in combination with CBT-I. The results from the investigation suggest that modafinil as a monotherapy did not produce significant effects on sleep continuity; the linear trends, however, were in the predicted direction. Dual therapy also did not result in improved efficacy but clearly resulted in an attenuation of sleepiness and enhanced compliance. The conceptual basis for this study (along with the mean trends) lead to the hypothesis that an alteration to the treatment regimen (one which promoted a longer duration of action) might result in independent effects for modafinil and additive effects when combined with CBT-I. Future studies are needed to assess the potential of this novel treatment paradigm.

Techniques for dealing with client non-compliance

CBT techniques for insomnia can be challenging for both the client and the practitioner. This may be particularly true early in the therapeutic process as the client will be asked to accept a difficult regimen of behavioral change and concomitant sleep deprivation. Sleep loss alone may try the patience of a client and this makes compliance with any therapeutic modality a problematic issue. There are, however, some strategies (most based in clinical experience) which may enhance the likelihood of a successful clinical outcome. Examples of these techniques include using:

1. Good salesmanship (a motivational approach to therapy) – There is no more important a method than the demonstration of a good knowledge base regarding (in general) sleep medicine and (in specific) the principles behind the behavioral interventions. Patients will often have challenging questions and concerns regarding the procedures. Simply providing a laundry list of techniques will not likely lead to good adherence, especially as sleep deprivation gets worse in the early stages. Clear and compelling explanations, provision of rationale, and setting of expectancies will go a long way towards gaining patient trust and compliance. Sharing information about the clinical efficacy and effectiveness of treatment can also be a powerful aid in obtaining compliance.

2. A Socratic versus pedantic approach to patient education – It is important to both educate and work collaboratively with the client throughout the treatment process. Whenever possible clients should be led to answers that they discover, rather than being simply told what to do and why to do it. This process will reduce patient resistance, particularly in reactant patients or in patients that are not treatment naive.

3. Realistic goal setting – It is of great importance for the therapist to understand the goals of the client and determine if and how they can be realistically met. Such evaluation of the client should include a discussion of life circumstances as it would be unwise to start a client through treatment at a time where personal situations may make compliance an issue. Part of the psychoeducational process involves some discussion of the notion that even good sleepers do not necessarily sleep for 8 uninterrupted hours per night and that they do not necessarily sleep well every night. It also important to make clients aware from the very first session that CBT will be difficult and that their insomnia symptoms may get worse before they get better.

4. A scientific approach to treatment – Finally, it is quite helpful to keep graphs of client progress throughout treatment. Rewarding a client by showing them their progress graphically from week to week makes the process more tangible and has the effect of proving to the client that the treatment is working and that they are gaining control over their problem and achieving success.

Concluding remarks

Insomnia represents one of the more ubiquitous forms of sleep disturbance in psychiatric and medical disorders, and in its primary form. Unfortunately, despite its prevalence and associated negative sequelae, only a small fraction of patients seek out treatment or have access to behavioral sleep medicine specialists. This is especially unfortunate given the existence of multiple forms of effective therapy. We hope the material presented in this chapter highlights the need to treat insomnia and provides healthcare professionals with information on the techniques employed by behavioral sleep medicine specialists. While this chapter provides a good introduction to the CBT of insomnia, the chapter cannot provide a good substitute for a complete step-by-step protocol and mentored clinical experience. We would like to encourage those interested in developing an expertise in the CBT treatment of insomnia to seek out additional training in behavioral sleep medicine through accredited fellowships and CME programs offered through individual institutions, the American Academy of Sleep Medicine, and at various national meetings like those of the Associated Professional Sleep Societies, the American Psychological Association, the Society for Behavioral Medicine, and the Association for Behavioral and Cognitive Therapies.

Potential conflict of interests (first author only)

Consultancies/speakers panels/PI grants: Sanofi-Aventis; Takeda; Cephalon; Actelion; and Resperonics.

Federal grants: funding/support: this research activity was supported, in part, by R21MH067184 and R21NR009080.

Suggested reading

Hauri P. *Case studies in insomnia*. New York, NY: Plenum Publishers; 1991.

Morin CM, Espie C A. *Insomnia: a clinician's guide to assessment and treatment*. New York, NY: Kluwer Academic/Plenum Publishers; 2000.

Perlis M, Lichstein K, eds. *Treating sleep disorders: the principles and practice of behavioral sleep medicine*. Philadelphia, PA: Wiley & Sons; 2003.

Perlis M, Jungquist C, Smith M, Posner D. *Cognitive behavioral treatment of insomnia: a session by session guide*. New York, NY: Springer-Verlag; 2005.

References

1. Hohagen F, Kappler C, Schramm E, et al. Sleep onset insomnia, sleep maintaining insomnia and insomnia with early morning awakening – temporal stability of subtypes in a longitudinal study on general practice attenders. *Sleep*. 1994;**17**(6):551–554.

2. Mendelson WB. Long-term follow-up of chronic insomnia. *Sleep*. 1995;**18**(8):698–701.

3. Morin CM, Belanger L, LeBlanc M, et al. The natural history of insomnia: A population-based three-year longitudinal study. *Arch Intern Med*. 2009;**169**(5):447–453.

4. Young T B. Natural history of chronic insomnia. *J Clin Sleep Med*. 2005;**1**:e466–e467.

5. Carey TJ, Moul DE, Pilkonis P, Germain A, Buysse D J. Focusing on the experience of insomnia. *Behav Sleep Med*. 2005;**3**(2):73–86.

6. Roth T, Roehrs T. Insomnia: epidemiology, characteristics, and consequences. *Clin Cornerstone.* 2003;**5**(3):5–15.

7. Shochat T, Umphress J, Israel A, Ancoli-Israel S. Insomnia in primary care patients. *Sleep.* 1999;**22**: S359–365.

8. Orff HJ, Drummond SP, Nowakowski S, Perlis ML. Discrepancy between subjective symptomatology and objective neuropsychological performance in insomnia. *Sleep.* 2007;**30**(9):1205–1211.

9. Harvey A. A cognitive model of insomnia. *Behav Res Ther.* 2002;**40**:869–893.

10. Espie CA, Broomfield NM, MacMahon KM, Macphee LM, Taylor L M. The attention-intention-effort pathway in the development of psychophysiologic insomnia: a theoretical review. *Sleep Med Rev.* 2006; **10**(4):215–245.

11. Johnson L, Spinweber CL. Quality of sleep and performance in the navy: A longitudinal study of good and poor sleepers. In: Guilleminault C, Lugaresi E, eds. *Sleep/wake disorders: natural history, epidemiology, and long-term evaluation.* New York: Raven Press; 1983:13–28.

12. Kupperman M, Lubeck DP, Mazonson P D. Sleep problems and their correlates in a working population. *J Gen Intern Med.* 1995;**10**:25–32.

13. Leger D, Guilleminault C, Blader G, Levy E, Paillard M. Medical and socio-professional impact of insomnia. *Sleep.* 2002;**25**:625–629.

14. Fullerton DS. The economic impact of insomnia in managed care: a clearer picture emerges. *Am J Manag Care.* 2006;**12**(8 Suppl):S246–252.

15. Walsh JK, Engelhardt CL. The direct economic costs of insomnia in the United States for 1995. *Sleep.* 1999;**22** (Suppl 2):S386–393.

16. Ozminkowski RJ, Wang S, Walsh J K. The direct and indirect costs of untreated insomnia in adults in the United States. *Sleep.* 2007;**30**(3):263–273.

17. NIH. State-of-the-Science Conference Statement on manifestations and management of chronic insomnia in adults. *NIH Consens State Sci Statements.* 2005; **22**(2):1–30.

18. Phillips B, Mannino DM. Do insomnia complaints cause hypertension or cardiovascular disease? *J Clin Sleep Med.* 2007;**3**(5):489–494.

19. Suka M, Yoshida K, Sugimori H. Persistent insomnia is a predictor of hypertension in Japanese male workers. *J Occup Health.* 2003;**45**(6):344–350.

20. Schwartz S, McDowell Anderson W, Cole SR, et al. Insomnia and heart disease: a review of epidemiologic studies. *J Psychosom Res.* 1999;**47** (4):313–333.

21. Knutson KL, Ryden AM, Mander BA, Van Cauter E. Role of sleep duration and quality in the risk and severity of type 2 diabetes mellitus. *Arch Intern Med.* 2006;**166**(16):1768–1774.

22. Pigeon WR, Perlis ML. Insomnia and depression: birds of a feather? *Int J Sleep Disorders.* 2007; **1**(3):82–91.

23. Breslau N, Roth T, Rosenthal L, Andreski P. Sleep disturbance and psychiatric disorders: a longitudinal epidemiological study of young adults. *Biol Psychiatry.* 1996;**39**(6):411–418.

24. Chang PP, Ford DE, Mead LA, Cooper-Patrick L, Klag MJ. Insomnia in young men and subsequent depression: The Johns Hopkins Precursors Study. *Am J Epidemiol.* 1997;**146**(2):105–114.

25. Dryman A, Eaton WW. Affective symptoms associated with the onset of major depression in the community: findings from the US National Institute of Mental Health Epidemiologic Catchment Area Program. *Acta Psychiatr Scand.* 1991;**84**(1):1–5.

26. Ford D, Kamerow D. Epidemiologic study of sleep disturbance and psychiatric disorders: an opportunity for prevention? *JAMA.* 1989;**262**:1479–1484.

27. Hohagen F, Rink K, Kappler C, et al. Prevalence and treatment of insomnia in general practice: A longitudinal study. *Eur Arch Psychiatry Clin Neurosci.* 1993;**242**(6):329–336.

28. Kennedy GJ, Kelman HR, Thomas C. Persistence and remission of depressive symptoms in late life. *Am J Psychiatry.* 1991;**148**(2):174–178.

29. Livingston G, Blizard B, Mann A. Does sleep disturbance predict depression in elderly people? A study in inner London. *Br J Gen Pract.* 1993; **43**(376):445–448.

30. Livingston G, Watkin V, Milne B, Manela MV, Katona C. Who becomes depressed? The Islington community study of older people. *J Affect Disord.* 2000;**58**(2): 125–133.

31. Mallon L, Broman JE, Hetta J. Relationship between insomnia, depression, and mortality: a 12-year follow-up of older adults in the community. *Int Psychogeriatr.* 2000;**12**(3):295–306.

32. Paffenbarger RS Jr, Lee IM, Leung R. Physical activity and personal characteristics associated with depression and suicide in American college men. *Acta Psychiatr Scand Suppl.* 1994;**377**:16–22.

33. Perlis ML, Smith LJ, Lyness JM, et al. Insomnia as a risk factor for onset of depression in the elderly. *Behav Sleep Med.* 2006;**4**(2):104–113.

34. Roberts RE, Shema SJ, Kaplan GA, Strawbridge WJ. Sleep complaints and depression in an aging cohort:

A prospective perspective. *Am J Psychiatry*. 2000;**157** (1):81–88.

35. Vollrath M, Wicki W, Angst J. The Zurich study. VIII. Insomnia: association with depression, anxiety, somatic syndromes, and course of insomnia. *Eur Arch Psychiatry Neurol Sci*. 1989;**239**(2):113–124.

36. Weissman M, Greenwald S, Nino-Murcia G, Dement W. The morbidity of insomnia uncomplicated by psychiatric disorders. *Gen Hosp Psychiatry*. 1997;**19**:245–250.

37. Perlis ML, Giles DE, Buysse DJ, Tu X, Kupfer DJ. Self-reported sleep disturbance as a prodromal symptom in recurrent depression. *J Affect Disord*. 1997;**42** (2–3):209–212.

38. Pigeon WR, Hegel M, Unutzer J, et al. Is insomnia a perpetuating factor for late-life depression in the IMPACT cohort? *Sleep*. 2008;**31**(4):481–488.

39. Nowell PD, Mazumdar S, Buysse DJ, et al. Benzodiazepines and zolpidem for chronic insomnia: a meta-analysis of treatment efficacy. *JAMA*. 1997; **278**(24):2170–2177.

40. Glass J, Lanctot KL, Herrmann N, Sproule BA, Busto UE. Sedative hypnotics in older people with insomnia: meta-analysis of risks and benefits. *BMJ*. 2005;**331** (7526):1169.

41. Morin CM, Culbert JP, Schwartz MS. Non-pharmacological interventions for insomnia: a meta-analysis of treatment efficacy. *Am J Psychiatry*. 1994;**151**:1172–1180.

42. Murtagh DR, Greenwood KM. Identifying effective psychological treatments for insomnia: a meta-analysis. *J Consult Clin Psychol*. 1995;**63**:79–89.

43. Smith MT, Perlis ML, Park A, et al. Comparative meta-analysis of pharmacotherapy and behavior therapy for persistent insomnia. *Am J Psychiatry*. 2002;**159** (1):5–11.

44. Aldrich MS. Automobile accidents in patients with sleep disorders. *Sleep*. 1989;**12**(6):487–494.

45. Krystal A. Treating the health, quality of life, and functional impairments in insomnia. *J Clin Sleep Med*. 2007;**3**(1):63–72.

46. Morin CM. Measuring outcomes in randomized clinical trials of insomnia treatments. *Sleep Med Rev*. 2003;**7**(3):263–279.

47. Leger D, Quera-Salva MA, Philip P. Health-related quality of life in patients with insomnia treated with zopiclone. *Pharmacoeconomics*. 1996;**10** (Suppl 1):39–44.

48. Walsh JK, Krystal AD, Amato DA, et al. Nightly treatment of primary insomnia with eszopiclone for six months: effect on sleep, quality of life, and work limitations. *Sleep*. 2007;**30**(8):959–968.

49. Edinger JD, Wohlgemuth WK, Krystal AD, Rice JR. Behavioral insomnia therapy for fibromyalgia patients: a randomized clinical trial. *Arch Intern Med*. 2005; **165**(21):2527–2535.

50. Pigeon WR, Jungquist CR, Matteson SR, Perlis ML. Pain, sleep and mood outcomes in chronic pain patients following cognitive behavioral therapy for insomnia. *Sleep*. 2007; **30**:A255–A256.

51. Fava M, McCall WV, Krystal A, et al. Eszopiclone co-administered with fluoxetine in patients with insomnia coexisting with major depressive disorder. *Biol Psychiatry*. 2006;**59**(11):1052–1060.

52. Manber R, Edinger JD, San Pedro M. Combining escitalopram oxalate (ESCIT) and individual cognitive behavioral therapy for insomnia (CBTI) to improve depression outcome. *Sleep*. 2007; **30**:A232.

53. Taylor DJ, Lichstein KL, Weinstock J, Sanford S, Temple JR. A pilot study of cognitive-behavioral therapy of insomnia in people with mild depression. *Behav Ther*. 2007;**38**(1):49–57.

54. Ohayon MM, Roth T. What are the contributing factors for insomnia in the general population? *J Psychosom Res*. 2001;**51**(6):745–755.

55. Ohayon M. Epidemiology of insomnia: what we know and what we still need to learn. *Sleep Med Rev*. 2002;**6**:97–111.

56. American Academy of Sleep Medicine. *International classification of sleep disorders*, 2nd ed. Westchester, IL: American Academy of Sleep Medicine; 2005.

57. Spielman AJ, Caruso LS, Glovinsky PB. A behavioral perspective on insomnia treatment. *Psychiatr Clin North Am*. 1987;**10**(4):541–553.

58. Perlis ML, Smith MT, Pigeon WR. Etiology and pathophysiology of insomnia. In: Kryger M, Roth T, Dement WC, eds. *Principles and practice of sleep medicine*, 4th ed. Philadelphia, PA: Elsevier Saunders; 2005:714–725.

59. Morin C, Stone J, Trinkle D, Mercer J, Remsberg S. Dysfunctional beliefs and attitudes about sleep among older adults with and without insomnia complaints. *Psychol Aging*. 1993;8.

60. Perlis M, Giles D, Mendelson W, Bootzin R, Wyatt J. Psychophysiological insomnia: the behavioural model and a neurocognitive perspective. *J Sleep Res*. 1997;**6**:179–188.

61. Chesson AL Jr, Anderson WM, Littner M, et al. Practice parameters for the nonpharmacologic treatment of chronic insomnia. An American Academy of Sleep Medicine report. Standards of Practice Committee of the American Academy

of Sleep Medicine. *Sleep*. 1999;
22(8):1128–1133.

62. Lacks P, Morin CM. Recent advances in the assessment and treatment of insomnia. *J Consult Clin Psychol*. 1992;**60**:586–594.

63. Morin C. *Insomnia: psychological assessment and management*. New York: Guilford Press; 1996.

64. Shoham-Salomon V, Rosenthal R. Paradoxical interventions: a meta-analysis. *J Consult Clin Psychol*. 1987;**55**(1):22–28.

65. Harvey AG. Identifying safety behaviors in insomnia. *J Nerv Ment Dis*. 2002;**190**(1):16–21.

66. Morin CM, Colecchi C, Stone J, Sood R, Brink D. Behavioral and pharmacological therapies for late-life insomnia: a randomized controlled trial. *JAMA*. 1999;**281**:991–999.

67. Perlis ML, Smith MT, Orff H, et al. The effects of modafinil and cognitive behavior therapy on sleep continuity in patients with primary insomnia. *Sleep*. 2004;**27**(4):715–725.

Depressive disorders

Philip R. Gehrman, Michael E. Thase, Dieter Riemann and Michael Perlis

Introduction

Disturbed sleep is a central feature of depression. So it comes as no surprise that there has been a fair amount of research on how it is that sleep is abnormal in the context of depression and how this aspect of the disorder is related to the risk for, and clinical course of, the illness.

In the present chapter the various manifestations of disturbed sleep in depression are reviewed in terms of direct effects on sleep, sleep-related circadian abnormalities, and sleep-related neurobiological perturbations. The clinical implications of these findings are reviewed along with the major models put forth to explain the relationship between sleep and depression. Lastly, an overview of strategies for the treatment of sleep disturbance in depression is provided.

Sleep abnormalities in major depressive disorder

Sleep may be construed in terms of sleep continuity$^\epsilon$, sleep architecture, and sleep microarchitecture (EEG power spectral profile), as well as various subtypes of these patterns. Each of these domains is reliably altered in significant proportions of people suffering from major depressive disorder (MDD).

Sleep continuity disturbances

The DSM-IV diagnostic criteria for MDD include subjective sleep disturbance in the form of either insomnia (i.e. difficulty initiating or maintaining sleep) or hypersomnia [1]. Unfortunately, the definition of insomnia in MDD is not uniform among clinicians or researchers. Insomnia has traditionally been clinically described in terms of initial, middle, and late insomnia; in research,

including polysomnographic (PSG) assessments, insomnia is typically measured in terms of sleep latency (SL), wake after sleep onset (WASO), number of awakenings (NWAK), sleep efficiency (SE), and total sleep time (TST). Regardless of the classification schema used, disturbed sleep quality is one of the most commonly reported depressive symptoms, occurring in up to 90% of individuals seeking treatment (e.g. [2]). A smaller subset of depressed individuals report increased sleep or subjective hypersomnia, which is defined as prolonged sleep duration that extends more than 1 hour over habitual total sleep time. Rates of hypersomnia vary more widely across studies and are somewhat population-dependent, ranging from as low as 5% to as high as 36% of depressed persons. The prevalence of hypersomnia is higher in studies of younger age groups and tends to be highest in studies of individuals meeting criteria for atypical depression [3,4].

Unlike the DSM-IV, the *International Classification of Sleep Disorders*, 2nd edition (ICSD-2) delineates other forms of insomnia including: psychophysiological, paradoxical, and idiopathic insomnia [5]. Psychophysiological insomnia includes problems with sleep initiation and maintenance where there is evidence of sleep difficulty and/or heightened arousal in bed, which is thought to occur as a result of psychological, behavioral, and conditioning factors. Paradoxical insomnia (formerly referred to as sleep state misperception insomnia) manifests with a subjective complaint of sleep initiation and/or maintenance that is unusually severe and there is, by definition, a poor correspondence between subjective complaint and the severity of the complaint as measured by PSG. Currently, there is no widely accepted theory regarding the precipitation and/or perpetuation of this form of insomnia, although several have posited that sleep

Foundations of Psychiatric Sleep Medicine, ed. John W. Winkelman and David T. Plante. Published by Cambridge University Press. © Cambridge University Press 2010.

state "misperception" occurs in association with a heightened level of sensory and information processing at sleep onset and during NREM sleep and the attenuation of the normal mesograde amnesia of sleep [6,7]. Idiopathic insomnia refers to sleep initiation and maintenance problems that have a childhood onset. Little is known about the average severity of this type of insomnia, the extent to which sleep state misperception occurs in these subjects, or this form of the disorder's etiology and/or pathophysiology [8].

Interestingly, there has been no effort to classify sleep continuity disturbances associated with depression in terms of the aforementioned ICSD-2 diagnostic types. Instead, the focus has been on the insomnia "subtypes" or phenotypes (e.g. early, middle, and late). It is generally held that "late insomnia" is more characteristic of the severe forms of major depressive disorder (i.e. early morning awakenings are a cardinal sign of endogenous depression or melancholia, whereas "initial insomnia" is equally characteristic of generalized anxiety disorder). From our vantage point, there have only been a few studies that systematically assess the differential occurrence of the insomnia subtypes in depression (using contemporary classifications of mood and anxiety disorders) and the results from one of the largest such investigations suggests that all three subtypes of insomnia occur with an equal prevalence in patients with MDD [9].

In terms of the severity of insomnia as measured by self-report, there also are no large-scale studies that provide relevant descriptive data (i.e. mean, range, and standard deviation), especially in comparison to healthy ("good sleeper") or insomnia (without depression) control groups. Thus, it cannot be said with confidence that self-reported sleep continuity disturbances associated with depression are similar to, or different from, those which are seen in individuals with primary insomnia. In the absence of definitive data, the results from one very small-scale study suggests that sleep continuity disturbances are more severe in primary insomnia than major depressive disorder and that patients with primary insomnia also are more prone to sleep state misperception (see Table 15.1) [10].

In terms of PSG-measured insomnia severity, there is (to our knowledge) only one contemporary study that provides descriptive data comparing sleep continuity in patients with depression to good sleeper controls [11]. In this case, the MDD patients (N=178) differed modestly from good sleeper subjects (N=108) on PSG-measured sleep continuity. Sleep latency was increased by ~5 minutes, wake after sleep onset was increased by ~20 minutes, the frequency of awakenings was increased by ~6 episodes per night, early morning awakening was moved forward by ~15 minutes, total sleep time was reduced by ~35 minutes, and sleep efficiency was reduced by ~8%. Interestingly, time in bed differed only minimally (~5 minutes). While these findings suggest that the insomnia in depression may not be driven by the same perpetuating factors as primary insomnia (i.e. sleep extension [12]), it is possible that the similarity in time in bed is an artifact of the laboratory setting given that subjects in this study all were studied on a fixed 11 p.m. to 7 a.m. schedule in the sleep laboratory. In practice, depressed patients with insomnia often report spending increased time in bed even when they are not able to sleep.

Sleep architecture abnormalities

A significant proportion of patients with major depressive disorder exhibit altered sleep architecture as compared to good sleepers. These architectural abnormalities include: (1) an altered distribution of slow-wave sleep (lack the traditional attenuation pattern across the night) [13], (2) reduced slow-wave sleep (in minutes and/or percent) [9], (3) decreased latency to the first episode of REM sleep (i.e. reduced REM latency) [14,15], (4) a prolonged first REM period [14,15], (5) increased REM percent (if not REM time in minutes) [14,15], and (6) increased REM density (i.e. eye movements per minute of REM sleep) [14,15].

With the single exception of increased REM density, these effects are remarkably like what is seen with aging (i.e. in elderly subjects) [11] and this led Gillin and colleagues [16], amongst others, to suggest that depression may mimic the CNS aging process. Further, alterations of both NREM and REM sleep led to a vigorous ongoing debate within the sleep community about whether one set of the effects occurred actively while the other occurred only as a necessary consequence of the primary effects. One group speculated that the "primary defect" existed within the NREM system and was related to altered sleep homeostasis [17]. The other group argued that increased REM "pressure" was largely responsible for the sleep alterations [18]. For a time, this debate centered on whether reduced REM latency was a specific and sensitive biomarker for major depressive disorder. This aspect of the debate lessened

Table 15.1 Sleep continuity measures

	PI	MDD	C	ANOVA	PI vs. MDD	PI vs. C	C vs. MDD
PSG measures							
SL	21.8 (17.9)	9.5 (9.3)	7.9 (6.8)	0.05	p <0.05	p <0.05	NS
NUMA	9.3 (3.7)	2.1 (1.7)	4.7 (3.9)	0.0004	p <0.05	p <0.05	NS
WASO	72.9 (74.5)	24.1 (48.7)	21.0 (16.4)	0.08	NS	p <0.05	NS
TST	323.7 (82.6)	366.7 (63.0)	348.3 (32.5)	0.37	NS	NS	NS
Sleep diary measures							
S_SL	79.6 (89.0)	22.2 (28.1)	17.6 (18.1)	0.05	p <0.05	p <0.05	NS
S_NUMA	2.4 (1.3)	3.1 (2.3)	1.8 (1.0)	NS	NS	NS	NS
S_WASO	76.1 (98.1)	23.6 (40.3)	16.2 (23.7)	0.08	NS	p <0.05	NS
S_TST	278.9 (119.7)	363.13 (58.9)	370.0 (47.4)	0.05	p <0.05	p <0.05	NS
Difference scores							
DSL	57.78 (79.0)	12.50 (19.7)	9.7 (18.3)	0.09	NS	p <0.05	NS
DNUMA	−6.9 (3.8)	0.9 (2.5)	−2.8 (3.7)	0.0002	p <0.05	p <0.05	P<.05
DWASO	3.2 (42.4)	−2.3 (17.7)	−4.8 (22.5)	0.85	NS	NS	NS
DTST	−44.8 (54.7)	8.8 (41.0)	21.7 (48.1)	0.02	p <0.05	p <0.05	NS

PI, primary insomnia; MDD, major depressive disorder; C, controls; SL, sleep latency; NUMA, number of awakenings; WASO, wake after sleep onset; TST, total sleep time; anything starting with 'S_' is the same variables above for sleep diary. The "D" before the last set of variables stands for "difference in."
Data from Perlis M, et al. Beta/gamma EEG activity in patients with insomnia. *Sleep*. 2001;24(1):110–117.

after publication of the meta-analysis by Benca and colleagues [19], which concluded that reduced REM latency was not pathognomic for depression but that there was the possibility that the whole of the sleep architectural profile was unique to major depression.

Sleep microarchitecture

The term sleep microarchitecture was likely first coined by Armitage and colleagues [20] in the mid 1990s. The term refers to an alternative approach to examining the EEG that is complimentary to the visual scoring of sleep architecture using techniques such as power spectral analysis (PSA) or digital period analysis (DPA) to provide a "finer grain" analysis of the sleep EEG. For example, whereas visual scoring assesses presence or absence of slow-wave sleep (SWS) in a 30-second epoch based on a minimum proportion ($\geq$20%) of slow waves (delta frequency with amplitude $\geq$75μV), PSA and DPA allow for a continuous measure of delta activity per time unit (e.g. per NREM cycle or for average NREM), where frequency may be variably defined and assessed in terms of accumulated voltage.

Studies of major depressive disorder utilizing PSA and DPA have not only confirmed some of the sleep architectural findings in depression (e.g. reduced slow-wave activity or increased REM counts), but has generated novel findings, such as altered patterns of delta activity per NREM cycle [20–22]. These findings are not, however, without controversy, as several investigations have either failed to replicate the finding of abnormal SWS in depression [23,24] or found this pattern only in men [25]. This may be because the reduction in SWS in depression may occur at an earlier age in men than women and some studies may not have included a sufficient number of older women. While there is substantially less research in frequencies other than the delta band, at least two studies have shown that beta and/or gamma EEG activity is reduced in depression [26]. This observation is consistent with the notion that depression may be associated with broader diminution of cortical activity, which, if true, could provide further support for the view that the

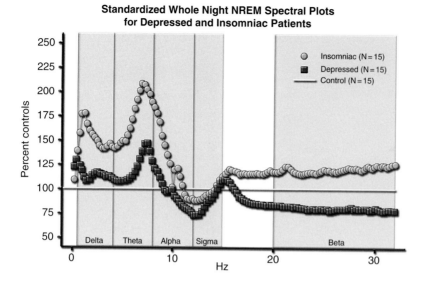

Figure 15.1 Standardized whole night NREM spectral plots for depressed and insomniac patients.

neurophysiological basis of insomnia in major depressive disorder is qualitatively different from that of primary insomnia. Figure 15.1, adapted from an unpublished figure by Nofzinger and colleagues, provides a depiction of the NREM EEG spectrum differences in good sleepers, patients with primary insomnia, and patients with major depressive disorder (i.e. that beta EEG is higher than normal in primary insomnia and lower than normal in patients with insomnia co-morbid with depression). This pattern is also evident in work by Perlis and colleagues [10].

Overall relationship between sleep and depression

One difficulty in studying the relationship between insomnia and depression is the sheer number of variables that can be used to describe sleep continuity, sleep architecture, and sleep microarchitecture. Further, depression can also be described in terms of myriad variables including clinical profile measures (age of onset, chronicity, subtype, or symptom severity) and symptom component measures (i.e. overall severity of specific measures of affective, behavioral, and cognitive dysfunction). This complexity in the measurement of both insomnia and depression has resulted in studies that have more narrow foci, such as studies that use single variables to differentiate between groups of interest (e.g. depressed and healthy subjects) or to predict clinical phenomena of interest (e.g. reduced REM latency as a biomarker for treatment response). This

approach, while productive, has not been able to answer questions like: (1) "What is the overall association between various sleep and depression measures?" (2) "Is the overall relationship moderated by specific variables or variable clusters?" or (3) "Are there aspects of sleep that are not related to depression and are there aspects of depression that are not related to sleep?" In order to address such issues, Perlis et al. [9] adopted a multivariate approach using a large archival data set from the Sleep and Depression research group at the University of Pittsburgh Medical Center. The data set included item responses from the Hamilton rating scale for depression and the Beck depression inventory (BDI) and polysomnographic measures from a sample of 361 unmedicated adult outpatients. Canonical correlation and serial multiple regression analyses were used to determine the associations between depressive symptoms and sleep measures. Canonical correlation showed that a single factor accounted for the majority of the relationship between depressive symptoms and sleep measures ($R = 0.55$, $p < 0.05$). Fifteen depression items and nine sleep measures accounted for 95% of the correlation. Depression variables encompassed a core set of mood, neurovegetative, and cognitive symptoms. Sleep variables were primarily related to SWS, including measures of delta EEG activity (see Figure 15.2). Taken together these data suggest that the severity of depressive illness is most related to factors that represent the initiation, density, and/or duration of SWS. Put differently, depressive illness seems to co-vary primarily with a marker of sleep homeostasis dysregulation.

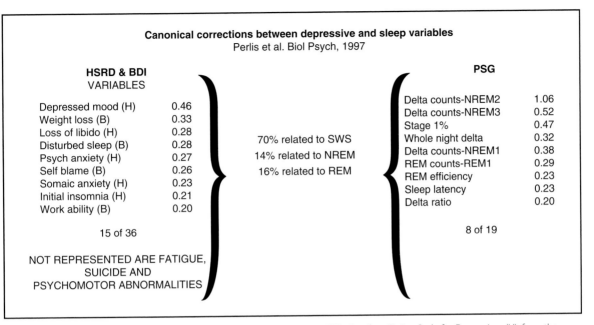

Canonical corrections between depressive and sleep variables
Perlis et al. Biol Psych, 1997

HSRD & BDI
VARIABLES

Depressed mood (H)	0.46
Weight loss (B)	0.33
Loss of libido (H)	0.28
Disturbed sleep (B)	0.28
Psych anxiety (H)	0.27
Self blame (B)	0.26
Somaic anxiety (H)	0.23
Initial insomnia (H)	0.21
Work ability (B)	0.20

15 of 36

NOT REPRESENTED ARE FATIGUE, SUICIDE AND PSYCHOMOTOR ABNORMALITIES

70% related to SWS
14% related to NREM
16% related to REM

PSG

Delta counts-NREM2	1.06
Delta counts-NREM3	0.52
Stage 1%	0.47
Whole night delta	0.32
Delta counts-NREM1	0.38
REM counts-REM1	0.29
REM efficiency	0.23
Sleep latency	0.23
Delta ratio	0.20

8 of 19

Figure 15.2 Canonical corrections between depressive and sleep variants. HSRD, Hamilton Rating Scale for Depression; (H), from the HRSD; (B), from the BDI. Reproduced from [9].

Interestingly, REM measures (including reduced REM latency) accounted for very little variance in that analysis. Parallel studies contrasting the sleep of depressed patients before and after treatment, recovered patients, and good sleeper healthy controls would be helpful to untangle state from trait variables.

Sleep-related circadian rhythm abnormalities

Investigation of the role of circadian rhythms in depression has generally supported a phase advance of the circadian rhythm. The reduction in REM latency once thought to be a cardinal sleep sign of depression was proposed to reflect an advance of the circadian rhythm of REM propensity [27]. Similarly, early morning awakenings could be the result of a phase advance such that the circadian alerting signal increases at an earlier hour. A number of studies found evidence of advances in the circadian rhythms of body temperature, cortisol, prolactin, norepinephrine, and melatonin, among others [28]. Interestingly, imposing a phase delay on non-depressed subjects creates REM sleep changes similar to those observed in depression [29]. Further support for the role of a phase advance came from studies that found that many antidepressants delay the phase of circadian rhythms [27]. This would suggest that these medications have circadian realignment as a mechanism of action. It should be noted, however, that many studies have failed to find any evidence of circadian misalignment in depression [30].

Souetre and colleagues [31] reported that it is the amplitude of circadian rhythms rather than the phase that is altered in depression. In their study, patients with depression had reduced amplitudes in body temperature, plasma cortisol, norepinephrine (NE), thyroid-stimulating hormone (TSH), and melatonin rhythms, with lower amplitude associated with greater severity of depression. Whether it is the phase position, the amplitude, or some other features of circadian rhythms at play, the data are mixed regarding the presence of specific abnormalities in depression. Further, it is unclear whether any abnormalities that do exist play a causative role or are merely epiphenomena.

Sleep-related neuroimaging and neuroendocrine abnormalities

An alternate approach to studying brain activity during sleep is through the use of neuroimaging, which has produced data that help to clarify the earlier REM and NREM findings. Neuroimaging studies during sleep are largely limited to PET studies due to the difficulty of sleeping during an fMRI (due to the noise generated by magnetic resonance imaging).

Nofzinger and colleagues [32] found that patients with depression demonstrated greater activation of structures involved in REM sleep as compared to healthy controls, including brainstem structures, the limbic and anterior paralimbic cortex, and the executive cortex. These data parallel the increased REM activity reported in sleep architectural studies. Group differences in NREM sleep were found in other studies, with the depressed group displaying higher overall brain metabolism and less of a decrease in activation in frontal areas in the transition from waking to NREM sleep [33,34]. These findings are similar to those from studies of primary insomnia compared to good sleepers [35] and suggest a failure of the mechanisms that normally dampen arousal during sleep, which in turn could be related to disturbance in sleep continuity.

In addition to the imaging findings, numerous studies have documented abnormalities of neuroendocrine systems in the sleep of depressed subjects with an overactivity of the hypothalamic-pituitary-adrenal (HPA) axis resulting in an increased output of cortisol (for an overview see [36]). Ehlers and Kupfer [37] as early as 1987 postulated that sleep architectural abnormalities commonly seen in depression are the result of a disturbance in the interaction of two hypothalamic peptides, growth hormone-releasing hormone (GRF) and corticotropin-releasing factor (CRF), and that this served as the neurochemical basis for the observed reduction of SWS and early onset of REM sleep in depression. This perspective has been revisited in recent years, and championed, by Richardson and colleagues [38].

Sleep deprivation in depression
Total sleep deprivation

Although sleep loss (insomnia) is a correlate of depression, it has long been known that total sleep deprivation (TSD) has therapeutic effects for a significant proportion of depressed people. Wu and Bunney [39] conducted a meta-analysis of sleep deprivation studies and concluded that 50–60% of depressed patients display at least a transient improvement of mood after TSD. As about 80% of unmedicated TSD responders relapse into depressed mood after the next night of sleep, the clinical usefulness of this particular intervention is limited. However, from a research point of view, TSD offers the opportunity to relate rapidly occurring changes in mood to simultaneous

changes of biological variables. It has consistently been shown that a diurnal variation of mood with a spontaneous improvement towards the afternoon and evening hours predicts a positive response to sleep deprivation [40,41]. Reduced REM latency may also predict a positive response to sleep deprivation.

Positron emission tomography (PET) studies reveal that depressed patients who subsequently respond to TSD have an elevated glucose metabolism in the cingulate gyrus, which normalizes after TSD [42–44]. Similar findings were reported by Ebert et al. [45,46] and Volk et al. [47,48] using single photon emission computed tomography (SPECT) before and after sleep deprivation. It is interesting to note that signal transduction in the cingulate gyrus is dominated by cholinergic neurotransmission [42], which is involved in REM sleep regulation.

Neurochemical hypotheses have been advanced to explain the effects of TSD on depression. One model focuses on the role of the inhibitory neuromodulator adenosine, which is now widely accepted to be involved in sleep regulation [49]. The cholinergic neurons that inhibit SWS appear to be particularly prone to inhibition by adenosine, which is mediated by adenosine A_1-receptors. Thus, agents that increase adenosine concentration in the brain or mimic its action at A_1-receptors promote SWS, while agents that block A_1-receptors, such as caffeine, inhibit SWS and increase wakefulness. Sleep deprivation not only increases adenosine concentration in the brain but also can upregulate adenosine A_1-receptors [50], which reinforces adenosine's sleep-promoting effect. Thus, it has been proposed that upregulation of A_1-receptors may play a role in mood regulation, including the antidepressant effects of both sleep deprivation and ECT, as well as the antimanic mechanism of action of carbamazepine, which acts as an A_1-antagonist and thus also upregulates A_1-receptors [51]. An obvious potential mechanism of the antidepressive effects of adenosine A_1-receptor activation is the inhibition of the cholinergic neurons in the basal forebrain, in striking agreement with the cholinergic–aminergic imbalance model of affective disorders [52] (see below).

Partial sleep deprivation

Although TSD is not a practical long-term clinical intervention, it is possible to deliver a more sustained effect through partial sleep deprivation. Specifically, individuals are asked to retire relatively early (i.e. 8 p.m.

or 10 p.m.) and permitted to sleep for an attenuated amount of time (e.g. 2–4 hours) before being awakened and asked to remain awake and active. Although the antidepressant effects of partial sleep deprivation tend to be less pronounced than those of TSD, they have been shown to meaningfully enhance the effects of other treatments, such as antidepressants [53]. Unfortunately, even partial sleep deprivation interventions are difficult to implement outside of hospital settings.

Selective deprivation of REM sleep

Based on the observation that all members of the tricyclic (TCA) and monoamine oxidase inhibitor (MAOI) classes of antidepressants significantly suppress REM sleep, the question arose whether this pharmacological effect may be a "conditio sine qua non" or even the basic underlying mechanism of action of antidepressant treatments. Vogel and colleagues [18] tested this hypothesis by depriving depressed individuals of REM sleep without pharmacological intervention by selective, PSG-monitored awakenings over a period of 3 weeks. This experimental therapy led to a 50% reduction in REM sleep and resulted in an antidepressant response comparable to that of the TCA imipramine. A control group, which was awakened during NREM sleep, did not show any clinical improvement.

Only one study [54] attempted to replicate the findings of Vogel and colleagues with a methodologically improved design. Selective REM sleep deprivation was compared to the same amount of well-balanced awakenings leading to NREM sleep deprivation in depressed inpatients. In accordance with the data of Vogel, REM deprivation was associated with a significant antidepressant effect. However, contrary to expectation, the group that was awakened from NREM sleep also exhibited an antidepressant effect, which tended to be larger in magnitude than observed with selective REM deprivation. In this study it was found that both experimental conditions increased the duration of NREM sleep cycles and it was therefore postulated that this might be the underlying mechanism of action.

Clinical correlates of disturbed sleep in depression

A number of investigators have examined the clinical correlates of sleep disturbance in depression. The evidence overwhelmingly supports the view that insomnia and sleep architecture perturbations are critically related to disease state and long-term outcome.

Clinical relevance of sleep continuity disturbance

Disturbances of sleep continuity have significant clinical implications that have been investigated across a number of studies. These studies indicate that disturbed sleep continuity is a prodromal symptom as well as a risk factor for new-onset illness and relapse.

Sleep continuity disturbance (insomnia) as a risk factor for new-onset depression. A number of longitudinal studies with time frames ranging from 6 months to 3 years have found that insomnia increases the risk of both new-onset and recurrent depression [55–73]. Studies with follow-up periods over decades have also found this relationship [56,63,64]. Averaged across studies, there is an approximately 3.5-fold increase in the risk of depression for people with persistent insomnia compared to those who do not complain of insomnia (see Figure 15.3). It is noteworthy that the measurement and definition of insomnia varied considerably across studies. The impact of age and sex interactions on this relationship has been examined in several studies. In those studies that controlled for age, the relative risk of insomnia for depressive onset was consistently higher than in those studies that did not control for age. This suggests that insomnia is not a uniform risk factor for all age cohorts; however, studies have not specifically examined the age groups for which risk is highest. In the studies that evaluated sex differences [57,63], the association between insomnia and depression was consistently more robust for women than men. Overall, these data strongly support the hypothesis that insomnia is a risk factor for depression.

Sleep continuity disturbance (insomnia) as a prodromal symptom of depression. In the natural history of individuals with recurrent illness, insomnia may be an early indicator of an impending major depressive episode. One retrospective study of depressed patients found that 40% reported a worsening of sleep prior to the onset of their first depressive episode [74]. In those subjects with recurrent depression, 56% reported that sleep disturbance preceded recurrence. In a prospective, 42-week study of remitted patients with a history of recurrent depression, weekly monitoring of depression symptoms was undertaken with the BDI, with increases in depressive symptoms resulting in a

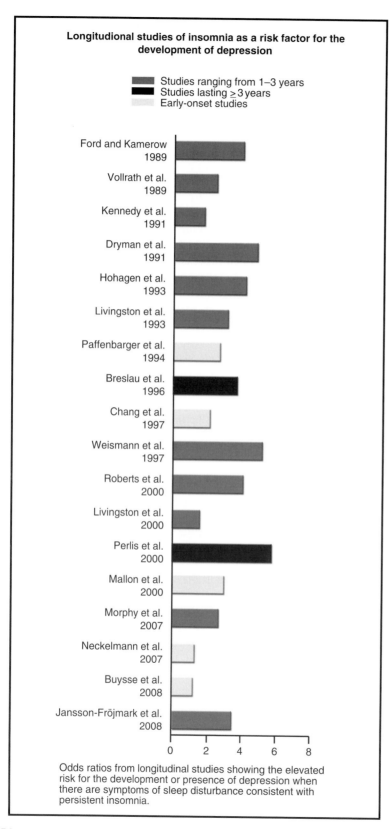

Figure 15.3 Longitudinal studies of insomnia as a risk factor for the development of depression.

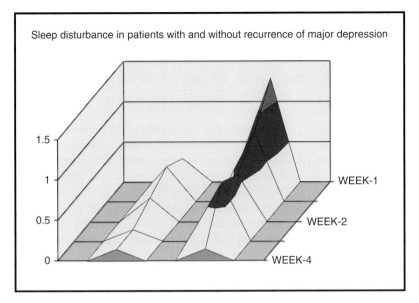

Sleep disturbance in patients with and without recurrence of major depression

Figure 15.4 Score on the sleep disturbance item from the BDI (y-axis) and time leading up to recurrence (z-axis). The pattern on the right is for patients who experienced a recurrence and who experienced an increase in sleep disturbance in leading up to recurrence. The pattern on the left is a matched group of patients who did not experience recurrence and who did not have an increase in sleep disturbance.

formal evaluation for recurrence [75]. The subgroup that experienced a syndromal recurrence of depression was compared to a subsample matched on age, sex, and clinical history by examining the single sleep item on the BDI (question 16) for the 5 weeks prior to the onset of the recurrent episode in the index group and for a temporally equivalent period in the subsample that did not suffer a recurrence. The time series data from this period showed, in distinction to the non-recurrent group, those who suffered a recurrence exhibited a progressively greater level of sleep disturbance that reached highest severity at the week of recurrence (see Figure 15.4). These data strongly suggest that insomnia is a prodromal symptom of depression, and lend weight to the possibility that worsening insomnia may trigger or precipitate new depressive episodes.

Sleep continuity disturbance (insomnia) is a residual symptom of depression and increases risk of depressive relapse. Although insomnia often occurs in the context of depression, remission of depression is not necessarily associated with improvement in sleep. Across studies of both cognitive behavioral and pharmacological treatment of depression, between 20% and 50% of patients continue to report insomnia despite clinical improvements in overall depression [76–79]. In one cohort study that assessed elderly patients with depression at baseline and 6 months later, patients with persistent insomnia were 10–12-fold less likely to have achieved remission or an improvement of ≥50% in depressive symptoms compared with patients with no insomnia [80]. Following resolution of a depressive

episode, the presence of residual insomnia symptoms increases the risk of recurrence of depression [77,81,82] whereas those whose sleep improves posttreatment have reduced rates of recurrence [83]. These studies demonstrate that insomnia is frequently a residual symptom of depression that is associated with both reduced likelihood of achieving remission and increased risk of recurrence.

Clinical relevance of sleep architecture findings

Similar to sleep continuity disturbance, sleep architecture abnormalities have important clinical impact on illness severity, response to treatment, and risk of relapse/recurrence.

Illness severity. The sleep architecture variables that have been most intensively studied with respect to illness severity are REM latency, REM density, and SWS time, with greater disturbances of sleep architecture typically associated with greater illness severity. REM latency has only been associated with illness severity to the extent that inpatients more reliably show this sleep abnormality compared to outpatients [84,85]. Most studies, however, show that REM latency tends to be stable within individuals across time (e.g. [14,86–89]). REM density tends to be correlated with severity of depression and this measure varies with clinical state [15,90–94]. Finally, there is some evidence that reduced SWS is associated with greater illness severity [9,95]. Thus, there are relationships between depression severity and both state (REM density and SWS) and trait (REM latency) sleep architecture parameters. As a stable trait measure, REM latency may confer risk for both new-onset and recurrence of depression [96], where state measures are more likely to be consequences of depression.

Response to treatment. REM-related measures, singly or aggregated with NREM measures such as SWS time, have substantial value for predicting treatment responders from non-responders. On balance, greater sleep architecture abnormalities are associated with a more robust response to pharmacotherapy and/ or ECT and a more mixed response to psychotherapeutic interventions [97–101].

Risk for relapse/recurrence. Reduced REM latency predicted clinical outcome among successfully treated patients who were monitored for variable periods after treatment. Reduced REM latency predicts a poorer outcome in patients with recurrent MDD and in at-risk subjects (e.g. [88,102,103]). This further supports the role of reduced REM latency as a trait vulnerability to depression. In one study, the loss of the normal exponential decline in delta activity between the first two NREM periods also predicted early recurrence (e.g. [104]).

In summary, sleep architecture abnormalities, like sleep continuity disturbance, are associated with important clinical outcomes including illness severity, treatment outcome, and risk for relapse.

Theories regarding the association of sleep disturbance with depression

Clearly, sleep disturbance and depression are intricately intertwined, although the direction of causation and potential interactions are less certain. Several theories have been proposed in this area, which are reviewed below.

Sleep continuity disturbance promotes depression

This perspective, proposed by Adrien et al. [105], suggests that insomnia is a systemic or autoregulatory response that is caused by deficit in serotonin neurotransmission that presumably triggers the syndrome of depression in predisposed individuals. The rationale is that: (1) the pathogenesis of depression is linked to CNS arousal and/or perturbed serotonin neurotransmission; and (2) insomnia is triggered by

increased serotonin synthesis and availability, which can increase countervailing homeostatic pressure that counteracts CNS arousal. The problem with the "insomnia response" is that, like partial or total sleep deprivation, it cannot be maintained at antidepressant levels for prolonged periods of time and, to the extent that the insomnia is persistent, it is thought to produce or exacerbate "secondary" depressive symptoms including anhedonia, loss of libido, fatigue, memory and concentration problems, and may also influence other neurovegetative phenomena like weight change [106]. These secondary symptoms may, in turn, give rise to tertiary symptoms that include interpersonal problems, social withdrawal, and/or cognitive distortions [107]. Sleeplessness also may increase opportunities for intrusive thoughts and ruminations that are laden with negative affect, further fueling the development of depression. This combined perspective is admittedly speculative but it has the conceptual advantage of fitting with the neurobiological and neuroendocrinological biological data, the sleep deprivation findings, and clear evidence that insomnia is related to the predisposition for, precipitation of, and perpetuation of depression.

Increased REM sleep is depressogenic

Given the heavy emphasis traditionally placed on REM sleep phenomena in depression, it is not surprising that one model proposes that REM sleep itself is depressogenic. According to this model, reduced REM latency, increased proportion of time spent in REM sleep, and higher REM density are all the result of an increased "pressure" for REM [18]. Perhaps the strongest early support for this model came from studies of REM sleep deprivation, which – as reviewed previously – led to improvement in depressive symptoms [108]. Also, many antidepressant medications suppress REM sleep [109,110]. Support for this model has waned over time, in part due to findings that TSD has more potent antidepressant effects than selective REM deprivation [111] and, in part, because several effective antidepressant medications were identified that did not have REM-suppressant effects (see below).

Primary defect hypothesis

Others have argued that REM-related phenomena in depression represent, not an increase of REM pressure, but a decrease in SWS sleep drive that is due to a deficiency in the homeostatic sleep process. This "primary defect hypothesis" [17] is supported by the reductions in SWS and delta activity found in some studies of depression, as described previously. Thus REM sleep is "released" earlier in the sleep cycle because of the reduced homeostatic drive. Sleep deprivation has its antidepressant effects by increasing homeostatic drive, and the relapse to depression seen after recovery sleep occurs because of the subsequent return to low levels of drive. As most antidepressant medications do not increase SWS, and some may even reduce SWS or delta activity, this would suggest that effective treatment does not remediate the proposed primary deficit associated with depressive vulnerability.

Phase advance hypothesis

Whereas the models described thus far have focused on sleep abnormalities, the phase advance hypothesis emphasizes circadian rhythm disturbance in the etiology of depression [112]. According to this hypothesis, the phase advance seen in circadian rhythms is a cause rather than a consequence of depression. A variation of the phase advance hypothesis called the internal phase coincidence model, argues that depression occurs because the phase advance leads to awakenings at a sensitive phase of the circadian period [113]. Riemann and colleagues tested the effects of imposing a phase advanced sleep schedule (5 p.m. to midnight) compared to a typical schedule (11 p.m. to 6 a.m.) in patients in remission from depression [114]. Individuals in the advanced schedule group had fewer relapses to depression, suggesting that realigning the sleep schedule to match endogenous circadian timing may have antidepressant effects. However, as described above, the evidence of a phase advance in depressed patients is mixed, with many studies failing to find any circadian rhythm abnormalities, reducing the likelihood that this circadian abnormality plays a significant role.

Shared neurobiology

Another possibility is that insomnia *per se* does not lead to depression, but a common neurophysiological substrate gives rise to both depression symptoms and sleep abnormalities. In normal sleep, the cyclical NREM–REM pattern within each sleep cycle is driven by patterns of activity of a large number of neurotransmitters, including norepinephrine, serotonin, and acetylcholine [115,116] (see Chapter 2: Neuroanatomy

and neurobiology of sleep and wakefulness). These three neuronal systems are most active during waking. During NREM, aminergic (norepinephrine and serotonin) neuronal tracts are less active and cholinergic tracts are virtually silent. This pattern is reversed in REM sleep, with cholinergic activity reaching near-waking levels and aminergic activity reaching minimal levels. Self-regulatory negative feedback loops orchestrate the interplay of NREM and REM sleep.

Increased cholinergic activity and/or decreased aminergic activity could disrupt this pattern and produce the altered REM architecture of depression. This has been called the cholinergic/aminergic imbalance hypothesis [52]. In support of this hypothesis, patients with depression have been found to have increased sensitivity to REM sleep induction by cholinergic agonists as compared to non-depressed controls [117]. Gillin and colleagues [118] administered scopolamine, a cholinergic agonist, to non-depressed participants and monitored sleep. Subjects exhibited the shortened REM latency and increased REM density seen in depressed patients, leading the authors to propose that cholinergic supersensitivity plays a primary role in the etiology of depression, including non-sleep symptoms [118]. Cholinergic–aminergic imbalance also has been linked to HPA axis activation, which is seen in more severe depressive states [119]. Thus, cholinergic/aminergic imbalance remains a plausible neurobiological substrate for both depression and sleep disturbance.

Treatment of insomnia in the context of depression

Antidepressant treatment alone

Before discussing treatment options specifically for insomnia in patients with depression, it is important to examine the impact of antidepressants on sleep in general as they can both promote and interfere with sleep. The effects of each antidepressant class on sleep can be summarized as follows:

- Tricyclic antidepressants, which are thought to exert their effects through the modulation of the monoamine neurotransmitter norepinephrine and, to a lesser extent, serotonin, are moderate REM sleep suppressors and, depending on other secondary effects (i.e. antagonism of histamine and serotonin type 2 receptors), have sedating properties

- Monoamine oxidase inhibitors, which decrease the intraneuronal degradation of norepinephrine, serotonin, and dopamine, are potent REM sleep suppressants and, for some patients, negatively impact sleep continuity [120]
- Selective serotonin reuptake inhibitors (SSRIs), which initially increase the availability of serotonin at the synapse, suppress REM sleep and, for some patients, decrease total sleep time, reduce sleep efficiency, and increase arousals [121]
- Serotonin and norepinephrine reuptake inhibitors, such as venlafaxine and duloxetine, have similar if not greater effects compared to the SSRIs [122]
- Bupropion, the only drug classified as a norepinephrine and dopamine reuptake inhibitor, has not been found in research studies to suppress REM sleep or appreciably affect sleep continuity [123], although clinical experience suggests it can interfere with sleep initiation in some people.

Aside from the more sedating TCAs (e.g. amitriptyline, doxepin, and trimipramine), trazodone, nefazodone, and mirtazapine are the only antidepressant medications that reliably improve sleep continuity [124]. Although these medications are not widely used in the USA for their antidepressant properties (in part because they are considered only modestly efficacious as antidepressants), trazodone is commonly used off-label for the treatment of insomnia, both alone and in combination with SSRIs and SNRIs. The widespread use of trazodone is somewhat puzzling. On the one hand, it is not a controlled substance; it does not have abuse liability, and is typically used in lower doses that do not have appreciable side-effects. On the other hand, its efficacy as a hypnotic has not been well studied (i.e. there are little to no data to suggest that it produces clinical outcomes, acutely or in the long term, that are comparable to traditional therapy with benzodiazepines and/or benzodiazepine receptor agonists) and the medication itself can have significant cardiovascular side-effects in vulnerable patients (such as the elderly) [125]. There is also the rare occurrence of priapism in men, which if not managed, can result in permanent structural and functional damage. For these reasons, the data suggest trazodone is less than ideal for the management of insomnia than is reflected by its extremely common use as a sedative-hypnotic. However, lack of evidence is not synonomous with evidence of inefficacy, and clinical experience suggests

trazodone does have a place in the pharmacological armamentarium for management of insomnia, particularly associated with depression; however, it is not clear that trazodone deserves its place as the de facto first-line agent.

Adjunctive treatment with sedative-hypnotics

Insomnia that occurs in the context of depression is frequently treated with adjunctive medication. The efficacy of benzodiazepines (e.g. temazepam) and benzodiazepine receptor agonists (BzRAs; e.g. zolpidem, eszopiclone) has been demonstrated in several studies [126–128]. Treatment has been shown to produce both objective and subjective improvements in sleep, as in patients with primary insomnia (see Chapter 13: Treatment of insomnia: pharmacotherapy). The BzRAs may have a safer side-effect profile and lower abuse potential compared to benzodiazepines and are approved for long-term use [129].

There have been concerns that adjunctive treatment with a sedative-hypnotic could interfere with antidepressant treatment response. The data, however, suggest just the opposite; adjunctive treatment with BzRAs can augment the efficacy of antidepressants, particularly in terms of daytime symptoms [126,127]. This is reasonable to expect since some of the daytime symptoms of depression, such as fatigue and irritability, can also be related to poor sleep. In fact, one treatment option is to intentionally focus on the daytime symptoms of depression rather than nocturnal sleep. The wake-promoting agent modafinil has been used to treat fatigue and sleepiness in patients with depression [130,131]. Treatment improved daytime fatigue and sleepiness and, in one study, was associated with improvements in depression as well. The benefits have been shown to be sustained over a period of 12 weeks [132], but longer-term treatment studies are needed.

In recent years there has been increased prescription of selected second-generation antipsychotic medications such as quetiapine and olanzapine in combination with antidepressants for relief of insomnia and concomitant anxiety. Although at least one of these medications has now been approved by the FDA for adjunctive treatment of depression use, this approval specifically pertains to patients who have had an inadequate response to adequate trials of antidepressants, not simply as a targeted therapy for persistent insomnia.

Although there is ample clinical evidence that adjunctive olanzapine or quetiapine can have sedative effects, there has been insufficient research to document the benefits of this strategy in relation to their medical risks. Specifically, the more sedating second-generation antipsychotics are associated with the greatest risks of weight gain, dyslipidemia, and hyperglycemia [133] and, although improvements over the first generation of medications, they are associated with some risk of extrapyramidal symptoms and, across extended courses of therapy, tardive dyskinesia. These medications also are extremely expensive options when compared to generic benzodiazepines.

Non-pharmacological treatments

Cognitive behavioral treatment of insomnia (CBT-I) has demonstrated efficacy and effectiveness for treatment of primary insomnia [134–136]. There is a growing body of evidence that CBT-I may be equally effective in patients with insomnia co-morbid with medical or psychiatric conditions [137]. CBT-I consists of several different strategies including stimulus control, sleep restriction, sleep hygiene, and cognitive restructuring. Other components may include training in relaxation exercises and cognitive strategies such as the use of behavioral experiments (see Chapter 14: Cognitive behavioral therapy for insomnia for more detail on CBT-I).

To date, there are only two small studies of CBT-I in patients with insomnia in the context of depression. In the first preliminary study, Taylor and colleagues delivered CBT-I to patients with mild depression in an individual format over six visits in a pilot study [138]. Despite the fact that there were no depression-focused intervention components, there were clinically significant improvements in sleep including sleep latency, total sleep time, wake after sleep onset, and sleep efficiency. These results (which were maintained at a 3-month follow-up) were paralleled by a decrease in depressive symptomatology such that 87.5% of patients enrolled in the trial were within normal limits on the BDI following treatment. In the second study, Manber and colleagues [139] delivered CBT-I or a control condition as an adjunct to escitalopram treatment in patients with depression and insomnia. The CBT-I group, compared to those in the control treatment, experienced greater rates of remission from insomnia (50.0% vs. 7.7%) and from depression (61.5% vs. 33.3%) by the end of the acute phase treatment protocol. While these studies represent initial ventures into this area of research, the results suggest that cognitive behavioral interventions that are sleep focused are effective in patients with depression, as adjunctive treatment or as a stand-alone intervention.

A second non-pharmacological treatment option is bright light exposure. Light therapy has been used primarily for seasonal affective disorder but there is growing evidence that it is effective in non-seasonal depression as well. For example, Benedetti and colleagues [140] used adjunctive morning bright light during the first 2 weeks of citalopram treatment and found a larger and more rapid treatment response compared to patients who received medication alone. Of note, the timing of the light treatment was chosen to produce a 2-hour phase advance in circadian rhythms. They also made use of light in the blue-green portion of the spectrum rather than full-spectrum white light since this color seems to be optimal for circadian phase shifting effects [141]. While this study focused on depression-related outcomes rather than sleep *per se*, the results suggest that bright light therapy may be an effective adjunctive treatment for depression.

Summary remarks: why treat insomnia in the context of depression?

There is a long history of research investigating the relationship between sleep disturbance and depression. Sleep abnormalities include disturbances in sleep continuity, sleep architecture, quantitative EEG, circadian rhythms, and CNS arousal. There is considerable consistency across these domains for increases in REM-related activity and decreases in slow-wave sleep. The role of sleep as a cause versus a consequence of depression has been considered in a number of theories and hypotheses. As is often the case, individual theories have emerged and then faded over time as contradictory evidence is uncovered. This is unfortunate since it is highly unlikely that depression is a homogenous condition. Thus there may be multiple mechanisms through which sleep and depression influence each other.

In concert with the development of etiological theories has been the development of options for treating disturbed sleep in the context of depression. Pharmacological treatment options include the use of sedating antidepressants and/or adjunctive sedative-hypnotic agents. Cognitive behavioral treatment of insomnia, whose efficacy and effectiveness are well proven in primary insomnia, may offer a non-pharmacological treatment option as well. Regardless of treatment option, the current strategy is to provide insomnia treatment in patients with depression. While this seems logical on the surface, management of sleep disturbance may offer a means for delaying or preventing an episode of depression from occurring in the first place. The evidence that insomnia is a risk factor for new-onset and recurrent depression suggests that successful treatment of insomnia in non-depressed individuals has the potential for preventing future depressive episodes. This is a virtually unexplored domain of clinical research that holds tremendous potential for the future.

References

1. American Psychiatric Association. *Diagnostic and statistical manual of mental disorders*, 4th ed. Washington, DC: American Psychiatric Association; 1994.

2. Tsuno N, Besset A, Ritchie K. Sleep and depression. *J Clin Psychiatry*. 2005;**66**(10):1254–1269.

3. Posternak MA, Zimmerman M. Symptoms of atypical depression. *Psychiatry Res*. 2001;**104**(2):175–181.

4. Roberts RE, Shema SJ, Kaplan GA, Strawbridge WJ. Sleep complaints and depression in an aging cohort: A prospective perspective. *Am J Psychiatry*. 2000; **157**(1):81–88.

5. American Academy of Sleep Medicine. *International classification of sleep disorders*, 2nd ed. Westchester, IL: American Academy of Sleep Medicine; 2005.

6. Mendelson W, Garnett D, Gillin J, Weingartner H. The experience of insomnia and daytime and nighttime functioning. *Psychiatry Res*. 1984;**12**:235–250.

7. Perlis M, Giles D, Mendelson W, Bootzin R, Wyatt J. Psychophysiological insomnia: The behavioural model and a neurocognitive perspective. *J Sleep Res*. 1997;**6**:179–188.

8. Hauri P, Olmstead E. Childhood-onset insomnia. *Sleep*. 1980;**3**(1):59–65.

9. Perlis ML, Giles DE, Buysse DJ, et al. Which depressive symptoms are related to which sleep electroencephalographic variables? *Biol Psychiatry*. 1997;**42**(10):904–913.

10. Perlis M, Smith M, Andrews P, Orff H, Giles D. Beta/gamma EEG activity in patients with primary and secondary insomnia and good sleeper controls. *Sleep*. 2001;**24**:110–117.

11. Riemann D, Hohagen F, Bahro M, Berger M. Sleep in depression: The influence of age, gender and diagnostic subtype on baseline sleep and the cholinergic REM induction test with RS 86. *Eur Arch Psychiatry Clin Neurosci*. 1994;**243**(5):279–290.

12. Spielman A, Caruso L, Glovinsky P. A behavioral perspective on insomnia treatment. *Psychiatr Clin North Am*. 1987;**10**:541–553.

13. Kupfer DJ, Reynolds CF 3rd, Ulrich RF, Grochocinski VJ. Comparison of automated REM and slow-wave sleep analysis in young and middle-aged depressed subjects. *Biol Psychiatry*. 1986;**21** (2):189–200.

14. Rush AJ, Erman MK, Giles DE, et al. Polysomnographic findings in recently drug-free and clinically remitted depressed patients. *Arch Gen Psychiatry*. 1986;**43**(9):878–884.

15. Kerkhofs M, Hoffmann G, De Martelaere V, Linkowski P, Mendlewicz J. Sleep EEG recordings in depressive disorders. *J Affect Disord*. 1985;**9**(1):47–53.

16. Gillin JC, Mendelson WB. Acetylcholine, sleep, and depression. *Human Neurobiol*. 1982;**1**:211–219.

17. Borbely AA, Wirz-Justice A. Sleep, sleep deprivation and depression: A hypothesis derived from a model of sleep regulation. *Hum Neurobiol*. 1982;**1**(3):205–210.

18. Vogel GW, Vogel F, McAbee RS, Thurmond AJ. Improvement of depression by REM sleep deprivation. *Arch Gen Psychiatry*. 1980;**37**:247–253.

19. Benca RM, Obermeyer WH, Thisted RA, Gillin JC. Sleep and psychiatric disorders: A meta-analysis. *Arch Gen Psychiatry*. 1992;**49**:651–670.

20. Armitage R. Microarchitectural findings in sleep EEG in depression: Diagnostic implications. *Biol Psychiatry*. 1995;**37**(2):72–84.

21. Borbely AA, Tobler I, Loepfe M, et al. All-night spectral analysis of the sleep EEG in untreated depressives and normal controls. *Psychiatry Res*. 1984; **12**(1):27–33.

22. Kupfer DJ, Ulrich RF, Coble PA, et al. Application of automated REM and slow wave sleep analysis: II. testing the assumptions of the two-process model of sleep regulation in normal and depressed subjects. *Psychiatry Res*. 1984;**13**(4):335–343.

23. Mendelson WB, Sack DA, James SP, et al. Frequency analysis of the sleep EEG in depression. *Psychiatry Res*. 1987;**21**:89–94.

24. Armitage R, Calhoun JS, Rush AJ, Roffwarg HP. Comparison of the delta EEG in the first and second non-REM periods in depressed adults and normal controls. *Psychiatry Res*. 1992;**41**(1):65–72.

25. Hoffmann R, Hendrickse W, Rush AJ, Armitage R. Slow-wave activity during non-REM sleep in men with schizophrenia and major depressive disorders. *Psychiatry Res*. 2000;**95**(3):215–225.

26. Perlis M, Merica H, Smith M, Giles D. Beta EEG activity and insomnia. *Sleep Med Rev.* 2001;**5**:365–376.

27. Goodwin FK, Wirz-Justice A, Wehr TA. Evidence that the pathophysiology of depression and the mechanism of action of antidepressant drugs both involve alterations in circadian rhythms. In: Costa E, Racagni G, eds. *Typical and atypical antidepressants: clinical practice.* New York: Raven Press; 1982:1–11.

28. Koenigsberg HW, Teicher MH, Mitropoulou V, et al. 24-h monitoring of plasma norepinephrine, MHPG, cortisol, growth hormone and prolactin in depression. *J Psychiatr Res.* 2004;**38**(5):503–511.

29. David MM, MacLean AW, Knowles JB, Coulter ME. Rapid eye movement latency and mood following a delay of bedtime in healthy subjects: Do the effects mimic changes in depressive illness? *Acta Psychiatr Scand.* 1991;**84**(1):33–39.

30. Gillin JC, Borbely AA. Sleep: A neurobiological window on affective disorders. *TINS.* 1985:537–541.

31. Souetre E, Salvati E, Belugou JL, et al. Circadian rhythms in depression and recovery: Evidence for blunted amplitude as the main chronobiological abnormality. *Psychiatry Res.* 1989;**28**(3):263–278.

32. Nofzinger EA, Nichols TE, Meltzer CC, et al. Changes in forebrain function from waking to REM sleep in depression: Preliminary analyses of [18F]FDG PET studies. *Psychiatry Res.* 1999;**91**(2):59–78.

33. Ho AP, Gillin JC, Buchsbaum MS, et al. Brain glucose metabolism during non-rapid eye movement sleep in major depression: A positron emission tomography study. *Arch Gen Psychiatry.* 1996;**53**(7):645–652.

34. Germain A, Nofzinger EA, Kupfer DJ, Buysse DJ. Neurobiology of non-REM sleep in depression: Further evidence for hypofrontality and thalamic dysregulation. *Am J Psychiatry.* 2004;**161**(10):1856–1863.

35. Nofzinger EA, Buysse DJ, Germain A, et al. Functional neuroimaging evidence for hyperarousal in insomnia. *Am J Psychiatry.* 2004;**161**(11):2126–2128.

36. Friess E, Wiedemann K, Steiger A, Holsboer F. The hypothalamic-pituitary-adrenocortical system and sleep in man. *Adv Neuroimmunol.* 1995;**5**(2):111–125.

37. Ehlers C, Kupfer D. Hypothalamic peptide modulation of EEG sleep in depression: A further application of the S-process hypothesis. *Biol Psychiatry.* 1987;**22**:513–517.

38. Richardson GS. Human physiological models of insomnia. *Sleep Med.* 2007;**8**(Suppl 4):S9–14.

39. Wu JC, Bunney WE. The biological basis of an antidepressant response to sleep deprivation and relapse: Review and hypothesis. *Am J Psychiatry.* 1990;**147**:14–21.

40. Reinink E, Bouhuys N, Wirz-Justice A, van den Hoofdakker R. Prediction of the antidepressant response to total sleep deprivation by diurnal variation of mood. *Psychiatry Res.* 1990;**32**(2):113–124.

41. Van den Hoofdakker RH. Total sleep deprivation: Clinical and theoretical aspects. In: Honig A, ed. *Depression.* London: John Wiley & Sons; 1997:563–589.

42. Wu JC, Gillin JC, Buchsbaum MS, et al. Effect of sleep deprivation on brain metabolism of depressed patients. *Am J Psychiatry.* 1992;**149**(4):538–543.

43. Wu J, Buchsbaum MS, Gillin JC, et al. Prediction of antidepressant effects of sleep deprivation by metabolic rates in the ventral anterior cingulate and medial prefrontal cortex. *Am J Psychiatry.* 1999;**156**(8):1149–1158.

44. Smith GS, Reynolds CF 3rd, Pollock B, et al. Cerebral glucose metabolic response to combined total sleep deprivation and antidepressant treatment in geriatric depression. *Am J Psychiatry.* 1999;**156**(5):683–689.

45. Ebert D, Feistel H, Barocka A. Effects of sleep deprivation on the limbic system and the frontal lobes in affective disorders: A study with tc-99m-HMPAO SPECT. *Psychiatry Res.* 1991;**40**(4):247–251.

46. Ebert D, Feistel H, Barocka A, Kaschka W. Increased limbic blood flow and total sleep deprivation in major depression with melancholia. *Psychiatry Res.* 1994; **55**(2):101–109.

47. Volk SA, Kaendler SH, Hertel A, et al. Can response to partial sleep deprivation in depressed patients be predicted by regional changes of cerebral blood flow? *Psychiatry Res.* 1997;**75**(2):67–74.

48. Volk S, Kaendler SH, Weber R, et al. Evaluation of the effects of total sleep deprivation on cerebral blood flow using single photon emission computerized tomography. *Acta Psychiatr Scand.* 1992;**86**(6):478–483.

49. Porkka-Heiskanen T, Strecker RE, McCarley RW. Brain site-specificity of extracellular adenosine concentration changes during sleep deprivation and spontaneous sleep: An in vivo microdialysis study. *Neuroscience.* 2000;**99**(3):507–517.

50. Basheer R, Halldner L, Alanko L, et al. Opposite changes in adenosine A1 and A2A receptor mRNA in the rat following sleep deprivation. *Neuroreport.* 2001;**12**(8):1577–1580.

51. Biber K, Fiebich BL, Gebicke-Harter P, van Calker D. Carbamazepine-induced upregulation of adenosine A1-receptors in astrocyte cultures affects coupling to the phosphoinositol signaling pathway. *Neuropsychopharmacology.* 1999;**20**(3):271–278.

52. Janowsky DS, El-Yousef MK, Davis JM. A cholinergic-adrenergic hypothesis of mania and depression. *Lancet.* 1972;**2**:632–635.

53. Svestka J. Sleep deprivation therapy. *Neuro Endocrinol Lett.* 2008;**29**(Suppl 1):65–92.

54. Grözinger M, Kögel P, Röschke J. Effects of REM sleep awakenings and related wakening paradigms on the ultradian sleep cycle and the symptoms in depression. *J Psychiatr Res.* 2002;**36**(5):299–308.

55. Breslau N, Roth T, Rosenthal L, Andreski P. Sleep disturbance and psychiatric disorders: A longitudinal epidemiological study of young adults. *Biol Psychiatry.* 1996;**39**(6):411–418.

56. Chang PP, Ford DE, Mead LA, Cooper-Patrick L, Klag MJ. Insomnia in young men and subsequent depression: the Johns Hopkins precursors study. *Am J Epidemiol.* 1997;**146**(2):105–114.

57. Dryman A, Eaton WW. Affective symptoms associated with the onset of major depression in the community: Findings from the US National Institute of Mental Health epidemiologic catchment area program. *Acta Psychiatr Scand.* 1991;**84**(1):1–5.

58. Ford D, Kamerow D. Epidemiologic study of sleep disturbance and psychiatric disorders: An opportunity for prevention? *JAMA.* 1989;**262**:1479–1484.

59. Hohagen F, Rink K, Kappler C, et al. Prevalence and treatment of insomnia in general practice: A longitudinal study. *Eur Arch Psychiatry Clin Neurosci.* 1993;**242**(6):329–336.

60. Kennedy GJ, Kelman HR, Thomas C. Persistence and remission of depressive symptoms in late life. *Am J Psychiatry.* 1991;**148**(2):174–178.

61. Livingston G, Blizard B, Mann A. Does sleep disturbance predict depression in elderly people? A study in Inner London. *Br J Gen Pract.* 1993;**43** (376):445–448.

62. Livingston G, Watkin V, Milne B, Manela MV, Katona C. Who becomes depressed? The Islington community study of older people. *J Affect Disord.* 2000; **58**(2):125–133.

63. Mallon L, Broman JE, Hetta J. Relationship between insomnia, depression, and mortality: A 12-year follow-up of older adults in the community. *Int Psychogeriatr.* 2000;**12**(3):295–306.

64. Paffenbarger RS Jr, Lee IM, Leung R. Physical activity and personal characteristics associated with depression and suicide in American college men. *Acta Psychiatr Scand Suppl.* 1994;**377**:16–22.

65. Perlis ML, Smith LJ, Lyness JM, et al. Insomnia as a risk factor for onset of depression in the elderly. *Behav Sleep Med.* 2006;**4**(2):104–113.

66. Vollrath M, Wicki W, Angst J. The Zurich study. VIII. Insomnia: Association with depression, anxiety, somatic syndromes, and course of insomnia. *Eur Arch Psychiatry Neurol Sci.* 1989;**239**(2):113–124.

67. Weissman M, Greenwald S, Nino-Murcia G, Dement W. The morbidity of insomnia uncomplicated by

psychiatric disorders. *Gen Hosp Psychiatry.* 1997;**19**:245–250.

68. Gregory AM, Rijsdijk FV, Lau JY, Dahl RE, Eley TC. The direction of longitudinal associations between sleep problems and depression symptoms: A study of twins aged 8 and 10 years. *Sleep.* 2009;**32**(2):189–199.

69. Buysse DJ, Angst J, Gamma A, et al. Prevalence, course, and comorbidity of insomnia and depression in young adults. *Sleep.* 2008;**31**(4):473–480.

70. Jansson-Frojmark M, Lindblom K. A bidirectional relationship between anxiety and depression, and insomnia? A prospective study in the general population. *J Psychosom Res.* 2008;**64**(4):443–449.

71. Morphy H, Dunn KM, Lewis M, Boardman HF, Croft PR. Epidemiology of insomnia: A longitudinal study in a UK population. *Sleep.* 2007;**30**(3):274–280.

72. Neckelmann D, Mykletun A, Dahl AA. Chronic insomnia as a risk factor for developing anxiety and depression. *Sleep.* 2007;**30**(7):873–880.

73. Gregory AM, Caspi A, Eley TC, et al. Prospective longitudinal associations between persistent sleep problems in childhood and anxiety and depression disorders in adulthood. *J Abnorm Child Psychol.* 2005;**33**(2):157–163.

74. Ohayon M, Roth T. Place of chronic insomnia in the course of depressive and anxiety disorders. *J Psychiatr Res.* 2003;**37**:9–15.

75. Perlis ML, Giles DE, Buysse DJ, Tu X, Kupfer DJ. Self-reported sleep disturbance as a prodromal symptom in recurrent depression. *J Affect Disord.* 1997;**42**(2–3): 209–212.

76. Carney CE, Segal ZV, Edinger JD, Krystal AD. A comparison of rates of residual insomnia symptoms following pharmacotherapy or cognitive-behavioral therapy for major depressive disorder. *J Clin Psychiatry.* 2007;**68**(2):254–260.

77. Dombrovski AY, Mulsant BH, Houck PR, et al. Residual symptoms and recurrence during maintenance treatment of late-life depression. *J Affect Disord.* 2007;**103**(1–3):77–82.

78. Manber R, Rush AJ, Thase ME, et al. The effects of psychotherapy, nefazodone, and their combination on subjective assessment of disturbed sleep in chronic depression. *Sleep.* 2003;**26**(2):130–136.

79. Thase ME, Fasiczka AL, Berman SR, Simons AD, Reynolds CF 3rd. Electroencephalographic sleep profiles before and after cognitive behavior therapy of depression. *Arch Gen Psychiatry.* 1998; **55**(2):138–144.

80. Pigeon WR, Hegel M, Unutzer J, et al. Is insomnia a perpetuating factor for late-life depression in the IMPACT cohort? *Sleep.* 2008;**31**(4):481–488.

81. Karp JF, Buysse DJ, Houck PR, et al. Relationship of variability in residual symptoms with recurrence of major depressive disorder during maintenance treatment. *Am J Psychiatry*. 2004;**161**(10):1877–1884.

82. Paykel ES, Ramana R, Cooper Z, et al. Residual symptoms after partial remission: An important outcome in depression. *Psychol Med*. 1995;**25**(6):1171–1180.

83. Buysse DJ, Frank E, Lowe KK, Cherry CR, Kupfer DJ. Electroencephalographic sleep correlates of episode and vulnerability to recurrence in depression. *Biol Psychiatry*. 1997;**41**(4):406–418.

84. Buysse DJ, Jarrett DB, Miewald JM, Kupfer DJ, Greenhouse JB. Minute-by-minute analysis of REM sleep timing in major depression. *Biol Psychiatry*. 1990;**28**(10):911–925.

85. Kupfer DJ, Reynolds CF 3rd, Grochocinski VJ, Ulrich RF, McEachran A. Aspects of short REM latency in affective states: A revisit. *Psychiatry Res*. 1986;**17**(1):49–59.

86. Coble PA, Kupfer DJ, Spiker DG, Neil JF, McPartland RJ. EEG sleep in primary depression: A longitudinal placebo study. *J Affect Disord*. 1979;**1**(2):131–138.

87. Giles DE, Etzel BA, Reynolds CF 3rd, Kupfer DJ. Stability of polysomnographic parameters in unipolar depression: A cross-sectional report. *Biol Psychiatry*. 1989;**25**(6):807–810.

88. Lee JH, Reynolds CF 3rd, Hoch CC, et al. Electroencephalographic sleep in recently remitted, elderly depressed patients in double-blind placebo-maintenance therapy. *Neuropsychopharmacology*. 1993;**8**(2):143–150.

89. Thase ME, Reynolds CF 3rd, Frank E, et al. Polysomnographic studies of unmedicated depressed men before and after cognitive behavioral therapy. *Am J Psychiatry*. 1994;**151**(11):1615–1622.

90. Buysse DJ, Kupfer DJ, Frank E, et al. Electroencephalographic sleep studies in depressed outpatients treated with interpersonal psychotherapy: I. Baseline studies in responders and nonresponders. *Psychiatry Res*. 1992;**42**(1):13–26.

91. Cartwright RD. Rapid eye movement sleep characteristics during and after mood-disturbing events. *Arch Gen Psychiatry*. 1983;**40**(2):197–201.

92. Nofzinger EA, Schwartz RM, Reynolds CF 3rd, et al. Affect intensity and phasic REM sleep in depressed men before and after treatment with cognitive-behavioral therapy. *J Consult Clin Psychol*. 1994;**62**(1):83–91.

93. Spiker DG, Coble P, Cofsky J, Foster FG, Kupfer DJ. EEG sleep and severity of depression. *Biol Psychiatry*. 1978;**13**(4):485–488.

94. Zarcone VP Jr, Benson KL. Increased REM eye movement density in self-rated depression. *Psychiatry Res*. 1983;**8**(1):65–71.

95. Simons AD, Thase ME. Biological markers, treatment outcome, and 1-year follow-up in endogenous depression: Electroencephalographic sleep studies and response to cognitive therapy. *J Consult Clin Psychol*. 1992;**60**(3):392–401.

96. Rao U, Hammen CL, Poland RE. Risk markers for depression in adolescents: Sleep and HPA measures. *Neuropsychopharmacology*. 2009;**34**(8):1936–1945.

97. Jarrett RB, Rush AJ, Khatami M, Roffwarg HP. Does the pretreatment polysomnogram predict response to cognitive therapy in depressed outpatients? A preliminary report. *Psychiatry Res*. 1990;**33**(3):285–299.

98. Kupfer DJ, Spiker DG, Coble PA, et al. Sleep and treatment prediction in endogenous depression. *Am J Psychiatry*. 1981;**138**(4):429–434.

99. Rush AJ, Giles DE, Jarrett RB, et al. Reduced REM latency predicts response to tricyclic medication in depressed outpatients. *Biol Psychiatry*. 1989;**26**(1):61–72.

100. Svendsen K, Christensen PG. Duration of REM sleep latency as predictor of effect of antidepressant therapy. A preliminary report. *Acta Psychiatr Scand*. 1981;**64**(3):238–243.

101. Thase ME, Simons AD, Reynolds CF 3rd. Abnormal electroencephalographic sleep profiles in major depression: Association with response to cognitive behavior therapy. *Arch Gen Psychiatry*. 1996;**53**(2):99–108.

102. Giles DE, Jarrett RB, Biggs MM, Guzick DS, Rush AJ. Clinical predictors of recurrence in depression. *Am J Psychiatry*. 1989;**146**(6):764–767.

103. Grunhaus L, Shipley JE, Eiser A, et al. Shortened REM latency postECT is associated with rapid recurrence of depressive symptomatology. *Biol Psychiatry*. 1994;**36**(4):214–222.

104. Kupfer DJ, Frank E, McEachran AB, Grochocinski VJ. Delta sleep ratio. A biological correlate of early recurrence in unipolar affective disorder. *Arch Gen Psychiatry*. 1990;**47**(12):1100–1105.

105. Adrien J. Neurobiological bases for the relation between sleep and depression. *Sleep Med Rev*. 2002;**6**(5):341–351.

106. Perlis M, Smith M, Orff H. Commentary. *Sleep Med Rev*. 2002;**6**(5):353–357.

107. Pigeon WR, Perlis ML. Insomnia and depression: Birds of a feather? *Int J Sleep Disorders*. 2007;**1**(3):82–91.

108. Wirz-Justice A, Van den Hoofdakker RH. Sleep deprivation in depression: What do we know, where do we go? *Biol Psychiatry*. 1999;**46**:445–453.

109. Vogel GW. Evidence for REM sleep deprivation as the mechanism of action of antidepressant drugs. *Prog Neuro-Psychopharmacol Biol Psychiatry*. 1983;7: 343–349.

110. Vogel GW, Buffenstein A, Minter K, Hennessey A. Drug effects on REM sleep and on endogenous depression. *Neurosci Biobehav Rev*. 1990;14:49–63.

111. Giedke H, Schwarzler F. Therapeutic use of sleep deprivation in depression. *Sleep Med Rev*. 2002;6(5): 361–377.

112. Wehr TA, Wirz-Justice A, Goodwin FK, Duncan W, Gillin JC. Phase advance of the circadian sleep-wake cycle as an antidepressant. *Science*. 1979;206:710–713.

113. Wehr TA, Wirz-Justice A. Internal coincidence model for sleep deprivation and depression. In: Koella WP, ed. *Sleep 1980*. Basel: Karger; 1981:26–33.

114. Riemann D, Hohagen F, Konig A, et al. Advanced vs. normal sleep timing: Effects on depressed mood after response to sleep deprivation in patients with a major depressive disorder. *J Affect Disord*. 1996;37(2–3):121–128.

115. Hobson JA, McCarley RW, Wyzinski PW. Sleep cycle oscillation: Reciprocal discharge by two brainstem neuronal groups. *Science*. 1975;4196:55–58.

116. McCarley RW, Hobson JA. Neuronal excitability modulation over the sleep cycle: A structural and mathematical model. *Science*. 1975;189:58–60.

117. Gillin JC, Sutton L, Ruiz C, et al. The cholinergic rapid eye movement induction test with arecoline in depression. *Arch Gen Psychiatry*. 1991;48(3):264–270.

118. Gillin JC, Sitaram N, Duncan WC. Muscarinic supersensitivity: A possible model for the sleep disturbance of primary depression? *Psychiatr Res*. 1979;1:17–22.

119. Risch SC, Janowsky DS, Mott MA, et al. Central and peripheral cholinesterase inhibition: Effects on anterior pituitary and sympathomimetic function. *Psychoneuroendocrinology*. 1986;11(2):221–230.

120. Mayers AG, Baldwin DS. Antidepressants and their effect on sleep. *Hum Psychopharmacol*. 2005;20(8): 533–559.

121. Jindal RD, Friedman ES, Berman SR, et al. Effects of sertraline on sleep architecture in patients with depression. *J Clin Psychopharmacol*. 2003;23(6): 540–548.

122. Guelfi JD, Ansseau M, Timmerman L, Korsgaard S, Mirtazapine-Venlafaxine Study Group. Mirtazapine versus venlafaxine in hospitalized severely depressed patients with melancholic features. *J Clin Psychopharmacol*. 2001;21(4):425–431.

123. Nofzinger EA, Berman S, Fasiczka A, et al. Effects of bupropion SR on anterior paralimbic function during waking and REM sleep in depression: Preliminary findings using [^{18}F]-FDG PET. *Psychiatry Res*. 2001;106(2):95–111.

124. Thase ME. Depression and sleep: Pathophysiology and treatment. *Dialogues Clin Neurosci*. 2006;8(2): 217–226.

125. James SP, Mendelson WB. The use of trazodone as a hypnotic: A critical review. *J Clin Psychiatry*. 2004; 65(6):752–755.

126. Asnis GM, Chakraburtty A, DuBoff EA, et al. Zolpidem for persistent insomnia in SSRI-treated depressed patients. *J Clin Psychiatry*. 1999;60(10):668–676.

127. Fava M, McCall WV, Krystal A, et al. Eszopiclone co-administered with fluoxetine in patients with insomnia coexisting with major depressive disorder. *Biol Psychiatry*. 2006;59(11):1052–1060.

128. Nowell PD, Buysse DJ. Treatment of insomnia in patients with mood disorders. *Depress Anxiety*. 2001; 14(1):7–18.

129. Walsh JK, Krystal AD, Amato DA, et al. Nightly treatment of primary insomnia with eszopiclone for six months: Effect on sleep, quality of life, and work limitations. *Sleep*. 2007;30(8):959–968.

130. Fava M, Thase ME, DeBattista C, et al. Modafinil augmentation of selective serotonin reuptake inhibitor therapy in MDD partial responders with persistent fatigue and sleepiness. *Ann Clin Psychiatry*. 2007; 19(3):153–159.

131. DeBattista C, Doghramji K, Menza MA, Rosenthal MH, Fieve RR, Modafinil in Depression Study Group. Adjunct modafinil for the short-term treatment of fatigue and sleepiness in patients with major depressive disorder: A preliminary double-blind, placebo-controlled study. *J Clin Psychiatry*. 2003;64(9): 1057–1064.

132. Thase ME, Fava M, DeBattista C, Arora S, Hughes RJ. Modafinil augmentation of SSRI therapy in patients with major depressive disorder and excessive sleepiness and fatigue: A 12-week, open-label, extension study. *CNS Spectr*. 2006;11(2):93–102.

133. Newcomer JW. Metabolic considerations in the use of antipsychotic medications: A review of recent evidence. *J Clin Psychiatry*. 2007;68(Suppl 1): 20–27.

134. Murtagh DR, Greenwood KM. Identifying effective psychological treatments for insomnia: A meta-analysis. *J Consult Clin Psychol*. 1995;63:79–89.

135. Morin CM, Culbert JP, Schwartz MS. Non-pharmacological interventions for insomnia: A meta-analysis of treatment efficacy. *Am J Psychiatry*. 1994;151:1172–1180.

136. Smith MT, Perlis ML, Park A, et al. Comparative meta-analysis of pharmacotherapy and behavior therapy

for persistent insomnia. *Am J Psychiatry*. 2002;
159(1):5–11.

137. Stepanski EJ, Rybarczyk B. Emerging research on the treatment and etiology of secondary or comorbid insomnia. *Sleep Med Rev*. 2006;**10**(1):7–18.

138. Taylor DJ, Lichstein KL, Weinstock J, Sanford S, Temple JR. A pilot study of cognitive-behavioral therapy of insomnia in people with mild depression. *Behav Ther*. 2007;**38**(1):49–57.

139. Manber R, Edinger JD, San Pedro M. Combining escitalopram oxalate (ESCIT) and individual cognitive behavioral therapy for insomnia (CBTI) to improve depression outcome. *Sleep*. 2007;**30**:A232.

140. Benedetti F, Colombo C, Pontiggia A, et al. Morning light treatment hastens the antidepressant effect of citalopram: A placebo-controlled trial. *J Clin Psychiatry*. 2003;**64**(6):648–653.

141. Horne JA, Donlon J, Arendt J. Green light attenuates melatonin output and sleepiness during sleep deprivation. *Sleep*. 1991;**14**:233–240.

Endnote

1. Sleep continuity for the purpose of this chapter encompasses multiple descriptive measures of sleep initiation and maintenance. While the term is not formally part of the sleep lexicon, it has the heuristic value of being a global term whose meaning may be contrasted with the class of variables that corresponds to "sleep architecture" and "sleep microarchitecture."

Chapter 6

Bipolar disorder

David T. Plante and John W. Winkelman

Introduction

Sleep disturbance has long been recognized as an essential aspect of bipolar disorder. Emil Kraepelin, who first distinguished the fluctuating course of manic depression from the unremitting progression of dementia praecox, noted nearly a century ago:

> The attacks of manic-depressive insanity are invariably accompanied by all kinds of bodily changes. By far the most striking are the disorders of sleep and general nourishment. In mania sleep is in the more severe states of excitement always considerably encroached upon; sometimes there is even almost complete sleeplessness, at most interrupted for a few hours, which may last for weeks, even months . . . In the states of depression in spite of great need for sleep, . . . the patients lie for hours, sleepless in bed, . . . although even in bed they find no refreshment [1].

Although Kraepelin's observations have greatly influenced modern day nosological classifications of major mental illness, including sleep-related criteria for manic and depressive episodes as defined by the *Diagnostic and Statistical Manual*, our understanding of the biology of sleep regulation and its relationship to bipolar disorder continues to advance. As detailed in previous chapters (see Chapter 2: Neuroanatomy and neurobiology of sleep and wakefulness), current models suggest that the interaction of a circadian clock and homeostatic sleep drive governs sleep onset and maintenance. Thus, abnormalities in either the circadian mechanism or sleep homeostat could theoretically manifest as a disorder of the sleep–wake cycle [2,3]. However, the vast majority of experiments, especially those designed to probe sleep in psychiatric illness, are not designed to uncouple homeostatic and circadian processes, and thus the mechanisms underlying an observed disturbance of sleep and wakefulness are often not clear. This caveat is of particular import when evaluating the literature regarding sleep in bipolar disorder, as disruptions in both sleep and circadian rhythms have been described in these patients [4,5].

This chapter will detail sleep–wake disturbances in the three primary states of bipolar disorder: mania, depression, and euthymia. Mixed states will not be a separate focus of discussion due to a dearth of available literature. Additionally, this chapter will focus on bipolar disorder in adults; for discussion of sleep in pediatric bipolar disorder, the reader is directed to other chapters in this volume (Chapter 22: Pediatric mood and anxiety disorders). In keeping with the aims of this volume to be a rigorous, yet clinically useful, text, particular attention will be paid to sleep in the course and treatment of bipolar disorder, including pharmacological and behavioral methods for maintaining adequate sleep quality and quantity in these patients.

Sleep in mania

The relationship between sleep and the manic phase of bipolar illness involves the following aspects: (1) decreased need for sleep is a marker of mania; (2) sleep deprivation can induce mania; (3) sleep duration may predict manic episodes; and (4) sleep time may be a marker of response (and target of treatment) in mania. Each of these relationships will be addressed in what follows.

Decreased need for sleep as a marker of mania

Decreased need for sleep is one of seven characteristic symptoms of the manic phase of bipolar disorder, and is of high diagnostic value since the ability to maintain wakefulness and energy without sufficient sleep is

Foundations of Psychiatric Sleep Medicine, ed. John W. Winkelman and David T. Plante. Published by Cambridge University Press.
© Cambridge University Press 2010.

not observed in many other psychiatric or medical disorders [6]. As evidence of its relatively high specificity for bipolar disorder, decreased need for sleep, along with euphoria and grandiosity, described one half of all clinically validated bipolar I cases in the National Co-morbidity Survey, and formed the only manic symptom profile that could be validly assessed with the Composite International Diagnositc Interview (CIDI), a fully structured interview developed to generate diagnoses according to the definitions and criteria of the DSM-III-R and ICD-10 [7].

Although the ability to maintain energy without sleep is characteristic of mania, it is noteworthy that manic patients still require sleep to sustain life. Prior to the advent of modern psychiatric treatments (e.g. neuroleptics and benzodiazepines), severe cases of florid mania characterized by almost no sleep were at times reported to result in death [8]. These observations are similar to animal models of sleep deprivation in which animals predictably die from prolonged total sleep deprivation, despite significantly increased food intake [9].

That decreased sleep is also characteristic of mania is corroborated by objective (e.g. polysomnographic and actigraphic) measures. Although polysomnography in manic patients is technically difficult, such studies of unmedicated manic patients demonstrate shortened total sleep time, increased time awake in bed, and shortened REM latency – similar to polysomnographic parameters seen in depressed patients [10,11]. Also, longitudinal studies utilizing actigraphy to measure rest–activity patterns in patients hospitalized with mania or mixed episodes demonstrate decreased total sleep time with increased nocturnal activity compared to euthymic periods [12]. It is worth noting that sleep measures in mania may be confounded by the effects of motor hyperactivity since sleep architecture can be affected by increased daytime activity in normal subjects [13]. Additionally, manic patients demonstrate increased nocturnal cortisol and an advanced (i.e. earlier) nadir of cortisol secretion compared to healthy subjects; however, similar alterations have been observed in sleep deprivation paradigms [14,15]. Thus, it is not clear if polysomnographic abnormalities seen in mania are caused by the manic state *per se*, are secondary to other associated abnormalities (e.g. increased physical activity levels, changes in metabolic and endocrine function, etc.), or are the sequelae of sleep deprivation itself.

Sleep reduction as a cause of mania

Potential triggers for mania are vast and have been reported to include drug use (licit and illicit), transmeridinal travel, post-partum states, bereavement, etc., all of which may be associated with sleep loss [16–22]. However, in most such cases, it is unclear whether sleeplessness was a cause or prodrome of mania. Thus cause and effect cannot be determined from case reports alone, especially if early manic symptoms may have spurred the behavior (e.g. drug use, travel, etc.) which subsequently produced sleep deprivation.

However, therapeutic studies of sleep deprivation in unipolar and bipolar depression do provide causal evidence for the propensity for sleep deprivation to induce manic switching. Recent work in this area has been performed in well-characterized subjects; however, the older literature (before definitions of rapid-cycling were established) includes mixtures of patients with both rapid and non-rapid cycling patterns, as well as those with unipolar depression. Further complicating interpretation of the older literature is that the majority of early sleep deprivation studies were not designed to detect mania, depressed unipolar and bipolar patients were not distinguished from one another in reported results, and hypomania and mania were often reported *post hoc* [23,24]. A comprehensive review of the older therapeutic sleep deprivation literature found 29% of bipolar depressed subjects and 25% of unspecified depressed subjects became hypomanic or manic after one night of total sleep deprivation (TSD) [25]. However, examination of sleep deprivation studies with experimental design that was better suited for predicting the frequency of manic switching has estimated a risk of hypomania and mania of 12% and 7%, respectively, with TSD [26]. More recently, Colombo et al. (1999), reviewed data from 206 patients who received TSD (frequently with supplemental medications intended to extend the duration of antidepressant response) for bipolar depression, finding only 4.9% and 5.8% of such patients switched into mania or hypomania, respectively [27]. Interestingly, one-third of subjects who switched into mania had resolution of symptoms within 3–5 days with nocturnal benzodiazepines; the remaining subjects required either mood stabilizers and/or antipsychotic medications [27]. One notable caveat when interpreting the sleep deprivation literature is that all such studies have been designed to treat depression (unipolar and/or bipolar type), and thus may not accurately reflect the likelihood of sleep

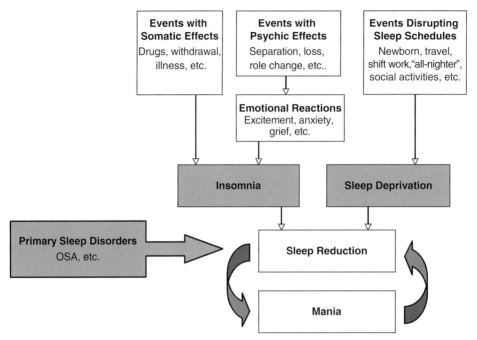

Figure 16.1 Sleep Reduction as a "final common pathway of mania" revisited. From Plante and Winkelman, 2008 [190], originally adapted from Wehr et al, 1987 [28]. Reprinted with permission from the American Journal of Psychiatry (Copyright 2008). American Psychiatric Association.

deprivation to induce manic switching in euthymic bipolar patients.

As a synthesis of experimental and observational studies, Wehr and colleagues proposed the "final common pathway" hypothesis, which posits sleep reduction as the fundamental proximal cause for manic switching (Figure 16.1) [28]. According to this model, all triggers of mania including biological causes (e.g. drugs, withdrawal), psychic effects (e.g. separation, bereavement), or direct disturbances of sleep schedules (e.g. newborn infants, shift work, transmeridian travel) act through sleep reduction [28]. This theory proposes that sleep deprivation is both a cause and consequence of mania, and thus mutually self-reinforcing sleep loss perpetuates the manic state. Prospective testing of the final common pathway hypothesis is logistically difficult since sleep deprivation is both a cause and prodromal symptom of mania. However, cases of bipolar inpatients switching into mania after sleep deprivation from varied etiologies have been reported, supporting the final common pathway hypothesis [29].

Of clinical import is the observation that primary sleep disorders, in particular obstructive sleep apnea, have been documented as causes of mania and/or

treatment resistance [30–32]. Thus, primary sleep disorders may be an additional cause of functional sleep deprivation leading to mania not originally included in Wehr's "final common pathway" model (Figure 16.1).

Sleep as a predictor of mania

If sleep deprivation can trigger mania, then perhaps sleep duration may anticipate and thus predict mania over the course of the illness. Recent analysis of self-reported sleep duration of participants in the Systemic Treatment Enhancement Program for Bipolar Disorder (STEP-BD) trial demonstrates an association between reported short sleep duration (<6 hours) in the week prior to enrollment and mood elevation, earlier age of onset, and longer illness duration compared to normal or long sleepers [33]. However, despite its impressive sample size (greater than 2000 subjects), this study can only suggest that current sleep duration is associated with mood and quality of life variables – inferences regarding a causal relationship between sleep and mood are not possible without longitudinal study.

There are unfortunately few longitudinal studies that examine the relationship between sleep and mood in bipolar patients. Wehr et al. (1982) followed inpatients with bipolar disorder (15 rapid-cycling and 52 non-rapid-cycling), and found that the majority experienced one or more consecutive nights without sleep each time they switched from depression to mania [34]. Leibenluft et al. (1996) followed 11 rapid-cycling bipolar subjects with sleep logs and mood ratings for 18 months, finding sleep duration predicted the subsequent day's mood, such that increased sleep was associated with decreased probability of hypomania or mania the following day in five of eight subjects who had a sufficient number of mood episodes for analysis [35]. Similarly, Bauer et al. (2008), building on previous pilot data, found a significant negative cross-correlation between sleep (defined as sleep or bed rest) and mood on the day of or before a mood change in 42% of a mixed population of 101 bipolar I and II outpatients such that decreased sleep (particularly of <3 hours) was more predictive of hypomanic or manic symptoms [36]. Notably, subjects who demonstrated a significant cross-correlation tended to be more symptomatic, with fewer euthymic days and more days with depression or mania. Furthermore, sleep duration, rather than time of sleep onset or offset, seemed to be most predictive of a mood change [37]. Perlman et al. (2006) examined self-reported sleep duration at monthly intervals in bipolar I subjects, finding sleep deficit predicted depressive symptoms at 6-month follow-up, but was not predictive of manic episodes [38]. Of note, manic patients were less likely to complete sleep measures and were more likely to drop out, and examining monthly intervals of self-reported sleep duration may have been too infrequent to detect a relationship between sleep and mania in this study [38].

There are also a few medication trials that examine the association of sleep disturbance in manic relapse. Klein et al. (1992), using actigraphy in a small, non-randomized, double-blind crossover study of lithium discontinuation, found relapsers did not differ from non-relapsers in estimated sleep efficiency or sleep activity either pre- or post-lithium discontinuation; however, significant differences were found in daytime motor activity [39]. In a *post hoc* analysis of Young Mania Rating Scale (YMRS) items in bipolar patients enrolled in a maintenance trial, Houston et al. (2005) found increased motor activity and energy was a strong marker of initial manic symptoms, and that decreased need for sleep occurred in

25% and 10.5% of patients in the 2 weeks preceding manic relapse in subjects maintained on olanzapine and lithium, respectively [40].

Although limited by recall bias, patient retrospective reports also provide insight into the role of sleep in the genesis of mania. Jackson et al. (2003) found sleep disturbance was the most commonly reported prodromal symptom (77% of patients) prior to a manic episode in a review of 11 studies [41]. Similarly, in a retrospective interview study of 127 women who developed bipolar affective post-partum psychosis, 48% of subjects reported not needing to sleep or being unable to sleep as the first symptoms of their episode [42]. Such observations are important as teaching patients to recognize early symptoms of a manic relapse and to seek early treatment may increase time to a manic episode, and improve occupational and social functioning [43].

Sleep as a marker of response and a therapeutic target in mania

There is some, albeit limited, evidence suggesting sleep duration may be a harbinger of response in mania. In a retrospective chart review, total sleep time on the first night of hospitalization was a predictor of rapid response (and discharge) for those admitted to an inpatient unit with mania [44]. Similarly, inpatient observations of sleep duration have correlated with ratings of cooperation and irritability among manic inpatients using the Nurses' Observation Scale for Inpatient Evaluation (NOSIE), but not using more standardized measures such as the YMRS [45].

Although there is no causal evidence that increased sleep improves the course of mania, clinicians have long used agents that can increase sleep and/or sedation in manic patients to achieve therapeutic effect. Sedating agents including bromides, chloroform, alcohol, and opium were utilized over a century ago to manage agitated psychiatric states. More recently, the sedating medications most frequently used in acute mania are benzodiazepines and antipsychotics, and clinical experience suggests that sedation alone caused by these agents may be valuable in managing manic behavior. Benzodiazepines (e.g. clonazepam and lorazepam) are as effective as neuroleptics as adjunctive medications when used with lithium in acute mania [46,47]. In fact, benzodiazepines are frequently used as rescue medications in clinical trials, and it is possible that a "placebo" response in some trials may be the result of benzodiazepine use [48]. All atypical anti-psychotics demonstrate efficacy in the management of acute mania, and it is noteworthy that these agents are often sedating and several increase total sleep time in healthy subjects [49–51]. Unfortunately, it is not clear to what degree these agents exert their effects via sleep-related systems, or to what degree sedation alone either masks manic symptoms or reverses underlying processes responsible for mania [24].

There is also evidence that improvement in sleep duration by manipulation of the circadian system may have some benefits in manic patients. In one open-label study, Bersani et al. (2000) found that melatonin (3 mg at bedtime) improved subjective sleep duration and manic symptoms in 11 outpatients with mania whose insomnia was resistant to benzodi-azepines [52]. Since melatonin is a relatively poor hypnotic but is an important neurohormone in the regulation of circadian rhythms, this result may have been mediated through circadian processes rather than homeostatic or sedating mechanisms [53].

In addition to pharmacological management, behavioral interventions designed to improve or extend sleep have been used in the treatment of mania for over 100 years [54]. During the nineteenth century, S. Weir Mitchell advocated that "rest cure" (prolonged bed rest) be used for a variety of neuropsychiatric disorders [54]. In modern times, similar techniques have shown prom-ise in treating patients with bipolar disorder. Wehr et al. (1998) used 14 hours of bed rest to stabilize a patient with treatment refractory rapid-cycling bipolar dis-order. Interestingly, prolonged bed rest did not increase total sleep time, but rather decreased variability of sleep duration [55]. Similarly, 14 hours of enforced darkness in hospitalized manic patients significantly decreased YMRS scores when treated within 2 weeks of onset of the manic episode, and patients treated with dark ther-apy also were discharged from the hospital more quickly and required lower doses of antimanic agents than those with standard care [56]. In this study, nursing observa-tion of sleep duration suggested enforced darkness did increase total sleep time; however, nursing observation of sleep duration can overestimate sleep duration [56,57]. Similar to the use of melatonin in mania, bed rest with enforced darkness may lead to improvement via a circadian manipulation, since light is the primary "zeitgeber" (timegiver) of the circadian clock, and patients may become better without clear improvement in sleep *per se*. Furthermore, more regulated light–dark cycles on inpatient units compared to outside the hospital could theoretically be responsible, at least in part, for the beneficial effects of the milieu on manic patients.

Sleep in bipolar depression

Although less is known about sleep disturbance in bipolar as compared to unipolar depression, in the following section we will highlight the phenomen-ology of sleep in bipolar depression and the potential of sleep deprivation as a theraputic strategy in the depressive phase of bipolar illness.

Objective and subjective sleep disturbance in bipolar depression

Sleep disturbance, either insomnia or hypersomnia, is a core diagnostic feature of depressive episodes in unipolar and bipolar depression [6]. Polysomno-graphic studies of sleep in bipolar depression have generally found similar abnormalities in unipolar and bipolar depression, with a lack of consensus regarding potential differences among studies [58]. However, the majority of studies did not carefully control for potential confounding variables, and recent data suggests that bipolar patients may have more early morning awakenings and greater total REM density than unipolar subjects when matched for age, gender, and severity of symptoms [59].

Some have argued that hypersomnia, rather than insomnia, either in isolation or as a component of atypical depression is more indicative of bipolar than unipolar depression [60,61]. Reported rates of hyper-somnia in studies of bipolar depression are highly variable, ranging from 17% to 78%, as are rates of insomnia, suggesting that neither can be relied upon solely to discriminate between bipolar and unipolar depression [58,62]. However, recent studies demon-strate that patients with bipolar disorder are more likely to report subjective hypersomnia during a depressive episode than unipolar subjects [63–65]. Additionally, hypersomnia, as part of the constell-ation of atypical depression, has been correlated with increased rates of family history of bipolar disorder, compared to depressed subjects without atypical features [66]. Thus the presence of subjective hyper-somnolence during a major depressive episode may be suggestive of an underlying bipolar diathesis, but is certainly not specific and must be considered in light of other current and past symptoms.

It is important for practicing clinicians to note that hypersomnolence that can occur in bipolar depression is different from that of narcolepsy and other disorders of central hypersomnolence (see Chapter 9: Hypersomnias of central origin). When evaluated using the multiple sleep latency test (MSLT), an objective measure of sleepiness, bipolar depressed subjects with subjective hypersomnia did not exhibit objective evidence of excessive daytime sleepiness, suggesting that bipolar hypersomnolence is more reflective of anergia/fatigue than true excessive sleepiness seen in some other primary sleep disorders [67]. This discrepancy between objective and subjective measures of hypersomnolence is important to consider when evaluating studies that examine relationships between sleep duration and depressed mood in bipolar subjects since self-reported long sleep duration could be due to an increased sleep propensity or to fatigue/anergia with increased time in bed without increased physiological sleep drive.

With this caveat in mind, there is some data to suggest that the subjective report of long sleep duration may correlate with depressed mood in bipolar disorder. Bauer et al. (2008) reported in their longitudinal sample of bipolar subjects that increased sleep from baseline (particularly >3 hours) was more predictive of a mood change to depression [36]. Additionally, self-reported average sleep duration that was either less than 6 hours or greater than 9 hours per night in the week prior to enrollment was associated with depressive symptoms, poorer life functioning, and quality of life compared to normal sleepers in the STEP-BD trial [33].

Sleep deprivation in bipolar depression

As discussed previously, the use of sleep deprivation as a treatment for depression significantly advanced our understanding of the relationship between sleep deprivation and mania. Although there is data suggesting that sleep deprivation may be an effective treatment for bipolar depression, the American Psychiatric Association considers it a novel approach, and sleep deprivation as a somatic therapy is currently not widely used or studied [68]. This is likely due to limited data compared to conventional treatments, concern about manic switching, logistical difficulties of sleep deprivation in controlled settings, frequent return of depressive symptoms after recovery sleep, and the dominance of other areas (e.g.

pharmacotherapy, neurochemistry, genetics) in mood disorders research [69]. Still, because sleep deprivation is the fastest known means of alleviating depressive symptoms, recent data suggest adjunctive treatments may prolong its antidepressant response, and bipolar depression can be clinically difficult to treat and lead to significant morbidity, some have called for renewed interest and study of sleep deprivation as a somatic therapy [70].

Although previous reviews of the older therapeutic sleep deprivation literature did not reveal differences in response to sleep deprivation among bipolar and unipolar subjects, more recent studies have suggested bipolar depressives may respond more robustly than unipolar subjects [25]. Szuba et al. (1990), in a small prospective study of 37 subjects with either unipolar, bipolar I, or bipolar II depression, found 8/9 (89%) bipolar I subjects responded to partial sleep deprivation (PSD), compared to 9/24 (38%) unipolar subjects [71]. Also, in a prospective study of 51 subjects using a repeated TSD paradigm, Barbini et al. (1998) found that although all subjects had improvement in depressive symptoms, bipolar I, bipolar II, and first-episode unipolar subjects had significantly greater response to TSD when compared to unipolar subjects with a prior history of depressive episodes [72]. Interestingly, whether depressive symptoms are amenable to sleep deprivation may also depend on the time course of the depressive episode as a small case series found little response to sleep deprivation early in the course of a depressive episode among rapid-cycling patients, but more significant responses later in the course of the mood episode [73].

Numerous approaches to augment and extend the antidepressant response to sleep deprivation have been examined. Several reports demonstrate lithium may improve response to sleep deprivation and sustain remission in unipolar and bipolar depressives [74–77]. Also, Smeraldi et al. (1999) demonstrated that pindolol, a $5-HT_{1A}$-beta adrenoreceptor blocking agent, improved the response rates of bipolar depressives to TSD and that remission could be maintained with lithium salts alone in nearly two-thirds of cases [78]. Additionally, bright light in the morning is also helpful in sustaining antidepressant response to sleep deprivation in bipolar subjects [79–81]. Also, phase advance (i.e. moving the sleep period several hours earlier than usual) after sleep deprivation sustains the antidepressant effects of sleep deprivation in both unipolar and bipolar subjects [82–85].

Increasingly, there is evidence that genetics, specifically genes important in neurotransmission and the molecular circadian mechanism, may play a role in the antidepressant response to sleep deprivation in bipolar disorder. Homozygotes for the long variant of a polymorphism in the transcriptional control region upstream of the coding sequence of the serotonin transporter 5-HTTLPR were more likely to respond to sleep deprivation than those who were heterozygotes or homozygotes for the short variant [86]. Additionally, bipolar depressives who were homozygotes for the T variant on the $5\text{-}HT_{2A}$ receptor gene polymorphism rs6313 had both perceived and observed benefits, as well as a higher final response rate, from a repeated TSD paradigm, than carriers of the C allele [87]. More recently, subjects with bipolar disorder who were homozygotes for a Val/Val variant in catechol-O-methyltransferase (COMT), which inactivates norepinephrine and dopamine, exhibited a decreased antidepressant response to sleep deprivation followed by bright light when compared to heterozygotes (Val/Met) or homozygotes (Met/Met) [88]. Additionally, a glycogen synthase kinase 3-beta (GSK3-β) promoter gene single nucleotide polymorphism (SNP) has an association with response to TSD in bipolar depression, which is noteworthy as GSK3-β is involved in the circadian molecular mechanism [89].

Sleep in euthymia

Euthymia, the absence of mood symptoms sufficient to warrant the diagnosis of a depressive, hypomanic, or manic episode, is the goal of treatment of bipolar disorder. However, most clinicians are well aware that this disease state is characterized by frequent subclinical symptomatology [90]. Although there is relatively little data about sleep in euthymic periods in bipolar disorder, it does appear that sleep disturbance is one of the more common forms of interepisode problems for these patients.

There are a limited number of studies that have utilized polysomnography in euthymic bipolar subjects. One study, using polysomnography over five nights, found the only difference between the ten remitted bipolar patients and age-matched controls was mildly elevated rates of arousals [91]. However, another study demonstrated increased REM density, percentage of REM sleep, and sensitivity to the REM latency reducing effects of arecoline (an acetylcholine agonist) compared to normal controls [92].

A few more recent studies have used actigraphy to monitor the sleep–wake patterns of remitted bipolar subjects. Using sleep diaries and actigraphy, Millar et al. (2004) demonstrated that remitted bipolar I patients had greater sleep onset latency, increased sleep duration, and more night-to-night variability of sleep patterns than healthy controls [93]. Jones et al. (2005) similarly compared the circadian activity patterns of bipolar subjects to healthy controls, finding greater variability of daytime activity patterns in bipolar subjects, but no significant differences in sleep parameters (e.g. sleep onset latency) between groups [94]. However, since subjects were only asked to record bedtime and getting up time, and the remaining sleep parameters were calculated using actigraphy, sleep latency and wake time after sleep onset may have been underestimated if subjects were awake in bed with little movement [94]. Finally, Harvey et al. (2005) compared euthymic bipolar patients, patients with insomnia, and subjects with good sleep, finding 70% of the euthymic bipolar patients exhibited a clinically significant sleep disturbance [95]. Interestingly, when compared to other groups, euthymic bipolar patients had diminished sleep efficiency, decreased daytime activity levels, increased anxiety and fear about poor sleep, and had levels of dysfunctional beliefs about sleep comparable to non-bipolar patients with insomnia [95].

As previously mentioned, it has been hypothesized that alterations in the circadian system may be involved in the pathophysiology of bipolar disorder. Of import is that sleep and/or circadian abnormalities are present in periods of euthymia as well as during mood episodes, suggesting that such abnormalities are trait markers of illness, rather than state dependent. Much of the older literature described abnormalities including blunting of the amplitude of the circadian rhythm, as well as phase advanced or non-24-hour rhythms; however, such conclusions were based on data from subjects with active mood symptoms, making it difficult to interpret whether such abnormalities are trait or state dependent [4,5]. More recently, two separate groups demonstrated that subjects with bipolar disorder are more likely to have an evening chronotype as measured by morningness/eveningness (M/E) scores, a stable, quantifiable self-report measure reflecting preferred circadian phase [96–98]. However, it is notable that data from one group suggested that frequent mood swings and higher scores on the Beck depression inventory (BDI) increased the likelihood of lower (i.e. evening preference) M/E scores, and thus it is not clear to what extent M/E reflects a state and/or trait marker of bipolar illness [96,97].

Alterations in the sensitivity to light have been proposed as potential trait markers for bipolar disorder. Indirect evidence for altered light sensitivity include seasonal patterns of symptoms, including the replicated finding of increased propensity for hospitalization for mania in the spring/summer months, although whether this is an effect of climate or sunlight exposure is debated [99–102]. Supporting the notion that bipolar patients may have altered sensitivity to light are studies that demonstrate decreased nocturnal melatonin levels and increased melatonin suppression in response to light exposure, both in euthymia and during mood episodes [103–105]. However, this finding has not been replicated across studies [106,107]. One potential explanation for inconsistent findings is that some, but not all, patients with bipolar disorder have altered sensitivity to light, suggesting potentially a different circadian endophenotype (discussed below).

Genetic influences: circadian clock genes and endphenotypes of bipolar disorder

It has long been appreciated that bipolar disorder tends to run in families, suggesting it is a heritable disorder. The estimated lifetime risk of bipolar disorder is 0.5–1.5% in the general population; however, the risk is 5–10% for first-degree relatives of bipolar probands, and 40–70% concordance in monozygotic twins [108]. However, despite extensive efforts to determine the genetics that underlies bipolar disorder, precise genetic loci remain unclear. This is likely due to several factors including a significant environmental influence in the development of the disease and multiple genes of small effect conferring genetic susceptibility [109]. Additionally, bipolar disorder has multiple phenotypes that may be related but have different underlying genetic susceptibilities. As a result, it has been proposed that reducing the complex behavioral and symptom patterns of bipolar disorder into putative endophenotypes may help tease out underlying genetic susceptibility and pathophysiology of the disease spectrum [110,111]. Endophenotypes are heritable, primarily state-independent biomarkers that are associated with an illness, with co-segregation of the illness and endophenotype

within families [112]. There are several proposed endophenotypes for bipolar disorder, and several involve sleep–wake mechanisms such as circadian rhythm instability, cholinergic sensitivity (and its effects on REM sleep), and response to sleep deprivation (previously discussed).

Several studies have evaluated genes involved in the molecular circadian mechanism (for review, see Chapter 2: Neuroanatomy and neurobiology of sleep and wakefulness) in bipolar subjects. Much of the work on relationships between circadian genes and bipolar phenotypes involve an SNP (311 T to C) in the CLOCK gene. In bipolar subjects, this SNP has been associated with increased evening activity levels, delayed sleep onset, reduced total sleep time, increased rates of recurrence, as well as increased insomnia and decreased need for sleep [113–116]. Further supporting the potential role for CLOCK in bipolar disorder are mouse models with a dominant-negative mutation of CLOCK that result in phenotypic traits that are akin to mania [117].

Besides CLOCK, other studies have found some small associations between bipolar disorder and haplotypes/polymorphisms in circadian genes including BMAL1 (ARNTL), TIMELESS, and PER3; however, associations for these genes are not consistent across studies [118–120]. Recently, a variable-number tandem-repeat (VNTR) polymorphism in PER3, which has been associated with diurnal preference, sleep homeostasis, and cognitive performance in response to sleep loss in healthy subjects, has been associated with age of onset of bipolar illness [121,122]. Of note, several other circadian genes including CRY1/2 and PER1/2 have failed to demonstrate association with bipolar illness [118,123,124].

As previously discussed, an SNP (-50T/C) in the promoter region of the gene coding for GSK3-β has been associated with improved antidepressant response to sleep deprivation in bipolar disorder [89]. This SNP has also been associated with a later age of onset of bipolar illness as well as efficacy of long-term lithium treatment [125,126]. Although the mechanism through which lithium provides mood stabilization remains unclear, there is growing theoretical interest in its effects on the circadian system via its interaction with GSK3-β, as lithium is a potent inhibitor of this enzyme [127,128]. GSK3-β also phosphorylates Rev-Erbα, a critical component of the stabilizing loop of the circadian clock, which is also sensitive to lithium [128]. Interestingly, a small study has recently demonstrated a nominal association of two polymorphisms in the Rev-Erbα gene with bipolar disorder in a population of Sardinian descent; however, these results are not definitive and require replication before more conclusive results can be drawn [129].

Evaluation of sleep complaints in bipolar disorder

Since sleep disturbance is common across all phases of bipolar illness, and as previously discussed, may play a role in the induction and maintenance of mood episodes, appropriate management of sleep complaints is an important clinical issue in bipolar disorder. Thus, it is essential that clinicians have an understanding of the disparate causes of sleep problems in bipolar patients, and employ a systematic approach to managing such complaints. The comprehensive evaluation of sleep complaints in patients with bipolar disorder is largely similar to the approach taken with other patients (for details, see Chapter 6: Taking a sleep history). A comprehensive sleep history that outlines the nature of the complaint and assesses potential causes of sleep disturbance including medical, neurological, psychiatric, and co-morbid primary sleep disorders is crucial. When identifiable, treatment should be directed towards the underlying cause of the sleep complaint, and potentially detrimental sleep-related effects of treatment directed towards the bipolar disorder itself should be considered in the differential diagnosis.

Primary sleep disorders and bipolar illness

We have previously alluded to the importance of primary sleep disorders as potential causes of sleep deprivation and manic relapse in bipolar disorder. Given that obstructive sleep apnea (OSA) and restless legs syndrome (RLS), two primary sleep disorders associated with sleep impairment, are common in the general population (roughly 2–4% and 2–7%, respectively), and potentially more so in psychiatric populations, we recommend all mental health practitioners screen for these disorders in patients with sleep complaints, and refer for further evaluation and management as required [130,131]. There is evidence that among bipolar and unipolar depressives, the presence of severe snoring, witnessed apneas, or excessive daytime sleepiness are of high predictive

value for OSA [132]. In addition, other clinical signs and symptoms that may suggest OSA include obesity, enlarged neck circumference, hypertension, morning dry mouth or headaches, or subjective report of restless sleep.

There have been few studies that examine prevalence of co-morbid OSA in bipolar disorder. One large telephone-based survey found that both bipolar disorder and OSA occurred more frequently among individuals with severe and moderate self-reported daytime sleepiness (6% and 3.9% for bipolar disorder; 6.7% and 4.8% for OSA) respectively, compared to proportions of the population without excessive somnolence; however, rates of co-occurrence of OSA and bipolar disorder were not reported [133]. In a cohort of OSA patients in the Veteran's Affairs system, 4.1% had co-morbid bipolar illness, while the prevalence of bipolar disorder in the non-apnea (control) population was 1.9% [134]. As previously discussed, there are case reports of treatment-resistant bipolar disorder related to OSA; however, there have also been isolated case reports of hypomania and mania induced by OSA treatment with positive airway pressure (PAP) therapy [135–138]. Although our clinical experience is that the majority of bipolar patients with OSA experience a positive benefit from PAP therapy, we recommend that clinicians continue to monitor their patients after starting PAP therapy, as effects on mood may theoretically be beneficial or detrimental.

Obesity, although not the *sine qua non* for OSA, is a major risk factor for sleep disordered breathing, and may be critically important in bipolar patients. Obese bipolar patients experience more lifetime mood episodes, and may have more severe and difficult to treat affective episodes, which may theoretically be related to OSA-induced mood destabilization [139]. In many cases, obesity in bipolar patients is iatrogenic as many psychotropic medications are associated with weight gain [140]. In fact, obesity, male gender, and chronic neuroleptic administration are risk factors for OSA among psychiatric patients, which is important for bipolar patients given the frequent use of atypical antipsychotics in the management of the disorder [141].

Restless legs syndrome (RLS) is a sensorimotor disorder in which the patient experiences an urge to move their legs (often associated with uncomfortable sensations) which is present at rest, temporarily relieved by movement, and most prominent at night, thus frequently interfering with sleep (see Chapter 8: Sleep-related movement disorders). RLS is often associated with periodic limb movements of sleep (PLMS), which are repetitive leg movements during sleep that may result in sleep fragmentation. Although RLS and PLMS are common in the general population, we know of no studies that have examined the prevalence of RLS in bipolar disorder. Still, there are a few aspects related to management of RLS and PLMS in bipolar disorder that merit discussion.

First, it is critical that practicing clinicians be aware that several types of psychotropic medications commonly used in the treatment of bipolar disorder, including atypical antipsychotics, lithium, and antidepressants, can cause RLS/PLMS, and thus inquiry about RLS symptoms prior to and in follow-up after starting these medications is recommended [50,142–148]. Second, since there is some limited evidence that carbamazepine, valproic acid, and lamotrigine may be at least somewhat effective in the management of RLS (although clearly not first-line agents), the use of these medications as mood stabilizers may be a reasonable strategy to minimize polypharmacy in bipolar patients with co-morbid RLS [149–153]. In a related point, dopamine agonists (pramipexole and ropinirole) are considered first-line agents in the treatment of RLS, and there is some data suggesting they may be useful and safe in the treatment of bipolar depression, with similar rates of treatment-emergent mania and hypomania compared to placebo in small studies [154]. However, it is noteworthy that these agents can rarely cause severe impulse control problems (i.e. compulsive gambling, shopping, etc.) in patients with RLS and Parkinson's disease (PD), and there is a case report of mania in a bipolar II patient treated with pramipexole [154,155]. Also, there is a theoretical risk of psychosis with dopamine agonists, which may lead to hesitancy in using these agents in psychiatric patients. A recent small retrospective study demonstrated that psychosis occurred in 13.7% of a cohort of patients with either PD or RLS treated with ropinirole; however, concurrent use of multiple dopaminergic medications, and not a history of an Axis I disorder, was significantly associated with the development of new or worsened psychosis [156]. Thus, based on the limited data available at present, we would recommend discussing the possible risks of impulse control difficulties and psychosis with all patients to whom these agents are prescribed, coupled with appropriate clinical follow-up, particularly in patients with bipolar disorder and/or a history of psychosis. However, these agents should not be universally excluded from use in the treatment of RLS in patients with psychiatric disorders, as they are highly effective and the potential benefits may frequently outweigh theoretical risks.

As previously discussed, the hypersomnia that is commonly associated with bipolar depression is objectively different (as measured by the MSLT) from that associated with disorders of central hypersomnolence. In the case of hypersomnolence associated with bipolar depression, we would not recommend the routine use of stimulant medications as these agents (including amphetamine, methylphenidate, and modafinil) have been associated with manic switching; however, the differential risk profiles of these agents are not entirely clear [157]. Based on retrospective chart review and one placebo-controlled trial, some have argued that modafinil may not induce manic switching [158,159]. However, there are several case reports in the literature of mania induced by modafinil, and in the placebo-controlled trial conducted by Frye et al. (2007), the modafinil group used significantly more sedative-hypnotic medication than the placebo group, which may have theoretically provided some protection against manic switching, for reasons previously discussed [159–162]. Thus, based on the available literature and our clinical experience, modafinil may be a safer alternative for the treatment of hypersomnia associated with bipolar depression than traditional stimulants; however, we would recommend that modafinil be used with caution in bipolar disorder. Similarly, on some rare occasions, patients may have bipolar disorder co-morbid with a disorder of central hypersomnolence, which can significantly complicate management. In such instances the risk/benefit decision-making process regarding the use of modafinil and/or stimulants must be carefully considered, weighing the morbidity associated with severe sleepiness (rather than anergia/fatigue) on the one hand versus the potential risks of mania on the other.

Management of insomnia in bipolar disorder

Insomnia, which can include difficulty falling asleep, multiple or prolonged awakenings from sleep, inadequate sleep quality, or short overall sleep duration when given enough time for sleep, is a common occurrence in bipolar disorder, and as previously discussed, may play a role in the disease across all phases of illness. In the absence of formal guidelines, potential treatments for bipolar insomnia include psychotherapeutic and pharmacological strategies that are similar to those used for primary insomnia and insomnia related to other psychiatric disorders, with some notable exceptions.

Psychotherapy for bipolar insomnia

Cognitive behavioral therapy for insomnia (CBT-I) is well established as the most efficacious psychotherapeutic treatment for primary insomnia (see Chapter 14: Cognitive behavioral therapy for insomnia). Unfortunately, there are currently no studies of CBT-I in bipolar insomnia, although the majority of CBT-I techniques could likely be employed without negative sequelae in bipolar patients. The exception is sleep restriction therapy, where time in bed is limited to the number of hours the patient believes they are sleeping, which would theoretically increase the likelihood of manic switching or reinforce hypo/manic states [163]. Unfortunately, sleep restriction is one of the more efficacious CBT-I techniques, potentially limiting the overall value of psychotheraputic strategies for managing bipolar insomnia [164]. CBT-I in bipolar patients may also be complicated by the fact that some bipolar patients (particularly rapid-cycling) often complain of difficulty arising in the morning and may have mild hypomanic symptoms intensify over the course of the day, potentially disrupting their ability to sleep at night or adhere to prescribed CBT-I-based interventions [165,166].

Although it is not possible to determine the extent that sleep-related components of common psychotherapeutic strategies to manage bipolar disorder contribute to the efficacy of the entire therapy, it is notable that many have components designed to improve or monitor sleep. Psychoeducational strategies that emphasize the identification of prodromal symptoms (including sleep disturbance) reduce the frequency of relapses to depressive, manic, hypomanic, and mixed episodes [167,168]. Interpersonal and social rhythm therapy (IPSRT), which is based on management of life stressors that disrupt patterns (including the sleep–wake cycle), can improve mood stability, prolong maintenance, and decrease affective relapse [169–170]. Similarly, cognitive behavioral treatments for bipolar disorder frequently stress maintenance of sleep–wake patterns through

cognitive behavioral approaches, and are an effective modality in bipolar disorder [171,172].

Pharmacotherapy for bipolar insomnia

Clinicians have a vast array of pharmacotherapies available to treat bipolar insomnia. These include: benzodiazepines and benzodiazepine receptor agonists (BzRAs), sedating antidepressants, sedating antipsychotics, antiepileptics, and melatonin receptor agonists. Although no medication is approved by the FDA specifically for management of bipolar insomnia, the practicing clinician should be aware of the potential benefits and pitfalls of these classes of medications in the context of bipolar disorder.

Benzodiazepines are a vast improvement over the barbiturates (that have a comparatively small therapeutic index), which had previously been the primary agents available as a treatment of insomnia. Benzodiazepines are highly effective in the treatment of insomnia and offer a wide range of half lives among the various compounds in this class. Although clinical experience suggests benzodiazepines are efficacious in the management of bipolar insomnia, there are no studies that demonstrate benzodiazepines specifically improve sleep or mood stability in bipolar patients. However, in both an uncontrolled retrospective chart review and prospective open trial (at the same institution), clonazepam was effective as a replacement for neuroleptics (as an adjunct to lithium) in the maintenance treatment of bipolar disorder, though this approach was not successful in two other studies [173–176].

Concerns regarding abuse, tolerance, withdrawal, daytime sedation, and motor/cognitive impairment limit the use of benzodiazepines for the treatment of insomnia. As a result, non-benzodiazepine benzodiazepine receptor agonists (BzRAs; zolpidem, zaleplon, eszopiclone), which are more selective for GABA-A receptors containing α-1 subunits than traditional benzodiazepines, are often the agents of choice. Marketed BzRAs have short to intermediate half lives, which reduce the likelihood of daytime carryover and resultant side-effects compared to agents with longer half lives. Although BzRAs also have potential for tolerance and withdrawal, there is data that suggests non-nightly use of BzRAs over 2–3 months is not associated with such problems [177,178]. Furthermore, newer agents have been studied for up to 6 months without evidence of tolerance or rebound insomnia on discontinuation [179,180]. Although they are commonly used agents in the management of bipolar insomnia, and clinical experience suggests they are useful, there are no known studies examining BzRAs in the management of bipolar disorder.

Since patients with bipolar spectrum disorders frequently have co-morbid drug and alcohol abuse or dependence, the use of benzodiazepines/BzRAs may be problematic in some patients, limiting their clinical viability in such "dual diagnosis" patients [181]. Additionally, substances of abuse (both licit and illicit) can have deleterious effects on sleep (see Chapter 19: Sleep in substance use disorders), and thus assessment for co-morbid substance use is an important component in the evaluation of bipolar insomnia. Although several agents (discussed below) with lower abuse potential than benzodiazepines are used off-label in the treatment of insomnia, there are several issues which must be considered when using these agents in patients with bipolar disorder.

The most commonly used medications to treat chronic insomnia are sedating antidepressants, despite a relative dearth of evidence for their efficacy [182]. However, lack of evidence is not synonymous with lack of efficacy, and certainly there is a place for these agents, based on clinical experience and well-understood safety profiles, in the treatment of insomnia. However, because trazodone and other sedating antidepressants, (e.g. TCAs) can induce mania in bipolar patients, we recommend these agents be used with caution (even at low doses) in patients with bipolar disorder, and should not be considered as first-line agents [183–185].

Atypical antipsychotics are increasingly utilized in the management of bipolar disorder. In addition to their approved uses as antimanic agents, mood stabilizers, and in some cases, antidepressants, they are frequently used as adjunctive sedative-hypnotics. The off-label use of neuroleptics primarily as sleeping medications has grown within psychiatric and general populations; however, this practice is somewhat controversial, especially given the potential for extrapyramidal symptoms, metabolic derangements, arrhythmogenesis, daytime sedation, and weight gain [186]. The atypical antipsychotic most commonly used as a sedative-hypnotic is quetiapine, typically in doses below those used in psychiatric illness (25–100 mg). It has been shown to increase total sleep time and improve subjective sleep quality in healthy subjects [50]. However, as previously discussed, clinicians should be cognizant that antipsychotics may

induce or worsen RLS and/or PLMS which may paradoxically diminish the quality of sleep in some patients.

Anticonvulsants that are not approved for the treatment of bipolar disorder (gabapentin, tiagabine) are also occasionally used off-label as hypnotics in bipolar patients. Although there is no specific evidence to support the use of these medications in this context, the rationale for this strategy is likely based on the fact that other antiepileptics have demonstrated mood stabilizing properties, and these agents have not been associated with manic switching. There is some evidence that gabapentin can improve subjective sleep quality, increase REM sleep, and increase SWS [187]. Similarly, tiagabine may increase SWS; however, its usefulness as a hypnotic in primary insomnia is very limited [188]. Sedating anticonvulsants are generally less effective than benzodiazepines and BzRAs in the treatment of insomnia, and the side-effects of these drugs (cognitive impairment, daytime sedation, etc.) must be considered when used as hypnotics in bipolar disorder.

Melatonin receptor agonists (including ramelteon or exogenous melatonin) may have some role in the management of bipolar insomnia; however, there is limited data to support their use. Although melatonin has shown some promise in treatment-refractory mania in rapid-cycling patients, melatonin receptor agonists have not been carefully studied as a maintenance drug in the treatment of bipolar disorder [52]. Exogenous melatonin had little effect on mood or sleep in a case series of five euthymic, rapid-cycling patients; however, melatonin withdrawal delayed sleep onset and may have had mild mood-elevating effects [189]. Thus, at present, the role for melatonin receptor agonists in bipolar insomnia is unclear.

Conclusion

It is clear that sleep disturbance is a clinically significant problem in all phases of bipolar disorder. However, specific cause and effect relationships are difficult to elucidate fully based on the current literature. There are few prospective studies of sleep disturbance in bipolar illness, and despite several lines of inferential evidence, there is no direct substantiation that treatment of sleep disturbance has significant effects on the course of the disorder. Additionally, individual variability of sleep–wake cycles, response to sleep deprivation, and circadian rhythms among patients with bipolar disorder complicate research in this area. However, some envision that this heterogeneity may be exploited to elucidate more fully the genetic underpinnings of bipolar disorder using sleep-related endophenotypes. For the time being, using a pragmatic approach to manage sleep disturbance in patients with bipolar disorder is warranted. Careful assessment of quality and quantity of sleep, thoughtful application of behavioral and pharmacological techniques for improving sleep, and screening for co-occurring sleep and medical disorders are crucial in the management of bipolar patients. Hopefully, further research will ultimately provide a broader evidence base for specific sleep-related modalities and treatments for bipolar disorder.

References

1. Kraepelin E. *Manic-depressive insanity and paranoia*. Translated by Barclay RM. Edinburgh: E&S Livingstone; 1921:44.

2. Dijk DJ, Lockley S W. Integration of human sleep-wake regulation and circadian rhythmicity. *J Appl Physiol*. 2002;**92**(2):852–862.

3. Richardson GS. The human circadian system in normal and disordered sleep. *J Clin Psychiatry*. 2005;**66**(Suppl 9):3–9; quiz 42–43.

4. Goodwin FK, Jamison KR. *Manic-depressive illness*. New York: Oxford University Press; 1990:541–574.

5. Wehr TA, Sack D, Rosenthal N, Duncan W, Gillin JC. Circadian rhythm disturbances in manic-depressive illness. *Fed Proc*. 1983;**42**(11):2809–2814.

6. American Psychiatric Association. *Diagnostic and statistical manual of mental disorders* 4th ed, Text Revision. Washington, DC: American Psychiatric Association; 2000.

7. Kessler RC, Rubinow DR, Holmes C, Abelson JM, Zhao S. The epidemiology of DSM-III-R bipolar I disorder in a general population survey. *Psychol Med*. 1997;**27**(5):1079–1089.

8. Bell LV. On a form of disease resembling some advanced states of mania and fever. *Am J Insanity*. 1849;**6**:97–127.

9. Rechtschaffen A, Bergmann BM, Everson CA, Kushida CA, Gilliland MA. Sleep deprivation in the rat: X. Integration and discussion of the findings. *Sleep*. 1989;**12**(1):68–87.

10. Hudson JI, Lipinski JF, Keck PE Jr, et al. Polysomnographic characteristics of young manic patients: Comparison with unipolar depressed patients and normal control subjects. *Arch Gen Psychiatry*. 1992;**49**(5):378–383.

11. Hudson JI, Lipinski JF, Frankenburg FR, Grochocinski VJ, Kupfer DJ. Electroencephalographic sleep in mania. *Arch Gen Psychiatry*. 1988;**45**(3):267–273.

12. Salvatore P, Ghidini S, Zita G, et al. Circadian activity rhythm abnormalities in ill and recovered bipolar I disorder patients. *Bipolar Disord*. 2008;**10**(2):256–265.

13. Horne JA, Moore VJ. Sleep EEG effects of exercise with and without additional body cooling. *Electroencephalogr Clin Neurophysiol*. 1985;**60**(1):33–38.

14. Linkowski P, Kerkhofs M, Van Onderbergen A, et al. The 24-hour profiles of cortisol, prolactin, and growth hormone secretion in mania. *Arch Gen Psychiatry*. 1994;**51**(8):616–624.

15. Banks S, Dinges DF. Behavioral and physiological consequences of sleep restriction. *J Clin Sleep Med*. 2007;**3**(5):519–528.

16. Jauhar P, Weller MP. Psychiatric morbidity and time zone changes: a study of patients from Heathrow airport. *Br J Psychiatry*. 1982;**140**:231–235.

17. Young DM. Psychiatric morbidity in travelers to Honolulu, Hawaii. *Compr Psychiatry*. 1995;**36**(3):224–228.

18. Peet M, Peters S. Drug-induced mania. *Drug Saf*. 1995;**12**(2):146–153.

19. Davenport YB, Adland ML. Postpartum psychoses in female and male bipolar manic-depressive patients. *Am J Orthopsychiatry*. 1982;**52**(2):288–297.

20. Reich T, Winokur G. Postpartum psychoses in patients with manic depressive disease. *J Nerv Ment Dis*. 1970;**151**(1):60–68.

21. Hollender MH, Goldin ML. Funeral mania. *J Nerv Ment Dis*. 1978;**166**(12):890–892.

22. Rosenman SJ, Tayler H. Mania following bereavement: a case report. *Br J Psychiatry*. 1986;**148**:468–470.

23. Wehr TA. Effects of wakefulness and sleep on depression and mania. In: Montplaisir J, Godbout R, eds. *Sleep and biological rhythms: basic mechanisms and applications to psychiatry*. New York: Oxford University Press; 1990:42–86.

24. Wehr TA. Sleep loss: a preventable cause of mania and other excited states. *J Clin Psychiatry*. 1989;**50**(Suppl):8–16; discussion 45–47.

25. Wu JC, Bunney WE. The biological basis of an antidepressant response to sleep deprivation and

relapse: review and hypothesis. *Am J Psychiatry*. 1990;**147**(1):14–21.

26. Kasper S, Wehr TA. The role of sleep and wakefulness in the genesis of depression and mania. *Encephale*. 1992;**18**(Spec No 1):45–50.

27. Colombo C, Benedetti F, Barbini B, Campori E, Smeraldi E. Rate of switch from depression into mania after therapeutic sleep deprivation in bipolar depression. *Psychiatry Res*. 1999;**86**(3):267–270.

28. Wehr TA, Sack DA, Rosenthal NE. Sleep reduction as a final common pathway in the genesis of mania. *Am J Psychiatry*. 1987;**144**(2):201–204.

29. Wehr TA. Sleep-loss as a possible mediator of diverse causes of mania. *Br J Psychiatry*. 1991;**159**:576–578.

30. Strakowski SM, Hudson JI, Keck PE Jr, et al. Four cases of obstructive sleep apnea associated with treatment-resistant mania. *J Clin Psychiatry*. 1991;**52**(4):156–158.

31. Fleming JA, Fleetham JA, Taylor DR, Remick RA. A case report of obstructive sleep apnea in a patient with bipolar affective disorder. *Can J Psychiatry*. 1985;**30**(6):437–439.

32. Blazer D. Hypersomnia in manic-depressive illness: a case of sleep apnea. *N C Med J*. 1981;**42**(11):781–782.

33. Gruber J, Harvey AG, Wang PW, et al. Sleep functioning in relation to mood, function, and quality of life at entry to the Systematic Treatment Enhancement Program for Bipolar Disorder (STEP-BD). *J Affect Disord*. 2009;**114**(1–3):41–49.

34. Wehr TA, Goodwin FK, Wirz-Justice A, Breitmaier J, Craig C. 48-hour sleep-wake cycles in manic-depressive illness: naturalistic observations and sleep deprivation experiments. *Arch Gen Psychiatry*. 1982;**39**(5):559–565.

35. Leibenluft E, Albert PS, Rosenthal NE, Wehr TA. Relationship between sleep and mood in patients with rapid-cycling bipolar disorder. *Psychiatry Res*. 1996;**63**(2–3):161–168.

36. Bauer M, Glenn T, Whybrow PC, et al. Changes in self-reported sleep duration predict mood changes in bipolar disorder. *Psychol Med*. 2008;**38**(7):1069–1071.

37. Bauer M, Glenn T, Grof P, et al. Comparison of sleep/wake parameters for self-monitoring bipolar disorder. *J Affect Disord*. 2009;**116**(3):170–175.

38. Perlman CA, Johnson SL, Mellman TA. The prospective impact of sleep duration on depression and mania. *Bipolar Disord*. 2006;**8**(3):271–274.

39. Klein E, Lavie P, Meiraz R, Sadeh A, Lenox RH. Increased motor activity and recurrent manic episodes: predictors of rapid relapse in remitted bipolar disorder

40. Houston JP, Lipkovich IA, Ahl J, et al. Initial symptoms of manic relapse in manic or mixed-manic bipolar disorder: Post hoc analysis of patients treated with olanzapine or lithium. *J Psychiatr Res*. 2007;**41**(7):616–621.

41. Jackson A, Cavanagh J, Scott J. A systematic review of manic and depressive prodromes. *J Affect Disord*. 2003;**74**(3):209–217.

42. Heron J, McGuinness M, Blackmore ER, Craddock N, Jones I. Early postpartum symptoms in puerperal psychosis. *Br J Obstet Gynaecol*. 2008;**115**(3):348–353.

43. Perry A, Tarrier N, Morriss R, McCarthy E, Limb K. Randomised controlled trial of efficacy of teaching patients with bipolar disorder to identify early symptoms of relapse and obtain treatment. *BMJ*. 1999;**318**(7177):149–153.

44. Nowlin-Finch NL, Altshuler LL, Szuba MP, Mintz J. Rapid resolution of first episodes of mania: sleep related? *J Clin Psychiatry*. 1994;**55**(1):26–29.

45. Barbini B, Bertelli S, Colombo C, Smeraldi E. Sleep loss, a possible factor in augmenting manic episode. *Psychiatry Res*. 1996;**65**(2):121–125.

46. Post RM, Ketter TA, Pazzaglia PJ, et al. Rational polypharmacy in the bipolar affective disorders. *Epilepsy Res Suppl*. 1996;**11**:153–180.

47. Modell JG, Lenox RH, Weiner S. Inpatient clinical trial of lorazepam for the management of manic agitation. *J Clin Psychopharmacol*. 1985;**5**(2):109–113.

48. Chengappa KN, Tohen M, Levine J, et al. Response to placebo among bipolar I disorder patients experiencing their first manic episode. *Bipolar Disord*. 2000;**2**(4):332–335.

49. Sharpley AL, Vassallo CM, Cowen PJ. Olanzapine increases slow-wave sleep: evidence for blockade of central 5-HT(2C) receptors in vivo. *Biol Psychiatry*. 2000;**47**(5):468–470.

50. Cohrs S, Rodenbeck A, Guan Z, et al. Sleep-promoting properties of quetiapine in healthy subjects. *Psychopharmacology (Berl)*. 2004;**174**(3):421–429.

51. Cohrs S, Meier A, Neumann AC, et al. Improved sleep continuity and increased slow wave sleep and REM latency during ziprasidone treatment: a randomized, controlled, crossover trial of 12 healthy male subjects. *J Clin Psychiatry*. 2005;**66**(8):989–996.

52. Bersani G, Garavini A. Melatonin add-on in manic patients with treatment resistant insomnia. *Prog Neuropsychopharmacol Biol Psychiatry*. 2000;**24**(2):185–191.

patients after lithium discontinuation. *Biol Psychiatry*. 1992;**31**(3):279–284.

53. Turek FW, Gillette MU. Melatonin, sleep, and circadian rhythms: rationale for development of specific melatonin agonists. *Sleep Med.* 2004; **5**(6):523–532.

54. Palmer HA. The value of continuous narcosis in the treatment of mental disorders. *J Ment Sci.* 1937;**83**:636–678.

55. Wehr TA, Turner EH, Shimada JM, et al. Treatment of rapidly cycling bipolar patient by using extended bed rest and darkness to stabilize the timing and duration of sleep. *Biol Psychiatry.* 1998; **43**(11):822–828.

56. Barbini B, Benedetti F, Colombo C, et al. Dark therapy for mania: a pilot study. *Bipolar Disord.* 2005; **7**(1):98–101.

57. Kupfer DJ, Wyatt RJ, Snyder F. Comparison between electroencephalographic and systematic nursing observations of sleep in psychiatric patients. *J Nerv Ment Dis.* 1970;**151**(6):361–368.

58. Harvey AG. Sleep and circadian rhythms in bipolar disorder: seeking synchrony, harmony, and regulation. *Am J Psychiatry.* 2008;**165**(7):820–829.

59. Riemann D, Voderholzer U, Berger M. Sleep and sleep-wake manipulations in bipolar depression. *Neuropsychobiology.* 2002;**45**(Suppl 1):7–12.

60. Detre T, Himmelhoch J, Swartzburg M, et al. Hypersomnia and manic-depressive disease. *Am J Psychiatry.* 1972;**128**(10):1303–1305.

61. Bowden CL. A different depression: clinical distinctions between bipolar and unipolar depression. *J Affect Disord.* 2005;**84**(2–3):117–125.

62. Kaplan KA, Harvey AG. Hypersomnia across mood disorders: a review and synthesis. *Sleep Med Rev.* 2009;**13**(4):275–285.

63. Benazzi F. Symptoms of depression as possible markers of bipolar II disorder. *Prog Neuropsychopharmacol Biol Psychiatry.* 2006; **30**(3):471–477.

64. Hantouche EG, Akiskal HS. Bipolar II vs. unipolar depression: psychopathologic differentiation by dimensional measures. *J Affect Disord.* 2005; **84**(2–3):127–132.

65. Forty L, Smith D, Jones L, et al. Clinical differences between bipolar and unipolar depression. *Br J Psychiatry.* 2008;**192**(5):388–389.

66. Akiskal HS, Benazzi F. Atypical depression: a variant of bipolar II or a bridge between unipolar and bipolar II? *J Affect Disord.* 2005;**84**(2–3):209–217.

67. Nofzinger EA, Thase ME, Reynolds CF 3rd, et al. Hypersomnia in bipolar depression: a comparison with narcolepsy using the multiple sleep latency test. *Am J Psychiatry.* 1991;**148**(9):1177–1181.

68. American Psychiatric Association. Practice guidelines for the treatment of patients with bipolar disorder (revision). *Am J Psychiatry.* 2002;**159**(4 Suppl):1–50.

69. Wirz-Justice A, Van den Hoofdakker RH. Sleep deprivation in depression: what do we know, where do we go? *Biol Psychiatry.* 1999;**46**(4):445–453.

70. Wirz-Justice A, Benedetti F, Berger M, et al. Chronotherapeutics (light and wake therapy) in affective disorders. *Psychol Med.* 2005;**35**(7):939–944.

71. Szuba MP, Baxter LR Jr, Fairbanks LA, Guze BH, Schwartz JM. Effects of partial sleep deprivation on the diurnal variation of mood and motor activity in major depression. *Biol Psychiatry.* 1991;**30**(8):817–829.

72. Barbini B, Colombo C, Benedetti F, et al. The unipolar-bipolar dichotomy and the response to sleep deprivation. *Psychiatry Res.* 1998;**79**(1):43–50.

73. Gill DS, Ketter TA, Post RM. Antidepressant response to sleep deprivation as a function of time into depressive episode in rapidly cycling bipolar patients. *Acta Psychiatr Scand.* 1993;**87**(2):102–109.

74. Baxter LR Jr, Liston EH, Schwartz JM, et al. Prolongation of the antidepressant response to partial sleep deprivation by lithium. *Psychiatry Res.* 1986; **19**(1):17–23.

75. Grube M, Hartwich P. Maintenance of antidepressant effect of sleep deprivation with the help of lithium. *Eur Arch Psychiatry Clin Neurosci.* 1990;**240**(1):60–61.

76. Szuba MP, Baxter LR Jr, Altshuler LL, et al. Lithium sustains the acute antidepressant effects of sleep deprivation: preliminary findings from a controlled study. *Psychiatry Res.* 1994;**51**(3):283–295.

77. Benedetti F, Colombo C, Barbini B, Campori E, Smeraldi E. Ongoing lithium treatment prevents relapse after total sleep deprivation. *J Clin Psychopharmacol.* 1999;**19**(3):240–245.

78. Smeraldi E, Benedetti F, Barbini B, Campori E, Colombo C. Sustained antidepressant effect of sleep deprivation combined with pindolol in bipolar depression: A placebo-controlled trial. *Neuropsychopharmacology.* 1999;**20**(4):380–385.

79. Benedetti F, Barbini B, Fulgosi MC, et al. Combined total sleep deprivation and light therapy in the treatment of drug-resistant bipolar depression: acute response and long-term remission rates. *J Clin Psychiatry.* 2005;**66**(12):1535–1540.

80. Colombo C, Lucca A, Benedetti F, et al. Total sleep deprivation combined with lithium and light therapy in the treatment of bipolar depression: replication of main effects and interaction. *Psychiatry Res.* 2000; **95**(1):43–53.

81. Benedetti F, Colombo C, Barbini B, Campori E, Smeraldi E. Morning sunlight reduces length of

hospitalization in bipolar depression. *J Affect Disord.* 2001;**62**(3):221–223.

82. Berger M, Vollmann J, Hohagen F, et al. Sleep deprivation combined with consecutive sleep phase advance as a fast-acting therapy in depression: an open pilot trial in medicated and unmedicated patients. *Am J Psychiatry.* 1997;**154**(6):870–872.

83. Riemann D, Konig A, Hohagen F, et al. How to preserve the antidepressive effect of sleep deprivation: A comparison of sleep phase advance and sleep phase delay. *Eur Arch Psychiatry Clin Neurosci.* 1999; **249**(5):231–237.

84. Neumeister A, Goessler R, Lucht M, et al. Bright light therapy stabilizes the antidepressant effect of partial sleep deprivation. *Biol Psychiatry.* 1996;**39**(1):16–21.

85. Benedetti F, Barbini B, Campori E, et al. Sleep phase advance and lithium to sustain the antidepressant effect of total sleep deprivation in bipolar depression: new findings supporting the internal coincidence model? *J Psychiatr Res.* 2001;**35**(6):323–329.

86. Benedetti F, Serretti A, Colombo C, et al. Influence of a functional polymorphism within the promoter of the serotonin transporter gene on the effects of total sleep deprivation in bipolar depression. *Am J Psychiatry.* 1999;**156**(9):1450–1452.

87. Benedetti F, Barbini B, Bernasconi A, et al. Serotonin 5-HT2A receptor gene variants influence antidepressant response to repeated total sleep deprivation in bipolar depression. *Prog Neuropsychopharmacol Biol Psychiatry.* 2008; **32**(8):1863–1866.

88. Benedetti F, Barbini B, Bernasconi A, et al. Acute antidepressant response to sleep deprivation combined with light therapy is influenced by the catechol-O-methyltransferase Val(108/158)Met polymorphism. *J Affect Disord.* 2010;**121**(1–2):68–72.

89. Benedetti F, Serretti A, Colombo C, et al. A glycogen synthase kinase 3-beta promoter gene single nucleotide polymorphism is associated with age at onset and response to total sleep deprivation in bipolar depression. *Neurosci Lett.* 2004; **368**(2):123–126.

90. Sachs GS. Unmet clinical needs in bipolar disorder. *J Clin Psychopharmacol.* 2003;**23**(3 Suppl 1):S2–8.

91. Knowles JB, Cairns J, MacLean AW, et al. The sleep of remitted bipolar depressives: comparison with sex and age-matched controls. *Can J Psychiatry.* 1986; **31**(4):295–298.

92. Sitaram N, Nurnberger JI Jr, Gershon ES, Gillin JC. Cholinergic regulation of mood and REM sleep: potential model and marker of vulnerability to affective disorder. *Am J Psychiatry.* 1982; **139**(5):571–576.

93. Millar A, Espie CA, Scott J. The sleep of remitted bipolar outpatients: a controlled naturalistic study using actigraphy. *J Affect Disord.* 2004; **80**(2–3):145–153.

94. Jones SH, Hare DJ, Evershed K. Actigraphic assessment of circadian activity and sleep patterns in bipolar disorder. *Bipolar Disord.* 2005;**7**(2):176–186.

95. Harvey AG, Schmidt DA, Scarna A, Semler CN, Goodwin GM. Sleep-related functioning in euthymic patients with bipolar disorder, patients with insomnia, and subjects without sleep problems. *Am J Psychiatry.* 2005;**162**(1):50–57.

96. Mansour HA, Wood J, Chowdari KV, et al. Circadian phase variation in bipolar I disorder. *Chronobiol Int.* 2005;**22**(3):571–584.

97. Wood J, Birmaher B, Axelson D, et al. Replicable differences in preferred circadian phase between bipolar disorder patients and control individuals. *Psychiatry Res.* 2009;**166**(2–3):201–209.

98. Ahn YM, Chang J, Joo YH, et al. Chronotype distribution in bipolar I disorder and schizophrenia in a Korean sample. *Bipolar Disord.* 2008; **10**(2):271–275.

99. Carney PA, Fitzgerald CT, Monaghan CE. Influence of climate on the prevalence of mania. *Br J Psychiatry.* 1988;**152**:820–823.

100. Mulder RT, Cosgriff JP, Smith AM, Joyce PR. Seasonality of mania in New Zealand. *Aust N Z J Psychiatry.* 1990;**24**(2):187–190.

101. Sayer HK, Marshall S, Mellsop GW. Mania and seasonality in the southern hemisphere. *J Affect Disord.* 1991;**23**(3):151–156.

102. Lee HC, Tsai SY, Lin HC. Seasonal variations in bipolar disorder admissions and the association with climate: a population-based study. *J Affect Disord.* 2007;**97**(1–3):61–69.

103. Lewy AJ, Nurnberger JI Jr, Wehr TA, et al. Supersensitivity to light: possible trait marker for manic-depressive illness. *Am J Psychiatry.* 1985; **142**(6):725–727.

104. Lewy AJ, Wehr TA, Goodwin FK, Newsome DA, Rosenthal NE. Manic-depressive patients may be supersensitive to light. *Lancet.* 1981; **1**(8216):383–384.

105. Kennedy SH, Kutcher SP, Ralevski E, Brown GM. Nocturnal melatonin and 24-hour 6-sulphatoxymelatonin levels in various phases of bipolar affective disorder. *Psychiatry Res.* 1996; **63**(2–3):219–222.

106. Whalley LJ, Perini T, Shering A, Bennie J. Melatonin response to bright light in recovered, drug-free, bipolar patients. *Psychiatry Res.* 1991;**38**(1):13–19.

107. Nurnberger JI Jr, Adkins S, Lahiri DK, et al. Melatonin suppression by light in euthymic bipolar and unipolar patients. *Arch Gen Psychiatry*. 2000; 57(6):572–579.

108. Craddock N, Jones I. Genetics of bipolar disorder. *J Med Genet*. 1999;36(8):585–594.

109. Taylor L, Faraone SV, Tsuang MT. Family, twin, and adoption studies of bipolar disease. *Curr Psychiatry Rep*. 2002;4(2):130–133.

110. Lenox RH, Gould TD, Manji HK. Endophenotypes in bipolar disorder. *Am J Med Genet*. 2002; 114(4):391–406.

111. Hasler G, Drevets WC, Gould TD, Gottesman II, Manji HK. Toward constructing an endophenotype strategy for bipolar disorders. *Biol Psychiatry*. 2006;60(2):93–105.

112. Gottesman II, Gould TD. The endophenotype concept in psychiatry: etymology and strategic intentions. *Am J Psychiatry*. 2003;160(4):636–645.

113. Benedetti F, Dallaspezia S, Fulgosi MC, et al. Actimetric evidence that CLOCK 3111 T/C SNP influences sleep and activity patterns in patients affected by bipolar depression. *Am J Med Genet B Neuropsychiatr Genet*. 2007;144B(5):631–635.

114. Benedetti F, Serretti A, Colombo C, et al. Influence of CLOCK gene polymorphism on circadian mood fluctuation and illness recurrence in bipolar depression. *Am J Med Genet B Neuropsychiatr Genet*. 2003;123B(1):23–26.

115. Serretti A, Benedetti F, Mandelli L, et al. Genetic dissection of psychopathological symptoms: insomnia in mood disorders and CLOCK gene polymorphism. *Am J Med Genet B Neuropsychiatr Genet*. 2003;121B(1):35–38.

116. Serretti A, Cusin C, Benedetti F, et al. Insomnia improvement during antidepressant treatment and CLOCK gene polymorphism. *Am J Med Genet B Neuropsychiatr Genet*. 2005;137B(1):36–39.

117. Roybal K, Theobold D, Graham A, et al. Mania-like behavior induced by disruption of CLOCK. *Proc Natl Acad Sci U S A*. 2007;104(15):6406–6411.

118. Mansour HA, Wood J, Logue T, et al. Association study of eight circadian genes with bipolar I disorder, schizoaffective disorder and schizophrenia. *Genes Brain Behav*. 2006;5(2):150–157.

119. Nievergelt CM, Kripke DF, Barrett TB, et al. Suggestive evidence for association of the circadian genes PERIOD3 and ARNTL with bipolar disorder. *Am J Med Genet B Neuropsychiatr Genet*. 2006; 141B(3):234–241.

120. Mansour HA, Talkowski ME, Wood J, et al. Association study of 21 circadian genes with bipolar I disorder, schizoaffective disorder, and schizophrenia. *Bipolar Disord*. 2009;11(7):701–710.

121. Benedetti F, Dallaspezia S, Colombo C, et al. A length polymorphism in the circadian clock gene Per3 influences age at onset of bipolar disorder. *Neurosci Lett*. 2008;445(2):184–187.

122. Viola AU, Archer SN, James LM, et al. PER3 polymorphism predicts sleep structure and waking performance. *Curr Biol*. 2007;17(7):613–618.

123. Shiino Y, Nakajima S, Ozeki Y, Isono T, Yamada N. Mutation screening of the human period 2 gene in bipolar disorder. *Neurosci Lett*. 2003;338(1):82–84.

124. Nievergelt CM, Kripke DF, Remick RA, et al. Examination of the clock gene Cryptochrome 1 in bipolar disorder: mutational analysis and absence of evidence for linkage or association. *Psychiatr Genet*. 2005;15(1):45–52.

125. Benedetti F, Bernasconi A, Lorenzi C, et al. A single nucleotide polymorphism in glycogen synthase kinase 3-beta promoter gene influences onset of illness in patients affected by bipolar disorder. *Neurosci Lett*. 2004;355(1–2):37–40.

126. Benedetti F, Serretti A, Pontiggia A, et al. Long-term response to lithium salts in bipolar illness is influenced by the glycogen synthase kinase 3-beta -50 T/C SNP. *Neurosci Lett*. 2005;376(1):51–55.

127. Gould TD, Manji HK. Glycogen synthase kinase-3: a putative molecular target for lithium mimetic drugs. *Neuropsychopharmacology*. 2005;30(7):1223–1237.

128. Yin L, Wang J, Klein PS, Lazar MA. Nuclear receptor Rev-erbalpha is a critical lithium-sensitive component of the circadian clock. *Science*. 2006; 311(5763):1002–1005.

129. Severino G, Manchia M, Contu P, et al. Association study in a Sardinian sample between bipolar disorder and the nuclear receptor REV-ERBalpha gene, a critical component of the circadian clock system. *Bipolar Disord*. 2009;11(2):215–220.

130. Flemons WW. Clinical practice: Obstructive sleep apnea. *N Engl J Med*. 2002;347(7):498–504.

131. Allen RP, Walters AS, Montplaisir J, et al. Restless legs syndrome prevalence and impact: REST general population study. *Arch Intern Med*. 2005;165(11): 1286–1292.

132. Hattori M, Kitajima T, Mekata T, et al. Risk factors for obstructive sleep apnea syndrome screening in mood disorder patients. *Psychiatry Clin Neurosci*. 2009;63(3): 385–391.

133. Ohayon MM, Caulet M, Philip P, Guilleminault C, Priest RG. How sleep and mental disorders are related to complaints of daytime sleepiness. *Arch Intern Med*. 1997;157(22):2645–2652.

134. Sharafkhaneh A, Giray N, Richardson P, Young T, Hirshkowitz M. Association of psychiatric disorders and sleep apnea in a large cohort. *Sleep*. 2005; **28**(11):1405–1411.

135. Berge D, Salgado P, Rodriguez A, Bulbena A. Onset of mania after CPAP in a man with obstructive sleep apnea. *Psychosomatics*. 2008;**49**(5):447–449.

136. Trakada G, Steiropoulos P, Bouros D. Continuous positive airways pressure treatment in a patient with sleep apnea-hypopnea syndrome and coexisting bipolar disorder. *Psychopharmacol Bull*. 2008; **41**(2):89–92.

137. Lahera Forteza G, Gonzalez Aguado F. Psychotic mania after introduction of continuous positive airway pressure (CPAP) in the treatment of obstructive sleep apnoea. *Actas Esp Psiquiatr*. 2007; **35**(6):406–407.

138. Hilleret H, Jeunet E, Osiek C, Mohr S, Blois R, Bertschy G. Mania resulting from continuous positive airways pressure in a depressed man with sleep apnea syndrome. *Neuropsychobiology*. 2001; **43**(3):221–224.

139. Fagiolini A, Kupfer DJ, Houck PR, Novick DM, Frank E. Obesity as a correlate of outcome in patients with bipolar I disorder. *Am J Psychiatry*. 2003; **160**(1):112–117.

140. Devlin MJ, Yanovski SZ, Wilson GT. Obesity: what mental health professionals need to know. *Am J Psychiatry*. 2000;**157**(6):854–866.

141. Winkelman JW. Schizophrenia, obesity, and obstructive sleep apnea. *J Clin Psychiatry*. 2001; **62**(1):8–11.

142. Pinninti NR, Mago R, Townsend J, Doghramji K. Periodic restless legs syndrome associated with quetiapine use: a case report. *J Clin Psychopharmacol*. 2005;**25**(6):617–618.

143. Kraus T, Schuld A, Pollmacher T. Periodic leg movements in sleep and restless legs syndrome probably caused by olanzapine. *J Clin Psychopharmacol*. 1999;**19**(5):478–479.

144. Wetter TC, Brunner J, Bronisch T. Restless legs syndrome probably induced by risperidone treatment. *Pharmacopsychiatry*. 2002;**35**(3):109–111.

145. Duggal HS, Mendhekar DN. Clozapine-associated restless legs syndrome. *J Clin Psychopharmacol*. 2007;**27**(1):89–90.

146. Heiman EM, Christie M. Lithium-aggravated nocturnal myoclonus and restless legs syndrome. *Am J Psychiatry*. 1986;**143**(9):1191–1192.

147. Yang C, White DP, Winkelman JW. Antidepressants and periodic leg movements of sleep. *Biol Psychiatry*. 2005;**58**(6):510–514.

148. Rottach KG, Schaner BM, Kirch MH, et al. Restless legs syndrome as side effect of second generation antidepressants. *J Psychiatr Res*. 2008;**43**(1):70–75.

149. Telstad W, Sorensen O, Larsen S, et al. Treatment of the restless legs syndrome with carbamazepine: a double blind study. *Br Med J (Clin Res Ed)*. 1984; **288**(6415):444–446.

150. Lundvall O, Abom PE, Holm R. Carbamazepine in restless legs: A controlled pilot study. *Eur J Clin Pharmacol*. 1983;**25**(3):323–324.

151. Zucconi M, Coccagna G, Petronelli R, et al. Nocturnal myoclonus in restless legs syndrome: effect of carbamazepine treatment. *Funct Neurol*. 1989; **4**(3):263–271.

152. Eisensehr I, Ehrenberg BL, Rogge Solti S, Noachtar S. Treatment of idiopathic restless legs syndrome (RLS) with slow-release valproic acid compared with slow-release levodopa/benserazid. *J Neurol*. 2004; **251**(5):579–583.

153. Youssef EA, Wagner ML, Martinez JO, Hening W. Pilot trial of lamotrigine in the restless legs syndrome. *Sleep Med*. 2005;**6**(1):89.

154. Aiken CB. Pramipexole in psychiatry: a systematic review of the literature. *J Clin Psychiatry*. 2007; **68**(8):1230–1236.

155. Sharma V, Smith A. A case of mania following the use of pramipexole. *Am J Psychiatry*. 2007;**164**(2):351.

156. Stoner SC, Dahmen MM, Makos M, et al. An exploratory retrospective evaluation of ropinirole-associated psychotic symptoms in an outpatient population treated for restless legs syndrome or Parkinson's disease. *Ann Pharmacother*. 2009; **43**(9):1426–1432.

157. Wingo AP, Ghaemi SN. Frequency of stimulant treatment and of stimulant-associated mania/hypomania in bipolar disorder patients. *Psychopharmacol Bull*. 2008;**41**(4):37–47.

158. Nasr S, Wendt B, Steiner K. Absence of mood switch with and tolerance to modafinil: A replication study from a large private practice. *J Affect Disord*. 2006; **95**(1–3):111–114.

159. Frye MA, Grunze H, Suppes T, et al. A placebo-controlled evaluation of adjunctive modafinil in the treatment of bipolar depression. *Am J Psychiatry*. 2007;**164**(8):1242–1249.

160. Ranjan S, Chandra PS. Modafinil-induced irritability and aggression? A report of 2 bipolar patients. *J Clin Psychopharmacol*. 2005;**25**(6):628–629.

161. Wolf J, Fiedler U, Anghelescu I, Schwertfeger N. Manic switch in a patient with treatment-resistant bipolar depression treated with modafinil. *J Clin Psychiatry*. 2006;**67**(11):1817.

162. Fountoulakis KN, Siamouli M, Panagiotidis P, et al. Ultra short manic-like episodes after antidepressant augmentation with modafinil. *Prog Neuropsychopharmacol Biol Psychiatry*. 2008; **32**(3):891–892.

163. Smith MT, Huang MI, Manber R. Cognitive behavior therapy for chronic insomnia occurring within the context of medical and psychiatric disorders. *Clin Psychol Rev*. 2005; **25**(5):559–592.

164. Morgenthaler T, Kramer M, Alessi C, et al. Practice parameters for the psychological and behavioral treatment of insomnia: an update. An American Academy of Sleep Medicine report. *Sleep*. 2006; **29**(11):1415–1419.

165. Ashman SB, Monk TH, Kupfer DJ, et al. Relationship between social rhythms and mood in patients with rapid cycling bipolar disorder. *Psychiatry Res*. 1999;**86**(1):1–8.

166. Feldman-Naim S, Turner EH, Leibenluft E. Diurnal variation in the direction of mood switches in patients with rapid-cycling bipolar disorder. *J Clin Psychiatry*. 1997;**58**(2):79–84.

167. Colom F, Vieta E, Martinez-Aran A, et al. A randomized trial on the efficacy of group psychoeducation in the prophylaxis of recurrences in bipolar patients whose disease is in remission. *Arch Gen Psychiatry*. 2003; **60**(4):402–407.

168. Colom F, Lam D. Psychoeducation: improving outcomes in bipolar disorder. *Eur Psychiatry*. 2005; **20**(5–6):359–364.

169. Frank E, Swartz HA, Kupfer D J. Interpersonal and social rhythm therapy: managing the chaos of bipolar disorder. *Biol Psychiatry*. 2000; **48**(6):593–604.

170. Frank E, Kupfer DJ, Thase ME, et al. Two-year outcomes for interpersonal and social rhythm therapy in individuals with bipolar I disorder. *Arch Gen Psychiatry*. 2005;**62**(9):996–1004.

171. Otto MW, Reilly-Harrington N, Sachs GS. Psychoeducational and cognitive-behavioral strategies in the management of bipolar disorder. *J Affect Disord*. 2003;73(1–2):171–181.

172. Lam DH, Watkins ER, Hayward P, et al. A randomized controlled study of cognitive therapy for relapse prevention for bipolar affective disorder: outcome of the first year. *Arch Gen Psychiatry*. 2003; **60**(2):145–152.

173. Sachs GS, Rosenbaum JF, Jones L. Adjunctive clonazepam for maintenance treatment of bipolar affective disorder. *J Clin Psychopharmacol*. 1990; **10**(1):42–47.

174. Sachs GS, Weilburg JB, Rosenbaum JF. Clonazepam vs. neuroleptics as adjuncts to lithium maintenance. *Psychopharmacol Bull*. 1990; **26**(1):137–143.

175. Aronson TA, Shukla S, Hirschowitz J. Clonazepam treatment of five lithium-refractory patients with bipolar disorder. *Am J Psychiatry*. 1989; **146**(1):77–80.

176. Winkler D, Willeit M, Wolf R, et al. Clonazepam in the long-term treatment of patients with unipolar depression, bipolar and schizoaffective disorder. *Eur Neuropsychopharmacol*. 2003;**13**(2):129–134.

177. Walsh JK, Roth T, Randazzo A, et al. Eight weeks of non-nightly use of zolpidem for primary insomnia. *Sleep*. 2000;**23**(8):1087–1096.

178. Perlis ML, McCall WV, Krystal AD, Walsh JK. Long-term, non-nightly administration of zolpidem in the treatment of patients with primary insomnia. *J Clin Psychiatry*. 2004;**65**(8):1128–1137.

179. Krystal AD, Walsh JK, Laska E, et al. Sustained efficacy of eszopiclone over 6 months of nightly treatment: results of a randomized, double-blind, placebo-controlled study in adults with chronic insomnia. *Sleep*. 2003;**26**(7):793–799.

180. Erman M, Krystal A, Zammit G, Soubrane C, Roth T. Zolpidem extended-release 12.5 mg, taken for 24 weeks "as needed" up to 7 nights/week, improves subjective measures of therapeutic global impression, sleep onset, and sleep maintenance in patients with chronic insomnia. *Int J Neuropsychopharmacol*. 2006; **9**(Suppl 1):S256.

181. Vornik LA, Brown ES. Management of comorbid bipolar disorder and substance abuse. *J Clin Psychiatry*. 2006;**67**(Suppl 7):24–30.

182. NIH. NIH State-of-the-Science conference statement on manifestations and management of chronic insomnia in adults. *NIH Consensus and State-of-the-Science Statements*. 2005;**22**(2):1–30. http://consensus. nih.gov/2005/2005InsomniaSOS026PDF.pdf. Accessed 30 October, 2009.

183. Peet M. Induction of mania with selective serotonin re-uptake inhibitors and tricyclic antidepressants. *Br J Psychiatry*. 1994;**164**(4):549–550.

184. Jabeen S, Fisher CJ. Trazodone-induced transient hypomanic symptoms and their management. *Br J Psychiatry*. 1991;**158**:275–278.

185. Terao T. Comparison of manic switch onset during fluoxetine and trazodone treatment. *Biol Psychiatry*. 1993;**33**(6):477–478.

186. Doghramji PP. Trends in the pharmacologic management of insomnia. *J Clin Psychiatry*. 2006; **67**(Suppl 13):5–8.

187. Foldvary-Schaefer N, De Leon Sanchez I, Karafa M, et al. Gabapentin increases slow-wave sleep in normal adults. *Epilepsia*. 2002; **43**(12):1493–1497.

188. Roth T, Wright KP Jr, Walsh J. Effect of tiagabine on sleep in elderly subjects with primary insomnia: a randomized, double-blind, placebo-controlled study. *Sleep*. 2006;**29**(3):335–341.

189. Leibenluft E, Feldman-Naim S, Turner EH, Wehr TA, Rosenthal NE. Effects of exogenous melatonin administration and withdrawal in five patients with rapid-cycling bipolar disorder. *J Clin Psychiatry*. 1997;**58**(9):383–388.

190. Plante DT, Winkelman JW. Sleep disturbance in bipolar disorder: therapeutic implications. *Am J Psychiatry*. 2008;**165**(7):830–843.

Sleep in anxiety disorders

Candice A. Alfano and Thomas A. Mellman

Introduction

Sleep disturbances including insomnia are frequently associated with and can comprise core features of anxiety disorders. The presence of anxiety poses risk for the later development of insomnia, with approximately 40% of adults reporting problems with insomnia following the onset of an anxiety disorder [1]. Similarly, sleep loss can exacerbate daytime symptoms of anxiety and persisting insomnia is a risk factor for the subsequent onset of anxiety disorders [2–6]. This bidirectional relationship implies a shared underlying pathophysiology and suggests the possibility of a progressive worsening of both disorders and associated impairments over time. The links between anxiety and sleep disturbances may therefore be relevant to understanding mechanisms and dysfunctions of arousal regulation that underlie both types of problems.

The senior author of this chapter (Dr. Mellman) has provided or contributed several relatively recent overviews of sleep aspects of anxiety disorders in adults [7,8]. Building on this work, emerging data indicate that not unlike adults, sleep problems during childhood are likely to co-occur with anxiety disorders. Since many adult sleep disorders originate during and persist from childhood [9], collectively, there is a clear need for a developmental framework in attempting to understand the interactions and ideal management of these problems at different stages across the life-span. Thus, in line with the clinical emphasis of the current volume, this chapter is distinguished by its inclusion and discussion of sleep aspects of anxiety disorders in children, made possible by the contribution of Dr. Alfano, a pediatric psychologist whose work focuses on sleep and anxiety in youth. Through this collaborative writing we hope to provide a more comprehensive overview and heighten awareness of the potential linkages between the regulation of sleep, arousal, and emotion in anxious adults as well as children.

While all types of anxiety disorders may co-occur with some form of sleep disruption, only post-traumatic stress disorder (PTSD), generalized anxiety disorder (GAD), and separation anxiety disorder (SAD) feature sleep disturbance among their diagnostic criteria in DSM-IV. Criteria for PTSD include nightmares with trauma-related content and difficulty initiating and maintaining sleep, which is a common definition of insomnia. Insomnia is also a symptom criterion and common feature of GAD. Although not a formal DSM-IV criterion, panic disorder (PD) has also been associated with complaints of difficulty initiating and maintaining sleep. Panic attacks that arise from sleep are not an uncommon occurrence with PD. All of the anxiety disorders that are diagnosed in adults can also be diagnosed in children, though PD prior to adolescence is rare. SAD is usually confined to childhood but may be a progenitor of adult panic disorder [10]. SAD criteria include both difficulty or refusal to sleep independently and separation-themed nightmares and, in many cases, sleep difficulties represent one of the more prominent features of the disorder. Lastly, data also are beginning to emerge suggesting that youth with obsessive-compulsive disorder (OCD) commonly experience sleep disruption, including difficulty falling asleep.

In adults and children there is considerable overlap between interventions that target insomnia and other sleep disturbances and those that are utilized in treating anxiety disorders. Overlapping approaches include medications, as well as behavioral modification and cognitive restructuring strategies. In children, attention to environmental and familial factors that serve to maintain both anxiety and sleep problems is

Foundations of Psychiatric Sleep Medicine, ed. John W. Winkelman and David T. Plante. Published by Cambridge University Press.
© Cambridge University Press 2010.

often necessary. For example, elimination of parental reinforcement of children's avoidant night-time behaviors that delay and/or interfere with sleep onset may be critical for treatment success [11,12]. Overall, however, optimal sequencing and/or integration of treatments targeting anxiety disorders and sleep problems are not well investigated. It is important for future research to address this deficiency. Meanwhile clinician's consideration of both sleep and anxiety symptoms in formulating their treatments is critical toward mitigating the chronicity, elevated relapse risk, and impairments associated with their co-occurrence.

Polysomnography (PSG) can provide objective indices of sleep initiation and maintenance, as well as information regarding sleep architecture. This tool and other laboratory methods applied to sleep can offer unique perspectives on the function of the neurobiological systems involved in arousal, sleep, and anxiety phenomena. However, the practicing clinician should be aware that PSG is not routinely indicated for the evaluation of an anxiety disorder unless a primary sleep disorder (e.g. obstructive sleep apnea) is suspected. In the following sections, clinical issues and sleep laboratory information (when available) regarding sleep aspects of specific anxiety disorders in adults and children are discussed, followed by a discussion of treatment issues that interface sleep and anxiety disorders.

Sleep in specific and social phobias

Intense fear and behavioral avoidance of certain things or situations are hallmark features of phobic disorders. Specific phobias often originate during childhood and fear and avoidance in general are not uncommon during childhood. For example, transient night-time fears such as the dark, monsters, or burglars are considered to be developmentally appropriate and occur in approximately 70% of young children [13,14]. Although most will overcome or outgrow these fears, a proportion of children experience persistent or severe enough fears that interfere with sleep and family functioning on an ongoing basis. In such cases, persistent night-time fears may be indicative of an underlying anxiety disorder. Muris et al. [14] found severe night-time fears to be related to one or more DSM anxiety disorders in more than 10% of children aged 4–12 years. Specific phobias, SAD, and GAD were the most common anxiety diagnoses. There is also some

evidence for associations between phobic and sleep disorders during adolescence. In one study specifically examining parasomnias, including sleep terrors and sleepwalking in adolescents, increased rates of co-morbidity with specific phobias and other anxiety disorders were reported [15]. Investigations relating sleep to specific phobias in adults are more limited. In one investigation by Clark et al. [16] sleep architecture was similar in depressed persons with and without phobias.

Similar to specific phobias, social phobia (SOC) can be an outgrowth of childhood shyness. In fact, modal age of onset occurs during adolescence [17]. The core feature of SOC includes a persistent fear of one or more social or performance situations in which a person may encounter unfamiliar people or possible scrutiny from others. Since these situations occur during interactions with the environment during wakefulness, sleep disturbances are not typically regarded as central to or commonly associated with this disorder. Nonetheless, persons with SOC may experience anticipatory anxiety prior to an event which then disrupts sleep. This may be particularly prominent when, for example, a SOC child begins a new school year or an adult with SOC must give a speech at work.

In a study among SOC adults, subjective report of poorer sleep quality, longer sleep latency, more frequent sleep disturbances, and increased daytime dysfunction were found compared to controls [18]. However, another study utilizing PSG recordings among SOC adults reported normal findings of sleep [19]. In a clinic sample of youth with SOC, SAD, and GAD, Alfano et al. [20] found that children with a diagnosis of SOC had significantly fewer parent-reported sleep problems (including insomnia, difficulty sleeping alone or away from home, and nightmares) than youth with SAD or GAD.

Sleep in obsessive-compulsive disorder

Obsessive-compulsive disorder (OCD) features recurring intrusive thoughts (obsessions) that seem excessive or irrational to the individual, and behavioral rituals (compulsions) that are also excessive and usually related to obsessive thoughts. Although onset of OCD may occur anytime from preschool age into adulthood, at least one-third of adults report an onset of symptoms prior to adolescence [21]. The disorder is generally characterized by a chronic course that causes significant distress and interference with daily life. Although sleep disturbances are not core syndromal manifestations or prominent associated features, it is not uncommon for individuals with OCD to get "stuck" on certain words, images, or thoughts or to engage in elaborate rituals at night which can interfere with sleep.

An early polysomnographic study reported impaired sleep maintenance and a reduced latency to rapid eye movement (REM) sleep in adults with OCD [22]. However, two other studies utilizing PSG failed to replicate these results, reporting the sleep patterns of adults with OCD as essentially normal [23,24]. More recently, Kluge and colleagues [25] compared 10 inpatients with OCD without co-morbid depression and 10 healthy matched controls on PSG variables. Sleep did not differ across the groups with the exception of reduced stage 4 sleep in OCD patients. Also, similar to previous findings [22], dramatically reduced sleep-onset REM latencies (<10 minutes) were found among patients with more severe forms of OCD.

Rapoport et al. [26] compared the sleep characteristics of a small sample of adolescents with OCD (aged 13–17 years) to healthy controls based on one night of PSG. Significantly reduced sleep efficiency and increased sleep latency were found among the OCD group. Adolescents with OCD required twice as long as controls to initiate sleep. Storch and colleagues [27] examined the presence of parent- and child-reported sleep problems among a larger sample (N=66) of youth with OCD, aged 8–17 years. More than 90% of the sample experienced at least one type of sleep problem; trouble sleeping and daytime tiredness were present in more than 50% of the sample. Sleep problems were more common among younger children and females and associated with a more severe form of illness. One limitation of this study, however, was that the majority of youth were taking selective serotonin reuptake inhibitors at the time of assessment, which may have affected sleep. Overall, available findings suggest that sleep disruption is more likely to co-occur with more severe forms of OCD and is more likely during childhood.

Sleep in generalized anxiety disorder

The core feature of generalized anxiety disorder (GAD) is persistent, uncontrollable worry. A unique pattern of distressing somatic symptoms also differentiates GAD from other anxiety disorders in adults

as well as children. DSM-IV requires the presence of (at least) three out of six symptoms in addition to worry, one of which is difficulty initiating or maintaining sleep or restless/unsatisfying sleep, for a diagnosis. Only one additional symptom is required in children. Two of the other symptoms, fatigue and irritability, are common consequences of sleep loss. In addition, the principal attribute of GAD, excessive worry or apprehensive expectation, is frequently implicated in the genesis and maintenance of insomnia. Thus, there is a high degree of overlap between the two disorders.

Ohayon et al. [4] found that the co-morbidity of GAD with insomnia was greater than for all of the other psychiatric disorders surveyed. Numerous studies utilizing objective sleep recordings corroborate these reports. Consistent findings of sleep disruption in GAD across PSG studies include reduced total sleep time, increased wake time after sleep onset, reduced sleep efficiency, decreased stage 4 sleep, and increased stage 2 latency [28–32]. Increases in stage 1 sleep and shorter REM latency also have been reported, albeit less consistently [31,32]. Findings for number of nocturnal awakenings have been somewhat inconsistent, with both significant increases [29,31] and decreases [30] reported. Overall, however, the data suggest sleep disruption in GAD to be a problem of impaired sleep initiation as well as maintenance.

Although no study has used PSG to specifically examine the sleep of youth with GAD, findings from a study by Forbes and colleagues [33] where 80% (N=19) of anxious children had a GAD diagnosis suggest that increased arousals, decreased slow-wave sleep, and greater sleep onset latency are characteristics of this population. Alfano et al. [34] compared rates of parent-reported sleep problems among children with GAD and children with other anxiety disorders (aged 8–16 years) and reported that 94% compared to 74% had at least one sleep-related problem, respectively. Nightmares, trouble sleeping, and daytime tiredness were most commonly reported. Using a larger sample (N=128) Alfano et al. [20] compared the prevalence of several sleep problems among anxious youth with and without a diagnosis of GAD. Children with GAD experienced significantly more sleep problems than children with SOC but not SAD. Similar to previous findings, nightmares, insomnia, and daytime tiredness were most common.

Consistent with their high degree of overlap and co-morbidity, there is also substantial overlap in treatment approaches for GAD and insomnia. Intervention strategies include the use of medications that target benzodiazepine receptors as well as psychotherapeutic interventions that target worry and cognitive arousal. Application of these approaches is discussed further in the final section of this chapter.

Sleep in panic disorder

The core feature of panic disorder (PD) is recurrent and unexpected periods of extreme fear that occur in a sudden, crescendo-like manner. Fear is accompanied by intense physical symptoms that may include chest pain, heart palpitations, shortness of breath, dizziness, or abdominal distress. Chronic anxiety related to anticipation of subsequent attacks and phobic avoidance (agoraphobia) are also common features. PD typically has its onset in early adulthood but can occur earlier or later in life. Perhaps as a consequence of its relative infrequency, research examining sleep in youth with PD is unavailable.

Panic attacks can emerge from sleep. Sleep panic attacks have been suggested to result in a conditioned fear and apprehension of sleep, resulting in secondary insomnia [35]. Surveys document that insomnia is more frequent in patients with PD than in control populations [36,37]. Most [38–41] but not all [42,43] published studies of patients with PD that have utilized objective methods of sleep recordings have found evidence of impaired sleep initiation and maintenance. One of these studies found increased motor activity during sleep [43]. While there appears to be an association between excess body movement during sleep and PD, two studies have found that, paradoxically, overall movement during sleep is reduced on nights when patients experience sleep panic attacks [38,44]. Survey data have noted associations between sleep complaints and co-morbid depression in persons with PD [42]. However, it is unclear whether sleep disturbances may be attributable to the presence of a depressive illness, which commonly co-exists with panic, or whether depression may be more likely to co-occur with a more severe variant of PD. As these studies are cross-sectional, and since insomnia is a risk factor for the subsequent onset of depression [2,3], depression also may be more likely to evolve as a co-morbid condition when PD features disturbed sleep.

Sleep panic attacks are not uncommon in persons with PD. In a study that prospectively monitored panic attacks, 18% occurred during sleep hours [45]. In surveys and clinical evaluations, 33–71% of PD populations reported having experienced sleep panic attacks [36,46–48]. As many as a third of patients will experience sleep panic as, or more frequently than, wake panic attacks [35,36]. It is not known how commonly patients experience sleep panic exclusively; however, in these authors' experience patients who only panic during sleep are rare. These episodes have been described as being awakened with a "jolt" and feature apprehension and somatic symptoms similar to panic attacks that are triggered during wake states. Studies that have captured sleep panic attacks during PSG recordings find that the episodes were preceded by either stage 2 or stage 3 non-REM sleep [38,49]. Mellman and Uhde [38] more specifically noted that sleep panic attacks originated during the transition from stage 2 into early slow-wave sleep, which is a period of diminishing arousal. Slow-wave sleep is also a state where cognitive activity is at its nadir [50]. The phenomenon of sleep panic indicates that in addition to panic attacks evolving from states of heightening arousal and apprehension, panic can also occur during states of diminishing arousal.

Studies have compared PD patients who experience sleep panic attacks with those who only experience panic attacks from wake states. Associations between sleep panic and early age of illness onset, higher symptom load, depression, and suicidal ideation suggest a relationship with a more severe variant of the illness [46,51]. Patients with sleep panic have also been noted to experience anxiety from relaxation and hypnosis, and to have less agoraphobic avoidance and fewer catastrophic cognitions compared with PD patients who do not experience sleep panic [36,47,52,53]. Thus, having sleep panic appears to mark a propensity for attacks triggered by lower levels of arousal and for attacks to occur relatively independently of situational and cognitive variables. The association with markers of severity may reflect a stronger disease diathesis.

Sleep panic attacks can present in a manner that mimics medical conditions. Holter cardiac monitoring or overnight PSG recordings may be indicated when associated symptomatology suggests cardiac arrhythmias or sleep-related breathing disorders. Patient education and informed reassurance are helpful to patients with these frequently upsetting occurrences. Sleep panic attacks have been anecdotally observed to respond to antidepressant types of antipanic medications but not necessarily benzodiazepines [35].

Sleep in separation anxiety disorder

Anxiety related to separating from parents or caretakers is a normal aspect of child development that for most children will subside by age 3. By comparison, separation anxiety disorder (SAD) includes excessive, age-inappropriate fear about being apart from family members, especially parents, and leads to problematic behavioral avoidance. Children with SAD frequently refuse to attend school, have difficulty making and maintaining friends, are unwilling to do even basic tasks independently, and develop other anxiety or phobic disorders. Not surprisingly, a significant proportion of children with SAD experience difficulty sleeping independently and experience recurrent nightmares. Although earlier case reports sometimes referred to these problems as a "sleep phobia" (e.g. [54]), closer examination of clinical descriptions and case studies generally reveal a more pervasive problem with separation anxiety.

Despite its high prevalence, surprisingly few studies have examined sleep disruption in children with SAD. Alfano et al. [20] compared the prevalence of sleep problems in anxious youth with and without an SAD diagnosis. Children with SAD experienced significantly more sleep problems than children with SOC but not GAD. Insomnia, refusal to sleep alone, and nightmares were most commonly reported by parents. In a study by Verduin and Kendall [55] where the occurrence of specific co-morbid diagnoses was examined among children with primary SAD, GAD, and SOC, enuresis and sleep terror disorder were significantly more common among youth with SAD. It is important to note, however, that children with SAD in both studies were younger on average than anxious youth in comparison groups and the ability to disentangle disorder-specific sleep problems from age-related differences is limited.

Sleep in post-traumatic stress disorder

Post-traumatic stress disorder is an anxiety disorder that develops in children and adults who are exposed to severely threatening events. While PTSD is common, it develops in a minority of individuals who are exposed to trauma. Factors that influence the development of PTSD include severity of the trauma, personal risk factors, and initial reactions to the traumatic event [56]. Sleep disturbances including trauma-related nightmares and difficulty initiating and maintaining sleep represent DSM-IV criteria and prominent symptoms of PTSD [57]. Nightmares and insomnia appear to be common also in the early aftermath of trauma, especially among those who develop PTSD [58–61]. Furthermore, sleep disruption leads to fatigue and irritability, which are daytime symptoms of the disorder. Sleep disruption also may interfere with healthy emotional regulation and thereby contribute to the early development of the disorder.

Sleep laboratory study results, most of which have featured male war veterans during the chronic phase of the disorder, have been mixed in terms of finding objective indices of impaired sleep initiation and maintenance [62]. A recent meta-analysis of 20 PSG studies indicates that patients with PTSD have lighter sleep (more stage 1, less stage 3) compared to controls [63]. It is possible that the perceived safety of the sleep laboratory environment has a salutary effect on sleep disturbance in research participants with PTSD. Two recent studies that utilized home monitoring methods found increased sleep onset latency and reduced sleep efficiency, supporting this hypothesis [64,65].

There is also some controversy as to whether PTSD is associated with sleep-related breathing abnormalities. Krakow et al. [66] found evidence for sleep disordered breathing in all but 4 of 44 treatment-seeking patients who were referred for PSG assessment. However, no increase in sleep disordered breathing in association with PTSD was found in a study of community-recruited participants [67].

There has been relatively consistent evidence for abnormalities related to REM sleep in PTSD. The aforementioned meta-analysis noted that increased REM density and increased phasic motor activity during REM have been found in combat veterans with PTSD [68]. Nightmares and other symptomatic awakenings disproportionately arise from REM sleep [69,70]. Breslau et al. reported more frequent transitions from REM sleep to stage 1 or wake in a community sample of subjects with either lifetime (i.e. remitted) or current PTSD compared with trauma-exposed and trauma-unexposed controls [67]. A recent clinical study from Japan noted "REM interruption" in association with PTSD [71]. In a unique study that applied PSG within a month of trauma exposure, Mellman et al. [72] found that the patients who later developed PTSD had shorter continuous periods of REM sleep prior to stage shifts or arousals. Thus, there is converging evidence for disruptions of REM sleep continuity (symptomatic awakenings, increased awakening/arousals, and motor activity) and increased REM activation with PTSD. Mellman and Pigeon [73] hypothesized that the disruption to REM sleep continuity in PTSD interferes with the normal and adaptive memory processing functions of REM.

Although well documented in adults, research has only begun to examine associations between childhood trauma exposure and sleep. Two studies have used actigraphy to examine the sleep patterns of abused children. Glod et al. [74] reported that abused children demonstrate significantly longer sleep onset latencies than controls and depressed youth, and poorer sleep efficiencies than controls. No differences in sleep parameters were found among abused children based on the presence/absence of a PTSD diagnosis, suggesting that the effects of early abuse on sleep occur irrespective of the development of the clinical disorder. Glodd and colleagues also reported poorer sleep efficiencies (measured using portable ambulatory monitoring) among children with a history of physical compared to sexual abuse; and this finding has been replicated by another study [75]. Lastly, children with a PTSD diagnosis without co-morbid depression exhibited significantly greater nocturnal activity, longer sleep onset latencies, and reduced sleep efficiencies compared to children with PTSD and depression. Although more research is needed, the possibility exists that a co-morbid depressive disorder may be protective of sleep by reducing hypervigilance and noradrenergic overactivation associated with PTSD [76].

The effects of early trauma on sleep extend into adulthood. Bader et al. [77] examined associations between childhood trauma and sleep in 39 adults with insomnia based on 1 week of actigraphy. After controlling for demographic characteristics, current levels of stress, and depression, childhood trauma was the strongest predictor of sleep onset latency, sleep efficiency, and nocturnal activity in adulthood. Noll et al. [78] examined the presence of sleep disturbances in 78 abused females 10 years after disclosure of sexual abuse occurring between the ages of 6 and 16 years. Compared to controls, sexually abused females reported significantly more sleep disturbances. Abuse was a unique predictor of sleep problems even after controlling for depressive symptoms. Curiously, participants experiencing relatively less severe forms of sexual abuse (e.g. abuse by a single perpetrator, minimal physical violence, shorter durations of abuse, etc.) displayed the highest levels of adult sleep disturbances. The authors propose that because these participants may have initially presented with only mild symptoms, appropriate treatment may not have been received. Despite striking concurrent and longitudinal associations, relationships between early trauma and adult sleep disturbances remain poorly understood.

Treatment of sleep problems associated with anxiety

Sleep disturbances including insomnia have been found to be a prospective risk factor for psychiatric disorders including depression and anxiety [2,3,5]. Therefore, in addition to alleviating distress associated with insomnia, amelioration of sleep disturbances could possibly serve to prevent relapse and exacerbation of symptoms. In contrast to melancholic subtypes of depression where mood can paradoxically improve, anxiety disorders do not benefit and can worsen from sleep deprivation [79–81]. These data suggest that intervention approaches need to be tailored to individual patients.

Behavioral treatments

Behavioral therapies for anxiety disorders and sleep disturbances overlap to a great extent. Similar to anxiety, cognitive behavioral treatments (CBT) developed for insomnia have well-established efficacy (see Chapter 14: Cognitive behavioral therapy for insomnia) [82]. A key intervention component includes instruction on sleep hygiene such as maintaining consistent bedtimes and wake times, avoiding maladaptive use of substances, and not spending excessive time awake in bed. Additional components include relaxation techniques and identifying and challenging dysfunctional beliefs that perpetuate insomnia (e.g. "If I only get five hours sleep I will not be able to function tomorrow"). Management of anxious arousal, reducing avoidance behaviors. and cognitive restructuring are also key components of CBT for anxiety disorders [83]. It would seem then that behavioral interventions designed for insomnia and anxiety can be synergistically applied.

One study documents improvement in insomnia symptoms in association with CBT for GAD [84]. In contrast, DeViva et al. [85] identified a group of patients with significant residual insomnia who had otherwise benefited from CBT for PTSD. They further describe a series of cases where residual insomnia was reduced by a subsequently administered CBT program focused specifically on sleep. These studies notwithstanding, development and evaluation of sequential or integrated treatments for insomnia and anxiety disorders is limited in adults as well as children.

A series of controlled trials indicate imagery rehearsal therapy (IRT) to be effective in reducing nightmares and insomnia symptoms as well as improving overall symptomatology in PTSD [86–89]. IRT is comprised of two main components: (1) educating patients about the impact of nightmares on sleep and how nightmares promote and condition insomnia; and (2) linking daytime imagery and dreams by selecting a specific nightmare, modifying its content (in either an individual or group setting) and rehearsing the new dream. The individual's perceived mastery over negative dream elements appears to be a key factor in the effectiveness of IRT [90].

Since little is known about the safety, tolerability, and efficacy of pharmacological sleep agents in youth, pediatric treatment guidelines designate behavioral interventions as treatments of choice for sleep problems co-occuring with anxiety and other psychiatric disorders [91]. Nonetheless, controlled behavioral treatment trials are lacking. A few case reports and controlled studies have reported significant reductions in sleep difficulties among night-time fearful children based on the use of behavioral interventions [92,93], but the generalizability of these data to youth with anxiety disorders is unclear.

Studies examining the impact of behavioral treatments for childhood anxiety on co-occurring sleep problems are equally limited. Storch et al. [27] found that 14 weeks of CBT resulted in an overall decrease in parent-reported sleep problems, including nightmares and trouble sleeping, among 41 youth with primary OCD. A reduction in sleep problems was not observed based on child report, however. These data underscore the need to gather information from multiple informants when assessing children's sleep and highlight a need to understand better the immediate and long-term effectiveness of CBT for co-morbid sleep disturbance in anxious youth.

Pharmacological treatments

Various benzodiazepine receptor agonist medications are approved and marketed for hypnotic indications and/or treatment of anxiety disorders, particularly GAD. Therefore if one is prescribing benzodiazepines, the use of the same agent for "24-hour coverage" with possible use of a higher dose at night would seem a reasonable strategy. In support of this, one study found that agents marketed and approved as hypnotics had benefits for daytime anxiety when used for the treatment of insomnia associated with GAD [94]. The novel agents pregabalin and tiagabine, which, like benzodiazepines, influence GABAergic neurotransmission, have been reported to improve insomnia symptoms associated with GAD. However, neither drug has FDA approval for GAD or insomnia [95,96].

The newer antidepressant medications, particularly those in the selective serotonin reuptake inhibitor (SSRI) and selective serotonin and norepinephrine inhibitor (SNRI) categories, are effective for a range of anxiety disorders. They also have advantages with respect to tolerance and dependence concerns relative to benzodiazepines and are now considered to be first-line treatments for most anxiety disorders. Effects on sleep vary among agents and among individuals and some have been noted to stimulate insomnia [97]. Among the novel antidepressants, mirtazapine, which is neither an SSRI nor an SNRI, tends to have sedating/sleep effects. Mirtazapine was recently reported to be beneficial for GAD patients in a preliminary open-label trial [98], although it is not FDA approved for this indication. A study utilizing the SSRI citalopram for late-life anxiety disorders indicated improved sleep with treatment in this subpopulation [99].

Studies examining pharmacological treatments (SSRIs) for childhood anxiety have generally failed to examine potential changes in sleep. In one study that did examine sleep-related outcomes, Alfano et al. [20] found that fluvoxamine produced significantly greater reductions in parent- and clinician-reported sleep problems compared to placebo in youth with SAD, SOC, or GAD after 8 weeks of treatment. Specifically, symptoms of insomnia and reluctance/refusal to sleep alone were significantly reduced. However, improvements in nightmares were not observed and long-term sleep-related outcomes were not examined.

Recently, augmentation of antidepressant therapy with the hypnotic medication eszopiclone (3 mg at bedtime) was shown to result in significant improvements in sleep, daytime functioning, and anxiety in a large sample of adults with GAD [100]. With regard to sleep characteristics specifically, adults treated with both escitalopram and eszopiclone evidenced significant reductions in sleep onset latency and increases in total sleep time (based on electronic diaries) compared to those treated with escitalopram and placebo across the 12-week treatment period. Co-therapy with escitalopram and eszopiclone also resulted in a greater magnitude and acceleration of anxiolytic effects, demonstrated from as early as week one of therapy. Although follow-up studies using objective measures of sleep are needed, these findings suggest that simultaneously targeting anxiety and sleep may result in greater treatment gains among adults with GAD.

Presently, SSRIs, specifically sertraline and paroxetine, are the only agents approved by the FDA for the treatment of PTSD. Benefits of these treatments tend to be modest and do not typically include reductions in sleep disturbance. Therefore, adjunctive interventions are often utilized to target sleep. There is now evidence from a small crossover study and a modest-sized placebo-controlled parallel groups designed trial supporting the efficacy of prazosin for nightmares and insomnia in combat-related PTSD [101,102]. Dosing was titrated gradually but aggressively with final doses averaging 9.5 and 13 mg at bedtime in the two studies, respectively. Prazosin is an older medication that is traditionally prescribed for treating hypertension and prostate outlet obstruction. Its mechanism of action is blockade of alpha-adrenergic receptors. Thus, its benefit may relate to the hypothesized role of noradrenergic signaling thought to disrupt REM sleep. A small controlled trial also reported sleep-related benefits from the second-generation antipsychotic medication (SGA) olanzapine, which was prescribed at a mean dose of 15 mg per day [103]. While to date there are no published controlled data, the SGA quetiapine appears to often be prescribed for sleep disturbances in PTSD. In choosing specific medications clinicians need to consider the spectrum of side-effects, most notably the metabolic risks associated with SGAs, as well as the fact that neither prazosin, olanzapine, nor quetiapine are FDA-approved for PTSD.

Summary

Sleep disturbances are commonly associated with anxiety disorders in adults as well as children, particularly GAD, SAD, and PTSD, and cause significant impairments in overall functioning. Evidence of a reciprocal relationship between anxiety and sleep is compelling such that sleep loss may contribute to the onset and relapse of these conditions. The underlying pathophysiology of these problems likely involves shared mechanisms including dysregulation of arousal, inability to inhibit negative cognition, and specific neurophysiological changes. In anxious youth, in particular, environmental contingencies, including inadvertent reinforcement of bedtime avoidance, can exacerbate both problems. Collectively, data suggest that effective treatment requires attention to both unique and common factors. Established treatments for anxiety disorders and insomnia overlap to a large extent, yet optimal sequencing and integration of these approaches remains underinvestigated and generally unknown.

References

1. Ohayon MM, Roth T. Place of chronic insomnia in the course of depressive and anxiety disorders. *J Psychiatr Res.* 2003;**37**:9–15.

2. Ford D, Kamerow D. Epidemiologic study of sleep disturbances and psychiatric disorders: An opportunity for prevention? *JAMA.* 1989;**262**:1479–1484.

3. Breslau N, Roth T, Rosenthal L, Andreski P. Sleep disturbance and psychiatric disorders: a longitudinal epidemiological study of young adults. *Biol Psychiatry.* 1996;**39**(6):411–418.

4. Ohayon M, Caulet M, Lemoine P. Comorbidity of mental and insomnia disorders in the general population. *Compr Psychiatry.* 1998;**39**:185–197.

5. Gregory AM, Caspi A, Eley TC, et al. Prospective longitudinal associations between persistent sleep problems in childhood and anxiety and depression disorders in adulthood. *J Abnorm Child Psychol.* 2005;**33**:157–163.

6. Ong HS, Wickramaratne P, Min T, Weissman MM. Early childhood sleep and eating problems as predictors of adolescent and adult mood and anxiety disorders. *J Affect Disord.* 2006;**96**:1–8.

7. Mellman TA. Sleep and anxiety disorders. *Psychiatric Clin North Am.* 2006; **29**:1047–1058.

8. Mellman TA. Sleep and anxiety disorders. *Sleep Med Clin.* 2008;**3**:261–268.

9. Philip P, Guilleminault C. Adult psychophysiologic insomnia and positive history of childhood insomnia. *Sleep.* 1996;**19**:S16–22.

10. Lewinsohn PM, Holm-Denoma JM, Small JW, Seeley JR, Joiner TE Jr. Separation anxiety disorder in childhood as a risk factor for future mental illness. *J Am Acad Child Adol Psychiatry.* 2008; **47**(5):548–555.

11. Kuhn BR, Elliott AJ. Treatment efficacy in behavioral pediatric sleep medicine. *J Psychosom Res.* 2003;**54**:587–597.

12. Mindell J, Kuhn B, Lewin D, Meltzer L, Sadeh A. Behavioral treatment of bedtime problems and night wakings in infants and young children. *Sleep.* 2006; **29**(10):1263–1276.

13. Friedman AG, Campbell TA. Children's nighttime fears: a behavioral approach to assessment and treatment. In: VandeCreek L, Knapp S, eds. *Innovations in clinical practice: a source book.* Sarasota, FL: Professional Resource Press/Professional Resource Exchange, Inc.; 1992:139–155.

14. Muris P, Merckelbach H, Ollendick TH, King NJ, Bogie N. Children's nighttime fears: parent-child ratings of frequency, content, origins, coping behaviors and severity. *Behav Res Ther.* 2001; **39**(1):13–28.

15. Gau S, Soong W. Psychiatric comorbidity of adolescents with sleep terrors or sleepwalking: a case-control study. *Aust N Z J Psychiatry.* 1999; **33**:734–739.

16. Clark C, Gillin J, Golshan S. Do differences in sleep architecture exist between depressives with comorbid simple phobia as compared with pure depressives? *J Affect Disord.* 1995;**33**:251–255.

17. Schneier FR, Johnson J, Hornig CD, Liebowitz MR, Weissman MM. Social phobia: Comorbidity and morbidity in an epidemiologic sample. *Arch Gen Psychiatry.* 1992;**49**:282–288.

18. Stein M, Kroft C, Walker J. Sleep impairment in patients with social phobia. *Psychiatry Res.* 1993; **49**(Suppl 3):251–256.

19. Brown T, Black B, Uhde T. The sleep architecture of social phobia. *Biol Psychiatry.* 1994;**35**(Suppl 6): 420–421.

20. Alfano CA, Ginsburg GS, Kingery JN. Sleep-related problems among children and adolescents with anxiety disorders. *J Am Acad Child Adol Psychiatry.* 2007; **46**(2):224–232.

21. Rasmussen SA, Eisen JL. The epidemiology and differential diagnosis of obsessive-compulsive disorder. *J Clin Psychiatry.* 1992;**53**(Suppl):4–10.

22. Insel T, Gillin J, Moore A, et al. The sleep of patients with obsessive-compulsive disorder. *Arch Gen Psychiatry.* 1982;**39**:1372–1377.

23. Robinson D, Walsleben J, Pollack S, Lerner G. Nocturnal polysomnography in obsessive-compulsive disorder. *Psychiatry Res.* 1998;**80**:257–263.

24. Hohagan F, Lis S, Krieger S, et al. Sleep EEG of patients with obsessive-compulsive disorder. *Eur Arch Psychiatry Clin Neurosci.* 1994;**243**:273–278.

25. Kluge M, Schussler P, Dresler M, Yassouridis A, Steiger A. Sleep onset REM periods in obsessive compulsive disorder. *Psychiatry Res.* 2007;**152**:29–35

26. Rapoport J, Elkins R, Langer DH, et al. Childhood obsessive-compulsive disorder. *Am J Psychiatry.* 1981;**138**(12):1545–1554.

27. Storch EA, Murphy TK, Lack CW, et al. Sleep-related problems in pediatric obsessive compulsive disorder. *J Anxiety Disord.* 2008;**22**:877–885.

28. Saletu-Zyhlarz G, Saletu B, Anderer P, et al. Nonorganic insomnia in generalized anxiety disorder: Controlled studies on sleep, awakening and daytime vigilance utilizing polysomnography and EEG mapping. *Neuropsychobiology.* 1997;**36**:117–129.

29. Arriaga F, Paiva T. Clinical and EEG sleep changes in primary dysthymia and generalized anxiety: a comparison with normal controls. *Neuropsychobiology.* 1990–1991;**24**:109–114.

30. Papadimitriou G, Kerkhofs M, Kempenaers C, Mendlewicz J. EEG sleep studies in patients with generalized anxiety disorder. *Psychiatry Res.* 1988;**26**:183–190.

31. Fuller KH, Waters WF, Binks PG, Anderson T. Generalized anxiety and sleep architecture: a polysomnographic evaluation. *Sleep.* 1997; **20**:370–376.

32. Rosa RR, Bonnet MH, Kramer M. The relationship of sleep and anxiety in anxious subjects. *Biol Psychiatry.* 1983;**16**:119–126.

33. Forbes EE, Bertocci MA, Gregory AM, et al. Objective sleep in pediatric anxiety disorders and major depressive disorder. *J Am Acad Child Adolesc Psychiatry.* 2007;**47**:148–155.

34. Alfano CA, Beidel DC, Turner SM, Lewin DS. Preliminary evidence for sleep complaints among children referred for anxiety. *Sleep Med.* 2006;**7**:467–473.

35. Mellman T, Uhde T. Patients with frequent sleep panic: clinical findings and response to medication treatment. *J Clin Psychiatry.* 1990;**51**:513–516.

36. Mellman T, Uhde T. Sleep panic attacks: new clinical findings and theoretical implications. *Am J Psychiatry.* 1989;**146**:1204–1207.

37. Stein M, Chartier M, Walker J. Sleep in nondepressed patients with panic disorder: I. Systematic assessment of subjective sleep quality and sleep disturbance. *Sleep.* 1993;**16**:724–726.

38. Mellman T, Uhde T. Electroencephalographic sleep in panic disorder: A focus on sleep-related panic attacks. *Arch Gen Psychiatry.* 1989;**46**:178–184.

39. Sloan E, Natarajan M, Baker B, et al. Nocturnal and daytime panic attacks: comparison of sleep

architecture, heart rate variablity, and response to sodium lactate challenge. *Soc Biol Psychiatry.* 1999;**45**:1313–1320.

40. Lydiard R, Zealberg J, Laraia M, et al. Electroencephalography during sleep of patients with panic disorder. *J Neuropsychiatry Clin Neurosci.* 1989;**1**:372–376.

41. Arriaga F, Paiva T, Matos-Pires A, et al. The sleep of non-depressed patients with panic disorder: a comparison with normal controls. *Acta Psychiatr Scand.* 1996;**93**:191–194.

42. Stein M, Enns M, Kryger M. Sleep in nondepressed patients with panic disorder. II. Polysomnographic assessment of sleep architecture and sleep continuity. *J Affect Disord.* 1993;**28**:1–6.

43. Uhde T, Roy-Byrne P, Gillin J, et al. The sleep of patients with panic disorder. *Psychiatry Res.* 1984;**12**:251–259.

44. Brown T, Uhde TW. Sleep panic attacks: a micro-movement analysis. *Depress Anxiety.* 2003;**18**(4):214–220.

45. Taylor C, Skeikh J, Agras S, et al. Ambulatory heart rate changes in patients with panic attacks. *Am J Psychiatry.* 1986;**143**:478–482.

46. Krystal J, Woods S, Hill C, Charney D. Characteristics of panic attack subtypes: assessment of spontaneous panic, situational panic, sleep panic, and limited symptom attacks. *Compr Psychiatry.* 1991;**32**:474–480.

47. Craske M, Lang A, Rowe M, et al. Presleep attributions about arousal during sleep: nocturnal panic. *J Abnorm Psychol.* 2002;**111**(1):53–62.

48. Shapiro C, Sloan E. Nocturnal panic: an underrecognized entity. *J Psychosom Res.* 1998;**44**:21–23.

49. Hauri P, Freidman M, Ravaris C. Sleep in patients with spontaneous panic attacks. *Sleep.* 1989;**12**:323–337. [Paper presented at 139th Annual Meeting American Psychiatric Association, Washington, DC, 1986.]

50. Hobson JA, Pace-Schott E, Stickgold R. Dreaming and the brain: Towards a cognitive neuroscience of conscious states. *Behav Brain Sci.* 2000;**23**:793–842.

51. Labbate L, Pollack M, Otto M, Langenauer S, Rosenbaum J. Sleep panic attacks: an association with childhood anxiety and adult psychopathology. *Biol Psychiatry.* 1994;**36**:57–60.

52. Tsao J, Craske M. Fear of loss of vigilance: development and preliminary validation of a self-report instrument. *Depress Anxiety.* 2003;**18**(4):177–186.

53. Craske M, Lang A, Mystkowski J, et al. Does nocturnal panic represent a more severe form of panic disorder? *J Nerv Ment Disease.* 2002;**190**(9):611–618.

54. Connell HM, Persley GV, Sturgess JL. Sleep phobia in middle childhood – a review of six cases. *J Am Acad Child Adol Psychiatry.* 1987;**26**(3):449–452.

55. Verduin TL, Kendall PC. Differential occurrence of comorbidity within childhood anxiety disorders. *J Clin Child Adol Psychol.* 2003;**32**:290–295.

56. American Psychiatric Association. *Diagnostic and statistical manual of mental disorders*, 4th ed. Text Revision. Washington, DC: American Psychiatric Press; 2000.

57. Neylan T, Marmar C, Metzler T, et al. Sleep disturbances in the Vietnam generation: findings from a nationally representative sample of male Vietnam veterans. *Am J Psychiatry.* 1998;**155**(7):929–933.

58. Green BL. Disasters and posttraumatic stress disorder. In: Davidson JRT, Foa EB, eds. *Posttraumatic stress disorder DSM-IV and beyond.* Washington, DC: American Psychiatric Press; 1993:75–97.

59. Mellman T, David D, Kulick-Bell R, Hebding J, Nolan B. Sleep disturbance and its relationship to psychiatric morbidity following Hurricane Andrew. *Am J Psychiatry.* 1995;**152**:1659–1663.

60. Koren D, Arnon I, Lavie P, Klein E. Sleep complaints as early predictors of posttraumatic stress disorder: a 1-year prospective study of injured survivors of motor vehicle accidents. *Am J Psychiatry.* 2002;**159**(5):855–857.

61. Mellman T, David D, Bustamante V, Torres J, Fins A. Dreams in the acute aftermath of trauma and their relationship to PTSD. *J Traumatic Stress.* 2001;**14**:241–247.

62. Lavie P. Current concepts: sleep disturbances in the wake of traumatic events. *NEJM.* 2001;**345**(25):1825–1832.

63. Kobayshi I, Boarts J, Delahanty D. Polysomnographically measured sleep abnormalities in PTSD: A meta-analytic review. *Psychophysiology.* 2007;**44**:660–669.

64. Germain A, Hall M, Shear KM, Nofzinger EA, Buysse DJ. Ecological study of sleep disruption in PTSD: a pilot study. *Ann N Y Acad Sci.* 2006;**1071**:438–441.

65. Calhoun PS, Wiley M, Dennis MF, et al. Objective evidence of sleep disturbance in women with posttraumatic stress disorder. *J Traum Stress.* 2007;**20**(6):1009–1018.

66. Krakow B, Melendrez D, Pederson B, et al. Complex insomnia: insomnia and sleep-disordered breathing in a consecutive series of crime victims with nightmares and PTSD. *Biol Psychiatry.* 2001;**49**:948–953.

67. Breslau N, Roth T, Burduvali E, et al. Sleep in lifetime posttraumatic stress disorder: a community-based polysomnographic study. *Arch Gen Psychiatry.* 2004;**61**:508–516.

68. Ross R, Ball W, Dinges D, et al. Motor dysfunction during sleep in posttraumatic stress disorder. *Sleep.* 1994;**17**:723–732.

69. Mellman T, Kulick-Bell R, Ashlock L, Nolan B. Sleep events among veterans with combat-related posttraumatic stress disorder. *Am J Psychiatry.* 1995;**152**:110–115.

70. Woodward S, Arsenault N, Santerre C, et al. *Polysomnographic characteristics of trauma-related nightmares.* Presented at Annual Meeting of Association of Professional Sleep Societies, Las Vegas, Nevada, June, 2000.

71. Habukawa M, Uchimura N, Maeda M, Kotorii N, Maeda H. Sleep findings in young adult patients with posttraumatic stress disorder. *Biol Psychiatry.* 2007;**62**:1179–1182.

72. Mellman T, Bustamante V, Fins A, Pigeon W, Nolan B. REM sleep and the early development of posttraumatic stress disorder. *Am J Psychiatry.* 2002;**159**(10): 1696–1701.

73. Mellman TA, Pigeon WR. Dreams and nightmares in posttraumatic stress disorder. In: Kryger M, Roth T, Dement W, eds (Section ed Stickgold R). *Principles and practices of sleep medicine,* 4th ed. Philadelphia, PA: Elsevier; 2005.

74. Glod CA, Teicher MH, Hartman CR, Harakal T. Increased nocturnal activity and impaired sleep maintenance in abused children. *J Am Acad Child Adol Psychiatry.* 1997;**36**:1236–1243.

75. Sadeh A, McGuire JP, Sachs H, et al. Sleep and psychological characteristics of children on a psychiatric inpatient unit. *J Am Acad Child Adol Psychiatry.* 1995;**34**(6):813–819.

76. Charney DS, Deutch AY, Krystal JH, Southwick SM, Davis M. Psychobiologic mechanisms of posttraumatic stress disorder. *Arch Gen Psychiatry.* 1993; **50**:294–305.

77. Bader K, Schafer V, Schenkel M, et al. Increased nocturnal activity associated with adverse childhood experiences in patients with primary insomnia. *J Nerv Ment Disease.* 2007;**195**:588–595.

78. Noll JG, Trickett PK, Susman EJ, Putnam FW. Sleep disturbances and childhood sexual abuse. *J Ped Psychol.* 2006;**31**:469–480.

79. Labbate L, Johnson M, Lydiard R, et al. Sleep deprivation in panic disorder and obsessive-compulsive disorder. *Can J Psychiatry.* 1997; **42**:982–983.

80. Labbate L, Johnson M, Lydiard R, et al. Sleep deprivation in social phobia and generalized anxiety disorder. *Biol Psychiatry.* 1998;**43**:840–842.

81. Roy-Byrne P, Uhde T, Post R. Effects of one night's sleep deprivation on mood and behavior in panic disorder: Patients with panic disorder compared with depressed patients and normal controls. *Arch Gen Psychiatry.* 1986;**43**:895–899.

82. Morin C, Culbert J, Schwartz S. Nonpharmacological interventions for insomnia: a meta-analysis of treatment efficacy. *Am J Psychiatry.* 1994; **151**:1172–1180.

83. Falsetti SA, Combs-Lane A, Davis JL. Cognitive behavioral treatment of anxiety disorders. In: Nutt DJ, Ballenger JC, eds. *Anxiety disorders.* Oxford, UK: Blackwell Science; 2003:425–444.

84. Belanger L, Morin CM, Langlois F, Ladouceur R. Insomnia and generalized anxiety disorder: effects of cognitive behavior therapy for gad on insomnia symptoms. *J Anxiety Disord.* 2004;**18**(4):561–571.

85. DeViva J, Zayfert C, Pigeon W, Mellman T. Treatment of residual insomnia after CBT for PTSD: Case studies. *J Traumatic Stress.* 2005;**18**:155–159.

86. Germain A, Nielsen T. Impact of imagery rehearsal treatment on distressing dreams, psychological distress and sleep parameters in nightmare patients. *Behav Sleep Med.* 2003;**1**:140–154.

87. Kellner R, Neidhardt EJ, Krakow BJ, Pathak D. Changes in chronic nightmares after one session of desensitization or rehearsal of instructions. *Am J Psychiatry.* 1992;**149**:659–663.

88. Krakow BJ, Hollifield M, Schrader R, et al. A controlled study of imagery rehearsal for chronic nightmares in sexual assault survivors with PTSD: a preliminary report. *J Trauma Stress.* 2000;**13**:589–609.

89. Krakow B, Hollifield M, Johnston L, et al. Imagery rehearsal therapy for chronic nightmares in sexual assault survivors with posttraumatic stress disorder: a randomized controlled trial. *JAMA.* 2001;**286**:537–545.

90. Germain A, Krakow B, Faucher B, et al. Increased mastery elements associated with imagery rehearsal treatment for nightmares in sexual assault survivors with PTSD. *Dreaming.* 2004;**14**:195–206.

91. Mindell JA, Emslie GE, Blumer J, et al. Pharmacological management of insomnia in children and adolescents: consensus statement. *Pediatrics.* 2006;**117**:1223–1232.

92. Graziano AM, Mooney KC. Family self-control instruction for children's nighttime fear reduction. *J Consult Clin Psychol.* 1980;**48**(2):206–213.

93. Ollendick TH, Hagopian LP, Huntzinger RM. Cognitive-behavior therapy with nighttime fearful children. *J Behav Ther Exp Psychiatry*. 1991;**22**(2): 113–121.

94. Fontaine R, Beaudry P, Le Morvan P, Beauclair L, Chouinard G. Zopiclone and triazolam in insomnia associated with generalized anxiety disorder: a placebo-controlled evaluation of efficacy and daytime anxiety. *Int Clin Psychopharmacol*. 1990;**5**(3): 173–183.

95. Rickels K, Pollack M, Feltner D, et al. Pregabalin for treatment of generalized anxiety disorder: a 4-week, multicenter, double-blind, placebo-controlled trial of pregabalin and alprazolam. *Arch Gen Psychiatry*. 2005;**62**:1022–1030.

96. Rosenthal M. Tiagabine for the treatment of generalized anxiety disorder: a randomized, open-label, clinical trial with paroxetine as a positive control. *J Clin Psychiatry*. 2003;**64**:1245–1249.

97. Winokur A, Gary KA, Rodner S, et al. Depression, sleep physiology, and antidepressant drugs. *Depress Anxiety*. 2001;**14**:19–28.

98. Gambi F, De Berardis D, Campanella D, et al. Mirtazapine treatment of generalized anxiety disorder: a fixed dose, open label study. *J Psychopharmacol*. 2005;**19**:483–487.

99. Blank S, Lenze E, Mulsant B, et al. Outcomes of late-life anxiety disorders during 32 weeks of citalopram treatment. *J Clin Psychiatry*. 2006;**67**:468–472.

100. Pollack MP, Kinrys G, Krystal A, et al. Eszopiclone co-administered with escitalopram in patients with generalized anxiety disorder. *Arch Gen Psychiatry*. 2008;**65**:551–562.

101. Raskind MA, Peskind ER, Kanter ED, et al. Reduction of nightmares and other PTSD symptoms in combat veterans by prazosin: a placebo-controlled study. *Am J Psychiatry*. 2003;**160**:371–373.

102. Raskind MA, Peskind ER, Hoff DJ, et al. A parallel group placebo controlled study of prazosin for trauma nightmares and sleep disturbances in combat veterans with posttraumatic stress disorder. *Biol Psychiatry*. 2007;**61**(8):928–934.

103. Stein M, Kline N, Matloff J. Adjunctive olanzapine for SSRI-resistant combat-related PTSD: a double-blind, placebo-controlled study. *Am J Psychiatry*. 2003;**160**:1189–1190.

Psychotic disorders

Allen C. Richert

Introduction

Schizophrenia, the archetypal psychotic disorder, is a chronic, currently incurable, prevalent, and devastating syndrome. While sleep disturbances are important aspects of psychotic illness, they are not primary symptoms of schizophrenia or any other psychotic disorder. Even so, sleep disturbances are frequently components of, influence quality of life in, and may exacerbate psychotic illnesses. A better understanding of sleep abnormalities associated with psychotic disorders may improve our understanding of the pathophysiology of these disorders.

For several reasons, succinctly summarizing the literature on sleep abnormalities associated with psychotic disorders is difficult. First, the DSM-IV-TR [1] category of psychotic disorders contains several disorders that are not necessarily syndromically or even pathophysiologically homogeneous. The disorders include schizophrenia, schizoaffective disorder, brief psychotic disorder, schizophreniform disorder, delusional disorder, shared psychotic disorder, and psychotic disorder not otherwise specified (NOS). Second, considerably more sleep research has focused on schizophrenia than any of the other psychotic disorders. Third, while some psychotic disorders (i.e. schizoaffective disorder and schizophreniform disorder) incorporate similar symptoms as schizophrenia, other psychotic disorders (i.e. delusional disorder, shared psychotic disorder, and brief psychotic disorder) differ from schizophrenia sufficiently to raise doubt that they spring from similar neurobiological abnormalities and therefore that their associated sleep abnormalities would be similar. Based upon the reasoning described above, this chapter will focus primarily on schizophrenia, and discuss other psychotic disorders when feasible.

It is important to additionally recognize that schizophrenia itself is a heterogeneous syndrome. The DSM-IV-TR acknowledges heterogeneity within schizophrenia by recognizing subtypes of schizophrenia, which include paranoid, disorganized, catatonic, undifferentiated, and residual types [1]. Because these variations within the diagnostic category of schizophrenia almost certainly arise as a result of variations in the neurological abnormalities underlying each type of schizophrenia, it would be short-sighted to assume that different types of schizophrenia would generate the same changes in sleep. It is with an appreciation of the above difficulties that the author endeavors to synthesize a coherent, clinically relevant, and pathophysiologically illuminating summary of the sleep abnormalities associated with psychotic disorders.

Subjective sleep disturbance in psychotic illness

Clinical lore and the author's experience suggest that sleep complaints frequently accompany schizophrenia and other psychotic disorders, just as they do many other psychiatric disorders. However, in contrast to the amount of research examining polysomnographic features of sleep in psychotic disorders (i.e. mostly schizophrenia), the literature examining subjective sleep complaints in psychotic disorders is small. The field lacks large-scale epidemiological studies addressing frequency, prevalence, and types of sleep complaints associated with psychotic disorders. But, a modest number of relatively small studies directly address or describe, as a secondary measure, sleep complaints in schizophrenia, schizophreniform disorder, schizoaffective disorder, and delusional disorder. Essentially no such studies exist for shared psychotic disorder. The author's experience as a psychiatrist who practices

Foundations of Psychiatric Sleep Medicine, ed. John W. Winkelman and David T. Plante. Published by Cambridge University Press.
© Cambridge University Press 2010.

mostly sleep medicine has not revealed any evidence to suggest that sleep disturbances occur more frequently in people with a shared psychotic disorder than they do in the general population, or that there is a higher incidence of shared psychotic disorder in people who have sleep complaints (e.g. insomnia) compared to the general population. However, the fact that shared psychotic disorder occurs infrequently [1] admittedly limits the reliability of personal clinical experience.

A handful of reports [2–4] have asked patients with psychotic disorders about their quality of sleep. Haffmans and colleagues [3] reported that 36.7% of a cohort of chronic medicated schizophrenics had "problems with their sleep," even though approximately half of the subjects reporting sleep difficulties were on antipsychotics. Of those reporting sleep difficulties, 37.5% had sleep-onset insomnia, 37.5% had middle insomnia, and 25% had late insomnia. Using a Japanese version of the Pittsburg sleep quality index, Doi and colleagues [2] found that patients with schizophrenia report having poor sleep quality, with decrements in global sleep quality, sleep latency, sleep disturbance, and sleep efficiency compared to control subjects but similar to patients with insomnia, major depression, and generalized anxiety disorder. Similarly, Serretti and colleagues [4] when examining depressive symptoms in psychotic disorders found a high incidence of insomnia in patients with schizophrenia and patients with delusional disorder. Even though the above studies are not definitive, they suggest that patients with schizophrenia and delusional disorder frequently feel that they do not sleep well.

The above reports do not explain why patients with psychotic disorders report subjective sleep disturbances. It is possible that co-morbid primary sleep disorders could cause the disturbances. A handful of investigators have explored the prevalence of primary sleep disorders in patients with psychotic disorders. Winkleman examined the frequency of obstructive sleep apnea (OSA; defined in this study as 10 or more apneas or hypopneas per hour) in psychiatric inpatients referred for polysomnography [5]. Within this group of referred psychiatric patients, OSA occurred more frequently in patients with schizophrenia or schizoaffective disorder compared to other psychiatric diagnoses. Logistic regression analysis revealed that elevated body mass index and male sex, both of which occurred more frequently in the schizophrenia/schizoaffective group, contributed more to the risk of having OSA than psychiatric diagnosis. Because the patients in this study were referred because they had symptoms of sleep disorders, we cannot draw conclusions from this study about the prevalence of sleep apnea in the general (i.e. unreferred) population with schizophrenia. Two studies have examined the prevalence of OSA in unreferred patients. Using ambulatory pulse oximetry alone, Takahashi and colleagues [6] examined the frequency of sleep-related respiratory disorders (SRRD; defined as greater than five desaturations per hour of sleep) in 101 patients with schizophrenia, finding SRRD in 22% of the men and 13% of the women in their sample. Ancoli-Israel and colleagues examined the frequency of OSA and periodic limb movements of sleep (PLMS) using a portable recording device to obtain unattended studies of breathing and movements during sleep in 52 elderly (i.e. mean age of 59) patients with schizophrenia or schizoaffective disorder [7]. Forty-eight percent of the elderly schizophrenic patients had 10 or more respiratory events per hour of sleep, which approximates results of other studies by this group in non-psychotic healthy elderly using the same recording device. Interestingly, the proportion of elderly patients with schizophrenia who had five or more limb movements during sleep (14%) was less than half of the proportion of non-psychotic elderly (45%), which suggests that something in the schizophrenia group protected it from the development of PLMS. Neuroleptic medication use did not explain the lower prevalence of PLMS in the schizophrenia group but the prevalence correlated inversely with the presence of tardive dyskinesia. In a related study, neuroleptic use was implicated in restless legs syndrome (RLS) in schizophrenic patients. In a study of 182 medicated inpatients with schizophrenia and 108 age- and sex-matched normal controls, RLS occurred more frequently in medicated patients (21.4%) than in controls (9.3%) [8].

In addition to primary sleep disorders, sleep-disrupting behaviors associated with schizophrenia (e.g. sleeping during the day, excessive time in bed, being active during the night, etc.) may lead to sleep disturbance. Such poor sleep hygiene behaviors and other psychological factors (e.g. conditioned arousal to lying in bed, worry about sleep, etc.) and environmental factors (e.g. television in the bedroom, uncomfortable bed, etc.) have a well-established role in maintaining primary insomnia not related to psychosis (see Chapter 12: Principles of insomnia). Though not well documented in the research literature, those same sleep-disrupting factors undoubtedly contribute to the subjective sleep complaints of patients with psychosis. The positive results of a handful of small trials of cognitive behavioral therapy for insomnia co-morbid with psychiatric disorders [9–12] suggest that the above sleep-disrupting factors contribute to insomnia co-morbid with psychiatric illness. But, only two of the studies enrolled subjects with psychotic disorders; one enrolled six [11] and the other two [12]. Dopke and others [11] were the only group to report on the presence of sleep-disrupting factors and they concluded that such factors contribute to the maintenance of insomnia co-morbid with severe mental illness.

The limitations of the above studies do not allow one to draw sweeping epidemiological conclusions, nor do they clarify the role of co-morbid primary sleep disorders or sleep-disrupting behaviors in the generation of poor sleep quality associated with psychotic disorders. Nevertheless, these studies suggest that patients with psychotic disorders may have subjective sleep disturbances due to primary sleep disorders like OSA and RLS or other behavioral factors. Thus, clinicians should be mindful and consider co-morbid primary sleep disorders and sleep-disrupting behaviors in the differential diagnosis of sleep complaints in patients with psychotic disorders.

Sleep-related diagnostic criteria

Sleep-related items are not specific criteria for any of the psychotic disorders, however, the DSM-IV-TR [1] discussion of sleep, behaviors related to sleep, and other sleep-related phenomena in the psychotic disorders merits discussion. The DSM-IV-TR clarifies that a hallucination "must occur in the context of a clear sensorium" to count as a criterion for the diagnosis of schizophrenia. Hallucinations that occur in association with either the onset of sleep, also known as hypnagogic hallucinations, or waking from sleep, also known as hypnopompic hallucinations, do not fulfill schizophrenia criteria for hallucinations. Criterion B for schizophrenia states that the disorder "involves dysfunction in one or more major areas of functioning" including self-care. The DSM-IV-TR explains that negative symptoms of schizophrenia could manifest as spending the bulk of one's time "in bed" and that the associated features of schizophrenia include, "disturbances in sleep pattern (e.g. sleeping during the day and night-time activity or restlessness)." As noted above, the inability to

maintain self-care including sleep hygiene coupled with the propensities toward unhealthy sleep behaviors, such as staying in bed during the day and being active during the night-time, probably contribute significantly to sleep complaints associated with schizophrenia and other psychotic disorders.

Of the remaining psychotic disorders, the DSM-IV-TR mentions sleep-related issues only in schizoaffective disorder. The DSM-IV-TR defines schizoaffective disorder as a syndrome of intermittent symptoms of major mood episodes superimposed upon persistent symptoms of schizophrenia. The schizoaffective section of the DSM-IV-TR contains only one reference to sleep-related issues, which is an example demonstrating mood symptoms that are "clearly the result of symptoms of schizophrenia (e.g. difficulty sleeping because of disturbing auditory hallucinations…)," and do not fulfill the criteria for a concurrent mood disorder. In summary, the DSM-IV-TR describes sleep-related phenomena and behaviors associated with schizophrenia and schizoaffective disorder, but the diagnostic criteria for psychotic disorders contain essentially no sleep-related issues.

Polysomnographic findings in psychotic disorders

Polysomnographic studies of sleep in psychotic disorders have examined schizophrenia and schizoaffective disorder almost exclusively. Most of those studies have identified abnormalities of sleep initiation and maintenance. Reports of abnormalities in rapid eye movement (REM) sleep and slow-wave sleep (SWS) have also frequently appeared in the literature but those findings are less consistent than abnormalities of sleep initiation and maintenance. Two meta-analyses of the available polysomnographic studies in schizophrenia by Benca and colleagues in 1991 [13] and Chouinard and colleagues in 2004 [14] succinctly summarize this literature.

Sleep disruption

Most of the sleep studies of schizophrenia demonstrate abnormalities in sleep initiation and maintenance. These findings include increased sleep latency, decreased total sleep time (TST), and decreased sleep efficiency. Even though much of this evidence comes from studies designed to examine SWS or REM sleep abnormalities, the findings are very reliable.

Table 18.1 Number of studies in Chouinard and colleagues' meta-analysis reporting sleep changes in unmedicated schizophrenia [14]

	Increase	Decrease	No difference	Not reported	Effect size (confidence interval)
Sleep latency	15	0	5	1	1.34
Total sleep time	0	12	6	3	−1.50
Sleep efficiency	0	11	3	7	−1.58

Table 18.2 Schizophrenia-related differences from normal sleep published after meta-analysis by Chouniard and colleagues [14]

	TST	SL	SE	%SWS	%REM	REML	Meds
Ferrarelli et al. [15]	NS	+	NS	NS	NR	NR	yes
Forest et al. [16]	NS	NR	NR	NS	NS	NR	no (naive)
Goder et al. [17]	NS	+	−	−	NS	NS	yes
Sekimoto et al. [18]	NS	NS	NS	−	NS	NS	mixed
Yang and Winkelman [19]	NS	+	−	−	NS	NS	no (2 wks)

TST, total sleep time; SL, sleep latency; SE, sleep efficiency; REML, REM latency; NS, non-significant; NR, not reported; +, increased; −, decreased.

Chouinard and colleagues' 2004 meta-analysis of sleep studies of schizophrenic patients provides a convenient summary of the findings (Table 18.1). All of the studies examined in this meta-analysis used normal subjects for controls and only unmedicated schizophrenics. Of 20 studies that reported on sleep latency 15 reported increased sleep latency, only 5 found no difference, and no studies identified reduced sleep latency in schizophrenia. Of 18 studies that reported on TST, 12 found decreased TST, 6 found no difference, and no studies found increased TST. For sleep efficiency, 11 of 14 studies found decreased sleep efficiency and the remaining 3 found no difference.

Since the publication of Chouinard and colleagues' meta-analysis, only five studies have reported TST, sleep latency, and sleep efficiency of polysomnographically recorded sleep in either medicated or unmedicated patients with schizophrenia or schizoaffective disorder in comparison to normal controls (Table 18.2). None of those studies found decreased total sleep time. Decreased sleep efficiency was found in two studies, was not present in two studies, and was not reported in one. The finding of increased sleep latency proved the most resilient with three of the five studies replicating it, one not finding a difference, and one not reporting this parameter. These findings support the reports from patients and family members and the DSM-IV-TR description of schizophrenia

that suggests that patients with schizophrenia have difficulty falling asleep and maintaining sleep. Increased sleep latency is the most common polysomnographic marker of impaired sleep initiation and/or maintenance in schizophrenic patients.

REM sleep

A significant literature on REM sleep in psychotic illness exists and is summarized in Table 18.3. Psychosis, an abnormal phenomenon, shares the hallucinatory experience that is an integral component of dreaming, a normal phenomenon. This observation led many in the early days of polysomnography to hypothesize that psychosis was a manifestation of a malfunctioning physiology of normal dreaming. Consequently, several of the earliest studies of REM sleep were performed on patients diagnosed with schizophrenia [20–22]. In fact, the second publication to describe rapid eye movements in sleep reported on the distribution, number, and quality of eye movements in schizophrenic patients [20]. The earliest of these studies did not uncover REM sleep abnormalities but later studies did. Feinberg and colleagues were the first to suggest that the REM sleep latency of schizophrenic patients differs from normal subjects and that this finding indicated "measurable differences in brain function"[31]. A host of other studies [23–26] that

Table 18.3 Summary of earlier studies examining REM sleep in psychotic disorders

Experimental state	Comparison group	Main finding	Date	Reference
Chronic unmedicated schizophrenics	Normal subjects	Quantity, quality, and distribution of REMs did not differ	1955	[20]
Hallucinating schizophrenics	Non-hallucinating schizophrenics	REM time not different	1963	[21]
Actively ill schizophrenics	Normal subjects	Fewer epochs of sleep with REMs but dream time not different	1964	[22]
Schizophrenics in remission	Normal subjects	No difference in number of epochs with REMs or dream time	1964	[22]
Actively ill schizophrenics	Schizophrenics in remission	No difference in number of epochs with REMs or dream time	1964	[22]
Actively ill schizophrenics	Normal subjects	Bimodal distribution of REM latencies in the actively ill schizophrenics	1965	[31]
Chronic schizophrenics near remission	Non-psychotic males	Shorter REM latency and higher REM percent	1967	[23]
Inactive schizophrenics	Psychiatric inpatients without schizophrenia	Elevated REM rebound following 2 nights of REM deprivation	1968	[32]
Actively ill schizophrenics	Psychiatric inpatients without schizophrenia	Reduced REM rebound following 2 nights of REM deprivation	1968 1969 1975	[32–34]
Acutely ill unmedicated schizophrenics	Normal subjects	Reduced REM latency with long sleep onset latency and reduced TST	1969	[24]
Acute schizophrenics in waxing phase	Normal subjects	Reduction in REM time and lengthening of REM latency	1970	[35]
Acute schizophrenics in waning phase	Normal subjects	Reduction in REM time and lengthening of REM latency	1970	[35]
Acute schizophrenics in post-psychotic and remission phases	Normal subjects	No difference	1970	[35]
Untreated long-term elderly schizophrenics	Age-matched controls	Short REM latencies and more frequent but shorter REM periods	1973	[25]
Acute schizophrenics	Chronic schizophrenics	Reduced absolute REM sleep	1975	[36]
Unmedicated, recently hospitalized schizophrenics	Normal controls	Short REM sleep latency	1985	[26]
Schizophrenia (and depression and schizoaffective)	Normal controls	Short REM latency	1987	[37]
Young (i.e. 23–31 years old) male schizophrenic inpatients	Group 1: Sex- and age-matched depressed inpatients & Group 2: Normal controls	No mean REM latency or REM time differences but distribution of schizophrenic REM latencies wider	1988	[28]

Table 18.3 (cont.)

Experimental state	Comparison group	Main finding	Date	Reference
Schizophrenic inpatients 2 weeks free of medicines	No controls	REM latencies bimodal with 16% of the patients having a REM latency <10 minutes	1991	[30]
Recently hospitalized schizophrenics with first episode or recent exacerbation, free of medicines for at least 3 months	Normal controls	No difference in REM latency or REM time	1997	[29]
Drug-naïve and previously medicated drug-free schizophrenics	Normal controls	Short REM latency in both schizophrenic groups	1992	[38]
4-week drug-free schizophrenics, manics, and depressed subjects	Normal controls	Short REM latency in all patient groups	1993	[39]
Schizophrenics after 1 year of treatment	Same patients when hospitalized and medication free for 2 weeks	Increase in REM latency, REM time, and average automated REM counts	1996	[40]

examined a heterogeneous group of patients (e.g. on and off medications, symptomatic and asymptomatic, old and young) with schizophrenia also reported shortened REM latencies.

However, not all studies that examined REM latency found differences [27–29]. In fact, neither Benca and colleagues' early [13] nor Chouinard and colleagues' later [14] meta-analyses identified significant abnormalities in REM latency or percent REM sleep. Some have argued that (1) the heterogeneity with regard to sex, age, clinical status, and medication use of the subjects studied and (2) the heterogeneity of schizophrenia itself (i.e. the various subtypes) have contributed to the relative inconsistency in the finding of schizophrenia-related REM sleep abnormalities. Some of the studies that did not find differences between group means did report greater variability and at times a bimodal distribution in REM latency [28–30]. This supports the hypothesis that heterogeneity among subjects might prevent identification of a true association between a specific phase or type of schizophrenia and REM sleep abnormalities. Other aspects of REM sleep such as the frequency of rapid eye movements during REM sleep (REM density) have been reported to be elevated and inversely correlated with cognitive deficits in schizophrenia [19]. However, thus far, purported abnormalities in REM sleep have done little to advance (1) our understanding of the pathophysiology or (2) the clinical management of schizophrenia (or other psychotic disorders).

Slow-wave sleep

In 1967 Cadwell and Domino [41] reported that a group of patients with schizophrenia had less SWS than a control group and that the patients with schizophrenia failed to show a SWS rebound after 85 consecutive hours of wakefulness [42]. Several researchers [26, 27, 43–46] but not all [25, 29, 38] have replicated the finding of decreased SWS in schizophrenic subjects. Chouinard and colleagues' meta-analysis of medication-free patients did not find significant deficits in either percent stage 4 sleep or percent SWS; however, this analysis included only visually scored measures of SWS. Keshavan and colleagues made the point that computerized analyses are free from several of the limitations of visual scoring and "can detect EEG changes missed by visual scoring" [45]. Of the 11 studies in Chouinard and colleagues' paper that did not find a difference, at least two had performed computerized period amplitude analysis or fast Fourier transform analysis that revealed reductions in power or amplitude of slow-wave frequencies [45, 47]. Additionally, two of the studies included in that analysis reported *increased* slow-wave sleep in patients with schizophrenia [48, 49]. In one of those studies [48] the control group's percent of SWS was unusually low (i.e. 8.1%), less than what other studies report for patients with schizophrenia (examples of schizophrenic SWS% reported in other studies: 13% [50], 17% [27], 16% [39], and 11% [51]). The unusually low control group SWS% made the SWS% of the subjects with schizophrenia (14.1%) appear high even though it was similar to the amount of SWS% in schizophrenia reported in other studies. Because of the above issues, Chouinard and colleagues' meta-analysis probably understates the magnitude of SWS deficits associated with schizophrenia. In the five studies that have been published since Chouinard and colleagues' analysis, three found reductions in visually scored SWS and two did not find significant differences (Table 18.2).

The SWS deficits associated with schizophrenia appear to differ from the reported REM sleep abnormalities in that the slow-wave deficits do not fluctuate over the course of the illness [40]; however, REM sleep abnormalities have been reported to do so [35–35]. Of note, young non-psychotic first-degree relatives of schizophrenia patients also have SWS deficits [52]. These trait-like aspects (e.g. temporal stability, apparent heritability) suggest that SWS deficits may be endophenotypes (i.e. genetically transmissible characteristics that are not apparent to the unaided eye) of schizophrenia. The normal decrease in SWS that occurs over the course of adolescence is exaggerated in these first-degree relatives at high risk for schizophrenia [52]. This exaggerated decrease of SWS may support a hypothesis put forth by Feinberg [53] that a disorder of the normal synaptic pruning process that occurs during adolescence causes schizophrenia. Keshavan has invoked dysfunction of thalamocortical circuits in the schizophrenia-related failure of SWS [54]. Similarly, others have begun to correlate SWS deficits with cognitive deficits in schizophrenia [19] and attempt to explain those cognitive deficits on the basis of thalamocortical dysfunction [17].

Other sleep and polysomnographic abnormalities

Researchers have identified other alterations in the sleep of schizophrenics that might provide insight into the pathophysiology of the illness. For instance, Manoach and colleagues demonstrated a failure of sleep-dependent motor learning in treated schizophrenic patients [55]. Others have noted decreased number, amplitude, duration, and integration of sleep spindle activity in patients with schizophrenia compared to depression and normal controls [15]. The authors suggest that these findings "may reflect dysfunction in thalamic-reticular and thalamocortical mechanisms and could represent a biological marker of illness." Others have found correlations suggesting that increased spindle activity and SWS improve attentional tasks, both among schizophrenics and normal controls [16]. Still others have used sophisticated mathematical analysis of the EEG to reveal "decreased nonlinear complexity of the EEG time series and diminished chaos in schizophrenia" that correlates with neurocognitive deficits [56]; however, it is not clear how such a finding relates to pathophysiology in schizophrenia.

Sleep disturbance in the course of schizophrenia

The only established risk factors for the development of schizophrenia are: (1) having first-degree relatives with schizophrenia, (2) being raised in an urban environment, (3) being an immigrant, (4) being exposed to a range of obstetric complications including infections, and (5) being born in late winter or early spring [57]. Disturbances of sleep have not been identified as risk factors for schizophrenia. However, as noted in the previous section, SWS deficits and exaggerated reduction in SWS during adolescence [52] might be expressions of a genetic predisposition to the development of schizophrenia. Prospective studies to test the value of SWS deficits in assessing risk for schizophrenia have not been performed.

As reviewed in the preceding sections, the sleep of schizophrenia patients is disturbed. The data reviewed above do not clarify if the sleep disturbances are either (1) consequences of schizophrenia's pathophysiology or (2) factors that cause or perpetuate schizophrenia. Some literature suggests that worsening sleep quality precedes schizophrenic exacerbations. Kumar and colleagues [58] asked 30 schizophrenics about prodramata of relapse, finding that sleep disruption was one of the most commonly reported prodromal symptoms along with slowness and underactivity. In a similar study Herz and Melville [59] gave a structured interview to 145 schizophrenia patients and 80 family members. Approximately 65% of patients and 69% of family members identified "difficulty sleeping" as a component of the pre-relapse syndrome.

Others have noted that sleep quality prospectively predicts psychotic symptomatology during withdrawal from psychotropic medicines. Chemerinski and colleagues observed that baseline total insomnia and terminal insomnia scores on the Hamilton depression rating scale respectively predicted increased psychotic symptomatology and disorganization during a 3-week medication-washout period [60]. Similarly, Mattai and colleagues found a positive correlation between sleep disturbance and symptom severity during a medication-washout period in childhood-onset schizophrenia [61]. Despite the above reports, Krystal and colleagues, who recently reviewed the effects of sleep disturbance on psychiatric illness, found "scant research on the effects of sleep disorders and the management of schizophrenia and that more research needs to be done" [64].

Interactions of sleep and psychotic illness

Sleep symptoms affect quality of life

The literature on the effects of primary sleep disorders on psychotic illnesses is small. However, primary sleep disorders (e.g. OSA and RLS) exacerbate the symptoms (e.g. cognitive deficits and daytime sleepiness) in psychotic disorders. More notable is the fact that poor subjective sleep quality, as measured by the Pittsburgh sleep quality index, is associated with a lower quality of life for patients with schizophrenia [62, 63]. The strong correlation between quality of sleep and quality of life in schizophrenia patients underscores the significance of Krystal and colleagues' assessment [64] that there is a relative paucity of research designed to improve sleep quality in schizophrenia, and the importance of further work in this area.

Clinical correlates of sleep deficits

Several researchers have investigated the clinical correlates of sleep disturbances associated with schizophrenia. Most of the studies contain small numbers of subjects and only some have been replicated. The following is a brief synopsis of the findings from these studies. Investigators have correlated sleep onset latency with the thinking disturbance subscale of the brief psychiatric rating scale (BPRS) [65]. Short REM latency has been associated with negative symptom severity [38, 66], REM latency has been inversely correlated with positive symptoms [51], and REM density and REM time have been negatively correlated with total BPRS, medication status [38], and poor

1-year outcomes in female patients [67]. REM density has also been both positively correlated with ratings of hallucinatory behavior [31] and inversely correlated with positive symptoms [19], as well as inversely correlated with cognitive symptoms, emotional discomfort symptoms, and total score on the positive and negative syndrome scale (PANSS) [19]. Within the same study, minutes of REM sleep and REM density in the first REM period of the night inversely correlated with neuropsychological performance, while REM minutes occurring after the first REM period correlated positively with neuropsychological performance. In a small study that did not correct for multiple statistical tests [42], REM activity and REM time both in the whole night data and in the first REM period correlated with suicidal behavior [68]. SWS has been inversely correlated with cognitive symptoms [19], negative outcomes at 1 and 2 years [69], and ventricular size [70]. While each of the above reports suggest that the sleep disturbance associated with schizophrenia and related disorders might provide insight into the pathophysiology of the illness or a marker for improved treatment approaches, none have done so yet.

Explanation of REM abnormalities

Understanding the biological mechanisms underlying the sleep disturbances associated with schizophrenia could provide further insight into the pathophysiology of the illness. Of the schizophrenia-related sleep disturbances, investigators have studied the mechanism underlying REM abnormalities the most. Tandon and colleagues demonstrated that an anticholinergic agent lengthens REM latency less in unmedicated schizophrenics than in normal controls [71]. They interpreted the muted response as evidence of increased cholinergic activity in the patients with schizophrenia. REM latency has also been demonstrated to inversely correlate with plasma acetylcholinesterase levels [72], that is higher acetylcholinesterase plasma levels (which suggests higher than normal levels of acetylcholinergic activity) are associated with shorter REM latency. Administration of a muscarinic agent also shortens REM latency in schizophrenia patients implying that muscarinic receptor supersensitivity might underlie short REM latency associated with schizophrenia [49]. A different line of research has also implicated nicotinic cholinergic receptors in the pathophysiology of schizophrenia. Patients with schizophrenia fail to suppress the P50 EEG potential in response to the second tone in a repeated paired auditory stimuli paradigm. It has been demonstrated that non-REM sleep, a state of relatively low central cholinergic tone, reverses the failed P50 suppression but only briefly [73], while REM sleep, a state of relatively high cholinergic tone, does not normalize the P50 suppression [74]. Interestingly, this normalization of P50 gating modulated by sleep can be reversed by exogenous exposure to nicotine [75].

Sleep and cognitive symptoms

Cognitive deficits are a core feature of schizophrenia, and recently researchers have begun to connect the characteristic sleep disturbances of schizophrenia with memory deficits. For instance, a group of patients with schizophrenia failed to show improvement on a newly learned finger-tapping motor-sequence task after a night of sleep, suggesting a failure of sleep-dependent procedural learning [55]. Goder and colleagues implicated the deficient SWS of schizophrenia patients with visuospatial memory impairments [17]. However, it is notable that impaired memory associated with decreased SWS is not specific to schizophrenia [76]. The same caveat is applicable to the connection of alteration of REM sleep measures and cognitive performance in schizophrenia, since altered REM sleep can occur in patients with depression, borderline personality disorder, and normal subjects [77].

Circadian rhythms and schizophrenia

Schizophrenics have been described as preferring to sleep during the day and stay active during the night [1]. Such behavior suggests that abnormalities in circadian rhythms might contribute to or arise from the pathophysiology underlying schizophrenia. A small study of two schizophrenia patients in an isolation unit suggested that they had an abnormally short (i.e. 23.7-hour) circadian period [78]. There is also a case report of a schizophrenia patient with an arrhythmic circadian rest-activity cycle while on haloperidol despite normal-amplitude but slightly phase-advanced melatonin and body temperature cycles [79]. Despite the apparent altered activity rhythms of some schizophrenia patients, their circadian rhythms of hormone secretion appear normal except for an exaggerated secretion of prolactin with sleep onset [80]. Older schizophrenia patients may have less robust circadian rhythms of activity associated with

age, that may also be affected by medications, lifestyle factors, and behavioral factors [81, 82]. Others have suggested that schizophrenics seem to be proverbial night owls and the severity of their nocturnal preference correlates with their quality of sleep, cognitions, and symptoms [83]. Unfortunately, the limited information on circadian rhythms in schizophrenia is not consistent. Nonetheless, the use of actigraphy to evaluate circadian rest–activity phases in schizophrenics has helped to facilitate psychosocial therapies (day structure) in one case report and thus could theoretically be applied to other patients [84].

Evaluation and treatment of co-morbid sleep disorders and psychotic illness
Obstructive sleep apnea

The available literature on the treatment of OSA in patients with psychotic disorders consists of four case reports of patients with either schizophrenia or schizoaffective disorder and sleep-related breathing disorders treated with continuous positive airway pressure (CPAP) therapy. Karanti and colleagues reported a case of a patient who had been diagnosed with hebephrenic schizophrenia and whose symptoms resolved completely upon treating the patient's obesity hypoventilation syndrome with CPAP [85]. However, it should be noted that resolution of psychotic symptoms as a result of treating a primary sleep disorder is highly unusual. Boufidis and colleagues [86] published a case report of a patient with schizophrenia and OSA whose positive symptoms and daytime sleepiness improved after 6 months of CPAP therapy; however, his cognitive deficits remained unchanged. This result is more similar to this author's clinical experience. Similarly, Dennis and Crisham [87] described the case of a patient with chronic schizoaffective disorder and treatment-resistant violent behavior whose aggressive behavior (but not all psychotic symptoms) dramatically decreased with treatment of previously unrecognized severe OSA. One additional case report described a 52-year-old patient with residual schizophrenia for whom CPAP therapy appeared to exacerbate psychotic symptoms [88]. Such a negative response to CPAP therapy seems as unlikely as the complete resolution of symptoms described previously [85]. It seems likely, as Ramos and Espinar have suggested [89], that psychosocial deficits accompany untreated OSA and improve with treatment of the sleep disorder in non-psychotic patients. It is therefore

37. Zarcone VP Jr, Benson KL, Berger PA. Abnormal rapid eye movement latencies in schizophrenia. *Arch Gen Psychiatry*. 1987;**44**:45–48.

38. Tandon R, Shipley JE, Taylor S, et al. Electroencephalographic sleep abnormalities in schizophrenia: Relationship to positive/negative symptoms and prior neuroleptic treatment. *Arch Gen Psychiatry*. 1992;**49**:185–194.

39. Hudson JI, Lipinski JF, Keck PE Jr, et al. Polysomnographic characteristics of schizophrenia in comparison with mania and depression. *Biol Psychiatry*. 1993;**34**:191–193.

40. Keshavan MS, Reynolds CF 3rd, Miewald JM, Montrose DM. A longitudinal study of EEG sleep in schizophrenia. *Psychiatry Res*. 1996;**59**:203–211.

41. Caldwell DF, Domino EF. Electroencephalographic and eye movement patterns during sleep in chronic schizophrenic patients. *Electroencephalogr Clin Neurophysiol*. 1967;**22**:414–420.

42. Taylor SF, Goldman RS, Tandon R, Shipley JE. Neuropsychological function and REM sleep in schizophrenic patients. *Biol Psychiatry*. 1992;**32**:529–538.

43. Feinberg I, Braun M, Koresko RL, Gottlieb F. Stage 4 sleep in schizophrenia. *Arch Gen Psychiatry*. 1969;**21**:262–266.

44. Kajimura N, Kato M, Okuma T, et al. A quantitative sleep-EEG study on the effects of benzodiazepine and zopiclone in schizophrenic patients. *Schizophr Res*. 1995;**15**:303–312.

45. Keshavan MS, Reynolds CF 3rd, Miewald MJ, et al. Delta sleep deficits in schizophrenia: evidence from automated analyses of sleep data. *Arch Gen Psychiatry*. 1998;**55**:443–448.

46. Benson KL, Zarcone VP Jr. Testing the REM sleep phasic event intrusion hypothesis of schizophrenia. *Psychiatry Res*. 1985;**15**:163–173.

47. Hoffmann R, Hendrickse W, Rush AJ, Armitage R. Slow-wave activity during non-REM sleep in men with schizophrenia and major depressive disorders. *Psychiatry Res*. 2000;**95**:215–225.

48. Nishino S, Mignot E, Benson KL, Zarcone VP Jr. Cerebrospinal fluid prostaglandins and corticotropin releasing factor in schizophrenics and controls: relationship to sleep architecture. *Psychiatry Res*. 1998;**78**:141–150.

49. Riemann D, Hohagen F, Krieger S, et al. Cholinergic REM induction test: muscarinic supersensitivity underlies polysomnographic findings in both depression and schizophrenia. *J Psychiatr Res*. 1994;**28**:195–210.

50. Benson KL, Faull KF, Zarcone VP Jr. Evidence for the role of serotonin in the regulation of slow wave sleep in schizophrenia. *Sleep*. 1991;**14**:133–139.

51. Poulin J, Daoust AM, Forest G, Stip E, Godbout R. Sleep architecture and its clinical correlates in first episode and neuroleptic-naive patients with schizophrenia. *Schizophr Res*. 2003;**62**:147–153.

52. Keshavan MS, Diwadkar VA, Montrose DM, Stanley JA, Pettegrew JW. Premorbid characterization in schizophrenia: the Pittsburgh High Risk Study. *World Psychiatry*. 2004;**3**:163–168.

53. Feinberg I. Schizophrenia: caused by a fault in programmed synaptic elimination during adolescence? *J Psychiatr Res*. 1982–1983;**17**:319–334.

54. Keshavan MS, Miewald J, Haas G, et al. Slow-wave sleep and symptomatology in schizophrenia and related psychotic disorders. *J Psychiatr Res*. 1995;**29**:303–314.

55. Manoach DS, Cain MS, Vangel MG, et al. A failure of sleep-dependent procedural learning in chronic, medicated schizophrenia. *Biol Psychiatry*. 2004;**56**:951–956.

56. Keshavan MS, Cashmere JD, Miewald J, Yeragani VK. Decreased nonlinear complexity and chaos during sleep in first episode schizophrenia: a preliminary report. *Schizophr Res*. 2004;**71**:263–272.

57. van Os J, Allardyce J. The clinical epidemiology of schizophrenia. In: Sadock BJ, Sadock VA, Ruiz P, eds. *Kaplan and Sadock's comprehensive textbook of psychiatry*. Philadelphia, PA: Lippincott Williams & Wilkins; 2009:1476–1487.

58. Kumar S, Thara R, Rajkumar S. Coping with symptoms of relapse in schizophrenia. *Eur Arch Psychiatry Neurol Sci*. 1989;**239**:213–215.

59. Herz MI, Melville C. Relapse in schizophrenia. *Am J Psychiatry*. 1980;**137**:801–805.

60. Chemerinski E, Ho BC, Flaum M, et al. Insomnia as a predictor for symptom worsening following antipsychotic withdrawal in schizophrenia. *Compr Psychiatry*. 2002;**43**:393–396.

61. Mattai AA, Tossell J, Greenstein DK, et al. Sleep disturbances in childhood-onset schizophrenia. *Schizophr Res*. 2006;**86**:123–129.

62. Ritsner M, Kurs R, Ponizovsky A, Hadjez J. Perceived quality of life in schizophrenia: relationships to sleep quality. *Qual Life Res*. 2004;**13**:783–791.

63. Hofstetter JR, Lysaker PH, Mayeda AR. Quality of sleep in patients with schizophrenia is associated with quality of life and coping. *BMC Psychiatry*. 2005;**5**:13.

64. Krystal AD, Thakur M, Roth T. Sleep disturbance in psychiatric disorders: effects on function and quality of life in mood disorders, alcoholism, and schizophrenia. *Ann Clin Psychiatry*. 2008;**20**: 39–46.

65. Zarcone VP, Benson KL. BPRS symptom factors and sleep variables in schizophrenia. *Psychiatry Res*. 1997;**66**:111–120.

66. Tandon R, Shipley JE, Eiser AS, Greden JF. Association between abnormal REM sleep and negative symptoms in schizophrenia. *Psychiatry Res*. 1989;**27**:359–361.

67. Goldman M, Tandon R, DeQuardo JR, et al. Biological predictors of 1-year outcome in schizophrenia in males and females. *Schizophr Res*. 1996;**21**:65–73.

68. Keshavan MS, Reynolds CF, Montrose D, et al. Sleep and suicidality in psychotic patients. *Acta Psychiatr Scand*. 1994;**89**:122–125.

69. Keshaven MS, Reynolds CF 3rd, Miewald J, Montrose D. Slow-wave sleep deficits and outcome in schizophrenia and schizoaffective disorder. *Acta Psychiatr Scand*. 1995;**91**:289–292.

70. Benson KL, Sullivan EV, Lim KO, et al. Slow wave sleep and computed tomographic measures of brain morphology in schizophrenia. *Psychiatry Res*. 1996;**60**:125–134.

71. Tandon R, Shipley JE, Greden JF, et al. Muscarinic cholinergic hyperactivity in schizophrenia: Relationship to positive and negative symptoms. *Schizophr Res*. 1991;**4**:23–30.

72. Keshavan MS, Mahadik SP, Reynolds CF 3rd, et al. Plasma cholinesterase isozymes and REM latency in schizophrenia. *Psychiatry Res*. 1992;**43**:23–29.

73. Griffith JM, Waldo M, Adler LE, Freedman R. Normalization of auditory sensory gating in schizophrenic patients after a brief period for sleep. *Psychiatry Res*. 1993;**49**:29–39.

74. Griffith JM, Freedman R. Normalization of the auditory P50 gating deficit of schizophrenic patients after non-REM but not REM sleep. *Psychiatry Res*. 1995;**56**:271–278.

75. Griffith JM, O'Neill JE, Petty F, et al. Nicotinic receptor desensitization and sensory gating deficits in schizophrenia. *Biol Psychiatry*. 1998;**44**:98–106.

76. Bodizs R, Lazar AS. Schizophrenia, slow wave sleep and visuospatial memory: sleep-dependent consolidation or trait-like correlation? *J Psychiatr Res*. 2006;**40**:89–90.

77. Cazzullo CL, Fornari MG, Maffei C, et al. Sleep, psychophysiological functioning and learning processes in schizophrenia. *Act Nerv Super*. 1977; **19**(Suppl 2):409–417.

78. Mills JN, Morgan R, Minors DS, Waterhouse JM The free-running circadian rhythms of two schizophrenics. *Chronobiologia*. 1977;**4**:353–360.

79. Wirz-Justice A, Cajochen C, Nussbaum P. A schizophrenic patient with an arrhythmic circadian rest-activity cycle. *Psychiatry Res*. 1997;**73**:83–90.

80. Van Cauter E, Linkowski P, Kerkhofs M, et al. Circadian and sleep-related endocrine rhythms in schizophrenia. *Arch Gen Psychiatry*. 1991;**48**:348–356.

81. Martin J, Jeste DV, Caliguiri MP, et al. Actigraphic estimates of circadian rhythms and sleep/wake in older schizophrenia patients. *Schizophr Res*. 2001;**47**:77–86.

82. Martin JL, Jeste DV, Ancoli-Israel S. Older schizophrenia patients have more disrupted sleep and circadian rhythms than age-matched comparison subjects. *J Psychiatr Res*. 2005;**39**:251–259.

83. Hofstetter JR, Mayeda AR, Happel CG, Lysaker PH. Sleep and daily activity preferences in schizophrenia: associations with neurocognition and symptoms. *J Nerv Ment Dis*. 2003;**191**:408–410.

84. Haug HJ, Wirz-Justice A, Rossler W. Actigraphy to measure day structure as a therapeutic variable in the treatment of schizophrenic patients. *Acta Psychiatr Scand Suppl*. 2000;**407**:91–95.

85. Karanti A, Landen M. Treatment refractory psychosis remitted upon treatment with continuous positive airway pressure: a case report. *Psychopharmacol Bull*. 2007;**40**:113–117.

86. Boufidis S, Kosmidis MH, Bozikas VP, et al. Treatment outcome of obstructive sleep apnea syndrome in a patient with schizophrenia: case report. *Int J Psychiatry Med*. 2003;**33**:305–310.

87. Dennis JL, Crisham KP. Chronic assaultive behavior improved with sleep apnea treatment. *J Clin Psychiatry*. 2001;**62**:571–572.

88. Chiner E, Arriero JM, Signes-Costa J, Marco J. Acute psychosis after CPAP treatment in a schizophrenic patient with sleep apnoea-hypopnoea syndrome. *Eur Respir J*. 2001;**17**:313–315.

89. Ramos Platon MJ, Espinar Sierra J. Changes in psychopathological symptoms in sleep apnea patients after treatment with nasal continuous positive airway pressure. *Int J Neurosci*. 1992;**62**:173–195.

90. DiPhillipo M, Fry J. Is schizophrenia a contraindication for nasal CPAP treatment? *Sleep Res*. 1990;**19**:212.

91. Cunningham S, Ellsworth S, Winkleman JW, et al. Compliance with nasal continuous positive airway pressure in psychiatric patients with obstructive sleep apnea. *Sleep Res*. 1994;**23**:192.

92. Shapiro B, Spitz H. Problems in the differential diagnosis of narcolepsy versus schizophrenia. *Am J Psychiatry*. 1976;**133**:1321–1323.

93. Douglass AB, Hays P, Pazderka F, Russell JM. Florid refractory schizophrenias that turn out to be treatable variants of HLA-associated narcolepsy. *J Nerv Ment Dis*. 1991;**179**:12–17.

94. Douglass AB, Shipley JE, Haines RF, et al. Schizophrenia, narcolepsy, and HLA-DR15, DQ6. *Biol Psychiatry*. 1993;**34**:773–780.

95. Nishino S, Ripley B, Mignot E, Benson KL, Zarcone VP. CSF hypocretin-1 levels in schizophrenics and controls: relationship to sleep architecture. *Psychiatry Res*. 2002;**110**:1–7.

96. Cadieux R, Kales J, Kales A, Biever J, Mann LD. Pharmacologic and psychotherapeutic issues in coexistent paranoid schizophrenia and narcolepsy: case report. *J Clin Psychiatry*. 1985;**46**(5):191–193.

97. Roy A. Psychiatric aspects of narcolepsy. *Br J Psychiatry*. 1976;**128**:562–565.

98. Ohayon MM, Priest RG, Caulet M, Guilleminault C. Hypnagogic and hypnopompic hallucinations: pathological phenomena? *Br J Psychiatry*. 1996;**169**:459–467.

99. Huang SS, Liao YC, Hsieh YY, et al. Combination antipsychotic therapy in psychiatric outpatient clinics in Taiwan. *Compr Psychiatry*. 2006;**47**:421–425.

100. Yamashita H, Mori K, Nagao M, et al. Effects of changing from typical to atypical antipsychotic drugs on subjective sleep quality in patients with schizophrenia in a Japanese population. *J Clin Psychiatry*. 2004;**65**:1525–1530.

101. Jus K, Jus A, Villeneuve A, Pires P, Fontaine P. The utilization of hypnotics in chronic schizophrenics: some critical remarks. *Biol Psychiatry*. 1979;**14**:955–960.

102. Kajimura N, Kato M, Okuma T, Onuma T. Effects of zopiclone on sleep and symptoms in schizophrenia: comparison with benzodiazepine hypnotics. *Prog Neuropsychopharmacol Biol Psychiatry*. 1994;**18**:477–490.

103. Klimke A, Klieser E. Sudden death after intravenous application of lorazepam in a patient treated with clozapine. *Am J Psychiatry*. 1994;**151**:780.

104. Shamir E, Laudon M, Barak Y, et al. Melatonin improves sleep quality of patients with chronic schizophrenia. *J Clin Psychiatry*. 2000;**61**:373–377.

105. Suresh Kumar PN, Andrade C, Bhakta SG, Singh NM. Melatonin in schizophrenic outpatients with insomnia: a double-blind, placebo-controlled study. *J Clin Psychiatry*. 2007;**68**:237–241.

106. Taylor SF, Tandon R, Shipley JE, Eiser AS. Effect of neuroleptic treatment on polysomnographic measures in schizophrenia. *Biol Psychiatry*. 1991;**30**:904–912.

107. Beasley CM Jr, Tollefson GD, Tran PV. Safety of olanzapine. *J Clin Psychiatry*. 1997;**58** (Suppl 10):13–17.

108. Angermeyer MC, Loffler W, Muller P, Schulze B, Priebe S. Patients' and relatives' assessment of clozapine treatment. *Psychol Med*. 2001;**31**: 509–517.

109. Gao K, Ganocy SJ, Gajwani P, et al. A review of sensitivity and tolerability of antipsychotics in patients with bipolar disorder or schizophrenia: focus on somnolence. *J Clin Psychiatry*. 2008;**69**:302–309.

110. Neylan TC, van Kammen DP, Kelley ME, Peters JL. Sleep in schizophrenic patients on and off haloperidol therapy: Clinically stable vs relapsed patients. *Arch Gen Psychiatry*. 1992;**49**:643–649.

111. Salin-Pascual RJ, Herrera-Estrella M, Galicia-Polo L, Laurrabaquio MR. Olanzapine acute administration in schizophrenic patients increases delta sleep and sleep efficiency. *Biol Psychiatry*. 1999;**46**:141–143.

112. Lee JH, Woo JI, Meltzer HY. Effects of clozapine on sleep measures and sleep-associated changes in growth hormone and cortisol in patients with schizophrenia. *Psychiatry Res*. 2001;**103**:157–166.

113. Cohrs S, Rodenbeck A, Guan Z, et al. Sleep-promoting properties of quetiapine in healthy subjects. *Psychopharmacology*. 2004;**174**:421–429.

114. Dursun SM, Patel JK, Burke JG, Reveley MA. Effects of typical antipsychotic drugs and risperidone on the quality of sleep in patients with schizophrenia: a pilot study. *J Psychiatry Neurosci*. 1999;**24**:333–337.

115. McEvoy JP, Lieberman JA, Perkins DO, et al. Efficacy and tolerability of olanzapine, quetiapine, and risperidone in the treatment of early psychosis: a randomized, double-blind 52-week comparison. *Am J Psychiatry*. 2007;**164**:1050–1060.

116. Twaites BR, Wilton LV, Shakir SA. The safety of quetiapine: results of a post-marketing surveillance study on 1728 patients in England. *J Psychopharmacol*. 2007;**21**:392–399.

117. Lindberg N, Virkkunen M, Tani P, et al. Effect of a single-dose of olanzapine on sleep in healthy females and males. *Int Clin Psychopharmacol*. 2002;**17**: 177–184.

118. Muller MJ, Rossbach W, Mann K, et al. Subchronic effects of olanzapine on sleep EEG in schizophrenic patients with predominantly negative symptoms. *Pharmacopsychiatry*. 2004;**37**:157–162.

119. Goder R, Fritzer G, Gottwald B, et al. Effects of olanzapine on slow wave sleep, sleep spindles and sleep-related memory consolidation in schizophrenia. *Pharmacopsychiatry*. 2008;**41**(3):92–99.

120. Cohrs S, Meier A, Neumann AC, et al. Improved sleep continuity and increased slow wave sleep and REM latency during ziprasidone treatment: a randomized, controlled, crossover trial of 12 healthy male subjects. *J Clin Psychiatry*. 2005;**66**(8):989–996.

Sleep in substance use disorders

Deirdre A. Conroy, J. Todd Arnedt, and Kirk J. Brower

Introduction

A survey conducted by the World Health Organization research consortium found that the USA had among the highest lifetime rates of tobacco and alcohol use and led the world in the proportion of citizens reporting marijuana or cocaine use at least once during their lifetime. Individuals using, abusing, or dependent on illicit drugs cost the USA half a trillion dollars per year and approximately 570 000 die each year due to substance-related deaths (NIDA, 2008).

Our current understanding of how substances affect sleep is influenced largely by factors related to the pharmacology of the substance, the population in which it is being studied, and the various methodologies used to measure sleep. Rarely are drugs studied across all populations and measures. Sleep complaints in the substance-using population are extremely common, but whether or not the sleep complaints are a consequence of substance use *per se* or a pre-existing complaint is a topic of increasing interest. For example, it is known that up to 91% of patients with a history of alcoholism have sleep complaints [1], but also that a pre-existing history of insomnia can increase the incidence of substance use disorders 3.5 years after the insomnia diagnosis has been made [2].

The diagnostic criteria for substance-induced sleep disorders are outlined in both the *Diagnostic and Statistical Manual* (DSM-IV) and the *International Classification of Sleep Disorders*, 2nd edition (ICSD-2). In DSM-IV, a substance-induced sleep disorder can be classified as insomnia, hypersomnia, parasomnia, or mixed with further specifications of onset during intoxication or onset during withdrawal. The ICSD-2 contains additional categories not found in DSM-IV, such as circadian rhythm sleep disorder and central sleep apnea due to a drug or substance. This chapter will explore the effects of both licit and illicit substances of abuse on sleep (see Table 19.1) and the reciprocal relationships among them. A greater understanding of this vicious cycle may help to reduce relapse rates by making informed treatment decisions of residual sleep disturbances during recovery from substance use. Early detection of sleep disturbance in children at high risk for developing a substance use disorder may help in the effort to prevent the onset of substance use disorders.

CNS sedating substances

Alcohol

Insomnia is an extremely common sleep complaint in patients who are actively drinking alcohol as well as in patients who have recently stopped drinking. The DSM-IV lists insomnia among its list of symptoms that can occur within several hours to a few days after cessation of alcohol use. Across seven studies of 1577 alcohol-dependent patients undergoing treatment, the average rate of self-reported insomnia was 58% (range = 36–91%) [1,3], substantially higher than rates of insomnia among the general population. One of the contributing factors to difficulty falling asleep in alcohol-dependent patients may be an underlying delay in the circadian sleep phase. One study revealed a delay of 1.5 hours in the onset of nocturnal melatonin secretion in alcohol-dependent patients compared to controls [4]. Another study suggested that alcohol-dependent patients may have less homeostatic drive (measured by EEG delta power after a night of partial sleep deprivation) for sleep than healthy controls [5].

Studies using polysomnography (PSG) have shown that when alcohol is consumed close to bedtime, it

Foundations of Psychiatric Sleep Medicine, ed. John W. Winkelman and David T. Plante. Published by Cambridge University Press.
© Cambridge University Press 2010.

Table 19.1 Effect of substances of abuse on sleep and wakefulness

Substance of abuse	Sleep continuity			Sleep architecture				Sleep disorders		MSLT[a]
	SOL	TST	SE	ROL	REM	SWS	S1	SDB	PLMS	MSLT
ALCOHOL										
Intoxication[b]	D[6–8]	D[8,146c]	I[8]	I[9]	D[7,9]	I[6–8]	D[8]	I[147d]	I[15]	I[148] D[149]
Withdrawal	I[12]D[11]	D[11] I[13e]	I[13]	D[12,14]	I[11]	D[10,12]	–	I[15,150]	I[18,19]	D[151f]
NICOTINE										
Intoxication	I[78,84]	D[84]	D[84]	D[85]	D[84]	NC[84]	NC[84]	NC[84]	D[82]	–
Withdrawal	I[88] D[78g]	I, D[86–88]	D[78,88]	D[88]	I[78,88]	I, D[86h] D[37] NC 36	D[88]NC[87i]	–	I[87j]	D[87]
CAFFEINE										
Intoxication	I[98,99]	D[98,100]	D[98,99]	I &D[98k]	NC 98k	D[99,100l]	I[100]	–	–	I[98,152]
Withdrawal	NC[98]	NC[98]	NC[98]	NC[98]	NC[98]	NC[98]	NC[98]	–	–	NC[98]
CANNABIS										
Intoxication	D[32]	I, D[32m]	I, D[32]	I[32]	D[33]	I[30,33]	I, D[33m]	D[32]	–	–
Withdrawal	I[31]	–	–	–	I[153]	D[31,153]	D[30]	–	–	–
OPIOIDS										
Intoxication	I[49]	NC[154] D[49]	NC[154] D[50]	I[155]	D[155]	D[154,155]	I[156] D[155]	I[155] NC[157] D[154]	–	–
Withdrawal	–	–	I[155]	–	I[52,155]	NC, I[52,155]	–	–	–	–
MDMA "ECSTASY"										
Intoxication	NC 158	D[108]	D[158] I[159]	–	D[158]	I[159]	I[160]	–	–	–
Withdrawal	I[160]	D[160]	D[160j]	D[160]	I[160j]	NC 160	–	I[160]	–	–
COCAINE										
Intoxication	I[161]	D[161]	D[161]	I[161]	D[161]	I[65]	NC[161]	–	–	–
Withdrawal	D[162g] NC[163] I[162e]	D[72,162e] I[162g]	D[70,71e] NC[164] I[162]	D[70] NC[71]	I[70,72] NC[71n]	D[162,163]	I[163]	–	–	D[68]
AMPHETAMINES										
Intoxication	–	–	–	–	–	–	–	–	–	I[75–77]
Withdrawal	I[72]	D[72]	D[72g]	D[72]	D[72g]	D[72]	I[72]	–	–	–

I = increase, D = decrease, NC = no change, – = no data.
Sleep onset latency = SOL, total sleep time = TST, sleep efficiency = SE, rapid eye movement sleep latency = ROL, rapid eye movement percentage = REM, slow-wave sleep = SWS, Stage 1 sleep = S1, sleep disordered breathing = SDB, periodic limb movements in sleep = PLMS, multiple sleep latency test = MSLT.
a = decrease in sleep onset on the MSLT indicates more sleepiness; b = alcohol's effects on sleep stages change from the 1st half to the 2nd half of the night; c = increased number of wake periods in sleep; d = only in men; e = late withdrawal (>3 weeks); f = increased SOL during first 75 min after consumption; g = early withdrawal (<3 weeks); h = Wetter et al. (2000) shows SWS decreases at day 3 but then increases from day 3–10 [86]; i = initially increased, but decreased over time; j = not significant; k = decreased shortly after caffeine intake but increase with late caffeine (see Table 1, p. 530 of Bonnet and Arand, 1992 [98]); l = during the first third of the sleep period; m = depending on dose of THC and CBD variables; include dose and time into withdrawal; n = Pace-Schott et al. (2005) is a binge abstinence protocol [71].

shortens sleep onset latency (SOL) [6–8], prolongs rapid eye movement onset latency (ROL) [9], and increases slow-wave sleep (SWS) in the first half of the night [6,7,10]. Sleep quality worsens in the second half of the night: stage 1 (S1) sleep, wakefulness, and the percentage of rapid eye movement (REM) sleep increase [6], and SWS decreases [6,7,10]. SOL, total sleep time (TST), and sleep efficiency (SE) have been shown to improve in those who remained abstinent during the first year, but arousals from sleep and stage changes remained elevated. REM sleep was disrupted (increased REM%, decreased REM sleep latency) even after 2 years of continued abstinence [11]. PSG findings have also been associated with rates of relapse. For example, abbreviated REM latency, less stage 4 sleep [12], increased REM density [13], and increases in REM% [14] have been shown to predict relapse.

Sleep-disordered breathing (SDB) has been shown to occur more frequently in alcohol-dependent patients, particularly in older males [15]. Moreover, results from an epidemiological investigation of the natural history of SDB show that men have a 25% greater chance of having SDB (defined as apnea-hypopnea index (AHI) ≥ 5) with every drink per day[16].

Movement disorders associated with sleep disruption, like restless legs syndrome (RLS) [17] and periodic limb movements in sleep, have been found in individuals who consume ≥ 2 drinks/day. Aldrich et al. (1993) found that twice as many women who reported high alcohol use had significant periodic limb movements of sleep (PLMS) (defined as >20 per hour), and were significantly more likely to be diagnosed with RLS, compared to women reporting normal levels of alcohol consumption [18]. Recovering alcohol-dependent patients were also shown to have significantly more periodic limb movements associated with arousals from sleep than controls, and the PLMS arousal index (number of PLMS per hour of sleep) was significantly elevated in relapsers compared to controls after 6 months of abstinence [19]. In fact, a discriminant function analysis based on PLMS arousal index correctly predicted the status of 55% of the overall sample, including 80% of abstainers and 44% of relapsers after 6 months of abstinence [19].

Sleep problems may predispose an individual to developing an alcohol use disorder or return to drinking alcohol once abstinent [20–22]. The Michigan Longitudinal Study, which has been following a cohort of children at high risk for alcoholism, found that mother-reported sleep difficulties in 3–5-year-old boys predicted earlier age of onset of drinking during early adolescence even after controlling for anxiety/depression, attention problems, and family history [23]. The onset of alcohol use is a robust indicator of problems with alcohol use in late adolescence, and it also is a strong predictor of an alcohol use disorder in adulthood. More recent work with a larger sample of the same cohort, which also included girls, replicated the male findings and also showed independent relationships of the early sleep difficulty to adolescent internalizing (e.g. anxiety/depression) and externalizing (e.g. impulsivity/acting out) problems [24]. This work suggests that sleep difficulties early in life may be a predisposing factor for later alcohol and behavioral problems.

In an epidemiological study of more than 10 000 adults, the incidence of alcohol abuse or dependence during a 1-year follow-up period was twice as likely in individuals with persistent complaints of insomnia compared to those without insomnia complaints, after controlling for baseline psychiatric disorders [25]. Given the sedating properties of alcohol, adults with sleep problems may be more likely to turn to alcohol as a way to self-medicate. In a forced choice paradigm across four nights in the sleep laboratory, when given the choice of color-coded cups prior to bedtime, insomnia subjects chose the cups containing alcohol on 67% of the nights versus the non-insomniacs who chose the cups with alcohol on only 22% of the nights [26].

In summary, both objective and subjective sleep problems may play a role in the development and course of alcohol use disorders. Insomnia complaints in alcohol-dependent patients are common and early treatment of insomnia, with pharmacological or behavioral treatments, may reduce the rate of relapse. Some evidence suggests that SDB, sleep-related movement disorders, and altered circadian rhythms may be more frequent in this patient population. Management of sleep problems in children may theoretically prevent the early onset of alcohol use during early adolescence, although data is currently insufficient to support this contention.

Cannabis

Most sleep complaints related to cannabis (marijuana) are documented to occur during withdrawal, and the DSM-IV includes insomnia as one of the diagnostic symptoms of cannabis withdrawal.

A study of 1735 frequent users of cannabis (>21 occasions in a single year), found that 235 (13.5%) reported difficulty sleeping during withdrawal [27]. Another study reported that 33% of cannabis users had difficulty sleeping during withdrawal [28]. The National Epidemiologic Survey on Alcohol and Related Conditions in the general US population revealed that of 2613 frequent cannabis users 24.5% of the sample reported subjective hypersomnia and 6.1% reported insomnia during cannabis withdrawal [29].

Cannabis taken at bedtime has been shown to increase (N=7) [30], decrease (N=2) [31], and have no effect (N=8) [32] on SWS and to decrease REM sleep [33]. Doses of 10, 20, and 30 mg of tetrahydrocannabinol (THC) prior to sleep have decreased SOL after subjects reported achieving a "high" subjectively [34]. Studies are more conclusive with respect to objective sleep disruption during cannabis withdrawal. Difficulty falling asleep and decreased SWS percentage have been documented by PSG during the first two nights of withdrawal [31], but no studies using PSG after prolonged abstinence have been conducted. Bolla et al. (2008) examined sleep of heavy cannabis users (104 +/− 51 joints/week) in the three nights prior to and after cannabis discontinuation. By the second night of withdrawal, cannabis users demonstrated lower sleep efficiency (SE), shorter total sleep time (TST), longer SOL, and shorter ROL compared to controls [35], supporting studies using subjective measures. Daytime consequences of cannabis use prior to bedtime are reported only following higher doses of THC (15 mg THC plus 15 mg cannabidiol) and include increased sleepiness, mood changes, and impaired memory [32].

Emerging research suggests that early sleep problems may be a pathway to cannabis use during the teenage years and into early adulthood. Wong et al. (2004) found that children with "trouble sleeping" or being "overtired" were almost three times more likely to use cannabis between the ages of 12 and 14 years old [23]. In teenagers entering treatment centers, cannabis is one of the most commonly reported illicit drugs. Because of teenagers' physiological tendency to exhibit a delayed circadian sleep phase, they are at greater risk for reporting difficulty falling asleep and morning tiredness. Therefore, the use of cannabis to self-medicate sleep problems has been explored in adolescents [36,37]. In a cross-sectional analysis of data from the National Longitudinal Study of Adolescent Health, Roane and Taylor (2008) found that

adolescents with insomnia were 1.32 to 2.05 times more likely than adolescents without insomnia to use cannabis [36].

These studies suggest that sleep disturbances even at a young age may be a risk factor to future cannabis use. Addressing sleep problems in children and teenagers may reduce the risk of drug use. Incorporating therapies to improve sleep into a continued care model, i.e. outpatient treatment services offered to teens after residential substance abuse treatment, may help to reduce risk of future substance use in adolescents [38].

Opioids

Subjective reports of opioids on sleep can vary. Many patients with pain report longer TST with opioids, presumably because of fewer pain-related arousals and awakenings [39]. Similarly, chronic pain patients with osteoarthritis reported sleeping better when their pain was relieved with tramadol [40]. On the other hand, Vella-Brincat et al. (2007) found an association between opioid use and reports of sleep disturbance, dreams, and nightmares in palliative care patients [41]. Subjective sleep quality is also impaired among treated opioid-dependent patients. Sleep assessments from 225 methadone-maintenance treatment (MMT) patients, for example, showed that 84% reported clinically significant sleep disturbances as defined by a score on the Pittsburgh Sleep Quality Index (PSQI) of >5 (mean score (SD) = 10.64 (4.9)) [42]. A separate study also found elevated PSQI scores in a group of 101 MMT patients (mean (SD) 9.4 (4.8)) which did not correlate with duration of MMT, gender, age, or recent abuse of opiates, cannabis, or cocaine [43]. Insomnia can be present during opioid withdrawal and is one of the symptoms in the DSM-IV diagnostic criteria for opioid withdrawal. Heroin-dependent patients detoxified with methadone reported even greater sleep problems than those maintained on methadone during the first months of heroin abstinence [44]. However, in an uncontrolled study, 57% of patients detoxified with a combination of buprenorphine and clonidine reported improved sleep [45].

Sleep laboratory studies suggest that opioids may affect sleep differently depending on whether or not the user is in pain and if the user is dependent on opioids. Opioids have also been associated with central sleep apnea in a dose-dependent fashion [46], occurring in about 24–30% of chronic users [47], a much higher rate than in the general population [48]. The latter study of consecutive patients from a pain clinic also found at least one type of sleep apnea (central, obstructive, mixed) in 85% of patients [48]. PSG findings in 10 MMT patients (dose range 50–120 mg/day) showed more central sleep apnea, more frequent awakenings [49], lower sleep efficiency, lower SWS, more stage 2 sleep, and less REM sleep than normal controls [50].

Sleep complaints often occur in association with psychiatric illness or chronic pain, which can in turn be a precipitating factor to opioid abuse or dependence. Peles et al. (2006) found that patients with a high score on the PSQI had higher rates of chronic pain, benzodiazepine abuse, psychiatric disorders, and had a longer duration of opiate abuse prior to entering treatment for opioid dependence. Moreover, patients who described themselves as "poor sleepers" used higher doses of methadone during their MMT compared to "normal sleepers" [43].

Few studies have evaluated sleep across prolonged periods of abstinence from opioids. Two early studies on male prisoners examined sleep across protracted methadone abstinence. Martin et al. (1973) found increased REM sleep and delta sleep after 10 weeks of methadone withdrawal [51]. Kay (1975) found increased TST, decreased wake time, decreased REM sleep, and increased SWS across the 22-week study period of methadone abstinence [52]. In contrast to studies with alcohol-dependent patients, sleep complaints in opioid-dependent patients predicted decreased relapse rates 1 month after detoxification in one recent study, although other related factors (e.g. increased attention by clinicians to subjects who had sleep disruption after detoxification) might have led to a spurious association [53]. Certainly, such findings require replication before concluding sleep disruption is protective of relapse in opioid dependence.

In summary, opioids can become deleterious to sleep with abuse or dependence. Early studies on prolonged methadone abstinence suggest that sleep may improve in MMT patients; however, studies longer than 22 weeks of abstinence are lacking. Additional risk factors such as benzodiazepine abuse, chronic pain, or psychiatric disorders may be precipitating or perpetuating factors.

Benzodiazepine receptor agonists (BzRAs)

Since approximately the 1990s, newer BzRAs (eszopiclone, zolpidem, zaleplon, and zolpidem CR) have been replacing benzodiazepines as the first-line pharmacological therapy for transient insomnia. Fewer prescriptions for the longer acting benzodiazepines (BZDs) (e.g. temazepam, flurazepam) are being written because the BzRAs carry fewer side-effects such as next day sedation, tolerance, and rebound insomnia. Two reviews have explored the abuse and dependence on BzRAs [54,55]. In a review of the literature between 1991 and 2002, nearly all reports of abuse and dependence on zolpidem and zopiclone (zopiclone is not sold in the USA) were reported in former drug or alcohol abusers or in patients with co-morbid psychiatric disorders. Another large review of the literature up to 2004 focused on the abuse liability of hypnotic drugs [54]. The authors generated a "likelihood of abuse score" for 19 hypnotics based on a cumulative score reflecting animal drug self-administration, human liking/reinforcement, and actual abuse. According to summary data of the BzRAs commonly used in the USA (e.g. zaleplon, zolpidem, and eszopiclone), the lowest likelihood of abuse score was found in zolpidem, for which abuse liability was rated as being similar to oxazepam and quazepam [54]. Zaleplon and eszopiclone had slightly higher likelihoods of abuse with abuse liability in the moderate range, more closely similar to temazepam and triazolam. Hypnotics not mediated through GABA receptor sites, like trazodone, ramelteon, and diphenhydramine, were reported to have the lowest likelihood of abuse.

Reports of abuse and dependence on BzRAs are relatively rare. In a 2003 review, for example, 36 cases for zolpidem and 22 cases for zopiclone had been reported in the medical literature [55]. Case studies have reported on patients without a substance use disorder history or co-morbid psychiatric illnesses. There have been three case studies on zolpidem dependence (10–15 mg) reporting anterograde amnesia with compulsive repetitive behaviors [56]. Another case study of zolpidem abuse reported a 27-year-old man who was taking zolpidem up to 800 mg. Upon withdrawal, he experienced extensive craving, withdrawal seizures, and life-threatening behavior [57]. Another study reported using diazepam to assist zolpidem detoxification [58]. Overdoses of eszopiclone have recently been reported [59]. In one study reported from the Texas Poison Center Network between 2005 and 2006, eszopiclone overdoses between 2 and 210 mg (in the absence of coingestants) were associated with mostly minor to moderate effects, e.g. drowsiness/lethargy, agitation/irritability, ataxia, tachycardia, slurred speech, hyperglycemia, and confusion. Guidelines from this report suggest that eszopiclone ingestions >6 mg be managed in a healthcare facility while <6 mg can be managed at home [59].

CNS stimulants

Sleep complaints with amphetamine, methamphetamine, and methylphenidate abuse or dependence are similar to those reported with cocaine use disorders [60,61]. According to the DSM-IV, insomnia or hypersomnia can occur during amphetamine or cocaine withdrawal. The milder yet more widely used stimulant, caffeine, prolongs sleep onset latency and leads to complaints of insomnia due to its antagonist effects at adenosine receptors [62]. Some people are more sensitive to caffeine-induced insomnia than others, which may reflect genotypic differences [63,64]. Tobacco smoking is also associated with poor sleep.

Cocaine

Sleep problems have been shown to be the second most common complaint, behind depression, of patients during cocaine withdrawal. In one study, nearly three-quarters of a group of 75 active cocaine users complained of sleep disturbance during withdrawal [65]. Another study found that 76% of 554 cocaine users had insomnia during withdrawal, and 49% reported vivid, unpleasant dreams [66]. During cocaine withdrawal, hypersomnia has been observed in up to 62% of users [66], presumably compensation for the extended sleep deprivation during binge use. Subjective insomnia during withdrawal, however, may improve despite worsening PSG abnormalities [67].

Self-administration of cocaine intranasally prior to sleep causes prolonged SOL, decreased SE, and decreased REM sleep [68]. Acute administration of cocaine to three abstinent abusers increased SOL by several hours, decreased SE, and decreased REM sleep percentage [68,69]. Subjective reports of sleep problems are a common side-effect of cocaine withdrawal, including hypersomnia and increased dreaming [65]. These complaints are reflected in PSG changes during withdrawal, including an initial increase in TST, shortened ROL, increased REM sleep percentage, and increased REM density [68,70]. After withdrawal, sleep quality worsens. After a 3-day binge period of smoked cocaine among dependent patients and 15 subsequent days of abstinence, TST, SE, and

SOL deteriorated [71]. Other studies have shown that SOL and wake time after sleep onset (WASO) remains elevated and sleep efficiency continues to be low in the 3 weeks post-abstinence [70,72]. Subjective reports of sleep quality, however, remained unchanged across the first 2 weeks of abstinence [71] and self-reported sleep parameters worsened 1 month after abstinence [73]. In sum, sleep is considerably disrupted objectively and subjectively for weeks after withdrawal from cocaine. The relationship between cocaine withdrawal symptoms and relapse to cocaine use following treatment is complex [66], and the effect of individual sleep-related symptoms on relapse is unknown.

Amphetamines and methylphenidate

Amphetamines enhance the release of dopamine (DA) and block the reuptake of norepinephrine (NE), serotonin, and DA which can lead to sleep complaints. TST may be decreased across protracted withdrawal and sleep quality has been shown to either become more disturbed [60] or to improve [61] during abstinence. In a randomized controlled trial of children treated for attention deficit disorder with hyperactivity (ADHD) with either methylphenidate three times daily or atomoxetine twice daily, treatment-emergent insomnia was more common with methylphenidate than atomoxetine (27% vs. 6%) [74].

In general, stimulants impair the quality of nocturnal sleep by increasing the amount of S1 sleep, decreasing S2 sleep, SWS and REM sleep, and by increasing ROL [69]. Stimulants also impede the ability to sleep during the day. Three studies have examined the effect of amphetamines or methylphenidate on daytime sleepiness using the MSLT. All three studies showed prolonged SOL on nap opportunities across the day [75–77], indicating decreased daytime sleepiness. Withdrawal from stimulants may result in rebound REM and hypersomnia, which is an important consideration in the sleep laboratory when evaluating multiple sleep latency test (MSLT) results from individuals discontinuing their stimulant medications, as some patients may be inappropriately diagnosed with a disorder of central hypersomnolence (see Chapter 9: Hypersomnias of central origin).

Sleep deprivation appears to increase the drug-seeking behaviors associated with some stimulants. For example, methylphenidate was chosen by healthy volunteers more often on days after a 4-hour time in bed (88%) compared to after an 8-hour time in bed (29%) [77]. Moreover, children with ADHD are known to be at higher risk of developing substance use disorders as adolescents and adults, although how or if this relationship is related to prescribed stimulants that disrupt sleep is not known.

Nicotine

In an early study on the effect of smoking status on sleep measured by PSG, Soldatos et al. (1980) found that 50 smokers had longer SOL compared to 50 matched non-smokers, but no differences were found between sleep stages' percentages [78]. In a more recent large-scale study of 779 smokers, PSG revealed increased sleep latency, decreased TST, and a shift to lighter stages of sleep characterized by decreased SWS and increased S1 sleep compared to never smokers [79]. Subjective sleep measures in 606 non-smokers and 163 smokers were compared in a study that controlled for demographic, health, behavioral, and psychological variables [80]. Chronic insomnia, as assessed by two weeks of sleep diaries and duration of sleep complaints, was reported by 39% of the 62 "light smokers" (<15 cigarettes/day), 33% of the 101 "heavy smokers" (>15 cigarettes/day), and 31% of the 606 non-smokers. Regression analyses showed that heavy smoking predicted chronic insomnia only in females. Phillips and Danner (1995) questioned students aged between 14 and 18 years (38% of who smoked) and adults aged between 20 and 84 years (20% of who smoked) about problems going to sleep, sleep disturbance, and daytime sleepiness. Results consistently showed that smoking was associated with poor sleep habits, poor sleep quality, and impairment of daytime functioning across a wide age range [81]. Another study found that smoking, particularly in females, was related both to frequent and infrequent difficulty getting to sleep [82]. Insomnia is a frequently encountered symptom of nicotine withdrawal among dependent smokers, which can last for 2–4 weeks [83]. Increased dreaming has also been reported [83].

Laboratory studies show that non-smokers with a nicotine patch took longer to fall asleep, had shorter TST, lower SE, and lower REM compared to participants with a placebo patch [84]. The effect of nicotine on non-smokers also varies with depression history. A randomized controlled trial found that depressed non-smokers wearing nicotine patches showed increased REM sleep and short-term mood improvements compared to non-depressed non-smokers [85]. The increased REM sleep persisted during withdrawal in depressed patients, while REM sleep in non-depressed patients decreased [86].

Among smokers, abstinence is associated with increases in sleep fragmentation [83]. Heavy smokers (mean smoking history of 24 years) were studied across a smoking week and a withdrawal week. During the withdrawal week, smokers had more arousals, awakenings, and stage changes compared to the smoking week [87]. Other studies have reported changes in sleep architecture and REM sleep during abstinence as well. In the first long-term study across 1 year of abstinence, seven former chronic smokers (>20 cigarettes/day for at least 10 years) who were not depressed underwent sleep studies at months 1, 2, 4, 6, 9, and 12. REM onset latency varied across the 12 months and then eventually decreased significantly from baseline. Interestingly, depression measures increased with abstinence and correlated with increased REM sleep, decreased ROL from sleep onset and S2, and increased stage shifts [88]. SWS also decreased significantly with abstinence. Although some evidence suggests that nicotine replacement therapy can disrupt sleep in non-smokers [89], withdrawal-related sleep fragmentation in smokers may be reversed by nicotine replacement therapy and slow-wave sleep may be increased [90].

A relationship between sleep problems in early childhood and early onset of occasional or regular smoking was observed in the Michigan Longitudinal Study. Toddlers reported by their mothers as having trouble sleeping were twice as likely (OR= 2.27 (1.05–4.91) to have occasional or regular cigarettes between 12 and 14 years of age [23].

In summary, the relationship between smoking and sleep disturbances in current smokers appears to be more variable than during smoking withdrawal. While some studies have found more sleep disturbance in smokers than non-smokers [78,81], one study found that the percentage of smokers who report insomnia is similar to non-smokers [80]. Methodological differences may be contributing, at least in part, to these discrepant findings (i.e. the use of PSG [78] versus sleep diaries [80] versus mail survey [81]). During nicotine withdrawal, sleep disturbances are common, have been demonstrated in the laboratory, and have been shown to predict relapse to smoking cigarettes [91].

However, no studies have been conducted to determine whether treatment of these sleep disturbances can decrease relapse rates.

Caffeine

Although caffeine dependence is not recognized in DSM-IV as a diagnosis, it is the most widely used stimulant in the world and it is reinforcing because it attenuates the progressive increase in sleepiness across the day [92]. At lower doses, the half life ranges from 2.5 to 4.5 hours in adults, but this can be reduced by about half in smokers [93]. Its effects can vary widely, however, depending on an individual's history of caffeine consumption [94] and genetic make-up [95]. According to a 2008 Sleep in America Poll, 58% of responders reported that they are at least somewhat likely to use caffeine when they are sleepy during the day [96].

Administration of caffeine at bedtime has been shown to prolong SOL, shorten TST, and reduce total SWS and S4 sleep in a dose-dependent manner [97–99]. During sleep deprivation, low to moderate caffeine doses (100–200 mg) have been found to increase S1 sleep and reduce the slow component of EEG power (0.75–2.0 Hz) relative to placebo; during recovery sleep, fast EEG components (11.25–20.0 Hz) were enhanced [99]. Higher caffeine doses during sleep deprivation (300 mg) reduce TST, increase S1 sleep, and reduce SWS in the first third of the night [100].

Low-dose caffeine improves daytime performance during extended wakefulness more than placebo [101]. Concomitant subjective sleepiness data has been more variable. For example, a recent double-blind parallel-group design using a forced desynchrony protocol found that low doses of repeated caffeine (0.3 mg per hour) across an extended 28.57 hour "day" reduced objective sleepiness compared to placebo, but increased subjective sleepiness [101].

Chronic caffeine use can lead to a physiological state of hyperarousal, a common characteristic of patients with insomnia. One study used caffeine to model insomnia by giving repeated doses of 400 mg of caffeine to healthy volunteers across 1 week. The study reported prolonged SOL, reduced S4, and shortened TST [98]. Metabolic rate measured via VO_2 also increased, consistent with the hyperarousal theory of insomnia. A later study by the same group examined electrocardiograms (ECGs) during sleep in 15 healthy volunteers who took 400 mg of caffeine a half-hour before bedtime. Heart rate variability, defined as the integration of the low frequency (LF)/ high frequency (HF) ratio band, was significantly higher during REM sleep in the caffeine group than in the placebo group. There was no difference between LF/HF ratios for wake-time and S2 sleep in the caffeine condition [102].

Withdrawal from chronic caffeine use is associated with distinct physiological and subjective withdrawal symptoms, due in large part to the hypersensitivity of adenosine receptors during abstinence [103]. Twelve to sixteen hours into caffeine withdrawal, sleepiness, lethargy, headaches, decreased alertness, depressed mood, irritability, and mental fogginess may occur [92,94]. Withdrawal symptoms usually dissipate within 3–5 days, but can last as long as 1 week [104].

In summary, the ability of caffeine to attenuate decrements in performance across prolonged wakefulness makes it a highly desired substance. However, caffeine can contribute to impairments in sleep if consumed in close proximity to bedtime (up to about 5 hours) and withdrawal can be associated with impairment in cognitive functioning.

Methylenedioxmethamphetamine (MDMA)

Among MDMA users, restless sleep persists for about 48 hours after last use [105]. Persistent use of the club drug "ecstasy" $(+/-)$ 3, 4-MDMA, which stimulates the release and inhibits the reuptake of serotonin (5HT) has been shown to shorten TST and impair S2 sleep [106,107]. An early study examined the effects of MDMA on the sleep of 23 MDMA abstinent users compared to age- and sex-matched controls with no history of use [108]. The MDMA users had a 19-minute reduction of TST and a slightly shorter ROL than controls (60 minutes versus 75 minutes). In a more recent study, alpha-methyl-para-tyrosine (AMPT), which decreases brain catecholamines, was administered to abstinent MDMA users to determine whether AMPT would differentially affect sleep and cognitive performance in abstinent users. Results showed that exposure to AMPT at 4 p.m. and 10 p.m. before a 12 a.m. bedtime resulted in a trend towards decreased TST, ROL, and significantly lower S2 sleep [109].

MDMA exposure has lasting effects on circadian rhythms in animal experiments. Rats exposed to MDMA had alterations in sleep and circadian pattern of activity (wheel running) for up to 5 days after dosage. In addition, SWS was still altered after 1 month [110]. *In vitro* administration of MDMA to rat brain slices impaired the resetting ability of cells in the suprachiasmatic nucleus (SCN) to a serotonin receptor agonist 20 weeks after initial exposure [111]. In sum, use of MDMA can decrease the duration and quality of the sleep period.

Treatment of insomnia in patients with substance use disorders

This topic, which has only recently become a subject of developing research, has been reviewed elsewhere, including recommended assessment and treatment guidelines [21,112,113]. The best-studied treatments to date are targeted towards patients with alcohol dependence and include both behavioral and pharmacological therapies.

Benzodiazepines and benzodiazepine receptor agonists (BzRAs)

Benzodiazepines and other benzodiazepine receptor agonists (e.g. zolpidem, zaleplon) are generally safe and efficacious sedative-hypnotics and often the medications of choice for treating transient insomnia in patients without a history of substance use disorders [114]. They also may have beneficial effects on sleep during subacute alcohol withdrawal [115]. However, in patients with a history of substance abuse or dependence there is an increased risk for sedative-hypnotic abuse [116–118], although some controversy endures and not all authors agree [119]. Most addiction treatment specialists recommend against the use of BzRAs in alcoholic patients as a first-line agent (except for benzodiazepines during acute alcohol withdrawal), because of their abuse potential, withdrawal effects, rebound insomnia, and potential for overdose when mixed with alcohol [120–123]. Whenever possible, medications with low abuse and overdose potential should be used in patients with substance use disorders [124]. If BzRAs are used, then a number of precautions are recommended, such as written informed consent about their abuse potential and permission to conduct urine drug screens as a condition for refills, limited prescriptions in terms of refills, more frequent clinic visits, pill counts, and possibly supervised administration when a support person is available.

Anticonvulsants

Selected anticonvulsants are commonly used in alcoholics for their sedative properties, in part because they do not lower the seizure threshold, an important issue given the risk of seizures in alcoholic-dependent patients. Carbamazepine, for example, reduced subjectively reported sleep problems more than lorazepam during treatment for alcohol withdrawal [125]. Gabapentin has a potentially desirable hypnotic profile for this population because it has minimal known abuse potential, is not metabolized by the liver, does not interfere with the metabolism of other medications, and does not require blood monitoring for toxicity. The effects of gabapentin on sleep have been studied both during acute withdrawal and after several weeks of abstinence. When used to treat alcohol withdrawal, gabapentin more effectively reduced sleep disturbance than lorazepam among patients with a history of multiple previous withdrawals [126], potentially due to its antikindling properties [127]. In an open-label pilot study of post-withdrawal insomnia, alcohol-dependent patients who were treated with gabapentin (mean dose (range) = 953 (200–1500) mg qhs), reported significantly improved sleep quality over a 4–6 week period [128]. When gabapentin (mean dose (range) = 888 (300–1800) mg qhs) was compared to trazodone (mean dose (range) = 105 (50–300) mg qhs) in another open pilot trial in patients at least 4 weeks post-withdrawal from alcohol, both medications were associated with significantly improved scores on the Sleep Problems Questionnaire, but the gabapentin-treated group was less likely to feel tired upon awakening [129]. In a randomized double-blind trial of gabapentin in recently abstinent alcoholic patients with insomnia, the gabapentin group (mean nightly dose range: 1218–1500 mg) had a delayed onset to heavy drinking across 6 weeks [130], although its effects on sleep could not be distinguished from placebo. In summary, gabapentin has shown some promise as an effective medication to improve sleep in alcohol-dependent patients and may delay the return to drinking.

The anticonvulsant tiagabine has been compared to lorazepam for its PSG effects in abstinent cocaine-dependent subjects [131]. Although lorazepam improved measures of sleep continuity, it did so at the expense of promoting lighter stages of sleep, whereas tiagabine was superior to lorazepam in increasing SWS. Moreover, lorazepam caused significantly more daytime impairment than tiagabine in terms of sleep-dependent learning and impulsivity.

Antidepressants

Trazodone is the most commonly prescribed anti-depressant medication for insomnia in the general population as well as for patients with alcohol use disorders [132]. Physicians tend to prescribe trazodone over other hypnotics because of its sedating side-effect and low abuse potential. One randomized, double-blind trial among alcohol-dependent patients with insomnia showed that trazodone was associated with greater sleep improvements than placebo when measured via PSG [133]. Another study also showed superior sleep outcomes of trazodone versus placebo over 12 weeks of treatment in alcohol-dependent patients, but indicated that problem drinking was higher in the trazodone-treated group compared to the placebo group [134]. The use of other sedating antidepressants, such as mirtazapine and doxepin, has not been studied specifically in patients with alcohol use disorders.

Mirtazapine has been compared to modafanil for its effects on sleep and other symptoms of amphetamine withdrawal [135]. Early day administration of modafinil was more effective than nightly administration of mirtazapine at decreasing daytime sleep and fatigue, but mirtazapine was more effective at increasing hours of night-time sleep. Unexpectedly, modafinil increased subjectively rated sleep depth and decreased the number of wake-ups compared to mirtazapine. Although the results of this study are limited by the absence of PSG to compare sleep differences, they do raise an important treatment issue regarding night-time effects on sleep versus daytime consequences.

Quetiapine is an atypical antipsychotic that is sometimes prescribed for sleep disturbance because of its sedating properties, likely due in part to antagonism of histamine, serotonin, and other CNS receptors, as well as reduction of nocturnal cortisol secretion [136,137]. In addition, several open-label pilot trials suggest that quetiapine may promote sleep and reduce relapse in alcohol and other substance-dependent (cocaine and methamphetamine) patients [138–140].

Behavioral treatment for substance-related insomnia

In a small randomized study with 22 alcohol-dependent patients, patients who underwent 1-hour sessions of progressive muscle relaxation found greater improvement in sleep quality compared to a waiting list control. However, the study failed to use validated sleep measures [141].

Two studies that have utilized cognitive behavioral therapy for insomnia (CBT-I) with alcohol-dependent patients found improvements in subjective reports of sleep [142,143]. Another study provided six sessions of CBT-I in a group setting to 55 adolescents (aged 13 to 19 years) with insomnia complaints and a history of substance abuse. The majority of the sample (51%) reported that cannabis was their drug of choice. By the fourth session, subjective reports of sleep improved. By the final session (Session 6), adolescents reported decreased drug problems (as measured by the Substance Problem Index), effects that were maintained at a 1-year follow-up assessment [144].

Summary

In general, drugs of abuse are associated with sleep disturbances when measured either subjectively or objectively. Some research indicates that sleep disturbance can precede and predict the development of substance use disorders, but whether this prospective relationship is or is not causal remains to be determined. Other research clearly demonstrates that drugs of abuse can disturb sleep in healthy subjects without any history of sleep or substance use disorders. Therefore, patients with substance use disorders may manifest symptoms that are a combination of both premorbid and substance-induced sleep disturbance. In addition, patients with substance use disorders have high rates of co-morbidity with psychiatric and medical disorders that can adversely impact sleep, particularly mood disorders. Moreover, they generally suffer from poor sleep hygiene.

When approaching patients with both substance use disorders and insomnia, clinicians should assume that substances may be only one of many causes of their sleep disturbance. To assess the effect of substances on sleep in the clinic, the clinician should ideally observe the course of sleep symptoms during a period of abstinence from the substance by using a sleep diary or questionnaires, and obtain a history of insomnia either during other periods of abstinence or prior to the onset of the substance use disorder [145]. Sleep disturbance that remits within approximately 4 weeks of abstinence may be regarded as substance-induced and not requiring further treatment.

Persistent sleep disturbance with ongoing abstinence suggests either substance-induced damage to sleep-regulation systems and/or other causes of sleep dysfunction that require assessment and treatment, including primary sleep disorders.

Treatment of insomnia in substance-abusing patients may both improve quality of life and daytime functioning as well as prevent relapse to substance use. Evidence-based research to guide treatment, however, is only emerging. Although benzodiazepine receptor agonists are safe and effective for treating insomnia in most patients, they are contraindicated in patients with substance use disorders, who are at risk of abusing alcohol and sedative-hypnotics. Conversely, some effective and commonly used treatments for substance use disorders (e.g. nicotine replacement therapy and methadone maintenance) may potentially disturb sleep. Therefore, further research examining the effect of medications on both sleep and relapse to substance use is needed. At present, sedating antidepressants and anticonvulsants show promise for some patients, but cannot be routinely recommended for all patients with both insomnia and substance use disorders. Behavioral therapy for insomnia in patients with substance use disorders also shows promise and should be considered.

References

1. Cohn T, Foster J, Peters T. Sequential studies of sleep disturbance and quality of life in abstaining alcoholics. *Addict Biol.* 2003;**8**:455–462.

2. Breslau N, Roth T, Rosenthal L, Andreski P. Sleep disturbance and psychiatric disorders: a longitudinal epidemiological study of young adults. *Biol Psychiatry.* 1996;**39**:411–418.

3. Brower KJ, Aldrich M, Robinson EAR, Zucker RA, Greden JF. Insomnia, self-medication, and relapse to alcoholism. *Am J Psychiatry.* 2001;**158**:399–404.

4. Kuhlwein E, Hauger R, Iriwn M. Abnormal nocturnal melatonin secretion and disordered sleep in abstinent alcoholics. *Soc Biol Psychiatry.* 2003;**54**:1437–1443.

5. Irwin M, Gillin J, Dang J, et al. Sleep deprivation as a probe of homeostatic sleep regulation in primary alcoholics. *Biol Psychiatry.* 2002;**51**(8):632–641.

6. MacLean A, Cairns J. Dose response effects of ethanol on the sleep of young men. *J Stud Alcohol.* 1982;**43**(5):434–444.

7. Williams D, MacLean A, Cairns J. Dose-response effects of ethanol on the sleep of young women. *J Stud Alcohol.* 1983;**44**(3):515–523.

8. Feige B, Gann H, Brueck R, et al. Effects of alcohol on polysomnographically recorded sleep in healthy subjects. *Alcohol Clinl Exp Res.* 2006;**30**(9):1527–1537.

9. Miyata S, Noda A, Atarashi M, et al. REM sleep is impaired by a small amount of alcohol in young women sensitive to alcohol. *Intern Med.* 2004;**43**: 679–684.

10. Allen R, Wagman A, Funderburk F. Slow wave sleep changes: alcohol tolerance and treatment implications. *Adv Exp Med Biol.* 1977;**85A**:629–640.

11. Drummond S, Gillin J, Smith T, DeModena A. The sleep of abstinent pure primary alcoholic patients: natural course and relationship to relapse. *Alcohol Clin Exp Res.* 1998;**22**:1796–1802.

12. Brower KJ, Aldrich MS, Hall JM. Polysomnographic and subjective sleep predictors of alcoholic relapse. *Alcohol Clin Exp Res.* 1998;**22**(8):1864–1871.

13. Clark C, Gillin J, Golshan S, et al. Increased REM sleep density at admission predicts relapse by three months in primary alcoholics with a lifetime diagnosis of secondary depression. *Biol Psychiatry.* 1998; **43**:601–607.

14. Gillin J, Smith T, Irwin M, et al. Increased pressure for rapid eye movement sleep at time of hospital admission predicts relapse in nondepressed patients with primary alcoholism at 3 month follow up. *Arch Gen Psychiatry.* 1994;**51**:189–197.

15. Aldrich MS, Brower KJ, Hall JM. Sleep-disordered breathing in alcoholics. *Alcohol Clin Exp Res.* 1999;**23**:134–140.

16. Peppard P, Austin D, Brown R. Association of alcohol consumption and sleep disordered breathing in men and women. *J Clin Sleep Med.* 2007;**3**(3):265–270.

17. Edinger J, Fins A, Sullivan R, et al. Sleep in the laboratory and sleep at home: Comparisons of older insomniacs and normal sleepers. *Sleep.* 1997; **20**(12):1119–1126.

18. Aldrich M, Shipley J. Alcohol use and periodic limb movements of sleep. *Alcohol Clin Exp Res.* 1993; **17**(1):192–196.

19. Gann H, Feige B, van Calker D, Voderholzer U, Riemann D. Periodic limb movements during sleep in alcohol dependent patients. *Eur Arch Psychiatry Neurosci.* 2002;**252**:124–129.

20. Blumenthal S, Fine T. Sleep abnormalities associated with mental and addictive disorders: implications for research and clinical practice. *J Prac Psychiatry Behav Health.* 1996;**2**:67–79.

21. Brower KJ. Alcohol's effects on sleep in alcoholics. *Alcohol Res Health.* 2001;**25**:110–125.

22. Brower KJ. Insomnia, alcoholism and relapse. *Sleep Med Rev.* 2003;**7**(6):523–539.

23. Wong M, Brower KJ, Fitzgerald H, Zucker R. Sleep problems in early childhood and early onset of alcohol and other drug use in adolescence. *Alcohol Clin Exp Res*. 2004;**28**(4):578–587.

24. Wong M, Brower K, Zucker R. Childhood sleep problems, early onset of substance use, and behavioral problems in adolescence. *Sleep Med*. 2009;**10**:787–796.

25. Weissman MM, Greenwald S, Nino-Murcia G, Dement W. The morbidity of insomnia uncomplicated by psychiatric disorders. *Gen Hosp Psychiatry*. 1997;**19**:245–250.

26. Roehrs T, Papineau K, Rosenthal L, Roth T. Ethanol as a hypnotic in insomniacs: self administration and effects on sleep and mood. *Neuropsychopharmacology*. 1999;**20**(3):279–286.

27. Wiesbeck G, Schuckit M, Kalmijn J, et al. An evaluation of the history of marijuana withdrawal syndrome in a large population. *Addiction*. 1996; **91**(10):1469–1478.

28. Copersino M, Boyd S, Tashkin D, et al. Cannabis withdrawal among non-treatment-seeking adult cannabis users. *Am J Addict*. 2006;**15**:8–14.

29. Hasin D, Keyes K, Alderson D, et al. Cannabis withdrawal in the United States: Results from NESARC. *J Clin Psychiatry*. 2008;**69**(9):1354–1363.

30. Pivik R, Zarcone V, Dement W, Hollister L. Delta-9-tetrahydrocannabinol and synhexyl; effects on human sleep patterns. *Clin Pharmacol Ther*. 1972;**13**:426–435.

31. Freemon F. The effect of chronically administered delta-9-tetrahydrocannabinol upon the polygraphically monitored sleep of normal volunteers. *Drug Alcohol Depend*. 1982;**10**(4):345–353.

32. Nicholson A, Turner C, Stone B, Robson P. Effect of delta-9-tetrahydrocannabinol and cannabidiol on nocturnal sleep and early morning behavior in young adults. *J Clin Psychopharmacol*. 2004;**24**(3):305–313.

33. Feinberg I, Jones R, Walker J, Cavness C, Floyd E. Effects of marijuana extract and tetrahydrocannabinol on electroencephalographic sleep patterns. *Clin Pharmacol Ther*. 1976;**19**:782–794.

34. Cousens K, Dimascio A. Delta-9-THC as an hypnotic. An experimental study of 3 dose levels. *Psychopharmacologia*. 1973;**33**:355–364.

35. Bolla K, Lesage S, Gamaldo C, et al. Sleep disturbance in heavy marijuana users. *Sleep*. 2008;**31**(6):901–908.

36. Roane B, Taylor D. Adolescent insomnia as a risk factor for early adult depression and substance abuse. *Sleep*. 2008;**31**(10):1351–1356.

37. Shibley HL, Malcolm RJ, Veatch LM. Adolescents with insomnia and substance abuse: consequences and comorbidities. *J Psychiatr Pract*. 2008;**14**(3):146–153.

38. Godley M, Godley S, Dennis M, Funk R, Passetti L. Preliminary outcomes from the assertive continuing care experiment for adolescents discharged from residential treatment. *J Subst Abuse Treat*. 2002; **23**:21–32.

39. Gillin J, Drummond S, Clark C, Moore P. Medication and substance abuse. In: Kryger M, Roth T, Dement WC, eds. *Principles and practice of sleep medicine*, 4th ed. Philadelphia: Elsevier Saunders; 2005: 1345–1358.

40. Kosinski M, Janagap C, Gajria K, Freedman J. Pain relief and pain related sleep disturbance with extended release tramadol in patients with osteoarthritis. *Curr Med Res Opin*. 2007;**23**(7):1615–1626.

41. Vella-Brincat J, Macleod A. Adverse effects of opioids on the central nervous systems of palliative care patients. *J Pain Palliat Care Pharmacother*. 2007; **21**(1):15–25.

42. Stein M, Herman D, Bishop S, et al. Sleep disturbances among methadone maintained patients. *J Subst Abuse Treat*. 2004;**26**(3):175–180.

43. Peles E, Schreiber S, Adelson M. Variables associated with perceived sleep disorders in methadone maintenance treatment (MMT) patients. *Drug Alcohol Depend*. 2006;**82**(2):103–110.

44. Shi J, Zhao L, Epstein D, Zhang X, Lu L. Long-term methadone maintenance reduces protracted symptoms of heroin abstinence and cue-induced craving in Chinese heroin abusers. *Pharmacol Biochem Behav*. 2007;**87**(1):141–145.

45. Wallen M, Lorman W, Gosciniak J. Combined buprenorphine and clonidine for short term opiate detoxification: patient perspectives. *J AddictDis*. 2006;**25**(1):23–31.

46. Walker J, Farney R, Rhondeau S, et al. Chronic opioid use is a risk factor for the development of central sleep apnea and ataxic breathing. *J Clin Sleep Med*. 2007; **3**(5):455–461.

47. Teicher M, Wang D. Sleep disordered breathing with chronic opioid use. *Expert Opin Drug Saf*. 2007; **6**(6):641–649.

48. Mogri M, Desai H, Webster L, Grant B, Mador MJ. Hypoxemia in patients on chronic opiate therapy with and without sleep apnea. *Sleep Breath*. 2009; **13**(1):49–57.

49. Staedt J, Wassmuth F, Stoppe G. Effects of chronic treatment with methadone and naltrexone on sleep in addicts. *Eur Arch Psychiatry Clin Neurosci*. 1996;**246**:305–309.

50. Teichtahl H, Prodromidis A, Miller B, Cherry G, Kronberg I. Sleep-disordered breathing in stable methadone programme patients: a pilot study. *Addiction*. 2001;**96**:395–403.

51. Martin W, Jasinki D, Haertzen C, et al. Methadone: a reevaluation. *Arch Gen Psychiatry.* 1973;**28**(2):286–295.

52. Kay D. Human sleep and EEG through a cycle of methadone dependence. *Electroencephalogr Clin Neurophysiol.* 1975;**38**(1):35–43.

53. Dijkstra B, De Jong C, Krabbe P, van der Staak C. Prediction of abstinence in opioid-dependent patients. *J Addict Med.* 2008;**2**(4):194–201.

54. Griffiths R, Johnson M. Relative abuse liability of hypnotic drugs: A conceptual framework and algorithm for differentiating among compounds. *J Clin Psychiatry.* 2005;**66**(Suppl 9):31–41.

55. Hajak G, Muller W, Wittchen H, Pittrow D, Kirch W. Abuse and dependence potential for the non-benzodiazepine hypnotics zolpidem and zopiclone: a review of case reports and epidemiological data. *Addiction.* 2003;**98**:1371–1378.

56. Tsai M, Tsai Y, Huang Y. Compulsive activity and anterograde amnesia after zolpidem use. *Clin Toxicol.* 2007;**45**:179–181.

57. Svitek J, Heberlein A, Bleich S, et al. Extensive craving in high dose zolpidem dependency. *Prog Neuropsychopharmacol Biol Psychiatry.* 2008; **32**:591–592.

58. Rappa L, Larose-Pierre M, Payne D, et al. Detoxification from high dose zolpidem using diazepam. *Ann Pharmacother.* 2004;**38**(4):590–594.

59. Forrester M. Eszopiclone ingestions reported to Texas poison control centers, 2005–2006. *Hum Exp Toxicol.* 2007;**26**:795–800.

60. Gossop M, Bradley B, Brewis R. Amphetamine withdrawal and sleep disturbance. *Drug Alcohol Depend.* 1982;**10**:177–183.

61. McGregor C, Srisurapanont M, Jittiwutikarn J, et al. The nature, time course and severity of methamphetamine withdrawal. *Addiction.* 2005;**100**:1320–1329.

62. Paterson L, Wilson S, Nutt D, Hutson P, Ivarsson M. Translational, caffeine-induced model of onset insomnia in rats and healthy volunteers. *Psychopharmacology.* 2007;**191**(4):943–950.

63. Retey J, Adam M, Khatami R, et al. A genetic variation in the adenosine A2A receptor gene (ADORA2A) contributes to individual sensitivity to caffeine effects on sleep. *Clin Pharmacol Ther.* 2007;**81**(5):692–698.

64. Luciano M, Zhu G, Kirk K, et al. "No thanks, it keeps me awake": the genetics of coffee-attributed sleep disturbance. *Sleep.* 2007;**30**:1378–1386.

65. Brower K, Maddahian E, Blow F, Beresford T. A comparison of self reported symptoms and DSM-III-R criteria for cocaine withdrawal. *Am J Drug Alcohol Abuse.* 1988;**14**(3):347–356.

66. Sofuoglu M, Dudish-Poulsen S, Poling J, Mooney M, Katsukami D. The effect of individual cocaine withdrawal symptoms on outcome in cocaine users. *Addict Behav.* 2005;**30**:1125–1134.

67. Schierenbeck T, Riemann D, Berger M, Hornyak M. Effect of illicit recreational drugs upon sleep: Cocaine, ecstasy, and marijuana. *Sleep Med Rev.* 2008;**12**(5):381–389.

68. Johanson C, Roehrs T, Schuh K, Warbasse L. The effects of cocaine on mood and sleep in cocaine-dependent males. *Exp Clin Psychopharmacol.* 1999;**7**(4):338–346.

69. Foral PA, Malesker MA, Hopkins H. Medication effects on sleep. In: Bowman TJ, ed. *Review of sleep medicine.* Burlington, MA: Butterworth Heinemann; 2003: 94–99.

70. Kowatch R, Schnoll S, Knisely J, Green D, Elswick R. Electroencephalographic sleep and mood during cocaine withdrawal. *J Addict Disorders.* 1992;**11**:21–45.

71. Pace-Schott E, Stickgold R, Mazur A, et al. Sleep quality deteriorates over a binge-abstinence cycle in chronic smoked cocaine users. *Psychopharmacology.* 2005;**179**:873–883.

72. Thompson P, Gillin J, Golshan S, Irwin M. Polygraphic sleep measures differentiate alcoholics and stimulant abusers during short term abstinence. *Biol Psychiatry.* 1995;**38**:831–836.

73. Weddington W, Brown B, Haertzen C, et al. Changes in mood, craving, and sleep during short term abstinence reported by male cocaine addicts: A controlled, residential study. *Arch Gen Psychiatry.* 1990;**47**:861–868.

74. Sangal R, Owens J, Allen A, et al. Effects of atomoxetine and methylphenidate on sleep in children with ADHD. *Sleep.* 2006;**29**(12):1573–1585.

75. Bishop C, Roehrs T, Rosenthal L, Roth T. Alerting effects of methylphenidate under basal and sleep deprived conditions. *Exp Clin Psychopharmacol.* 1997; 5(4):344–352.

76. Mitler M, Hajdukovic R, Erman M. Treatment of narcolepsy with methamphetamine. *Sleep.* 1993; **16**(4):306–317.

77. Roehrs T, Papineau K, Rosenthal L, Roth T. Sleepiness and the reinforcing and subjective effects of methylphenidate. *Exp Clin Psychopharmacol.* 1999; 7(2):145–150.

78. Soldatos C, Kales J, Scharf M, Bixler E, Kales A. Cigarette smoking associated with sleep difficulties. *Science.* 1980;**207**:551–552.

79. Zhang L, Samet J, Caffo B, Punjabi N. Cigarette smoking and nocturnal sleep architecture. *Am J Epidemiol.* 2006;**164**(6):529–537.

80. Riedel B, Durrence H, Lichstein K, Taylor D. The relation between smoking and sleep: the influence of smoking level, health, and psychological variables. *Behav Sleep Med*. 2004;**2**(1):63–78.

81. Phillips B, Danner F. Cigarette smoking and sleep disturbance *Arch Intern Med*. 1995;**155**(7):734–737.

82. Wetter DW, Young TB. The relation between cigarette smoking and sleep disturbance. *Prevent Med*. 1994;**23**:328–334.

83. Hughes J. Effects of abstinence from tobacco: valid symptoms and time course. *Nicotine Tob Res*. 2007;**9**(3):315–327.

84. Davila D, Hurt R, Offord K, Harris C, Shepard J. Acute effects of transdermal nicotine on sleep architecture, snoring, and sleep disordered breathing in nonsmokers. *Am J Resp Crit Care Med*. 1994;**150**:469–474.

85. Salin-Pascual R, de la Fuente J, Galicia-Polo L, Drucker-Colin R. Effects of transdermal nicotine on mood and sleep in nonsmoking major depressed patients. *Psychopharmacology (Berl)*. 1995;**121**(4):476–479x.

86. Wetter DW, Carmack C, Anderson C, et al. Tobacco withdrawal signs and symptoms among women with and without a history of depression. *Exp. Clin Psychopharmacol*. 2000;**8**(1):88–96.

87. Prosise G, Bonnet M, Berry R, Dickel M. Effects of abstinence from smoking on sleep and daytime sleepiness. *Chest*. 1994;**105**(4):1136–1141.

88. Moreno-Coutino A, Calderon-Ezquerro C, Drucker-Colin R. Long-term changes in sleep and depressive symptoms of smokers in abstinence. *Nicotine Tob Res*. 2007;**9**:389–396.

89. Colrain I, Trinder J, Swan G. The impact of smoking cessation on objective and subjective markers of sleep: review, synthesis, and recommendations. *Nicotine Tob Res*. 2004;**6**(6):913–925.

90. Aubin H, Luthringer R, Demazieres A, Dupont C, Lagrue G. Comparison of the effects of a 24-hour nicotine patch and a 16-hour nicotine patch on smoking urges and sleep. *Nicotine Tob Res*. 2006; **8**(2):193–201.

91. Boutou A, Tsiata E, Pataka A, et al. Smoking cessation in clinical practice: predictors of six-month continuous abstinence in a sample of Greek smokers. *Prim Care Respir J*. 2008;**17**:32–38.

92. Roehrs T, Roth T. Caffeine: Sleep and daytime sleepiness. *Sleep Med Rev*. 2008;**12**(2):153–162.

93. Nehlig A. Are we dependent upon coffee and caffeine? A review on human and animal data. *Neurosci Biobehav Rev*. 1999;**23**:563–576.

94. James J, Keane M. Caffeine, sleep, and wakefulness: implications of new understanding about withdrawal reversal. *Human Psychopharmacol*. 2007;**22**:549–558.

95. Luciano M, Zhu G, Kirk K. "No thanks, it keeps me awake": the genetics of coffee-attributed sleep disturbance. *Sleep*. 2007;**30**(10):1378–1386.

96. Sleep in America Poll 2008. Available at http://www.sleepfoundation.org.

97. Nicholson A, Stone B. Heterocyclic amphetamine derivative and caffeine on sleep in man. *Br J Clin Pharmacol*. 1980;**9**:195–203.

98. Bonnet M, Arand D. Caffeine use as a model of acute and chronic insomnia. *Sleep*. 1992;**15**:526–536.

99. Landolt H, Retey J, Tonz K, et al. Caffeine attenuates waking and sleep electroencephalographic markers of sleep homeostasis in humans. *Neuropsychopharmacology*. 2004;**29**(10):1933–1939.

100. LaJambe C, Kamimori G, Belenky G, Balkin T. Caffeine effects on recovery sleep following 27 hours of total sleep deprivation. *Aviat Space Environ Med*. 2005;**76**(2):108–113.

101. Wyatt J, Cajochen C, Ritz-De Cecco A, Czeisler C, Dijk D. Low-dose repeated caffeine administration for circadian-phase dependent performance degradation during extended wakefulness. *Sleep*. 2004;**27**(3):374–381.

102. Bonnet M, Tancer M, Uhde T, Yeragani V. Effects of caffeine on heart rate and QT variability during sleep. *Depress Anxiety*. 2005;**22**:150–155.

103. Biaggioni I, Paul S, Puckett A, Arzubiaga C. Caffeine and theophylline as adenosine receptor antagonists in humans. *J Pharmacol Exp Therapeut*. 1991;**258**(2): 588–593.

104. Hughes J, Oliveto A, Bickel W, Higgins S, Badger G. Caffeine self-administration and withdrawal: incidence, individual differences and interrelationships. *Drug Alcohol Depend*. 1993; **32**:239–246.

105. Huxster J, Pirona A, Morgan M. The sub-acute effects of recreational ecstasy (MDMA) use: a controlled study in humans. *J Psychopharmacol*. 2006;**20**(2):281–290.

106. Jansen K. Ecstasy (MDMA) dependence. *Drug Alcohol Depend*. 1999;**53**:121–124.

107. Parrott A. Human psychopharmacology of Ecstasy (MDMA): a review of 15 years of empirical research. *Human Psychopharmacol*. 2001;**16**:557–577.

108. Allen R, McCann U, Ricaurte G. Persistent effects of 3, 4-Methylenedioxymethamphetamine (MDMA, "Ecstasy") on human sleep. *Sleep*. 1993;**16**(6):560–564.

109. McCann U, Peterson S, Ricaurte G. The effect of catecholamine depletion by alpha-methyl-para-tyrosine on measures of cognitive performance

and sleep in abstinent MDMA users. *Neuropsychopharmacology*. 2007;**32**:1695–1706.

110. Balogh B, Molnar E, Jakus R, et al. Effects of a single dose of 3,4 methylenedioxymethamphetamine on circadian patterns, motor activity and sleep in drug naive rats and rats previously exposed to MDMA. *Psychopharmacology (Berl)*. 2004;**173**: 296–309.

111. Biello S, Dafters R. MDMA and fenfluramine alter the response of the circadian clock to a serotonin agonist in vitro. *Brain Res*. 2001;**920**:202–209.

112. Arnedt J, Conroy D, Brower K. Treatment options for sleep disturbances during alcohol recovery. *J Addict Dis*. 2007;**26**(4):41–54.

113. Casola P, Goldsmith R, Dalter J. Assessment and treatment of sleep problems. *Psychiatric Annals*. 2006;**36**(12).

114. Roehrs T, Roth T. Hypnotics: an update. *Curr Neurol Neurosci Rep*. 2003;**3**(2):181–184.

115. Aubin H-J, Goldenberg F, Benoit O, et al. Effects of tetrabamate and of diazepam on sleep polygraphy during subacute withdrawal in alcohol-dependent patients. *Hum Psychopharmacol*. 1994;**9**:191–195.

116. Graham AW. Sleep disorders. In: Graham AW, Schultz T, eds. *Principles of addiction medicine*. Chevy Chase, MD: American Society of Addiction Medicine; 1998:793–808.

117. Ciraulo DA, Nace EP. Benzodiazepine treatment of anxiety or insomnia in substance abuse patients. *Am J Addict*. 2000;**9**:276–284.

118. Hajak G, Müller WE, Wittchen HU, Pittrow D, Kirch W. Abuse and dependence potential for the non-benzodiazepine hypnotics zolpidem and zopiclone: a review of case reports and epidemiological data. *Addiction*. 2003;**98**:1371–1378.

119. Posternak M, Mueller T. Assessing the risks and benefits of benzodiazepines for anxiety disorders in patients with a history of substance abuse or dependence. *Am J Addict*. 2001;**10**:48–68.

120. Johnson B, Longo LP. Considerations in the physician's decision to prescribe benzodiazepines to patients with addiction. *Psychiatric Annals*. 1998;**28**:160–165.

121. Kranzler HR. Evaluation and treatment of anxiety symptoms and disorders in alcoholics. *J Clin Psychiatry*. 1996;**57**:15–21.

122. Schuckit MA. Recent developments in the pharmacotherapy of alcohol dependence. *J Consult Clin Psychol*. 1996;**64**:669–676.

123. Swift RM. Pharmacologic treatment for drug and alcohol dependence: experimental and standard therapies. *Psychiatric Annals*. 1998;**28**:697–702.

124. Connery HS, Kleber HD. Practice guideline for the treatment of patients with substance use disorders. In: Deborah J, Hales MD, Hyman M, Rapaport MD, eds. *Focus*, Vol V, 2nd ed. American Psychiatric Publishing, Inc; 2007:163–166.

125. Malcolm R, Myrick H, Roberts J, Wang W, Anton R. The differential effects of medication on mood, sleep disturbance, and work ability in outpatient alcohol detoxification. *Am J Addict*. 2002;**11**(2): 141–150.

126. Malcolm R, Myrick L, Veatch L, Boyle E, Randall P. Self-reported sleep, sleepiness, and repeated alcohol withdrawals: a randomized, double blind, controlled comparison of lorazepam vs gabapentin. *J Clin Sleep Med*. 2007;**32**:24–32.

127. Zullino D, Khazaal Y, Hattenschwiler J, Borgeat F, Besson J. Anticonvulsant drugs in the treatment of substance withdrawal. *Drugs Today (Barc)*. 2004; **40**(7):603–619.

128. Karam-Hage M, Brower K. Gabapentin treatment for insomnia associated with alcohol dependence. *Psychiatry Clin Neurosci*. 2000;**157**:151.

129. Karam-Hage M, Brower K. Open pilot study of gabapentin versus trazodone to treat insomnia in alcoholic patients. *Psychiatry Clin Neurosci*. 2003;**57**:542–544.

130. Brower K, Kim HM, Strobbe S, et al. A randomized double-blind pilot trial of gabapentin versus placebo to treat alcohol dependence and comorbid insomnia. *Alcohol Clin Exp Res*. 2008;**32**(8):1–10.

131. Morgan P, Malison R. Pilot study of lorazepam and tiagabine effects on sleep, motor learning, and impulsivity in cocaine abstinence. *Am J Drug Alcohol Abuse*. 2008;**34**(6):692–702.

132. Friedmann P, Herman D, Freedman S, et al. Treatment of sleep disturbance in alcohol recovery: a national survey of addiction medicine physicians. *J Addict Dis*. 2003;**22**(2):91–103.

133. Le Bon O, Murphy J, Staner L, et al. Double-blind, placebo controlled study of the efficacy of trazodone in alcohol post-withdrawal sydrome: polysomnography and clinical evaluations. *J Clin Psychopharmacol*. 2003;**23**:377–383.

134. Friedmann P, Rose J, Swift R, et al. *Trazodone for sleep disturbance after detoxification from alcohol dependence: a double-blind, placebo-controlled trial*. Paper presented at 18th Annual Meeting and Symposium of the American Academy of Addiction Psychiatry, Coronado, CA, 2007.

135. McGregor C, Srisurapanont M, Mitchell A, Wickes W, White J. Symptoms and sleep patterns during inpatient treatment of methamphetamine withdrawal: a comparison of mirtazapine and modafinil with

treatment as usual. *J Subst Abuse Treat.* 2008; **35**(3):334–342.

136. Cohrs S, Pohlmann K, Guan Z, et al. Quetiapine reduces nocturnal urinary cortisol excretion in healthy subjects. *Psychopharmacologia.* 2004;**174**:414–420.

137. Cohrs S, Rodenbeck A, Guan Z, et al. Sleep-promoting properties of quetiapine in healthy subjects. *Psychopharmacology.* 2004;**174**:421–429.

138. Sattar SP, Bhatia S, Petty F. Potential benefit of quetiapine in the treatment of substance dependence disorders. *J Psychiatry Neurosci.* 2004;**29**(6):452–457.

139. Croissant B, Klein O, Gehrlein L, et al. Quetiapine in relapse prevention in alcoholics suffering from craving and affective symptoms: a case series. *Eur Psychiatry.* 2006;**21**:570–573.

140. Monnelly E, Ciraulo D, Knapp C, LoCastro J, Sepulvda I. Quetiapine for treatment of alcohol dependence. *J Clin Psychopharmacol.* 2004;**24**:532–535.

141. Greeff A, Conradie W. Use of progressive relaxation training for chronic alcoholics with insomnia. *Psychol Rep.* 1998;**82**:407–412

142. Arnedt J, Conroy D, Rutt J, et al. An open trial of cognitive-behavioral treatment for insomnia comorbid with alcohol dependence. *Sleep Med.* 2007; **8**(2):176–180.

143. Currie S, Clark S, Hodgins D, El-Guebaly N. Randomized controlled trial of brief cognitive-behavioural interventions for insomnia in recovering alcoholics. *Addiction.* 2004;**99**(9):1121–1132.

144. Bootzin RR, Stevens SJ. Adolescents, substance abuse, and the treatment of insomnia and daytime sleepiness. *Clin Psychol Rev.* 2005;**25**:629–644.

145. Sullivan JT, Sykora K, Schneiderman J, Naranjo CA, Sellers EM. Assessment of alcohol withdrawal: the revised clinical institute withdrawal assessment for alcohol scale (CIWA-Ar). *Br J Addict.* 1989;**84**:1353–1357.

146. Van Reen E, Jenni O, Carskadon M. Effects of alcohol on sleep and the sleep electroencephalogram in healthy young women. *Alcohol Clin Exp Res.* 2006; **30**(6):974–981.

147. Prinz P, Roehrs T, Vitaliano P, Linnoila M, Weitzman E. Effect of alcohol on sleep and nighttime plasma growth hormone and cortisol concentrations. *J Clin Endocrinol Metab.* 1980;**51**(4):759–764.

148. Roehrs T, Zwyghuizen-Doorenbos A, Knox M, Moskowitz H, Roth T. Sedating effects of ethanol and time of drinking. *Alcohol Clin Exp Res.* 1992; **16**(3):553–557.

149. Roehrs T, Claiborue D, Knox M, Roth T. Residual sedating effects of alcohol. *Alcohol Clin Exp Res.* 1994;**18**(4):831–834.

150. Aldrich M, Shipley J, Tandon R, Kroll P, Brower K. Sleep-disordered breathing in alcoholics: Association with age. *Alcohol Clin Exp Res.* 1993;**17**(6):1179–1183.

151. Papineau K, Roehrs T, Petrucelli N, Rosenthal L, Roth T. Electrophysiological assessment (The Multiple Sleep Latency Test) of the biphasic effects of ethanol in humans. *Alcohol Clin Exp Res.* 1998;**22**(1):231–235.

152. Zwyghuizen-Doorenbos A, Roehrs T, Lipschutz L, Timms V, Roth T. Effects of caffeine on alertness. *Psychopharmacology (Berl).* 1990;**100**(1):36–39.

153. Feinberg I, Jones R, Walker J, Cavness C, March J. Effects of high dosage delta-9-tetrahydrocannabinol on sleep patterns in man. *Clin Pharmacol Ther.* 1975; **17**(4):458–466.

154. Dimsdale J, Norman D, DeJardin D, Wallace MS. The effect of opioids on sleep architecture. *J Clin Sleep Med.* 2007;**3**(1):33–36.

155. Wang D, Teichtahl H, Drummer O, et al. Central sleep apnea in stable methadone maintenance treatment patients. *Chest.* 2005;**128**:1348–1356.

156. Kay D, Pickworth W, Neider G. Morphine-like insomnia from heroin in nondependent human addicts. *Br J Clin Pharmacol.* 1981;**11**(2):159–169.

157. Shaw I, Lavigne G, Mayer P, Choiniere M. Acute intravenous administration of morphine perturbs sleep architecture in healthy pain-free young adults: a preliminary study. *Sleep.* 2005;**28**(6):677–682.

158. Gouzoulis E, Steiger A, Ensslin M, Kovar A, Hermle L. Sleep EEG effects of 3, 4-methylenedioxymethamphetamine (MDE;"eve") in healthy volunteers. *Biol Psychiatry.* 1992;**32**(12):1108–1117.

159. Ricaurte G, McCann U. Experimental studies on 3, 4-methylenedioxymethamphetamine (MDMA, "Ecstasy") and its potential to damage brain serotonin neurons. *Neurotox Res.* 2001;**3**(1):85–99.

160. McCann U, Ricaurte G. Effects of (+/−) 3, 4-methylenedioxymethamphetamine (MDMA) on sleep and circadian rhythms. *The Scientific World Journal.* 2007;**7**(S2):231–238.

161. Watson R, Bakos L, Compton P, Gawin F. Cocaine use and withdrawal: Effect on sleep and mood. *Am J Drug Alcohol Abuse.* 1992;**18**:21–28.

162. Morgan P, Pace-Schott E, Sahul Z, et al. Sleep, sleep-dependent procedural learning and vigilance in chronic cocaine users: Evidence for occult insomnia. *Drug Alcohol Depend.* 2006;**82**:283–249.

163. Valladares E, Eljammal S, Lee J, et al. Sleep dysregulation in cocaine dependence during acute abstinence. *Sleep.* 2006;**29**(Suppl):A334.

164. Valladares E, Irwin M. Polysomnographic sleep dysregulation in cocaine dependence. *The Scientific World Journal.* 2007;**7**(S2):213–216.

Sleep in dementias

Aimee L. Pierce and Alon Y. Avidan

Introduction

Sleep disorders, such as insomnia, circadian rhythm disturbances, obstructive sleep apnea, and rapid eye movement (REM) sleep behavior disorder (RBD) are common in healthy older adults and even more so in older patients with dementia. The presentation, pathophysiology, diagnosis, and treatment of sleep disorders in dementia will be discussed, including the emerging concept of RBD as a pre-clinical marker for a class of neurodegenerative diseases, the "synucleinopathies." Sleep disorders may worsen cognitive and behavioral symptoms in dementia, and are a source of stress for caregivers, thus recognition and adequate treatment are important.

Changes in sleep associated with aging

The quest for a good nights' sleep is truly life-long, with up to 50% of older Americans suffering from chronic sleep complaints [1], including difficulty with sleep initiation, decreased total sleep time, increased night-time awakenings, increased daytime napping, and increased early morning awakenings. Many members of the general public, and even physicians, suffer from the misconception that older adults "require" less sleep than the middle-aged, and sleep complaints may be unasked, unmentioned, or minimized in geriatric patients. However, to do so misses a prime opportunity to ameliorate both quality of health and quality of life.

Several qualitative and quantitative changes in the polysomnogram occur with aging. One notes a reduction in or absence of slow-wave sleep (stages 3 and 4 of non-REM), a decrease in REM sleep in proportion to total sleep time, and reduced sleep efficiency [2].

Sleep complaints in the elderly may be due to a primary sleep disorder or secondary to another medical condition. Both primary and secondary causes of sleep disorders are more common in older adults. The causes of secondary sleep disorders in older adults are vast and include medical, psychiatric, and psychosocial difficulties, as well as polypharmacy (Figure 20.1). Furthermore, the increased prevalence of primary sleep disorders in older patients may reflect age- or disease-related neurodegeneration of brain structures important for maintenance of the circadian rhythm.

Insomnia is a very common problem in the older population; a large epidemiological study by Foley et al. in patients 65 years and older found that 28% suffered from chronic insomnia and few patients were satisfied with their sleep [3].

Older adults are also more prone to circadian rhythm disturbances, wherein they may experience abnormal and irregular sleep–wake cycles. This occurs when there is desynchrony between the activity of the brain's pacemaker, the suprachiasmatic nucleus (SCN) of the anterior hypothalamus, and the demands of the environment. Both pathophysiological and environmental hypotheses have been proposed to account for circadian rhythm disturbances in older adults. For example, the SCN deteriorates with age, and its rhythms become progressively disrupted or weaker [4]. Furthermore, there is noted to be a predictable reduction in nocturnal melatonin secretion with aging [5]. Aside from, or synergistic with, these neurohormonal changes, older adults have decreased external cues to reset their circadian

Foundations of Psychiatric Sleep Medicine, ed. John W. Winkelman and David T. Plante. Published by Cambridge University Press.
© Cambridge University Press 2010.

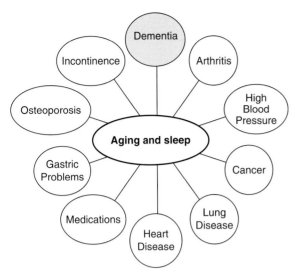

Figure 20.1 The causes of secondary sleep disorders in older adults are many and include medical, psychiatric, polypharmacy, and psychosocial difficulties. Sleep disorders related to dementias such as Parkinson's disease and Alzheimer's disease are the focus of this chapter.

pacemaker daily. For example, older adults are more prone to be homebound, thus have decreased exposure to bright light and physical activity [6]. A common circadian rhythm disturbance in older adults is advanced sleep phase syndrome, in which patients feel sleepy and go to bed early in the evening, then wake up too early in the morning. They are unable to return to sleep, and consequently spend the remainder of the day feeling tired, potentially napping later in the day, and thus perpetuating the process.

Several other sleep disorders are also more prevalent in older adults, including sleep disordered breathing, REM sleep behavior disorder (RBD), and periodic limb movements of sleep (PLMS). PLMS are limb (usually leg) movements that occur every 20–40 seconds during sleep, and may be associated with night-time arousals, changes in sleep architecture, and excessive daytime sleepiness (Figure 20.2). The prevalence of PLMS is much greater in older adults (5% in adults, 44% in a population over 65 years) [7]. PLMS is also associated with restless legs syndrome (RLS). Secondary causes of PLMS and RLS may account for a significant degree of the increased incidence with age; these include renal failure, iron-deficiency anemia, diabetes, and peripheral neuropathy, but an age-related reduction in dopaminergic function may also play an important role.

Sleep disturbance in dementia

The *Diagnostic and Statistical Manual of Mental Disorders*, 4th edition (DSM-IV) describes dementia as a progressive cognitive disorder composed of memory impairment in addition to at least one other cognitive disturbance (aphasia, agnosia, apraxia, or disturbance in executive functioning), not exclusively during the course of a delirium [8]. The underlying cause of dementia may be a neurodegenerative disease, a vascular or structural insult, trauma, toxic-metabolic effects, infection, or inflammation. In the USA, the most common causes of dementia are Alzheimer's disease, vascular dementia, mixed Alzheimer-type and vascular dementia, and dementia with Lewy bodies.

Most of the dementias studied have been associated with sleep–wake disturbances beyond those associated with aging alone. There are several potential causes of sleep disturbances in patients with dementia. These include primary causes such as degeneration in brain regions important for generating and maintaining sleep, and a multitude of secondary causes including decreased exposure to external circadian rhythm cues, medication side-effects, psychiatric disorders, psychosocial difficulties, and sundowning.

Sundowning is a very common behavioral disturbance in patients with dementia, whereby they have a tendency to become more confused and agitated in the evening, in comparison to their daytime baseline. This can lead to wandering behaviors and prevent them from sleeping. The condition can be very challenging to control in the home, in a nursing home, or in the hospital. It is extremely important to recognize and manage this problem, as well as other sleep disturbances in patients with dementia, because they may be an immediate precipitant, or an underlying factor, in nursing home placement.

The following sections will highlight the important sleep disturbances co-morbid with some of the key neurodegenerative disorders, utilizing clinical cases to illustrate pertinent diagnostic and management issues.

Sleep disturbance in Alzheimer's disease

Case 1: Mr. R.S. is a 78-year-old man who has had a 10-year slowly progressive course of memory loss, followed by language disturbance, and mild paranoia. He was diagnosed with Alzheimer's disease 8 years

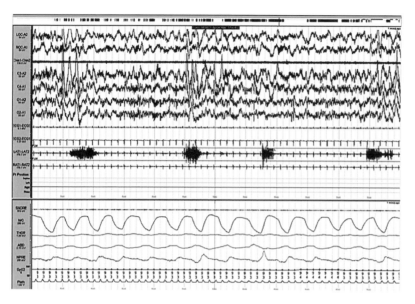

Figure 20.2 A 1-minute sleep epoch from a diagnostic polysomnogram of a 69-year-old man with Parkinson's disease who experiences difficulties initiating and maintaining sleep, excessive daytime sleepiness, and uncomfortable sensation in his legs associated with an irresistible urge to move his legs. His wife describes night-time kicking and jerking movements which disrupt his sleep. Illustrated in this figure is a succession of periodic limb movements occurring in the left anterior tibialis muscles. Channels are as follows: electrooculogram (left: LOC-A2, right: ROC-A1), chin EMG (chin-chin), EEG (left central (C3-A2), right central (C4-A1), left occipital (O1-A2), right occipital (O2-A1)), electrocardiogram (ECG), limb EMG (left leg (LAT), right leg (RAT)), patient position, snoring (SNORE), nasal–oral airflow (N/O), respiratory effort (thoracic (THOR), abdominal (ABD)), nasal pressure (NPRE), and oxygen saturation (SpO$_2$) and plethysmography channel.

earlier, and is currently prescribed donepezil. He is still living in his home with his wife; however, for the past 6 months he has become agitated and confused in the evening: he has been unable to find his way around his house to the restroom (although during the day he can do so), and has also accused his wife of being an intruder when she tries to comfort him in the evening. He stays up past midnight most nights, and then wakes up at 6 a.m. and spends most of his waking hours sitting in a chair languidly, drifting between sleep and wakefulness. *What is the underlying sleep disturbance, what are the contributing factors, and what are the treatment options?*

Alzheimer's disease (AD) is the most common cause of dementia in the USA: there are currently estimated to be 4.5 million people with AD in the USA [9]. The incidence of AD increases dramatically with age: about 5% of people between the ages of 65 and 74 years have the disease; however, nearly 50% of people over the age of 85 years have the disease [10]. AD typically presents with deficits in short-term memory, but as the disease progresses, deficits in language and executive function become more prominent. Patients with AD also may suffer from psychiatric symptoms such as depression, apathy, agitation, and psychosis. The majority of cases are sporadic, however 2–5% of cases are inherited in an autosomal dominant fashion, due to mutations in genes encoding the amyloid precursor protein, presenilin 1, and

presenilin 2 [10]. In sporadic cases, presence of the E4 allele of the apolipoprotein gene confers a threefold increased risk of AD. The pathological findings associated with AD include amyloid plaques, neurofibrillary tangles, and cerebral atrophy. AD is a progressive disease, and there is no cure as of yet.

The most common sleep disturbances in AD are related to circadian rhythm abnormalities, commonly presenting as fragmentation of the sleep–wake cycle (night-time wakefulness and frequent daytime naps) or sundowning. Polysomnographic changes in patients with AD include increased time awake in bed, frequent awakenings, and less time in both slow-wave sleep and REM sleep [11]. Furthermore, circadian rhythm disruptions worsen with disease severity. In addition to sleep–wake fragmentation, patients with AD have disruptions of other circadian rhythms. For example, body temperature, cortisol release, and melatonin rhythms are less robust, with lower amplitude or less coordination, in patients with AD [12].

The mechanism of these abnormalities may be primary neurodegeneration in the suprachiasmatic nucleus (SCN). In fact, amyloid plaques have been discovered in the SCN in pathological examination of brains of patients with AD [13]. Furthermore, there is reduced number and function of neurons in the SCN in both aging and AD [14] and reduced melatonin production by the pineal gland in AD [15]. Secondary causes of circadian rhythm disturbances in patients with AD include reduced exposure to ambient light and diminished daytime activity.

The majority of patients with AD are prescribed an acetylcholinesterase inhibitor, memantine, or the combination, as symptomatic treatment for dementia. These medications, particularly the acetylcholinesterase inhibitors, may also have beneficial effects upon sleep. Donepezil has been shown to increase REM sleep in both young adults and patients with AD [16,17]. In patients with AD, the degree of increase in REM sleep seems to correlate with the degree of cognitive improvement on donepezil [18]. The other acetylcholinesterase inhibitors (galantamine and rivastigmine) are not as well studied, although small studies suggest they have similar effects [19,20]. Data in laboratory animals indicated that while galantamine had no significant influence on the sleep pattern, donepezil and memantine showed significant alterations in sleep architecture consisting of increases in sleep latency and total waking time and a decrease in total non-REM sleep time. In addition these data show that memantine decreased total REM sleep time [21]. The effects of memantine on sleep architecture in humans have not been studied to date.

Treatments for AD circadian rhythm abnormalities include standard sleep hygiene practices and pharmacological treatments for insomnia and agitation. As for most aspects of their life, patients with AD respond well to routines. It is useful to keep a regular bedtime and awakening time. In addition, it is important to reduce environmental noise and light in the bedroom and minimize night-time awakenings for administration of medications, vital signs collection, or bedchecks (this is mainly an issue in a hospital or nursing home setting).

To date, none of the FDA-approved medications for insomnia have undergone large-scale controlled trials in patients with AD; however, standard and new medications for insomnia are used widely. When treating sleep disturbances in AD, two principles should guide use of these medications. First, antipsychotics should be used sparingly and with full attention to risks and benefits of use, especially in light of the FDA black box warning: "both conventional and atypical antipsychotics are associated with an increased risk of mortality in elderly patients treated for dementia-related psychosis." [22] Furthermore, although they have not been tested for improving sleep and sundowning in patients with dementia, in a randomized double-blind, placebo-controlled trial, olanzipine, quetiapine, and risperidone did not improve psychosis, aggression, or agitation in patients with AD, and all were associated with increased rate of adverse events [23]. As for sleep-related adverse events, patients on antipsychotics experienced a higher incidence of sedation (15–24%) than patients on placebo (5%). However, in all groups, 5% of patients experienced sleep disturbance as an adverse event.

Second, in treating sleep disturbances in AD, pertinent mechanisms of action and side-effects of hypnotics must be attended to, including anticholinergic properties of tricyclic antidepressants which may worsen confusion in patients with dementia, and the fact that many hypnotics can cause daytime sedation which may further compromise cognitive performance.

Bright light therapy and melatonin therapy are appealing potential treatments for circadian rhythm disturbances in patients with AD, because they theoretically may target the underlying environmental and pathophysiological causes of circadian rhythm disturbances in this population.

The results of several studies of bright light therapy (open-label and small controlled trials) have varied. Some have shown that light exposure (of varying times and intensities) benefits rest–activity rhythms in patients with AD, but others have not [24,25]. The difference in results is not unexpected, given the different patient populations, study location, light regimen, and outcome measures.

Abnormalities in melatonin receptor expression and beneficial effects of melatonin in *in vitro* and rodent models of Alzheimer's disease have been described. Levels of melatonin receptor subtypes are decreased in the retina, pineal gland, and cortex of humans with AD [26–28]. *In vitro*, melatonin has been demonstrated to reduce hyperphosphorylation of tau [29] and reduce amyloid pathology in a transgenic mouse model of AD [30].

While theoretically plausible, melatonin's role in AD as either a sleep aid or a cognitive enhancer is unclear. Although an open-label study and one small trial suggested that melatonin may improve sleep measures in patients with AD [31,32], the largest randomized controlled trial to date, performed by the Alzheimer's Disease Cooperative Study, was negative [33]. In this study a total of 157 patients who slept less than 7 hours per night and had frequent nocturnal awakenings were assigned to one of three groups: placebo, 2.5 mg slow-release melatonin, or

10 mg melatonin. Patients were observed for 2 months with wrist actigraphy. There were no statistically significant differences in nocturnal total sleep time, sleep efficiency, wake-time after sleep onset, and day–night sleep ratio. The only randomized controlled trial for melatonin as a cognitive enhancer contained just 20 patients; however, those receiving active drug (3 mg) had small, statistically significant improvements in their scores on the Alzheimer's disease assessment scale (ADAS), both in cognitive and non-cognitive domains [32].

The second sleep disturbance that is common in AD is obstructive sleep apnea (OSA). It has been hypothesized that there may be cell loss in the brainstem respiratory center in AD that predisposes these patients to sleep apnea. Conversely, nightly hypoxemia of sleep apnea could worsen the neuronal degeneration of AD [34]. Another relationship between the two conditions was illuminated by recent results that showed that the APOE4 allele, the only known genetic risk factor in sporadic AD, was also associated with an increased risk of OSA [35]. This result was not found in earlier studies, however the population background and ages differed [36,37]. Despite this genetic result, at a population level there does not appear to be an increased prevalence of OSA in patients with AD compared to age-matched controls, and the high comorbidity may be due to an increasing prevalence of both disorders with age, rather than any underlying mechanistic interdependence. However, clinicians must still be sensitive to the problems of diagnosis and management of both diseases in the same patient. For example, OSA has been associated with cognitive impairment on neuropsychological testing in both normal adults and patients with AD. Among patients with dementia, those with severe sleep apnea have more cognitive impairment than those with mild or no apnea [38]. Those areas of cognition most affected by OSA include attention, initiation, perseveration, conceptualization, and memory. In both normal adults and patients with AD, treatment of OSA with CPAP has been shown to ameliorate some of these cognitive changes [39, 40].

Treatment of sleep apnea in patients with dementia may be challenging, because patients may find their CPAP mask to be uncomfortable and incomprehensible, and there may be nightly battles over its use. If CPAP is worsening night-time agitation and preventing sleep, this may outweigh any benefit in daytime cognition, and use of CPAP may need to be modified. For example, if the patient suffers from mild supine-related OSA, the use of positional therapy (by avoiding sleep in the supine position) may be a reasonable alternative.

The chronic mental and physical health burdens upon caregivers of patients with dementia are becoming more evident to the medical profession. These include elevations in stress hormones and inflammatory markers, depression, and sleep disturbance [41]. Sleep disturbances in caregivers of patients with dementia are multifactorial and include insomnia due to depression, anxiety, appropriate worry, or circadian rhythm disturbance due to ongoing caregiving duties during the night. Sleep disturbance in patients with dementia is a strong predictor of subsequent sleep disturbance in caregivers and may predict institutionalization. Thus, strategies such as night-time hired caregivers and temporary respite care may allow the patient to remain in their home longer.

Case 1, discussion: This patient has advanced AD and is now manifesting circadian rhythm disturbances including an altered sleep–wake cycle and sundowning. Aside from potential degeneration of the SCN and reduced production of melatonin by the pineal gland, a low level of physical activity and exposure to ambient light may worsen these symptoms. Possible treatments include daytime bright light therapy, increase in daily outdoor physical activity (supervised, during daylight hours), strict regulation of bedtime and awakening time, and consideration of a night-time caregiver (to reduce burden on his wife.) If these conservative measures do not resolve the situation, some consideration may be given to melatonin therapy, control of evening agitation and delusions with an atypical antipsychotic (with attention to current black box warnings in the elderly), or a low dose of a hypnotic such as zolpidem.

Sleep disturbance in vascular dementia

Vascular dementia is the second most common form of dementia in the USA. Vascular pathology frequently overlaps with AD pathology, which is known as dementia of mixed vascular and Alzheimer's pathology. Because of this overlap, exact estimates of prevalence are difficult, however vascular dementia likely accounts for between 10% and 33% of cases of dementia [10]. The pathology of vascular dementia is heterogeneous and may include a single or multiple large cortical strokes, multiple lacunar infarcts or confluent white matter disease, or a single, strategically placed stroke (such as in the angular gyrus). Clinical criteria include cognitive decline in memory and at least one other domain of cognition, interfering with activities of daily living, and a time course that is usually stepwise or abrupt. Symptoms are typically those of subcortical frontal dementia, such as apathy, impaired executive function, psychomotor slowing, and impaired gait. Alternatively, symptoms may be attributable to the location of the stroke, such as a receptive aphasia resulting from a left temporal stroke. The risk factors for vascular dementia are the same as those for stroke, and include hypertension, diabetes, hyperlipidemia, and cigarette smoking. Treatment focuses on prevention and management of risk factors, but both cholinesterase inhibitors and memantine have been used with some benefit.

There has been very little published research on sleep disturbance in vascular dementia, though a small actigraphic study found that patients with multi-infarct dementia (a subtype of vascular dementia) had disrupted sleep–wake cycles compared to both controls and ambulatory patients with AD [42].

More striking are the interactions between sleep and stroke, which are beginning to be elucidated. It remains to be determined whether sleep disordered breathing is an independent risk factor for stroke. However, the blood pressure-lowering effects of CPAP may lead to a reduction in risk of stroke of up to 20% in patients with OSA [43]. Sleep disorders post-stroke are common and can worsen outcomes; a recent study found that OSA was a risk factor for death after stroke [44]. Other post-stroke sleep disorders include central sleep apnea and failure of automatic breathing (Ondine's curse), Cheyne-Stokes breathing, and REM sleep behavior disorder associated with pontine tegmental infarct. Treatment of sleep disordered breathing has been shown to improve subjective well-being and mood in stroke patients [45, 46]. Finally, it is important to remember that the consequences of stroke such as depression, immobilization, and pain may also negatively impact sleep.

Sleep disturbance in dementia with Lewy bodies

Dementia with Lewy bodies (DLB) is the third most common cause of dementia in the USA. The cardinal clinical features include a fluctuating course, visual hallucinations, and parkinsonism. The pathological diagnosis requires cortical Lewy bodies, which are intracellular synuclein inclusions. DLB exists on a spectrum with both Parkinson's disease and AD. In a patient with parkinsonism and dementia, the clinical diagnosis depends upon which symptom developed first (DLB requires dementia at onset; in contrast, patients with idiopathic Parkinson's disease (PD) usually do not develop dementia until late in their disease). Ultimately, both patients with DLB and Parkinson's disease dementia will develop substantia nigra and cortical Lewy bodies. In the case of AD, there is a "Lewy body variant" with slight clinical differences, but most often diagnosed post-mortem, with the classic Alzheimer's pathology of plaques and tangles co-existent with cortical Lewy bodies. Current treatment for DLB includes: cholinesterase inhibitors and memantine, dopamine or dopamine agonists for severe parkinsonism (with attention to any worsening psychosis), and avoidance of neuroleptics when possible (patients with DLB tend to be very sensitive to these medications and can develop severe parkinsonism.)

In the 1990s, physicians began to report a high incidence of REM sleep behavior disorder (RBD) in their patients with DLB [47] and other "synucleinopathies" – diseases associated with either mutations in or abnormal accumulations of the protein synuclein. These synucleinopathies include DLB, Parkinson's disease, and multiple system atrophy. Increasing awareness of RBD and its association with synucleinopathies has led the DLB consortium to include RBD as a "suggestive feature" for the diagnosis [48].

RBD is characterized by absence of normal muscle atonia during REM sleep (Figure 20.3). Thus, patients enact their dreams, resulting in vigorous, complicated, and sometimes dangerous motor activity during sleep. Both the patient themselves and the bed partner are at risk for injury during violent or thrashing dreams. RBD is idiopathic in 40% of cases, and associated with a neurodegenerative disease in 60% of cases [49]. There is a much higher incidence of RBD in men, though the reason for this is unknown. There may be an underlying pathophysiological difference between the sexes, or RBD may be under diagnosed in women, as they may have less violent or active dream content, and may be less likely to have a bed partner (because of womens' longer life-span.)

The diagnosis of RBD is suggested by history and confirmed by overnight polysomnography with multiple limb electromyography and continuous video monitoring, which demonstrates electromyographic

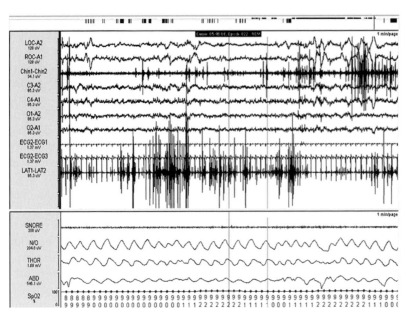

Figure 20.3 A 60-second epoch of a diagnostic polysomnogram of an 80-year-old man who was referred to the sleep disorders clinic for evaluation of recurrent violent night-time awakenings. Illustrated in this figure is a typical spell that this patient was experiencing. He was noted to yell, jump from bed, and have complex body movements. Channels are as follows: electrooculogram (left: LOC-A2, right: ROC-A1), chin electromyogram (EMG), electroencephalogram (left central, right central, left occipital, right occipital), two ECG channels, limb EMG (LAT), snore channel, nasal–oral airflow, respiratory effort (thoracic, abdominal), and oxygen saturation (SaO$_2$).

bursts in the chin or limbs during REM sleep (see Figure 20.3 for a typical polysomnogram in RBD). Treatment requires ensuring a safe sleeping environment for the patient and bed partner, such as locked windows and doors, removal of dangerous objects or weapons from the bedroom, lowering the bed or placing the mattress on the ground, and, if necessary, separate beds. In addition, clonazepam (0.25 to 1 mg orally at bedtime) is effective in 90% of cases of RBD [50].

Research in cats implicates the pons and medulla as regions involved in muscle atonia during REM sleep. The peri locus coeruleus of the pontine tegmentum activates the medullary inhibitory zone by way of the tegmentoreticular tract. Then, the medullary inhibitory zone inhibits the reticulospinal tract of the spinal cord, leading to REM-associated atonia (Figure 20.4). In humans, some cases of RBD have occurred after focal lesions in the pontine tegmentum [51], and it is hypothesized that RBD may develop in neurodegenerative disorders due to neuron loss in this region.

When associated with neurodegenerative disorders, RBD may predate diagnosis of PD, DLB, etc. by up to 20 years. In a study of 44 patients with RBD in Spain, 45% of patients developed a neurodegenerative disorder a mean of 11.5 years after onset of RBD [52]. The most common disorder was PD and the second most common was DLB. Studies are now underway to

determine if and how RBD may be used as a "preclinical marker" for these diseases, to allow early diagnosis and treatment which may be disease-modifying, rather than only symptomatic, which is currently the state of treatment for neurodegenerative diseases.

Sleep disturbance in Parkinson's disease

Case 2: Ms. M.O. is a 60-year-old woman who developed a resting tremor in her right hand, and has had some slowing of her movements. She was diagnosed with idiopathic Parkinson's disease and was started on ropinirole. She is concerned because she has fallen asleep twice during meetings at work and feels sluggish throughout the day. In contrast, she has trouble falling asleep at night. In addition, her husband has moved out of their bedroom, after having been hit and kicked inadvertently during her sleep. *What are the etiologies of her sleep disturbances, what are the contributing factors, and what are the treatment options?*

Parkinson's disease (PD) is the most common movement disorder in the USA, afflicting approximately 500 000 people [34]. Diagnosis is clinical, based upon the presence of the cardinal features of tremor, rigidity, bradykinesia, and postural instability. Pathologically, it is characterized by Lewy bodies and dopaminergic cell loss in the substantia nigra. Dementia occurs late in the disease in up to 32% of

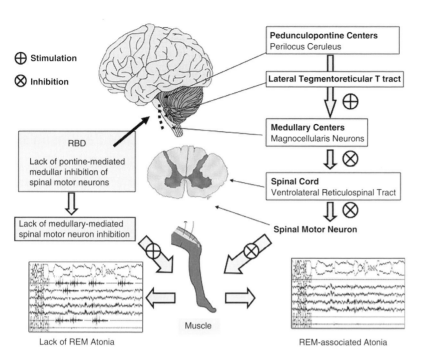

⊕ Stimulation

⊗ Inhibition

Pedunculopontine Centers
Perilocus Ceruleus

Lateral Tegmentoreticular T tract

Medullary Centers
Magnocellularis Neurons

Spinal Cord
Ventrolateral Reticulospinal Tract

Spinal Motor Neuron

RBD
Lack of pontine-mediated medullar inhibition of spinal motor neurons

Lack of medullary-mediated spinal motor neuron inhibition

Muscle

Lack of REM Atonia

REM-associated Atonia

Figure 20.4 Muscle atonia during REM sleep results from pontine-mediated perilocus ceruleus inhibition of motor activity. This pontine activity exerts an excitatory influence on medullary centers (magnocellularis neurons) via the lateral tegmentoreticular tract. These neuronal groups, in turn, hyperpolarize the spinal motor neuron post-synaptic membranes via the ventrolateral reticulospinal tract. In REM sleep behavior disorder (RBD), the brainstem mechanisms generating muscle atonia become disrupted. Understanding of the pathophysiology of RBD in humans is based on the cat model. In the cat model, bilateral pontine lesions result in a persistent absence of REM atonia associated with prominent motor activity during REM sleep, similar to that observed in RBD in humans. The pathophysiology of the idiopathic form of RBD in humans is still not very well understood but may be related to reduction of striatal presynaptic dopamine transporters. Modified from Avidan AY. Sleep disorders in the elderly. *Primary Care: Clinics in Office Practice on Sleep Disorders.* 2005;32(2):536–587.

patients, at which time it is called Parkinson's disease dementia (PDD) [53].

Sleep disturbances are myriad and very common in PD, and tend to occur early in the course of the disorder. Nearly two-thirds of patients with PD reported a sleep disorder in a community-based survey of 245 patients [54]. The most commonly reported problems include fragmented sleep, frequent arousals, and trouble going back to sleep. The polysomnogram in PD reveals a reduction in sleep efficiency; increased wake-time after sleep onset; increased sleep fragmentation; reduction of slow-wave sleep and REM sleep; disruption of non-REM-to-REM cyclicity; loss of muscle atonia (suggestive of REM sleep behavior disorder); and increased electromyographic activity due to tremor or periodic leg movements of sleep (PLMS) [34].

Pathological daytime sleepiness including sleep attacks is a common problem in PD. A common cause is the use of dopamine agonists such as pramipexole and ropinirole. Another cause may be sleep debt related to sleep fragmentation and/or circadian rhythm disturbances which can result in difficulties with sleep initiation and maintenance, as well as spontaneous daytime dozing.

A second common sleep disorder in PD is sleep fragmentation related to motor abnormalities. These include nocturnal immobility, rest tremor, eye blinking, dyskinesias, periodic limb movements of sleep (PLMS), restless legs syndrome, and fragmentary myoclonus [34]. Many of these motor phenomena can be treated by adjusting the evening dose of levodopa/carbidopa, depending upon the symptom. For example, if the patient is waking up because they cannot roll over in bed or because of tremor, they may benefit from a bedtime dose of immediate-release or long-acting levodopa/carbidopa, depending upon the time the symptoms occur. If they are waking up due to dyskinesias, the evening dose of levodopa/carbidopa should be reduced.

Patients with PD are also prone to sleep disordered breathing including central sleep apnea, OSA, and alveolar hypoventilation. They may also have a restrictive pulmonary defect due to abnormal muscle tone or respiratory incoordination [55].

RBD is frequently encountered in PD, as in other synucleinopathies. Just as in DLB, interest is developing in attempting to use RBD as a potential preclinical marker for PD. RBD may begin before or after PD is diagnosed. In a study of 80 patients with idiopathic PD, over 8 years, 27 patients were diagnosed with RBD [56].

Patients with PD may suffer from hypnagogic hallucinations and vivid dreams, noted particularly in the middle-to-late stages of illness. These symptoms can disturb sleep and may be worsened by or secondary to medications for PD.

When evaluating sleep disorders in a patient with PD, it is very important to review the quality and timing of symptoms as well as the medication list. Many medications used to treat PD have sleep-related side-effects including: daytime sleep attacks (e.g. dopamine agonists), hypnagogic hallucinations/vivid dreams (e.g. dopamine agonists, levodopa/carbidopa, MAO-B inhibitors), and insomnia (e.g. dopamine agonists, MAO-B inhibitors, amantadine). If these symptoms are occurring, one option is to give medications earlier in the day or reduce the dose. Conversely, if the patient is having motor symptoms related to inadequate dopamine repletion keeping them awake, such as tremor or stiffness, a bedtime dose of immediate-release or long-acting levodopa/carbidopa is appropriate. Evaluation should also include attention to co-existing psychiatric symptoms, such as anxiety and depression, which are both common in PD and can alter sleep. If RBD, PLMS, or sleep-disordered breathing are suspected, evaluation should include an overnight polysomnogram. Treatment for these disorders in PD is similar to treatment in other patients. Finally, attention to the quality of sleep in caregivers of patients with PD is also warranted, as the decision to hospitalize or institutionalize patients is frequently due to nightly sleep disturbance of the caregiver.

Case 2, discussion: This patient likely has REM sleep behavior disorder associated with Parkinson's disease; however, periodic limb movements of sleep is another possibility. Diagnosis may be confirmed with overnight polysomnogram. Treatment should attend to ensuring the safety of the patient and her husband in their bedroom. Treatment may also include clonazepam (0.25–1 mg) before bedtime if RBD is diagnosed, but, given the existing daytime sleepiness, a shorter acting benzodiazepine (e.g. lorazepam) would be a reasonable alternative. In addition, she is describing daytime somnolence and sleep attacks, which may be side-effects of dopamine agonists such as ropinirole. Hypersomnia may also be due to sleep-disordered breathing, or may be related to a sleep deficit from insomnia. A nocturnal polysomnogram would be helpful for diagnosis of sleep apnea. In any case, with this level of daytime somnolence, she should be advised not to drive, and ropinirole should be tapered or removed, if another treatable cause of somnolence is not found. Finally, the cause of her initiation insomnia should be further investigated: are stiffness and pain preventing her from falling asleep? This may be improved by a later dose of ropinirole or levodopa/carbidopa. Does she have symptoms of restless legs syndrome? Is she anxious or depressed with ruminative thoughts keeping her awake? If no other cause is found, again consider tapering, removing, or giving the dose of ropinirole earlier in the day.

Sleep disturbance in other Parkinson's plus syndromes

Parkinson's plus syndromes are neurodegenerative diseases which cause parkinsonism "plus" symptoms such as autonomic dysfunction, ataxia, eye movement abnormalities, apraxia, early falls, or dementia. They are usually divided into categories based upon the pathogenic protein: "synucleinopathies" such as multiple system atrophy and DLB, and "tauopathies" such as progressive supranuclear palsy and corticobasal degeneration. Using this schema, AD and some forms of frontotemporal dementia may also be classified as tauopathies; please see Figure 20.5 for a taxonomic visualization of the main synucleinopathies and tauopathies.

Multiple system atrophy (MSA) is a synucleinopathy that requires at least two of the following: autonomic dysfunction, parkinsonism, or cerebellar ataxia. Depending upon the initial and most prominent system involved, it is designated as MSA-A (autonomic, formerly Shy-Drager syndrome), MSA-P (parkinson, formerly striatonigral degeneration), or MSA-C (cerebellar, formerly olivopontocerebellar atrophy.)

As in other synucleinopathies (such as PD and DLB), REM sleep behavior disorder is frequently seen in up to 90% of patients with MSA and may pre- or post-date diagnosis of MSA [34]. In addition, patients with MSA are prone to a unique and serious form of sleep disordered breathing: inspiratory stridor associated with upper airway obstruction. This is audibly distinct from typical OSA, in that the stridor is high pitched and whining rather than low pitched and snoring. This stridor may be due to vocal cord abductor paralysis and may lead to sudden death during sleep. In order to make the diagnosis, polysomnogram and larygoscopy during sleep must be performed. Although CPAP may be useful in some patients, tracheostomy is the most reliable treatment for respiratory disturbances caused by vocal cord abductor paralysis.

Progressive supranuclear palsy (PSP) is a tauopathy with clinical features of vertical supranuclear

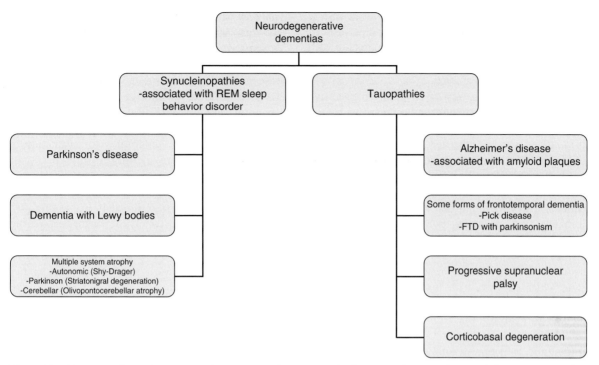

Figure 20.5 Taxonomy of neurodegenerative disease: recent advances in molecular genetics have greatly expanded our knowledge of gene/protein pathophysiology which results in neurodegenerative diseases. Today, neurodegenerative diseases are believed to be caused by excessive protein misfolding and protein aggregation. They are largely classified into tauopathies and synucleinopathies. Tau proteins belong to the family of microtubule-associated proteins involved in maintaining the cell shape, and serve as tracks for axonal transport. The main tauopathies include Alzheimer's disease (AD), progressive supranuclear palsy (PSP), and corticobasal degeneration (CBD). The main synucleinopathies consist of Parkinson's disease, DLB, and MSA. The function of the alpha-synuclein protein is unknown.

gaze palsy, early falls, and axial rigidity. Patients with PSP also develop a dementia of the frontal-subcortical type. Although RBD and sleep disordered breathing are not common features in PSP, sleep disturbances are very common, particularly sleep maintenance insomnia related to immobility in bed. The polysomnogram in PSP is unique: ocular EMG reveals absence of vertical eye movements during REM sleep. In addition, sleep architecture demonstrates an increased sleep latency, increased arousal and awakening frequency, decreased stage 2 sleep, reduced REM sleep, and reduced REM latency [34].

Corticobasal degeneration (CBD) is a tauopathy characterized by parkinsonism, dystonia, apraxia, and alien limb phenomenon. Because of its rarity, few studies have been published on sleep in CBD. However, it is believed that RBD is not prominent in CBD. A recent small case series of five patients with CBD found that all five had insomnia and four of the five had either PLMS or restless legs syndrome. None had RBD or excessive daytime sleepiness [57].

Sleep disturbance in other dementias

Frontotemporal dementia is a neurodegenerative dementia characterized by some combination of personality or behavior change, executive dysfunction, and aphasia. It may be the most common form of dementia in patients during middle age. However, there has been very little published literature on sleep disturbance in frontotemporal dementia.

Huntington's disease (HD) is an autosomal dominant disease caused by an expanded triplet nucleotide repeat in the gene encoding huntingtin. The disease is characterized by progressive chorea, dementia, and psychiatric problems. The characteristic sleep disturbances in HD are insomnia, sleep fragmentation, and circadian rhythm abnormalities. Polysomnography in HD reveals increased sleep-onset latency, reduced sleep efficiency, increased arousals and sleep fragmentation, decreased slow-wave sleep, frequent nocturnal awakenings, increased time spent awake, and reduced sleep efficiency [34].

Interestingly, patients with HD have also shown higher density of sleep spindles in comparison to controls, the significance of which is uncertain [58]. Whether patients with HD have a higher prevalence of OSA has not been studied.

Prion diseases are very rare, rapidly progressive dementias, which are thought to be caused by a misfolded prion protein which is able to propagate itself. Prion diseases can be inherited, sporadic, or transmissible. The most common prion disease is Creutzfelt-Jacob disease (CJD), which is characterized by dementia and startle myoclonus. A recent study of sleep in patients with CJD found that all had sleep–wake disturbances and interesting polysomnogram findings: loss of sleep spindles, very low sleep efficiency, and virtual absence of REM sleep [59]. Fatal familial insomnia (FFI) is an autosomal dominant prion disease, which presents with insomnia and then progresses to dementia and eventually death. Prion plaques form in the thalamus. The polysomnogram in FFI demonstrates dramatic sleep rhythm disorganization and reduction in total sleep time. In addition there is a reduction in sleep spindles and K complexes, a complete abolition of NREM sleep, and only brief residual periods of REM sleep without atonia [60].

Diagnostic approach to sleep disturbance in dementia

As in most medical specialties, a thorough and detailed history is crucial to uncover the diagnosis of a sleep disorder in a patient with dementia. Because the patient's underlying impaired cognition may make explaining their own symptoms difficult, and because critical clues are collected while the patient is asleep, it is essential to also obtain a history from a bed partner or caregiver. Important questions in the history include: when did the problem start, what are the exacerbating and alleviating factors, what are the daily and nightly activity and sleep patterns, what medications and non-medical stimulants and sedatives are being taken, and what breathing, movement, or behavioral abnormalities are noted before or during sleep?

Important aspects of the physical exam include a complete neurological exam with mental status (as patients in early stages of dementia have problems different from those in later stages), motor exam (to evaluate for parkinsonism or other movement disorders which may impair sleep), and oropharyngeal exam for Mallampati score (see Figure 6.5).

Some of the common indications for polysomnogram in patients with dementia are for evaluation of suspected sleep disordered breathing, RBD, or PLMS. Additional diagnostic tests may be useful, depending upon the clinical situation, such as a multiple sleep latency test (for evaluation of daytime somnolence), actigraphy (for evaluation of insomnia or circadian rhythm disturbances), or brain imaging (if there are unexplained neurological deficits on examination).

When evaluating sleep disorders in patients with dementia, attention must always be paid to sleep-related side-effects caused by current medications. In addition, many medications used in sleep medicine can be sedating and can worsen some aspects of cognition, so they must be used with care. Conversely, patients with dementia respond very well to a regulated schedule and environment, so attention to good sleep hygiene can be productive and is often the best treatment.

Because inadequate sleep can impair many aspects of cognition, the diagnosis and appropriate treatment of sleep disorders in patients with dementia is rewarding in that both sleep symptoms and cognitive symptoms can potentially be improved. Furthermore, adequately treating sleep disturbances in patients with dementia can prolong the time to nursing home placement and improve the interaction and relationship between patients and their caregivers. Until a cure for these diseases is found, supportive care will be the rule, and adequate sleep can truly improve quality of life for these patients.

References

1. Foley DJ, Monjan AA, Brown SL, et al. Sleep complaints among elderly persons: an epidemiologic study of three communities. *Sleep*. 1995;**18**:425–432.

2. Cohen-Zion M, Gehrman PR, Ancoli-Israel S. Sleep in the elderly. In: Lee-Chiong TL, Sateia MJ, Carskadon MA, ed. *Sleep medicine*. Philadelphia: Hanley & Belfus; 2002:115–123.

3. Foley DJ, Monjan A, Simonsick EM, et al. Incidence and remission of insomnia among elderly adults: an epidemiologic study of 6,800 persons over three years. *Sleep*. 1999;**22**:S366–S372.

4. Lydic R, Schoene WC, Czeisler CA, Moore-Ede MC. Suprachiasmatic region of the human hypothalamus: homolog to the primate circadian pacemaker? *Sleep*. 1980;**2**:355–361.

5. van Coevorden A, Mockel J, Laurent E, et al. Neuroendocrine rhythms and sleep in aging men. *Am J Physiol*. 1991;**260**:E651–E661.

6. Shochat T, Martin J, Marler M, Ancoli-Israel S. Illumination levels in nursing home patients: effects on sleep and activity rhythms. *J Sleep Res*. 2000;**9**:373–379.

7. Ancoli-Israel S, Kripke DF, Klauber MR, et al. Periodic limb movements in sleep in community-dwelling elderly. *Sleep*. 1991;**14**:486–495.

8. American Psychiatric Association. *Diagnostic and statistical manual of mental disorders*, 4th ed. Washington, DC: American Psychiatric Publishing; 1994.

9. National Institute on Aging. *Alzheimer's disease fact sheet*, 2006. http://www.nia.nih.gov/Alzheimers/Publications/adfact.htm. Accessed 7 November, 2008.

10. Daffner KR, Wolk DA. Behavioral neurology and dementia. In: Samuels MA, ed. *Manual of neurologic therapeutics*, 7th ed. Philadelphia: Lippincott Williams & Wilkins; 2004:410–448.

11. Prinz PN, Peskind E, Raskind M, et al. Changes in the sleep and waking EEG in nondemented and demented elderly. *J Am Geriatr Soc*. 1982;**30**:86–93.

12. Van Someren EJ. Circadian rhythms and sleep in human aging. *Chronobiol Int*. 2000;**17**(3):233–243.

13. Swaab DF, Fliers E, Partiman TS. The suprachiasmatic nucleus of the human brain in relation to sex, age and senile dementia. *Brain Res*. 1985;**342**:37–44.

14. Hoffman MA. The human circadian clock and aging. *Chronobiol Int*. 2000;**17**(3):245–260.

15. Srinivasan V, Pandi-Perumal SR, Cardinali DP, Poeggeler B, Hardeland R. Melatonin in Alzheimer's disease and other neurodegenerative disorders. *Behav Brain Funct*. 2006;**2**:1–23.

16. Kanbayashi T, Sugiyama T, Aizawa R, et al. Effects of donepezil (Aricept) on the rapid eye movement sleep of normal subjects. *Psychiatry Clin Neurosci*. 2002;**56**:307–308.

17. Moraes W. dos S, Poyares D, Guilleminault C, et al. The effect of donepezil on sleep and REM sleep EEG in patients with Alzheimer disease: a double-blind placebo-controlled study. *Sleep*. 2006;**29**(2):199–205.

18. Mizuno S, Kameda A, Inagaki T, Horiguchi J. Effects of donepezil on Alzheimer's disease: The relationship between cognitive function and rapid eye movement sleep. *Psychiatry Clin Neurosci*. 2004;**58**:660–665.

19. Schredl M, Weber B, Braus D, Heuser I. The effect of rivastigmine on sleep in elderly healthy subjects. *Exp Gerontol*. 2000;**35**:243–249.

20. Cooke J, Loredo J, Liu L, et al. Acetylcholinesterase inhibitors and sleep architecture in patients with Alzheimer's disease. *Drugs Aging*. 2006;**23**(6):503–511.

21. Ishida T, Kamei C. Characteristic effects of anti-dementia drugs on rat sleep patterns. *J Pharmacol Sci*. 2009;**109**(3):449–455.

22. Center for Drug Evaluation and Research. FDA public health advisory: deaths with antipsychotics in elderly patients with behavioral disturbances, 11 April, 2005. Available at http://www.fda.gov/Drugs/DrugSafety/PublicHealthAdvisories/ucm051200.htm.

23. Schneider L, Tariot P, Dagerman K, et al. Effectiveness of atypical antipsychotic drugs in patients with Alzheimer's disease. *N Engl J Med*. 2006;**355**(15):1525–1538.

24. Ancoli-Israel S, Gehrman P, Martin J, et al. Increased light exposure consolidates sleep and strengthens circadian rhythms in severe Alzheimer's disease patients. *Behav Sleep Med*. 2003;**1**(1):22–36.

25. Dowling G, Burr R, Van Someren E, et al. Melatonin and bright-light treatment for rest-activity disruption in institutionalized patients with Alzheimer's disease. *J Am Geriatr Soc*. 2008;**56**(2):239–246.

26. Savaskan E, Jockers R, Ayoub M. The MT2 melatonin receptor subtype is present in human retina and decreases in Alzheimer's disease. *Curr Alzheimer Res*. 2007;**4**(1):47–51.

27. Brunner P, Sozer-Topcular N, Jockers R, et al. Pineal and cortical melatonin receptors MT1 and MT2 are decreased in Alzheimer's disease. *Eur J Histochem*. 2006;**50**(4):311–316.

28. Wu YH, Zhou JN, Van Heerikhuize J, et al. Decreased MT1 melatonin receptor expression in the suprachiasmatic nucleus in aging and Alzheimer's disease. *Neurobiol Aging*. 2007;**28**(8):1239–1247.

29. Wang JZ, Wang ZF. Role of melatonin in Alzheimer-like neurodegeneration. *Acta Pharmacol Sin*. 2006;**27**(1):41–49.

30. Matsubara E, Bryant-Thomas T, Pacheco Quinto J, et al. Melatonin increases survival and inhibits oxidative and amyloid pathology in a transgenic model of Alzheimer's disease. *J Neurochem*. 2003;**85**(5):1101–1108.

31. Brusco LI, Fainstein I, Marquez M, Cardinali DP. Effect of melatonin in selected populations of sleep-disturbed patients. *Biol Signals Recept*. 1999;**8**(1–2):126–131.

32. Asayama K, Yamadera H, Ito T, et al. Double blind study of melatonin effects on the sleep-wake rhythm, cognitive and non-cognitive functions in Alzheimer type dementia. *J Nippon Med Sch*. 2003;**70**(4):334–341.

33. Singer C, Tractenberg R, Kaye J, et al. A multicenter, placebo-controlled trial of melatonin for sleep

disturbance in Alzheimer's disease. *Sleep.* 2003;**26**(7): 893–901.

34. Avidan AY. Sleep and neurologic problems in the elderly. *Sleep Med Clin.* 2006;**1**:273–292.

35. Punjabi NM, Shahar E, Redline S, et al. Sleep-disordered breathing, glucose intolerance, and insulin resistance: the Sleep Heart Health Study. *Am J Epidemiol.* 2004;**160**:521–530.

36. Foley DJ, Masaki K, White L, et al. Relationship between apolipoprotein E epsilon4 and sleep-disordered breathing at different ages. *JAMA.* 2001;**286**:1447–1448.

37. Saarelainen S, Lehtimaki T, Kallonen E, et al. No relation between apolipoprotein E alleles and obstructive sleep apnea. *Clin Genet.* 1998;**53**:147–148.

38. Ancoli-Israel S, Klauber MR, Butters N, et al. Dementia in institutionalized elderly: relation to sleep apnea. *J Am Geriatr Soc.* 1991;**39**:258–263.

39. Ferini-Strambi L, Baietto C, Di Gioia M, et al. Cognitive dysfunction in patients with obstructive sleep apnea (OSA): partial reversibility after continuous positive airway pressure (CPAP). *Brain Res Bull.* 2003;**61**(1):87–92.

40. Ancoli-Israel S, Palmer B, Cooke J, et al. Cognitive effects of treating obstructive sleep apnea in Alzheimer's disease: a randomized controlled study. *J Am Geriatr Soc.* 2008;**56**(11):2076–2081.

41. Mills PJ, Ancoli-Israel S, Kanel RV, et al. Effects of gender and dementia severity on Alzheimer's disease caregivers' sleep and biomarkers of coagulation and inflammation. *Brain Behav Immun.* 2009;**23** (5):605–610.

42. Aharon-Peretz J, Masiah A, Pillar T, et al. Sleep-wake cycles in multi-infarct dementia and dementia of the Alzheimer type. *Neurology.* 1991;**41**(10): 1616–1619.

43. Pepperell JC, Ramdassingh-Dow S, Crosthwaite N, et al. Ambulatory blood pressure after therapeutic and subtherapeutic nasal continuous positive airway pressure for obstructive sleep apnoea: a randomised parallel trial. *Lancet.* 2002;**359**(9302): 204–210.

44. Sahlin C, Sandberg O, Gustafson Y, et al. Obstructive sleep apnea is a risk factor for death in patients with stroke: a 10-year follow-up. *Arch Intern Med.* 2008; **168**(3):297–301.

45. Sandberg O, Franklin KA, Bucht G, et al. Nasal continuous positive airway pressure in stroke patients with sleep apnoea: a randomized treatment study. *Eur Respir J.* 2001;**18**(4):630–634.

46. Wessendorf TE, Wang YM, Thilmann AF, et al. Treatment of obstructive sleep apnoea with nasal

continuous positive airway pressure in stroke. *Eur Respir J.* 2001;**18**(4):623–629.

47. Boeave B, Silber M, Ferman T, et al. REM sleep behavior disorder and degenerative dementia: an association likely reflecting Lewy body disease. *Neurology.* 1998;**51**(2):363–370.

48. McKeith IG, Dickson DW, Lowe J, et al. Diagnosis and management of dementia with Lewy bodies: third report of the DLB Consortium. *Neurology.* 2005;**65**(12): 1863–1872.

49. Olson E, Boeve B, Silber M. Rapid eye movement sleep behaviour disorder: demographic, clinical and laboratory findings in 93 cases. *Brain.* 2000;**123**(Pt 2): 331–339.

50. Mahowald MW, Schenck CH. *REM sleep behavior disorder.* Philadelphia: WB Saunders; 1994.

51. Xi Z, Luning W. REM sleep behavior disorder in a patient with pontine stroke. *Sleep Med.* 2009; **10**(1):143–146.

52. Iranzo A, Molinuevo J, Santamaria J, et al. Rapid-eye-movement sleep behaviour disorder as an early marker for a neurodegenerative disorder: a descriptive study. *Lancet Neurol.* 2006;**5**(7):572–577.

53. Wallin A, Jennersjo C, Graneras AK. Prevalence of dementia and regional brain syndromes in long-standing Parkinson's disease. *Parkinsonism Relat Disord.* 1999;**5**(3):103–110.

54. Tandberg E, Larsen JP, Karlsen K. A community-based study of sleep disorders in patients with Parkinson's disease. *Mov Disord.* 1998;**13**(6):895–899.

55. Aldrich MS. Parkinsonism. In: Kryger MH, Roth T, Dement WC, eds. *Principles and practice of sleep medicine.* Philadelphia: WB Saunders; 2000:1051–1057.

56. Onofrj M, Thomas A, D'Andreamatteo G, et al. Incidence of RBD and hallucination in patients affected by Parkinson's disease: 8-year follow-up. *Neurol Sci.* 2002;**23**(Suppl 2):S91–94.

57. Roche S, Jacquesson JM, Destee A, et al. Sleep and vigilance in corticobasal degeneration: a descriptive study. *Neurophysiol Clin.* 2007;**37**(4):261–264.

58. Emser W, Brenner M, Stober T, Schimrigk K. Changes in nocturnal sleep in Huntington's and Parkinson's disease. *J Neurol.* 1988;**235**(3):177–179.

59. Landolt HP, Glatzel M, Blättler T, et al. Sleep-wake disturbances in sporadic Creutzfeldt-Jakob disease. *Neurology.* 2006;**66**(9):1418–1424.

60. Sforza E, Montagna P, Tinuper P, et al. Sleep-wake cycle abnormalities in fatal familial insomnia: Evidence of the role of the thalamus in sleep regulation. *Electroencephalogr Clin Neurophysiol.* 1995;**94**(6):398–405.

Chapter 2

Sleep in attention-deficit/hyperactivity disorder (ADHD)

Samuele Cortese and Michel Lecendreux

Introduction

Problems of inattention, hyperactivity, and/or impulsivity represent one of the most common reasons for referral to child neuropsychiatric services. According to the *Diagnostic and statistical manual of mental disorders*, 4th edition (DSM-IV) [1] and its updated version (Text Revision, TR) [2], attention-deficit/hyperactivity disorder (ADHD) is defined by a persistent and age-inappropriate pattern of symptoms of impaired attention, hyperactivity–impulsivity, or both. Moreover, onset before the age of seven and impaired functioning in two or more settings (e.g. school/work, home, extracurricular activities) are currently required for the diagnosis. The DSM-IV defines four types of ADHD: "predominantly inattentive," "predominantly hyperactive−impulsive," "combined," and "not otherwise specified." ADHD is estimated to affect 5–10% of school-aged children worldwide [3].

The *International Classification of Diseases*, 10th edition (ICD-10) [4] defines a more narrow and severe syndrome, i.e. the hyperkinetic disorder (HKD). Although the list of symptoms of inattention, hyperactivity, and impulsivity are the same as DSM-IV-defined ADHD, the diagnosis of HKD requires all three types of symptoms together (impairing in two or more settings) and discourages the use of multiple diagnoses (but allowing for a diagnosis of hyperkinetic conduct disorder). Thus, HKD is ostensibly equivalent to the combined type of ADHD. The prevalence of HKD is believed to range from 40 to 140 per 10 000 children [5].

Deficits in executive functions (defined as the set of cognitive skills that are necessary to plan, monitor, and execute a sequence of goal-directed complex actions including inhibition, working memory, planning, and sustained attention) are commonly, although not always, found in patients with ADHD/ HKD [6]. Impairing symptoms of inattention, restlessness, and impulsivity may persist into adulthood in about 40–60% of cases [7].

Stimulants (methylphenidate and amphetamines) are the first-line FDA-approved pharmacological treatment for ADHD, followed by the non-stimulant atomoxetine [8]. This is similar to European Guidelines for the treatment of ADHD and HKD [9,10]. Behavioral therapy may be recommended as an initial treatment if the patient's ADHD symptoms are mild with minimal impairment, the diagnosis of ADHD is uncertain, or parents reject medication treatment [8].

Evidence from a large body of clinical as well as epidemiological studies has established that ADHD is frequently co-morbid with other psychiatric and neurodevelopmental disorders, including oppositional defiant disorder (ODD; co-morbid with ADHD in about 54−84% of cases, a significant portion of which will develop conduct disorder, CD)[11,12], smoking or other substance abuse disorders (15−19%)[13,14], learning or language problems (25−35%)[8], anxiety disorders (about 30%)[8], mood disorders (5−30%)[8], and Tourette syndrome (10−30%)[15], while the prevalence of pediatric bipolar disorder (BPD) among patients with ADHD remains a contentious issue [8].

Conversely, the relationship between ADHD and sleep disturbances has been largely overlooked, both in the scientific literature as well as in clinical practice by child and adult psychiatrists, neurologists, and pediatricians assessing and treating patients for ADHD symptoms. For example, although the item "moves about excessively during sleep" was included as a criterion of ADHD in DSM-III [16], this item was removed from DSM-III-R [17] diagnostic criteria

Foundations of Psychiatric Sleep Medicine, ed. John W. Winkelman and David T. Plante. Published by Cambridge University Press. © Cambridge University Press 2010.

because teachers lacked adequate knowledge of this behavior [18]. However, prompted in part by the frequent complaints of sleep disturbances associated with ADHD symptoms in clinical practice, an increasing number of studies on the relationship between ADHD and sleep have been published in recent years, examining sleep in both children and adults with ADHD.

Gaining insight into the relationship between ADHD and sleep is paramount both from a theoretical and a practical standpoint. A large body of research has shown that sleep disturbances may lead to or contribute to symptoms of inattention, irritability, impulsivity, and, paradoxically, at least in children, to hyperactivity [19], thus mimicking ADHD symptoms in children referred for ADHD evaluation but who actually have a primary sleep disturbance [20]. Clearly, this is of relevance for the differential diagnosis and clinical management of the patient.

Conversely, sleep complaints are frequently reported by parents of children diagnosed with ADHD (by formal evaluation) or by adults with ADHD themselves. According to a review of the literature by Corkum et al. [21], 25–55% of parents complain of sleep problems in their children diagnosed with ADHD. Sleep problems may represent a significant source of distress for the patient and/or the family. As stated by Laufer and Denhoff [22] in 1957: "Generally the parents of hyperkinetic children are so desperate over the night problems that the daytime ones pale in significance." As sleep problems may also worsen symptoms of ADHD (described above), the appropriate assessment and treatment of sleep problems might improve the quality of life of patients with ADHD and their families and reduce the severity as well as the impairment of ADHD.

Finally, a better understanding of the relationship between sleep/alertness alterations and ADHD might provide useful insights into the pathophysiology of ADHD, with the ultimate goal of developing specific pathophysiologically oriented treatments.

It has been correctly pointed out that sleep complaints reported by patients with ADHD are multifactorial [20], meaning they may be ascribed to different underlying sleep/alertness alterations or other factors associated with ADHD itself. Therefore, the appropriate management of sleep problems in patients with ADHD is based on the correct identification and treatment of sleep disorder(s) or alterations underlying these problems.

In the first part of this chapter, we provide an overview of the most frequent causes of sleep complaints in patients with ADHD, discussing the most relevant data from the literature. Given that most of the studies used DSM criteria, we will refer to ADHD, not to HKD. Although literature on sleep in adults with ADHD is growing, it is still limited and this prevents clear conclusions on this topic in adulthood. Therefore, we discuss only data from studies conducted in children and adolescents. However, preliminary data from adult studies seem to parallel quite well those reported in pediatric literature. The reader who is particularly interested in sleep disturbances in adults with ADHD can consult the review by Philipsen et al. [23] which provides a thoughtful overview of the topic, as well as the articles by Sobanski et al. [24], Boonstra et al. [25], Gau et al. [26], and Schredl et al. [27] published after the above-mentioned review. We will then discuss the management of sleep disturbances in patients with ADHD or referred for symptoms of inattention, impulsivity, and/or hyperactivity. Finally, we will suggest future avenues of research in the field.

Causes of sleep complaints in patients with ADHD
Psychiatric co-morbidities

As previously stated, most patients (up to two-thirds) with ADHD present with one or more co-morbid psychiatric disorders, which are associated with and possibly contribute to several sleep disturbances. Although intrinsic alterations of ADHD may underlie sleep complaints in these patients, as we will point out below, we start from the potential, but often overlooked, role of psychiatric co-morbidities to stress that they should be considered by the clinician when managing sleep disturbances in patients with ADHD.

Since the relationship between sleep alterations and psychiatric disorders other than ADHD is described in detail in other chapters of this book, in this section we provide a general and concise overview, focusing in particular on those psychiatric disorders which co-occur more frequently with ADHD in childhood.

Oppositional defiant disorder (ODD), the disorder most commonly co-morbid with ADHD, may be associated with limit-setting disorder, characterized by non-compliant behavior in response to parental requests to get ready for bed, bedtime resistance, and delayed sleep onset [20]. In fact, the high concurrence of ODD with ADHD can complicate the interpretation of the scientific literature (discussed in further detail in later sections).

Subjective sleep disturbances, including difficulty falling asleep, sleep continuity problems (waking at night), and daytime sleepiness have been reported in children with major depressive disorder (MDD) [28], paralleling problems reported by adults with MDD. On the other hand, as discussed in a comprehensive review of the literature by Ivanenko et al. [29], the findings from objective studies are still equivocal, possibly because some of the EEG sleep changes associated with depression in adults emerge gradually across adolescence [30] (see Chapter 22: Sleep in pediatric mood and anxiety disorders).

Available data on pediatric anxiety disorders, although largely limited to generalized anxiety disorder (GAD) and using non-specific subjective measures of sleep, suggest that most children with GAD report at least one sleep-related problem, and more than half experience three or more sleep-related problems [31]. Evidence on sleep problems associated with BPD is still very limited, in part because the consensus definition of pediatric BPD is still actively debated in the field. However, preliminary evidence suggests that children with a profile at risk for pediatric BPD reported poorer sleep efficiency and more awakenings after sleep onset, less rapid eye movement (REM) sleep, and longer periods of slow-wave sleep (SWS) than matched controls, as well as significantly more sleep problems, including difficulty initiating sleep, restless sleep, nightmares, and morning headaches, than controls [32]. As for Tourette syndrome, available data suggest a longer sleep period time, longer sleep latency, reduced sleep efficiency, and prolonged wakefulness after sleep onset, more time awake and less sleep stage 2, increased epochs with short arousal-related movements, and increased frequency of sleepwalking, night terrors, trouble getting to sleep, and early awakenings [33–35]. Finally, although evidence on the effect of substance abuse on sleep in children and adolescents is limited, available data suggest a dose-dependent relationship between sleep problems and use of illicit drugs, alcohol, and cigarettes [36].

Medications used to treat the aforementioned co-morbid conditions may also contribute to sleep disturbances. For example, selective serotonin reuptake inhibitors (SSRIs), used to treat co-morbid mood and anxiety disorders, may increase sleep onset latency, cause daytime sedation, and suppress REM sleep [20]. Antipsychotics used to treat aggression associated with ADHD when stimulants alone are not effective, as well as co-morbid tics or bipolar disorder, may have a sedative effect, decrease sleep onset latency, increase sleep continuity, and suppress REM sleep [20].

Medications used to treat ADHD

Clinical experience suggests that stimulants, which, as previously stated, are the first-line pharmacological treatment of ADHD, may negatively impact on sleep, but the effect varies markedly among patients. As noted by Brown and McMullen [37], while some patients with ADHD are able to get to sleep easily just a few hours after taking a stimulant, others need an interval of 6−8 hours. Data from the literature are mixed and inconclusive. As reviewed by Sangal et al. [38], while some investigators have reported polysomnographically determined *lengthened total sleep time, increased sleep-stage shifts, increased number of rapid eye movement (REM) periods, elevated indexes of REM activity* and *REM period fragmentation, parent-reported longer latencies to sleep onset* or *higher rates of "insomnia"* in ADHD children treated with stimulants versus healthy controls, others did not confirm these findings. It is possible that the inconsistency in results is linked, at least in part, to the different stimulant formulations, dose, and dose-scheduling used in the available studies. As for dose-scheduling in particular, some studies assessed the effect of stimulants given in two doses (morning and noon). Since stimulants are associated with the so-called "rebound effect" (increase over baseline values in ADHD symptoms when the medication wears off [39]), it is possible that sleep problems reported in these studies may be linked to restlessness linked to the rebound effect more than to the direct action of stimulants. However, other studies [40,41] using a third dose (to avoid the rebound effect) did indeed find a more significant sleep onset delay in children treated with stimulants versus untreated subjects. On the other hand, some authors have reported that a small dose of methylphenidate taken before bedtime can facilitate sleep [42,43]. The different formulations, dose and dose-scheduling used in the available studies also make it difficult to develop evidence-based clinical guidelines on the impact of stimulants on sleep. However, on the basis of clinical experience, as well as data reported in the literature, it is possible to state that stimulants may, although not necessarily, negatively impact on sleep, either due to a direct effect or due to a secondary "rebound" effect as medications wear off.

With regard to atomoxetine, which is considered a second-line treatment for ADHD, in a randomized, double-blind, crossover study comparing the effect of methylphenidate (given thrice daily) and atomoxetine (given twice daily) on the sleep of the children with ADHD, Sangal et al. [38] found that methylphenidate increased sleep onset latency significantly more than did atomoxetine, using both actigraphy and polysomnography. Moreover, both child diaries and parental report indicated a better quality of sleep (easier to get ready in the morning, less resistance to getting ready for bed, less difficulty falling asleep) with atomoxetine compared with methylphenidate. Both medications decreased night-time awakenings, but the decrease was greater for methylphenidate. Clearly, these results need to be replicated before definitive conclusions can be drawn.

Primary sleep disorders associated with ADHD

As previously stated, primary sleep disorders may lead to or contribute to diurnal inattention, irritability, impulsivity, and, in children, restlessness, thus mimicking the cardinal symptoms of ADHD. However, recent evidence seems to suggest that some primary sleep disorders, such as restless legs syndrome (and associated periodic limb movements in sleep), sleep disordered breathing, and, possibly, circadian rhythm disorders might actually be co-morbid with "real" ADHD, thus worsening its symptoms. We discuss here data from the literature on the relationship between ADHD and these three categories of primary sleep disorders.

Restless legs syndrome and periodic limb movements in sleep

Restless legs syndrome (RLS) is a sensorimotor disorder characterized by an irresistible urge to move the legs, which is often accompanied by uncomfortable sensations in the legs (or, less frequently, other body parts such as the arms), which are relieved by movement and are worse in the evening or at night and at rest. The diagnosis of RLS is based on the revised criteria developed by the International Restless Legs Syndrome Study Group (IRLSSG) [44]. An increasing body of research including evidence from biopsy, imaging, and supplementation studies shows that iron deficiency is involved in the pathophysiology of RLS [45] (see Chapter 8: Sleep-related movement disorders).

Since, as suggested by several case reports and by one epidemiological study [46], RLS may occur also in children, although with different characteristics, the IRLSSG has proposed a set of criteria for the diagnosis of RLS in childhood [44]. Recognizing that the diagnosis of childhood RLS may be hampered by several issues, including the limited verbal ability of children to describe RLS sensations and the progressive and sometimes intermittent manifestation of RLS symptoms during development, the IRLSSG proposed three sets of criteria, respectively, for the diagnosis of definite, probable, and possible RLS in childhood. Previous studies on the relationship between ADHD and RLS used somewhat different RLS diagnostic criteria, thus complicating interpretation of the literature. However, several interesting observations have been reported. In a review of the literature [47] completed in 2005, we concluded that a relationship between RLS and ADHD symptoms was evidenced in the literature, although not all available studies included representative samples and state of the art assessment of ADHD. Some studies reported that RLS is associated with ADHD symptoms, without a formal diagnosis of ADHD [47]. To explain these results, we speculated that sleep disruption associated with RLS might lead to inattentiveness, moodiness, and paradoxical overactivity. Moreover, diurnal manifestations of RLS, such as restlessness and inattention, might be mistaken for ADHD symptoms. However, some studies reported an association between RLS and "real" ADHD (i.e. diagnosed according to formal criteria) [47]. In these cases, RLS might be co-morbid with idiopathic ADHD. We [47] and others [48] hypothesized that subjects with RLS and a subset of subjects with ADHD might share a common dopaminergic dysfunction. This is in part because, in our clinical practice, we often diagnose RLS in parents or siblings of children diagnosed with "real" ADHD. When associated with ADHD, RLS symptoms may exacerbate ADHD symptoms. Also, in our clinical experience, we have found that children with RLS may develop bedtime refusal, probably because they associate bedtime with the occurrence of the unpleasant RLS sensations. Parents may consider this refusal as the expression of a general oppositional attitude, ignoring the real cause of the child's behavior [49]. Therefore, RLS may be frequently overlooked in children with ADHD and oppositional behavior.

Not only might unrecognized RLS present with ADHD-type symptoms, it is also possible that ADHD worsens RLS symptoms. Chervin et al. [50] noticed that adult patients with RLS sometimes report that increased daytime activity worsens their nocturnal symptoms. In the study of Wagner et al. [48] RLS symptoms were more severe in RLS patients with ADHD symptoms than in RLS patients without ADHD symptoms.

It is important to point out that the previously discussed hypotheses are based on the results of studies largely conducted in units with a special interest in both ADHD and RLS, thus leading to a possible selection bias. Therefore at present, the prevalence of RLS in patients with ADHD is unclear due to the lack of large epidemiological surveys using formal criteria for the diagnosis of both ADHD and RLS.

Over the last few years sleep specialists interested in ADHD have also studied the relationship between ADHD and periodic limb movements in sleep (PLMS), which are defined as a series of four or more consecutive movements lasting 0.5–5 seconds separated by intervals of 4–90 seconds [51]. It is difficult to summarize data on PLMS in children with ADHD diagnosed according to DSM criteria, since available studies reported different indices to quantify periodic limb movements and their impact on sleep fragmentation. Some utilize the PLM index (PLMI, i.e. the number of PLMS per hour of sleep), others report prevalence of periodic limb movement disorder (PLMD, i.e. a sleep disorder characterized by PLMS, associated with clinical sleep disturbance which cannot be accounted for by another primary sleep disorder). A descriptive analysis of the available studies indicates that three of them reported no significant differences in PLMI between children with ADHD and controls [52–54]. One [54] study reported no significant differences in the prevalence of PLMD, while in four reports [54–57], the prevalence of PLMS >5 (which is considered pathological in children) was higher in children with ADHD compared to controls. Therefore, preliminary data suggest that children with "real" ADHD may have a pathological number of PLMS.

Sleep disordered breathing (SDB)

According to the *International Classification of Sleep Disorders*, 2nd edition [51], the most common form of pediatric sleep disordered breathing (SDB) is obstructive sleep apnea, which is characterized by prolonged partial upper airway obstruction, intermittent complete or partial obstruction (obstructive apnea or hypopnea), or both prolonged and intermittent obstruction that disrupts normal ventilation during sleep, normal sleep patterns, or both. It has been extensively demonstrated that SDB may lead to symptoms mimicking those of ADHD (in particular, inattention, irritability, and hyperactivity) [58].

Whether or not children with ADHD diagnosed according to formal criteria and without other co-morbidities have significantly higher prevalence of SDB compared to normal controls is still debated. In part, this is due to the lack of consensus on the exact definition of the characteristics of SDB in children, in particular what apnea-hypopnea index (AHI) (i.e. the number of apneas or hypopneas per hours of sleep) should be considered pathological in children. We were able to find only three studies [52,54,55] analyzing AHI in children with ADHD diagnosed according to formal criteria and without co-morbid disorders. One study [52] reported no significant differences in AHI between children with ADHD and controls, while two [54,55] reported significantly higher AHI in ADHD versus controls. The mean AHI values in ADHD children in the three objective studies were not very elevated (1.0, 5.8, and 3.57, respectively [52,54,55]). However, if one assumes that moderate values of AHI between 1 and 5 deserve clinical attention in children (which is still controversial [59,60]), all the previous data concur to suggest that SDB may be more frequent in children with ADHD than controls. According to Chervin [59], mild SDB, in an AHI range of 1 and 5 and sometimes less, rather than more severe SDB, may be particularly common in children with ADHD, perhaps because more severe SDB may cause enough daytime sleepiness or other problems to mask hyperactivity.

The causal contribution of SDB to ADHD, if any, remains to be established in detail. It has been reported that adenotonsillectomy can significantly reduce rates of ADHD (diagnosed according to DSM criteria) in children referred for adenotonsillectomy [61]. Therefore, it is possible that some children with ADHD could benefit from adenotonsillectomy, although, at present, given the limited number of studies and the methodological issues relating to the definition of pediatric "pathological" AHI, it is not possible to accurately estimate the prevalence of children with ADHD who have SDB and might benefit from adenotonsillectomy.

Circadian rhythm disorders

Circadian rhythm disorders include a series of conditions characterized by a persistent and recurrent pattern of sleep disturbance due primarily to alterations of the circadian timekeeping system or a misalignment between the endogenous circadian rhythm and exogenous factors that affect the timing or duration of sleep (see Chapter 11: Circadian rhythm disorders).

In a series of elegant studies examining dim light melatonin onset (DLMO) in children with ADHD, Van der Heijden et al. [62] showed that the endogenous circadian pacemaker may be fixed at a later phase than the desired sleep–wake schedule in children with ADHD and sleep-onset insomnia (SOI), independent of co-morbid ODD or inappropriate parental educative attitude. In particular, when comparing DLMO in 87 children with rigorously diagnosed ADHD and SOI (ADHD-SOI) and 33 children with ADHD without SOI (ADHD-noSOI), the authors found that DLMO was significantly later in ADHD-SOI (20:32 +/−0:55 hours) compared with ADHD-noSOI (19:47 +/−0:49 hours) (p <0.001) [62]. It is notable that the possible alteration does not concern all children with ADHD but only those with a sleep onset delay. This finding is interesting but it needs to be replicated in other larger samples including healthy controls. Moreover, the clinical impact of a delay of roughly 45 minutes on sleep onset should be better understood in children with ADHD.

The independent effects of ADHD on sleep

The question whether ADHD itself, independently from the effect of associated psychiatric co-morbidities or medication status, is associated with intrinsic sleep alterations is an interesting but quite difficult question to answer definitively. Sleep in children with ADHD has been investigated in *subjective* and *objective* studies. The former have used sleep questionnaires (including several sleep items) filled out by the parents or, less frequently, by the children/

adolescents themselves. The latter have used the gold standard for the objective and standardized assessment of sleep, i.e. multichannel polysomnography (PSG), as well as other techniques such as actigraphy (a wristwatch-like device that measures sleep/wake periods), infrared video camera, and the multiple sleep latency test (MSLT, used to assess daytime sleepiness by means of polysomnographic recording). Data from subjective and, in particular, objective studies on sleep and ADHD are quite inconsistent [63]. While some authors found that specific subjective sleep items or objective sleep parameters were abnormal in children with ADHD compared with controls, others failed to replicate these results. It is possible that the discrepancy in the results is linked, at least in part, to the fact that not all studies excluded or controlled for psychiatric co-morbidities and medication status, which can clearly impact on sleep variables.

In order to reach evidence-based conclusions on sleep in ADHD, in 2005 our group conducted a systematic review [64] of subjective and objective studies and a meta-analysis of objective sleep parameters. We included only studies assessing children with a rigorous diagnosis of ADHD, drug-naïve, and without psychiatric co-morbidities (depressive and mood disorders; children with ODD were included because ODD represents a very frequent co-morbidity in children with ADHD and thus we felt that the exclusion of studies assessing children with ADHD plus ODD would have been inappropriate). We concluded that children with ADHD had significantly greater daytime sleepiness (on both MSLT and parental reports) and a higher AHI, as well as more movements during sleep compared with controls, while no significant alterations of sleep macroarchitecture or continuity were found. In the last 3 years since that meta-analysis, there have been a series of new publications in the field. Therefore, we felt it useful to update the results of our previous work and to extend the meta-analysis to subjective sleep measures. We used the same selection criteria of our previous systematic review. Our updated meta-analysis [65] included nine subjective sleep items and fifteen objective parameters from sixteen studies published between 1987 and 2008 (total pooled sample: 722 children with ADHD vs. 638 controls).

The parameters examined in the subjective studies were: (1) bedtime resistance (BR); (2) sleep onset difficulties (SOD); (3) night awakenings (NA); (4) sleep duration (SD); (5) difficulties with morning awakenings (DMA); (6) daytime sleepiness (DS); (7) sleep disordered breathing (SDB); (8) restless sleep (RS); and (9) parasomnia (PA).

The parameters examined in the objective studies were: (1) sleep onset latency evaluated with polysomnography (SOL-PSG); (2) sleep onset latency evaluated with actigraphy (SOL-a); (3) number of stage shifts in total sleep time (SHIFTS); (4) number of stage shifts/hour sleep (SHIFTS/h); (5) percentage of stage 1 (ST1%); (6) percentage of stage 2 (ST2%); (7) percentage of slow-wave sleep (SWS%); (8) rapid eye movement (REM) sleep latency (REML); (9) percentage of REM (REM%); (10) sleep efficiency (SE, i.e. the ratio of total sleep time to nocturnal time in bed) assessed with polysomnography (SE-PSG); (11) SE assessed with actigraphy (SE-a); (12) true sleep on actigraphy (TS); (13) night wakings on actigraphy (NW); (14) average time to fall asleep during MSLT (MSLT); and (15) apnea-hypopnea index (AHI) (i.e. the number of apneas or hypopneas per hours of sleep).

With regards to subjective items, we found that, according to parental reports, children with ADHD had significantly higher bedtime resistance (z = 6.94, p <0.001), more sleep onset difficulties (z = 9.38, p <0.001), night awakenings (z = 2.15, p = 0.031), difficulties with morning awakenings (z = 5.19, p <0.001), sleep disordered breathing (z = 2.05, p = 0.04), and daytime sleepiness (z = 1.96, p = 0.05) compared to controls. The significantly higher sleep disordered breathing item is in line with data from PSG studies on sleep disordered breathing previously discussed. We will discuss the finding about "daytime sleepiness" later in this section, along with the objective findings on MSLT studies. Several explanations may be considered as to why *bedtime resistance, sleep onset difficulties, night awakenings,* and *difficulties with morning awakenings* were more problematic for children with ADHD. It is possible that the difficulties reported as significantly higher in children with ADHD refer to inappropriate behavior in the context of problematic parent–child interactions [66]. Another possible explanation is that symptoms of ADHD, such as restlessness in the evening and poor organization, contribute to difficult behavior during the evening and early morning, even in the context of appropriate sleep habits established by the parents. As we previously mentioned, some of the children with ADHD included in the meta-analysis presented with co-morbid ODD, which can contribute to problematic behavior during the evening and

early morning. Therefore, the inclusion of children with ADHD plus ODD prevented us from teasing out the effect of ODD and ADHD itself on difficult sleep behaviors. As clinicians, we would like to point out that it is sometimes very difficult in day-to-day practice to understand if difficult behaviors in the evening or early morning are due to ODD, ADHD itself, or to a combination of both. Another explanation for the significantly higher rate of difficult sleep behaviors in children with ADHD is that parents of children with ADHD may be more likely to report high levels of daytime and sleep-related problematic behaviors in a sort of "negative halo effect" [66]. However, it is also possible that objective sleep alterations contribute to difficult behaviors around sleep time. Parents may consider the difficult behaviors around sleep time as the expression of a general oppositional attitude, thus ignoring the cause of the child's behavior which may be the expression of an underlying real sleep disturbance which manifests itself with behavioral difficulties.

Indeed, the analysis of objective parameters revealed that children with ADHD do present with significantly more objective sleep alterations compared to controls. We found that sleep onset latency (on actigraphy) was significantly higher in ADHD versus controls. However, *sleep onset latency measured with polysomnography* (SOL-PSG) did not differ between children with ADHD and controls. While this discrepancy deserves further study, we point out that sleep onset latency tends to be the least reliable sleep parameter measured by actigraphy [66,67]. On the other hand, SOL-PSG has some limitations as well. In fact, since it has been reported that a structured environment may modify the expression of the child's ADHD symptoms, we wonder to what extent a structured environment such as the one provided by a sleep laboratory may modify sleep parameters in children with ADHD. Moreover, it has been suggested that children with ADHD present with night-to-night variability in sleep patterns [68]. Therefore, it is possible that the measure of SOL during one single night or few nights, which occurred in most studies, does not capture SOL variability in an appropriate way.

We also found that children with ADHD presented with a significantly higher number of stage shifts/hour sleep and lower sleep efficiency on PSG, suggesting that their sleep is more fragmented compared to controls. It is possible that abnormal movements in sleep may contribute to this fragmentation.

It was not possible to combine data on general sleep movements since the two selected studies [56,69] used different parameters and techniques. However, the descriptive analysis of these two studies suggests that children with ADHD present a significantly higher number of general sleep movements compared to controls.

On the other hand, the parameters ST1%, ST2%, SWS%, REM%, and REML did not significantly differ between ADHD and controls. Sleep architecture in ADHD has been the subject of investigations dating back to the 1970s [70], with inconsistent results. It has been reported that a reduction in REM latency associated with an increased REM duration might be characteristic of sleep in ADHD [56]. However, the pooled analysis of all data on sleep architecture suggested no alterations in REM sleep. This is a major finding, confirming the conclusions of our previous meta-analysis [47] as well as those of Sadeh et al. [71], indicating that sleep macroarchitecture is not substantially altered in children with ADHD.

Finally, with regard to data from MSLT studies, the average time to fall asleep (considering all MSLT nap opportunities) was significantly shorter in children with ADHD than controls (mean MSLT score of 21.9 ± 5.5 minutes versus 27.9 ± 2.0 minutes, $p < 0.005$) [19,55], indicating that children with ADHD display a tendency to be sleepier than normal controls during the daytime. According to the hypoarousal theory of ADHD first defined by Weinberg et al. [72] and further confirmed with MSLT for the first time by our group [19], children with ADHD are sleepier than controls and might use excessive motor activity as a strategy to stay awake and alert. Interestingly, recent data on cyclic alternating pattern in subjects with ADHD confirmed that they may present with a hypoaroused state [73]. The nature of excessive daytime sleepiness has to be determined: excessive daytime sleepiness might be a primary disorder or the consequence of some other sleep alteration.

Management of sleep disturbances in patients with ADHD

Based on data reported in the above overview, we suggest that clinicians should systematically inquire about sleep disturbances and disorders not only in patients with diagnosed ADHD, but also in patients referred for symptoms of inattention, impulsivity, and/or hyperactivity, since sleep disturbances may mimic ADHD symptoms. Simple questions addressed to parents as well as age-appropriate questions for children or adolescents should be used. Based on the results of our meta-analysis, inquiry should focus on bedtime resistance, sleep onset difficulty, night awakenings, difficulty with morning awakenings, sleep disordered breathing, and daytime sleepiness. If possible, specific questionnaires, such as the one by Bruni et al. [74] and that by Owens et al. [75] for children, assessing sleep and/or alertness as well as sleep diaries filled out by parents and patients should be used to complement the clinical interview. We dedicate particular attention to a systematic inquiry for RLS in children with ADHD, particularly if one or both parents present with diagnosed RLS or with symptoms suggestive of this disorder. Given the role of iron deficiency in RLS, we suggest the systematic measurement of peripheral iron markers (such as serum ferritin) in children with ADHD, particularly if the clinician suspects RLS. The cut-off value used for low ferritin differs across centers, limiting its accuracy for detecting the presence of iron deficiency. When iron stores are depleted, typically below the widely accepted cut-off for serum ferritin of 12 µg/L, there is decreased hemoglobin synthesis [76]. However, a "normal" ferritin level for hemoglobin and myoglobin synthesis could be insufficient for neurotransmitter function in the brain [76]. Therefore, Allen and Earley [45] suggest a cut-off of about 45 µg/L to indicate low peripheral iron stores with negative impact on CNS function in adults, although no empirical data are available for children.

An all night polysomnographic recording would be warranted if the clinician suspects sleep disordered breathing or seeks to evaluate potential sleep-related causes of excessive daytime sleepiness or sleep fragmentation due to frequent nocturnal arousals (including periodic limb movement disorder). Finally, MSLT preceded by all-night polysomnography is useful to evaluate daytime sleepiness secondary to sleep alterations or as an expression of a primary alteration of arousal. MSLT is also recommended to rule out the presence of sleep-onset REM periods (REM latency of less than 20 minutes) which would suggest specific disorders of alertness such as narcolepsy without cataplexy.

Once the specific sleep disorder underlying parental or personal complaints is diagnosed, the clinician should start the appropriate specific treatment. Given the lack of empirical data, no evidence-based guidelines are available, particularly in children. Therefore, we discuss the treatment strategies for the most common sleep disorders underlying subjective complaints on the basis of data provided by case report, case series, and personal experience of our group as well as that of our colleagues in the field.

Sleep disturbances associated with RLS/PLMS

Case reports [77,78] suggest the efficacy of dopaminergic agents (levodopa/carbidopa, pergolide, and ropinirole) in children diagnosed with both ADHD and RLS and previously treated with psychostimulants with limited efficacy or intolerable side-effects. However, to date, the limited number of patients treated and the absence of double-blind, placebo-controlled, randomized trials do not allow evidence-based recommendations for treatment to be made. No studies on iron supplementation for RLS in children have been published to date. On the other hand, Simakajornboon et al. [79] reported a decrease in periodic limb movements in sleep in children treated with iron sulphate (3 mg/kg of elemental iron per day for 3 months). Non-pharmacological management of RLS includes consistent and appropriate sleep schedule, limit-setting techniques, exercise program, and restriction of caffeinated beverages.

Excessive nocturnal motricity

Late afternoon methylphenidate doses may reduce nocturnal activity both during sleep and prior to sleep onset and improve sleep quality by consolidating sleep [80,81]. However, while some studies have shown that thrice daily methylphenidate does not impact sleep [82] or causes only a slight decrease in sleep duration [40], others have reported that a third dose of methylphenidate does worsen sleep [41,83]. Given these contrasting findings, at present, late afternoon stimulant treatment cannot be recommended for ADHD patients with high nocturnal activity.

Circadian rhythm disorders

To date, one open-label study [84] and two randomized, double-blind, placebo-controlled studies [85,86] have assessed the efficacy and tolerability of melatonin for the management of SOI, presumably due to circadian rhythm disorder, in children with ADHD, using doses of 3 mg/day for a body weight <40 kg and 6 mg/day

for a body weight >40 kg (Van der Heijden et al. [85]), and a unique dose of 5 mg/day (Weiss et al. [87]), respectively. In the two randomized studies, in spite of improvements in sleep onset after 4 weeks, melatonin given 20 minutes before bedtime by Weiss and colleagues [87] and at 7 p.m. by Van der Heijden and co-workers [85] demonstrated no effect on behavior, cognitive performance, or quality of life. Although the number of acute adverse events did not differ significantly between melatonin and placebo, since data on possible long-term effects, such as on the gonadotropic system and onset of puberty are not available, further evidence is needed before recommending melatonin systematically for SOI in children with ADHD.

Bearing in mind that a delayed evening increase in endogenous melatonin levels might explain SOI in children with ADHD, some authors investigated the efficacy of light therapy (LT). In an open trial, Rybak et al. [88] administered 3 weeks of morning bright LT to 29 adults with ADHD. They found a significant phase advance in circadian preference, as well as a significant improvement in both subjective and objective measures of ADHD. To our knowledge, no controlled study has been conducted to assess the efficacy of LT in children with ADHD. Therefore, we think that research in this field should be encouraged.

Sleep problems associated with sleep disordered breathing

Growing empirical evidence shows a significant improvement not only of breathing parameters, but also of ADHD symptoms in children diagnosed with ADHD plus SDB, after adenotonsillectomy [61,89]. As previously stated, it is not possible to estimate accurately the prevalence of children with ADHD who have SDB and might benefit from adenotonsillectomy. However, these promising results should prompt further studies to assess the effectiveness of surgery for sleep disorders and for core ADHD symptoms in patients with SDB and ADHD. They also suggest that appropriate recognition and surgical treatment of underlying SDB in children with ADHD might prevent long-term stimulant treatment.

Sleep disturbances associated with ADHD medications

A panel of ADHD experts [90] proposed several strategies to deal with sleep alterations caused by stimulants

Table 21.1 Possible strategies to deal with sleep alterations caused by stimulants

1. Simply wait (generally insomnia caused by stimulants attenuates after 1–2 months) [90,96]

2. Adjustment in dose or dosing schedules (e.g. avoid evening stimulant dose) [90]

3. Switch to another stimulant formulation (in our clinical experience, different formulations of the same stimulant may impact sleep differently)

4. Switch to another stimulant (there are some data suggesting that amphetamines may impact sleep more significantly than methylphenidate) [97]

5. Switch to a non-stimulant: e.g. atomoxetine (initiate at the lowest available dose (10 mg) and titrate slowly to minimize side-effects, up to 1.8 mg/kg/day [90]), bupropion (daily maximum dose to obtain sleep improvement: 50–150 mg [98])

6. Add antihistamines (diphenhydramine (25–50 mg orally [90,99]) and cyproheptadine (2–4 mg orally [90]), trazodone (25–50 mg [90,100]), mirtazapine (30–45 mg in adolescents [101]), or melatonin (1–6 mg [84,85,87])

7. Use clonidine

(Table 21.1). As for clonidine in particular, a relatively large case series [91] (N = 62; 42 children and 20 adolescents) showed that 85% of children with ADHD treated with clonidine (average dose 4.4 μg/kg/h.s.; range 50–800 μg/h.s.) for ADHD-associated sleep disturbances were considered to be much to very much improved. Children and adolescents with ADHD with baseline, medicine-induced, or medicine-exacerbated sleep disturbances responded equally well to clonidine treatment. Thirty-one percent of patients reported mild adverse effects (fatigue, morning sedation). One patient discontinued clonidine because of depression, which resolved after discontinuation. To our knowledge, this is the largest case series on the use of clonidine for sleep disorders in children with ADHD.

If, on the other hand, the impact on sleep is caused by a "rebound effect" (rebound hyperactivity leading to sleep onset difficulties), in our, as well as in others', clinical experience, giving a low dose of methylphenidate in late afternoon or evening could be helpful. Doses in late evening could also be considered if the rebound effect persists (rebound hyperactivity can be distinguished from other causes of sleep onset difficulties since it strictly depends on the schedule of medication, manifesting itself when the medication wears off).

Sleep disturbances caused by medications used to treat co-morbid conditions

If sleep disturbances are accounted for by drugs used to treat co-morbid disorders, the clinician should use alternative drugs with a reduced impact on sleep or modify the doses of the current treatment. In particular, among antidepressants, citalopram, a new SSRI, has been reported to have fewer negative effects on sleep continuity [92] and may actually improve sleep in depressed patients [93]. Nefazodone (not available in Europe) and mirtazapine may cause significantly less insomnia than other SSRIs, although their use may be associated with daytime sleepiness [20]. However, clinicians should consider that mirtazapine can induce RLS [94].

Future perspectives

In recent years, there have been significant improvements in study methodology in research examining sleep in ADHD, but given the still limited amount of data, it is clear that the field needs more methodologically sound studies.

As for studies investigating subjective measures of sleep, most of these used parental reports. However, older children, and in particular adolescents, can provide information on sleep difficulties not detected by parents (e.g. older children and adolescents may lie in bed quietly after "lights out" and parents may not even be aware of the sleep onset difficulties). Therefore, we encourage the use of sleep and somnolence questionnaires adapted for children and adolescents as complementary to data provided by parents.

As for objective studies, we suggest ecologically sound PSG and standardized actigraphic recordings during several days, assessing both weekday and weekend sleep time, in order to capture the potential variability in sleep patterns in ADHD. Although sleep macroarchitecture seems not to be altered, it has been reported that children with ADHD may present more subtle sleep alterations (i.e. alteration of the cyclic alternating pattern; CAP) not captured with routine PSG scoring. However, to date only one study [73] assessed CAP in ADHD and so studies exploring CAP in patients with ADHD should be encouraged.

Sleep alterations should be studied in relation to the developmental and pubertal phase (Tanner stages were assessed in only two studies [19,69]) as well as in relation to the subtype of ADHD. Since all the available studies in childhood included school-aged subjects, it would be of interest to assess possible differences in sleep patterns in preschool children with ADHD versus healthy controls, and to better understand the potential relationship between sleep alterations and symptoms of ADHD in very young children.

With regard to specific issues, we encourage further studies using similar methodology to assess general movement and PLMS in ADHD children, by means of PSG or actigraphy with ankle or feet placement. This may provide insights into sleep alterations in ADHD, given that the sleep fragmentation induced by sleep movements may lead to sleep disruption with possible daytime consequences. Moreover, we suggest the systematic measure of iron markers and to study their potential correlations with abnormal sleep movements and, possibly, other sleep parameters. As for sleep disordered breathing, we suggest that BMI should systematically be reported in future studies assessing SDB in children with ADHD in order to assess the potential effect of obesity on SDB. We strongly encourage replication studies using MSLT, both in children and adults. Our group has suggested that excessive daytime sleepiness may be a paramount and primary alteration in at least a subsample of ADHD children. We have also speculated [95] that alterations of the hypocretin/orexin system, which is involved in alertness and other major functions (which may also be altered in ADHD) such as food seeking, weight control, and motor activity regulation, may contribute to excessive daytime sleepiness in ADHD children. Future studies should address this issue promptly due to the potential therapeutic implications (use of specific wake-promoting agents for ADHD patients with excessive daytime sleepiness). Finally, and perhaps most importantly, we strongly encourage large, multi-site and randomized treatment studies, including pharmacological and psychotherapeutic trials, for sleep disorders in patients with ADHD, especially in pediatric patients, given the paucity of empirical-based data.

This body of future research will advance our knowledge of subjective and objective sleep alterations in patients with ADHD and on the mechanisms by which objective alterations contribute to subjective complaints, as well as on the most effective and safe treatment strategies. This will form the theoretical basis for a better assessment and management of sleep disturbances in patients with ADHD, thus allowing a better quality of life for these individuals and their families.

References

1. American Psychiatric Association. *Diagnostic and statistical manual of mental disorders*, 4th ed. Washington, DC: American Psychiatric Association; 1994.

2. American Psychiatric Association. *Diagnostic and statistical manual of mental disorders*, 4th ed. Text Revision. Washington, DC: American Psychiatric Association; 2000.

3. Faraone SV, Sergeant J, Gillberg C, Biederman J. The worldwide prevalence of ADHD: is it an American condition? *World Psychiatry*. 2003;**2**:104–113.

4. WHO. *The ICD-10 classification of mental and behavioral disorders: Clinical descriptions and diagnostic guidelines 1992; diagnostic criteria for research 1993*. Geneva: WHO; 1992.

5. Taylor E, Sandberg S, Thorley G, Giles S. *The epidemiology of childhood hyperactivity*. London: Maudsley Monographs; 1991.

6. Biederman J, Faraone S. Attention-deficit/hyperactivity disorder. *Lancet*. 2005;**366**:237–248.

7. Kessler RC, Adler LA, Barkley R, et al. Patterns and predictors of attention-deficit/hyperactivity disorder persistence into adulthood: results from the national comorbidity survey replication. *Biol Psychiatry*. 2005;**57**:1442–1451.

8. Pliszka S. Practice parameter for the assessment and treatment of children and adolescents with attention-deficit/hyperactivity disorder. *J Am Acad Child Adolesc Psychiatry*. 2007;**46**:894–921.

9. Banaschewski T, Coghill D, Santosh P, et al. Long-acting medications for the hyperkinetic disorders: A systematic review and European treatment guideline. *Eur Child Adolesc Psychiatry*. 2006;**15**:476–495.

10. Taylor E, Dopfner M, Sergeant J, et al. European clinical guidelines for hyperkinetic disorder: first upgrade. *Eur Child Adolesc Psychiatry*. 2004;**13** (Suppl 1):17–30.

11. Barkley RA. *Attention deficit hyperactivity disorder: a clinical handbook*, 3rd ed. New York: Guilford; 2006.

12. Faraone SV, Biederman J, Jetton JG, Tsuang MT. Attention deficit disorder and conduct disorder: longitudinal evidence for a familial subtype. *Psychol Med*. 1997;**27**:291–300.

13. Biederman J, Wilens T, Mick E, et al. Is ADHD a risk factor for psychoactive substance use disorders? Findings from a four-year prospective follow-up study. *J Am Acad Child Adolesc Psychiatry*. 1997; **36**:21–29.

14. Milberger S, Biederman J, Faraone SV, Chen L, Jones J. ADHD is associated with early initiation of cigarette smoking in children and adolescents. *J Am Acad Child Adolesc Psychiatry*. 1997;**36**:37–44.

15. Spencer T, Biederman J, Coffey B, et al. Tourette disorder and ADHD. *Adv Neurol*. 2001;**85**:57–77.

16. American Psychiatric Association. *Diagnostic and statistical manual of mental disorders*, 3rd ed. Washington, DC: American Psychiatric Association; 1980.

17. American Psychiatric Association. *Diagnostic and statistical manual of mental disorders*, 3rd ed. Revised. Washington, DC: American Psychiatric Association; 1987.

18. Sherman DK, Iacono WG, McGue MK. Attention-deficit hyperactivity disorder dimensions: a twin study of inattention and impulsivity-hyperactivity. *J Am Acad Child Adolesc Psychiatry*. 1997;**36**:745–753.

19. Lecendreux M, Konofal E, Bouvard M, Falissard B, Mouren-Simeoni MC. Sleep and alertness in children with ADHD. *J Child Psychol Psychiatry*. 2000;**41**:803–812.

20. Mindell JA, Owens JA. *Diagnosis and management of sleep problems*. Philadelphia: Lippincott Williams & Wilkins; 2003.

21. Corkum P, Tannock R, Moldofsky H. Sleep disturbances in children with attention-deficit/hyperactivity disorder. *J Am Acad Child Adolesc Psychiatry*. 1998;**37**:637–646.

22. Laufer MW, Denhoff E. Hyperkinetic behavior syndrome in children. *J Pediatr*. 1957;**50**:463–474.

23. Philipsen A, Hornyak M, Riemann D. Sleep and sleep disorders in adults with attention deficit/hyperactivity disorder. *Sleep Med Rev*. 2006;**10**:399–405.

24. Sobanski E, Schredl M, Kettler N, Alm B. Sleep in adults with attention deficit hyperactivity disorder (ADHD) before and during treatment with methylphenidate: a controlled polysomnographic study. *Sleep*. 2008;**31**:375–381.

25. Boonstra AM, Kooij JJ, Oosterlaan J, et al. Hyperactive night and day? Actigraphy studies in adult ADHD: a baseline comparison and the effect of methylphenidate. *Sleep*. 2007;**30**:433–442.

26. Gau SS, Kessler RC, Tseng WL, et al. Association between sleep problems and symptoms of attention-deficit/hyperactivity disorder in young adults. *Sleep*. 2007;**30**:195–201.

27. Schredl M, Alm B, Sobanski E. Sleep quality in adult patients with attention deficit hyperactivity disorder (ADHD). *Eur Arch Psychiatry Clin Neurosci*. 2007;**257**:164–168.

28. Ryan ND, Puig-Antich J, Ambrosini P, et al. The clinical picture of major depression in children and adolescents. *Arch Gen Psychiatry*. 1987;**44**:854–861.

29. Ivanenko A, Crabtree VM, Gozal D. Sleep and depression in children and adolescents. *Sleep Med Rev*. 2005;**9**:115–129.

30. Bertocci MA, Dahl RE, Williamson DE, et al. Subjective sleep complaints in pediatric depression: a controlled study and comparison with EEG measures of sleep and waking. *J Am Acad Child Adolesc Psychiatry*. 2005;**44**:1158–1166.

31. Alfano CA, Ginsburg GS, Kingery JN. Sleep-related problems among children and adolescents with anxiety disorders. *J Am Acad Child Adolesc Psychiatry*. 2007;**46**:224–232.

32. Mehl RC, O'Brien LM, Jones JH, et al. Correlates of sleep and pediatric bipolar disorder. *Sleep*. 2006;**29**:193–197.

33. Kirov R, Banaschewski T, Uebel H, Kinkelbur J, Rothenberger A. REM-sleep alterations in children with co-existence of tic disorders and attention-deficit/hyperactivity disorder: impact of hypermotor symptoms. *Eur Child Adolesc Psychiatry*. 2007;**16** (Suppl 1):45–50.

34. Kirov R, Kinkelbur J, Banaschewski T, Rothenberger A. Sleep patterns in children with attention-deficit/hyperactivity disorder, tic disorder, and comorbidity. *J Child Psychol Psychiatry*. 2007;**48**:561–570.

35. Kostanecka-Endress T, Banaschewski T, Kinkelbur J, et al. Disturbed sleep in children with Tourette syndrome: a polysomnographic study. *J Psychosom Res*. 2003;**55**:23–29.

36. Ivanenko A, Crabtree VM, Gozal D. Sleep in children with psychiatric disorders. *Pediatr Clin North Am*. 2004;**51**:51–68.

37. Brown TE, McMullen WJ Jr. Attention deficit disorders and sleep/arousal disturbances. *Ann N Y Acad Sci*. 2001;**931**:271–286.

38. Sangal RB, Owens J, Allen AJ, et al. Effects of atomoxetine and methylphenidate on sleep in children with ADHD. *Sleep*. 2006;**29**:1573–1585.

39. Carlson GA, Kelly KL. Stimulant rebound: how common is it and what does it mean? *J Child Adolesc Psychopharmacol*. 2003;**13**:137–142.

40. Ahmann PA, Waltonen SJ, Olson KA, et al. Placebo-controlled evaluation of Ritalin side-effects. *Pediatrics*. 1993;**91**:1101–1106.

41. Stein MA, Blondis TA, Schnitzler ER, et al. Methylphenidate dosing: twice daily versus three times daily. *Pediatrics*. 1996;**98**:748–756.

42. Jerome L. Can methylphenidate facilitate sleep in children with attention deficit hyperactivity disorder? *J Child Adolesc Psychopharmacol*. 2001;**11**:109.

43. Kinsbourne M. Stimulants for insomnia. *N Engl J Med.* 1973;**288**:1129.

44. Allen RP, Picchietti D, Hening WA, et al. Restless legs syndrome: diagnostic criteria, special considerations, and epidemiology: A report from the restless legs syndrome diagnosis and epidemiology workshop at the National Institutes of Health. *Sleep Med.* 2003;**4**: 101–119.

45. Allen RP, Earley CJ. The role of iron in restless legs syndrome. *Mov Disord.* 2007;**22**(Suppl 18):S440–S448.

46. Picchietti D. Is iron deficiency an underlying cause of pediatric restless legs syndrome and of attention-deficit/hyperactivity disorder? *Sleep Med.* 2007;**8** (7–8):693–694.

47. Cortese S, Konofal E, Lecendreux M, et al. Restless legs syndrome and attention-deficit/hyperactivity disorder: a review of the literature. *Sleep.* 2005;**28**:1007–1013.

48. Wagner ML, Walters AS, Fisher BC. Symptoms of attention-deficit/hyperactivity disorder in adults with restless legs syndrome. *Sleep.* 2004;**27**:1499–1504.

49. Cortese S, Lecendreux M, Mouren MC, Konofal E. ADHD and insomnia. *J Am Acad Child Adolesc Psychiatry.* 2006;**45**:384–385.

50. Chervin RD, Archbold KH, Dillon JE, et al. Associations between symptoms of inattention, hyperactivity, restless legs, and periodic leg movements. *Sleep.* 2002;**25**:213–218.

51. American Academy of Sleep Medicine. *The international classification of sleep disorders: diagnostic and coding manual*, 2nd ed. Westchester, IL: American Academy of Sleep Medecine; 2005.

52. Cooper J, Tyler L, Wallace I, Burgess KR. No evidence of sleep apnea in children with attention deficit hyperactivity disorder. *Clin Pediatr (Phila).* 2004;**43**:609–614.

53. Gruber R, Tong X, Frenette S, et al. Sleep disturbances in pre-pubertal children with attention deficit hyperactivity disorder: a home polysomnography study. *Sleep.* 2008;**32**(3):343–350.

54. Huang YS, Chen NH, Li HY, et al. Sleep disorders in Taiwanese children with attention deficit/hyperactivity disorder. *J Sleep Res.* 2004;**13**:269–277.

55. Golan N, Shahar E, Ravid S, Pillar G. Sleep disorders and daytime sleepiness in children with attention-deficit/hyperactive disorder. *Sleep.* 2004;**27**:261–266.

56. Kirov R, Kinkelbur J, Heipke S, et al. Is there a specific polysomnographic sleep pattern in children with attention deficit/hyperactivity disorder? *J Sleep Res.* 2004;**13**:87–93.

57. Picchietti DL, England SJ, Walters AS, Willis K, Verrico T. Periodic limb movement disorder and restless legs syndrome in children with

58. attention-deficit hyperactivity disorder. *J Child Neurol.* 1998;**13**:588–594.

58. Guilleminault C, Pelayo R. Sleep-disordered breathing in children. *Ann Med.* 1998;**30**:350–356.

59. Chervin RD. How many children with ADHD have sleep apnea or periodic leg movements on polysomnography? *Sleep.* 2005;**28**:1041–1042.

60. Sangal RB, Owens JA, Sangal J. Patients with attention-deficit/hyperactivity disorder without observed apneic episodes in sleep or daytime sleepiness have normal sleep on polysomnography. *Sleep.* 2005;**28**:1143–1148.

61. Dillon JE, Blunden S, Ruzicka DL et al. DSM-IV diagnoses and obstructive sleep apnea in children before and 1 year after adenotonsillectomy. *J Am Acad Child Adolesc Psychiatry.* 2007;**46**:1425–1436.

62. Van der Heijden KB, Smits MG, Van Someren EJ, Gunning WB. Idiopathic chronic sleep onset insomnia in attention-deficit/hyperactivity disorder: a circadian rhythm sleep disorder. *Chronobiol Int.* 2005;**22**:559–570.

63. Cohen-Zion M, Ancoli-Israel S. Sleep in children with attention-deficit hyperactivity disorder (ADHD): a review of naturalistic and stimulant intervention studies. *Sleep Med Rev.* 2004;**8**:379–402.

64. Cortese S, Konofal E, Yateman N, Mouren MC, Lecendreux M. Sleep and alertness in children with attention-deficit/hyperactivity disorder: a systematic review of the literature. *Sleep.* 2006;**29**:504–511.

65. Cortese S, Faraone S, Konofal E, Lecendreux M. Sleep in children with attention-deficit/hyperactivity disorder: meta-analysis of subjective and objective studies. *J Am Acad Child Adolesc Psychiatry.* 2009;**48** (9):894–908.

66. Owens JA. Sleep disorders and attention-deficit/ hyperactivity disorder. *Curr Psychiatry Rep.* 2008;**10**:439–444.

67. Sadeh A, Hauri PJ, Kripke DF, Lavie P. The role of actigraphy in the evaluation of sleep disorders. *Sleep.* 1995;**18**:288–302.

68. Gruber R, Sadeh A, Raviv A. Instability of sleep patterns in children with attention-deficit/ hyperactivity disorder. *J Am Acad Child Adolesc Psychiatry.* 2000;**39**:495–501.

69. Konofal E, Lecendreux M, Bouvard MP, Mouren-Simeoni MC. High levels of nocturnal activity in children with attention-deficit hyperactivity disorder: a video analysis. *Psychiatry Clin Neurosci.* 2001;**55**: 97–103.

70. O'Brien LM, Gozal D. Sleep in children with attention deficit/hyperactivity disorder. *Minerva Pediatr.* 2004;**56**:585–601.

71. Sadeh A, Pergamin L, Bar-Haim Y. Sleep in children with attention-deficit hyperactivity disorder:

a meta-analysis of polysomnographic studies. *Sleep Med Rev.* 2006;**10**:381–398.

72. Weinberg WA, Brumback RA. Primary disorder of vigilance: a novel explanation of inattentiveness, daydreaming, boredom, restlessness, and sleepiness. *J Pediatr.* 1990;**116**:720–725.

73. Miano S, Donfrancesco R, Bruni O, et al. NREM sleep instability is reduced in children with attention-deficit/hyperactivity disorder. *Sleep.* 2006;**29**:797–803.

74. Bruni O, Ottaviano S, Guidetti V, et al. The Sleep Disturbance Scale for Children (SDSC): Construction and validation of an instrument to evaluate sleep disturbances in childhood and adolescence. *J Sleep Res.* 1996;**5**:251–261.

75. Owens JA, Maxim R, Nobile C, McGuinn M, Msall M. Parental and self-report of sleep in children with attention-deficit/hyperactivity disorder. *Arch Pediatr Adolesc Med.* 2000;**154**:549–555.

76. Picchietti D. Is iron deficiency an underlying cause of pediatric restless legs syndrome and of attention-deficit/hyperactivity disorder? *Sleep Med.* 2007;**8**:693–694.

77. Konofal E, Arnulf I, Lecendreux M, Mouren MC. Ropinirole in a child with attention-deficit hyperactivity disorder and restless legs syndrome. *Pediatr Neurol.* 2005;**32**:350–351.

78. Walters AS, Mandelbaum DE, Lewin DS, et al. Dopaminergic therapy in children with restless legs/periodic limb movements in sleep and ADHD. Dopaminergic Therapy Study Group. *Pediatr Neurol.* 2000;**22**:182–186.

79. Simakajornboon N, Gozal D, Vlasic V, et al. Periodic limb movements in sleep and iron status in children. *Sleep.* 2003;**26**:735–738.

80. Konofal E, Lecendreux M, Bouvard M, Mouren MC. Effects of vesperal methylphenidate (MPH) administration on diurnal and nocturnal activity in ADHD children: an actigraphic study. *Sleep.* 2001; Abstract Supplement **24**:G363.

81. Kooij JJ, Middelkoop HA, van GK, Buitelaar JK. The effect of stimulants on nocturnal motor activity and sleep quality in adults with ADHD: an open-label case-control study. *J Clin Psychiatry.* 2001;**62**:952–956.

82. Kent JD, Blader JC, Koplewicz HS, Abikoff H, Foley CA. Effects of late-afternoon methylphenidate administration on behavior and sleep in attention-deficit hyperactivity disorder. *Pediatrics.* 1995; **96**:320–325.

83. Pelham WE, Gnagy EM, Chronis AM, et al. A comparison of morning-only and morning/late afternoon Adderall to morning-only, twice-daily, and three times-daily methylphenidate in children with attention-deficit/hyperactivity disorder. *Pediatrics.* 1999;**104**:1300–1311.

84. Tjon Pian Gi CV, Broeren JP, Starreveld JS, Versteegh FG. Melatonin for treatment of sleeping disorders in children with attention deficit/hyperactivity disorder: a preliminary open label study. *Eur J Pediatr.* 2003;**162**:554–555.

85. Van der Heijden KB, Smits MG, Van Someren EJ, Ridderinkhof KR, Gunning WB. Effect of melatonin on sleep, behavior, and cognition in ADHD and chronic sleep-onset insomnia. *J Am Acad Child Adolesc Psychiatry.* 2007;**46**:233–241.

86. Weiss M, Tannock R, Kratochvil C, et al. A randomized, placebo-controlled study of once-daily atomoxetine in the school setting in children with ADHD. *J Am Acad Child Adolesc Psychiatry.* 2005;**44**:647–655.

87. Weiss MD, Wasdell MB, Bomben MM, Rea KJ, Freeman RD. Sleep hygiene and melatonin treatment for children and adolescents with ADHD and initial insomnia. *J Am Acad Child Adolesc Psychiatry.* 2006;**45**:512–519.

88. Rybak YE, McNeely HE, Mackenzie BE, Jain UR, Levitan RD. An open trial of light therapy in adult attention-deficit/hyperactivity disorder. *J Clin Psychiatry.* 2006;**67**:1527–1535.

89. Huang YS, Guilleminault C, Li HY, et al. Attention-deficit/hyperactivity disorder with obstructive sleep apnea: a treatment outcome study. *Sleep Med.* 2007;**8**:18–30.

90. Kratochvil CJ, Lake M, Pliszka SR, Walkup JT. Pharmacological management of treatment-induced insomnia in ADHD. *J Am Acad Child Adolesc Psychiatry.* 2005;**44**:499–501.

91. Prince JB, Wilens TE, Biederman J, Spencer TJ, Wozniak JR. Clonidine for sleep disturbances associated with attention-deficit hyperactivity disorder: a systematic chart review of 62 cases. *J Am Acad Child Adolesc Psychiatry.* 1996;**35**:599–605.

92. van Bemmel AL, van den Hoofdakker RH, Beersma DG, Bouhuys AL. Changes in sleep polygraphic variables and clinical state in depressed patients during treatment with citalopram. *Psychopharmacology (Berl).* 1993;**113**:225–230.

93. Lader M, Andersen HF, Baekdal T. The effect of escitalopram on sleep problems in depressed patients. *Hum Psychopharmacol.* 2005;**20**:349–354.

94. Kim SW, Shin IS, Kim JM, et al. Factors potentiating the risk of mirtazapine-associated restless legs syndrome. *Hum Psychopharmacol.* 2008;**23**:615–620.

95. Cortese S, Konofal E, Lecendreux M. Alertness and feeding behaviors in ADHD: does the hypocretin/

orexin system play a role? *Med Hypotheses.* 2008;**71**:770–775.

96. Golinko BE. Side-effects of dextroamphetamine and methylphenidate in hyperactive children – a brief review. *Prog Neuropsychopharmacol Biol Psychiatry.* 1984;**8**:1–8.

97. Efron D, Jarman F, Barker M. Side-effects of methylphenidate and dexamphetamine in children with attention deficit hyperactivity disorder: a double-blind, crossover trial. *Pediatrics.* 1997;**100**:662–666.

98. Simeon JG, Ferguson HB, Van Wyck FJ. Bupropion effects in attention deficit and conduct disorders. *Can J Psychiatry.* 1986;**31**:581–585.

99. Merenstein D, Diener-West M, Halbower AC, Krist A, Rubin HR. The trial of infant response to

diphenhydramine: the TIRED study – a randomized, controlled, patient-oriented trial. *Arch Pediatr Adolesc Med.* 2006;**160**:707–712.

100. Kallepalli BR, Bhatara VS, Fogas BS, Tervo RC, Misra LK. Trazodone is only slightly faster than fluoxetine in relieving insomnia in adolescents with depressive disorders. *J Child Adolesc Psychopharmacol.* 1997;**7**:97–107.

101. Haapasalo-Pesu KM, Vuola T, Lahelma L, Marttunen M. Mirtazapine in the treatment of adolescents with major depression: an open-label, multicenter pilot study. *J Child Adolesc Psychopharmacol.* 2004;**14**: 175–184.

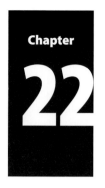

Chapter

22

Sleep in pediatric mood and anxiety disorders

Valerie McLaughlin Crabtree and Anna Ivanenko

Introduction

Sleep complaints such as difficulty initiating and maintaining sleep, restless sleep, daytime sleepiness, and bedtime anxieties are highly prevalent among children with psychiatric disorders. In particular, children with mood and anxiety disorders have significantly more night-time awakenings than children with other psychiatric disorders [1]. Recent attention has been paid to the relationship between mood disorders and sleep, particularly in adults with major depressive disorder (MDD). An extension of this work has been made investigating sleep in children and adolescents with depression and anxiety. Some of the work has involved assessing subjective complaints in children and adolescents with mood and anxiety disorders, while others have studied objective sleep disruption in this population. Objective studies have globally assessed sleep architecture differences between children with mood and anxiety disorders and healthy peers, while others have looked at the microarchitecture of sleep in children and adolescents with depression.

Dahl [2] has posited a bidirectional theory of the relationship between emotional and behavioral difficulties and sleep in children. Support for his theory comes from five primary bodies of evidence. First, pediatric patients with emotional disorders have shown increased rates of sleep disturbance. Correspondingly, children with sleep disturbance have a significantly higher prevalence of psychiatric problems. Third, even in the short term a stressful event may induce sleep disruption in children, while insufficient sleep may directly lead to disruptive behavior during the day. Fourth, significant overlap in symptoms is present between those with sleep disorders and those with psychiatric disorders, particularly in

relation to depressive symptomatology. Finally, the similar neurobehavioral systems related to both sleep and mood regulation provide evidence of this bidirectional relationship between these regulatory systems.

While the majority of focus on sleep disruption in children with mood disorders has been on depression, some investigations have examined the sleep of children and adolescents with bipolar disorder and anxiety disorders. In the following sections, we will review the nature of sleep disturbance in pediatric mood and anxiety disorders, focusing on both subjective and objective data, and when available, discuss treatment options, with the caveat that the vast majority of treatments are based on clinical experience rather than evidence-based medicine.

Sleep and pediatric depression
Subjective sleep complaints in depressed pediatric patients

Subjective sleep disturbance is extremely common in pediatric depression. Early studies investigating subjective complaints of pediatric patients with depression revealed that approximately two-thirds of children with MDD reported difficulty initiating and maintaining sleep, and half reported early morning awakenings [3]. Ivanenko and colleagues compared parental report of children's behavior with sleep complaints and found that those with delayed sleep onset and shorter sleep duration tended to experience more negative mood during the day. Difficulty maintaining sleep was also associated with anxiety, depressive, and somatic symptoms. Parental report of excessive daytime sleepiness was significantly more likely to be associated with depressive and somatic symptoms than with hyperactivity [1].

Foundations of Psychiatric Sleep Medicine, ed. John W. Winkelman and David T. Plante. Published by Cambridge University Press.
© Cambridge University Press 2010.

In an assessment of sleep complaints in 7- to 14-year-old children diagnosed with depression, Liu and colleagues [4] closely examined both insomnia and subjective hypersomnia (report of sleeping more than usual, napping in the afternoon/after dinner, or have trouble waking up) in this population. While slightly over half of the sample had experienced insomnia alone in the past month, 9% reported hypersomnia alone, and 10% reported experiencing both hypersomnia and insomnia over the previous month. Children with any sleep disturbance exhibited more significant depression than those without sleep disturbance. Children who exhibited both hypersomnia and insomnia were significantly more likely to experience a recurrent episode of depression, to have had a longer course of depression, and to have the most severe depressive symptomatology as compared to children with either insomnia or hypersomnia alone. Additionally, children with any sleep disturbance were significantly more likely to have co-morbid anxiety disorders but were significantly less likely to have oppositional defiant disorders than depressed children without sleep disturbance [4].

In a comparison of depressive symptoms between prepubertal children (mean age = 9 years) and adolescents (mean age = 14 years) with MDD, symptoms of insomnia were equally prevalent across age groups, with nearly three-quarters of the sample reporting significant insomnia. Subjective hypersomnia, on the other hand, was significantly more prevalent in adolescents than in prepubertal children (34% vs. 16%). When the age groups were combined, hypersomnia and fatigue were more prevalent in those with endogenous depression subtype, while insomnia was related more to anxious depression [5].

A recent longitudinal clinical assessment of neurobehavioral factors in pediatric affective disorder demonstrated that adolescents with MDD reported significantly longer time to initiate sleep, more frequent nocturnal awakenings, more difficulty with morning awakening, and poorer subjective sleep quality than adolescents without depression. Those with co-morbid anxiety disorders exhibited more nocturnal awakenings, increased difficulty with morning awakening, and poorer subjective sleep quality than those without co-morbid depression [6].

Genetic influences may be important contributors to the relationship of sleep disturbance and depressive symptoms. In a study of 8-year-old twins, those with self-reported depressive symptoms were significantly more likely to have their parents report bedtime problems, such as resisting bedtime and delaying sleep onset [7]. Monozygotic twins were significantly more likely to have concordance with both depressive symptoms and sleep problems and a higher bivariate correlation, indicating sleep problems in one twin and depressive symptoms in the other, than dizygotic twins. Thus, the association between sleep problems and depression was due, at least to some extent, to genetic factors, and there was substantial overlap between the genes influencing sleep problems and those influencing depression. The authors also investigated the relationship between child self-reports of anxiety and sleep disturbance and noted that this relationship was far less robust than that between depression and sleep problems [7].

There are few studies that examine the effects of treatment of pediatric depression on co-occurring sleep complaints. Across an 8-week course of treatment that included selective serotonin reuptake inhibitors and/or cognitive behavioral therapy, adolescents with MDD exhibited a significant reduction in caffeine use but did not have improvements in their sleep [6]. One year after initial assessment of subjective sleep complaints, Puig-Antich and colleagues [8] reassessed a subset of children whose depression had remitted, and only 10% continued to experience symptoms of insomnia after their remission. However, the children in this study tended to maintain a similar rise time while having a significantly later bedtime and sleep onset time. As a result, the children obtained approximately 30 minutes less sleep each night following their recovery than while experiencing their depressive episode, though they subjectively reported improved sleep [8].

Predictive value of sleep complaints and future depression

Several longitudinal studies probe the relationship between sleep disturbance and depression. Early sleep complaints have been posited to be related to later development of depression and anxiety; while, conversely, there is some evidence that early depressive symptoms may predict persistent sleep difficulties. In a longitudinal study investigating sleep complaints and depressive symptoms in adolescents, 75% of those who initially reported some symptoms of depression (but did not meet diagnostic criteria for MDD) in addition to sleep disturbances eventually met criteria for MDD over the course of 12 months [9]. To more specifically assess the role of sleep disturbance in anxiety and depression in children, Johnson and colleagues [10], using data from a large study examining the psychiatric sequelae of low birth weight, correlated sleep disturbance, and anxious/depressive symptoms in children at the age of 6, as well as the predictive value of sleep disturbance in anxious/depressive symptoms at the age of 11. At both ages 6 and 11, maternal report of difficulty sleeping was significantly related to anxious/depressive symptoms in the children, though the relationship was somewhat stronger at age 11. Trouble sleeping at age 6 was not predictive of anxious/depressive symptoms at age 11 in children who were not anxious/depressed at age 6. Unfortunately, this study is limited by the fact that only one question of difficulty sleeping was used in the analysis.

In a very long-term longitudinal study of children who were 6–23 years of age (mean age = 16 years) at baseline data collection, Ong and colleagues [11] found that those whose parents reported that they had poor sleep rhythmicity as young children, defined as having non-regular sleep habits prior to age 6, were significantly more likely to have adolescent-onset MDD or anxiety disorders, such as generalized anxiety disorder, obsessive-compulsive disorder, post-traumatic stress disorder (PTSD), panic disorder, agoraphobia, simple phobia, or social phobia when interviewed with the Schedule for Affective Disorders and Schizophrenia-Lifetime Version (SADS-L) or the Kiddie-SADS, depending upon the age of the participant. On the other hand, no early childhood temperament domain was predictive of adult-onset mood disturbance.

In a large (>2000 subjects) longitudinal study in Holland, 14 years after being rated as sleeping less than others, being overtired, and having difficulty sleeping as children (mean age = 9), young adults were significantly more likely to report symptoms of anxiety and depression than their peers who had not evidenced such sleep difficulties in childhood. Parental reports of sleeping less than other children also predicted aggressive behavior in young adulthood and remained the most robust predictor of future emotional difficulties [12]. Similarly, using computer-assisted personal interviews and self-administered questionnaires from managed care enrollment rosters, adolescents with self-reports of insomnia were significantly more likely to have symptoms of

depression 1 year later, even when controlling for insomnia at the second time point [13]. Also, in a longitudinal twin study, sleep problems in 8-year-old children were predictive of depressive symptoms at age 10. Conversely, depressive symptoms at age 8 were not predictive of sleep problems at age 10. Thus, the authors suggest early treatment of sleep disturbance may provide a protection against later development of depressive symptoms [14].

There is some evidence that depressive symptoms in adolescents may be predictive of persistent sleep problems. In a very large cohort of adolescents, those with depressive symptoms at both the initial interview and 4 years later had the highest rate of sleep problems, while those with no depressive symptoms at either time point had the lowest rates. Those who had depressive symptoms at baseline that were no longer present at the 4-year follow-up also had higher rates of sleep problems at the follow-up time point than those who had not experienced depressive symptoms at baseline [15].

Sleep architecture in pediatric depression

While adults with depression tend to show consistent differences in their sleep architecture from healthy adults, including reduced slow-wave sleep (SWS), shortened REM latency, and increased sleep fragmentation [16], depressed children and adolescents tend to show very discrepant findings with respect to sleep architecture. In this section, we will provide a pertinent overview of sleep architecture in pediatric depression. For a detailed review of polysomnographic findings in this population, the reader is directed to the review by Ivanenko and colleagues [17].

Several studies have failed to show any significant differences in sleep architecture between children with depression and their healthy peers [3,18–20]. However, when subgroups in one study were analyzed, prepubertal children with more severe depression had reduced REM latency, a higher percentage of REM sleep, and less stage 4 sleep, similar to findings in depressed adults [19]. To explain these findings, Dahl and colleagues have hypothesized that sleep in children and adolescents with depression may be more "protected" than the sleep of depressed adults due to their greater likelihood of having more SWS and greater sleep efficiency than adults, and thus changes in sleep architecture are seen only in more severe cases of pediatric depression [19].

On the other hand, other polysomnographic studies found depressed children have significantly more sleep disturbance than healthy peers, including increased sleep onset latency, more stage 1 sleep, decreased REM latency, increased REM density (number of eye movements/time in REM sleep), increased percentage of REM sleep, and more frequent arousals [21–24]. Furthermore, as depressed children and adolescents age, REM density may decrease [21]. Sleep in children after remission of depressive symptoms has also revealed shorter REM latency and increased REM periods than when they were depressed (and in comparison to healthy peers) which is opposite the trend seen in adults in which REM latency increases towards the normal range with resolution of depressive symptoms [8].

In a meta-analysis of 27 polysomnographic studies of children and adolescents with depression, Knowles and MacLean [25] conclude that polysomnographically measured sleep disruption appears to increase as a function of age in this population. In their analysis, a linear relationship emerged between age and sleep architecture differences (total sleep time, minutes awake, sleep efficiency, percentage of SWS, and REM latency) between depressed patients and healthy controls.

Most likely as a function of these age-related increases in sleep disruption, depressed adolescents have sleep architecture more similar to that of depressed adults with reduced REM latency [26–30] and delayed sleep onset [29,31–33]. Analyses of subgroups of these patients have revealed that those who are suicidal and/or hospitalized as psychiatric inpatients have longer sleep latencies, shortened REM latency, increased REM density, and increased percentage of REM sleep than normal controls [34]. Those with psychotic features also had increased sleep latency in comparison to outpatient depressed adolescents [35], and those with non-endogenous depression exhibited increased wake after sleep onset (WASO) and lower sleep efficiency [32]. Although the imposed sleep schedules of the inpatient environment may directly influence REM latency in hospitalized depressed adolescents [28], when all adolescent patients studied had imposed schedules, increased sleep onset latency and decreased REM latency remained in the more severely depressed adolescents, supporting the hypothesis that these are true sleep-related features of adolescent depression [34].

Additional data explaining the inconsistent findings in sleep architecture differences between depressed and healthy children and adolescents reveal an interaction of gender and age. In a large study of 8- to 18-year-old pediatric patients with depression and their healthy peers, depressed adolescent males had the most sleep disturbance in comparison to the other groups, with more stage 1 sleep, decreased REM latency, decreased percentage of SWS, and increased frequency of arousals. Girls with depression did not appear to differ significantly from their healthy peers. Interestingly, chronological age appeared to explain the differences in sleep architecture better than did Tanner staging [36].

Corroboration between depressed children's subjective report of sleep quality and polysomnographic findings revealed inconsistencies between subjective and objective measures of sleep. Depressed children aged 8–17 years self-reported significantly poorer sleep quality, more difficulty rising in the morning, more nocturnal awakenings, and greater WASO than healthy peers. However, polysomnography demonstrated subjects with MDD had fewer awakenings and less WASO than their healthy peers, in contrast to their subjective report of more frequent and longer awakenings. When the authors performed spectral analysis (quantification of EEG frequencies) on a subset of the children's EEG data, there were no differences between the depressed and healthy groups on any measure. The authors hypothesized that this subjective–objective disparity may have been related to the children's depressogenic negative bias regarding the quality of their sleep or to their increased sensitivity to sleep disruptions. A complementary explanation provided by the authors was that children may exhibit an increased need for sleep during a depressive episode, thereby worsening their perception of sleep that appears "normal" in relation to healthy controls [37].

Predictive value of sleep architecture in future depression

As sleep complaints have been hypothesized to predict future development of depression (discussed above), alterations in sleep architecture have also been posited as a predictor of future depressive episodes. Rao and colleagues [38] found that healthy controls who developed depression 7 years after their initial polysomnography exhibited significantly higher REM density at baseline than those who did not develop depression. When investigating the premorbid sleep of adolescents who had no history of depression at the time of their polysomnography but developed depression 10–15 years later, Goetz and colleagues [39] found that latent depressive subjects had longer sleep onset latencies and sleep period time (similar to adolescents with depression at baseline) than those who did not later develop depression. Finally, in a cohort of depressed children and adolescents, increased sleep onset latency and decreased sleep efficiency at baseline were predictive of earlier recurrence of depression after remission [40].

Sleep microarchitecture in pediatric depression

Several studies utilizing power spectral analysis to examine EEG microarchitecture, which allows for a more detailed analysis of the sleep EEG by analyzing its component frequencies, show changes in adults with depression. Similarly, newer studies of microarchitecture of depressed children's and adolescents' sleep reveal distinctions. Specifically, these studies examine the degree to which the brain is organized by examining the correlation of brain activity across regions of the brain and across EEG rhythms. While children and adolescents with depression demonstrate lower intrahemispheric beta and delta coherence than their healthy peers [24,41–42], only depressed adolescents show lower interhemispheric coherence [24,41]. Depressed females, in particular, have lower temporal coherence than depressed males [24,41–42]. Depressed adolescent girls have lower right hemisphere coherence than their healthy counterparts; whereas, depressed adolescent boys do not differ from their peers [24]. Furthermore, intrahemispheric coherence values have greater variability among the depressed children and adolescents than healthy controls. When looking specifically at left hemisphere coherence, adolescent depressed girls had lower coherence than their healthy peers. This is interesting, given the previously discussed sleep macroarchitectural (e.g. using standard polysomnographic variables) differences noted more in depressed boys than in girls [36].

Predictive value of sleep microarchitecture in future depression

Temporal coherence of EEG findings may predict recovery or recurrence in depressed children and adolescents. In a 1-year naturalistic study of children

and adolescents with MDD, those who did not recover from their depressive episode 1 year after their initial polysomnography had the lowest degree of temporal coherence, followed by those who recurred within a year, while those who recovered and did not recur 1 year later had the greatest degree of temporal coherence [43]. More specifically, temporal coherence was more strongly related to time to recurrence of depression in boys; whereas, in girls it was more strongly related to time to recovery [43]. Adolescent females without a history of depression, but who were considered at high risk given a maternal history of depression, demonstrated lower temporal EEG coherence than healthy counterparts. As a result, Morehouse and colleagues [44] hypothesized that EEG coherence may be useful in predicting the onset and course of depression.

Alteration of circadian rhythms in adolescent depression

Markers of circadian rhythmicity, including rest–activity patterns assessed using actigraphy and hormonal markers, may be altered in pediatric depression. Circadian rhythm amplitude has also been shown to be disrupted in pediatric depression with both preadolescent and adolescent depressed girls having lower amplitude circadian rhythms, even when controlling for total activity level, indicating poorer entrainment to the 24-hour day and/or decreased exposure to environmental cues; while depressed adolescent boys showed higher circadian rhythm amplitude. As a group, depressed adolescents have decreased activity levels and lower light exposure than their healthy peers. As a result, it is possible that increasing light exposure may serve to improve the circadian rhythm and activity level of depressed pediatric patients [45].

While depressed children and adolescents overall have similar nocturnal cortisol secretion patterns to their healthy peers [46,47], the findings related to cortisol secretion in specific groups of depressed children and adolescents is less clear. In one study, suicidal and inpatient depressed adolescents were more likely to show a disrupted pattern of evening cortisol secretion during the typical quiescent period and significantly later cortisol nadir than non-suicidal patients [48]. However, another study demonstrated no difference in cortisol secretion between suicidal and non-suicidal children and adolescents during sleep; however, depressed adolescents did exhibit higher cortisol secretion in the hour preceding sleep onset than depressed children [49].

Sleep and pediatric bipolar disorder

Subjective sleep complaints in children with bipolar disorder

Pediatric bipolar disorder remains a somewhat poorly understood phenomenon. While the criteria utilized to diagnose bipolar disorder are consistent across pediatric and adult populations, the symptoms expressed in children are often very different from those seen in adults. Children frequently exhibit more rapid-cycling mood changes and are more likely to present with mixed states of depression and mania [50]. Fewer studies have clearly delineated sleep disruption in pediatric bipolar disorder compared to pediatric depression and anxiety. This may be in part due to the difficulty diagnosing bipolar disorder in children, as children and adolescents who eventually develop bipolar disorder are often initially diagnosed with either ADHD or unipolar depression.

Decreased need for sleep is a hallmark feature of manic episodes in both adults and children. In fact, a decreased need for sleep may be a symptom of high diagnostic value in pediatric bipolar disorder [51] with approximately 40–72% of children experiencing a manic episode reporting a significantly decreased need for sleep during a manic episode in comparison to only 6% of children with ADHD and 1% of healthy children [52–54]. As a result, sleep disruption has been proposed as an effective tool for discriminating between ADHD and bipolar disorder in children [52,55].

Insomnia is a significant symptom of concern during depressive episodes of bipolar disorder, with 82% of families reporting sleep problems during their child's worst depressive episode [53]. Almost all children with bipolar disorder report moderate to severe sleep problems, including bedtime resistance, difficulty initiating sleep, sleep-related anxiety, nocturnal awakenings, parasomnias, excessive daytime sleepiness, and decreased need for sleep, either at the time of the assessment or during their worst manic or depressive episode, with 96–99% of children and/or parents reporting sleep disruption [53,56]. Sleep disruption is most commonly reported during mixed depressive-manic states, with 89% reporting sleep

disruption during this time. Interestingly, in childhood bipolar disorder, parents' and children's reports of sleep problems are very discrepant, with children reporting sleep problems that parents do not report almost a third of the time [53], underscoring the importance of obtaining child self-report when assessing sleep in this population.

Objective assessment of sleep in bipolar disorder

Very few studies have directly assessed the objective sleep of children with diagnosed bipolar disorder. In an attempt to characterize the sleep of adolescents with incident depression who were later diagnosed with bipolar disorder, Rao and colleagues [30] reassessed the sleep of 24 depressed adolescents 7 years following their initial polysomnography. Of those, 5 had converted to bipolar disorder over the course of the 7 years, while 19 maintained a unipolar depression diagnosis. Upon re-analysis of the polysomnography data, those who converted to bipolar disorder had significantly more stage 1 sleep than healthy controls or adolescents who maintained a unipolar depression diagnosis. Interestingly, those who developed bipolar disorder maintained an REM sleep profile more similar to the healthy controls than did the adolescents with unipolar depression.

Sleep and pediatric anxiety

Subjective sleep complaints in anxiety

Anxiety is closely tied to hypervigilance and hyperarousability, which inhibit sleep [57]. As a result, anxiety clearly is related to sleep disruption in children. A reciprocal relationship between anxiety and sleep has been posited, in which increased anxiety contributes to sleep disruption, which then exacerbates the anxiety, further disrupting sleep [58].

Anxious children tend to report broad-based sleep difficulties with problems initiating and maintaining sleep, as well as sleep-related anxieties, such as bedtime fears and nightmares. Sleep-related fears are also common in children without anxiety disorders, and up to 75% of healthy children between the ages of 4 and 12 report bedtime fears [59]. Parent-reported sleep problems significantly correlate with child self-reports of environmental fears [60]. While parents tend to report significant relationships between their child's anxiety and experience of nightmares, children do not mirror this report. In fact, there has been no difference found in children's self-report of anxiety between those who reported experiencing nightmares and those who did not. Instead, children report a significant relationship between anxiety and the distress caused by their nightmares, rather than the experience of the nightmare itself [61].

When specific sleep complaints are assessed, 83–92% of children with anxiety disorders report at least one sleep-related complaint [58,62–63]. Among those with generalized anxiety disorder (GAD), 42–56% of children and 49–57% of adolescents report trouble sleeping [64,65]. The most common sleep complaints noted by parents of children with GAD include nightmares, being overtired, and trouble sleeping [62]. Two-thirds of a general population of children with anxiety disorders report insomnia, and over half report frequent nightmares. Sixty-one percent of anxious children aged 6–11 reported refusing to sleep alone, and they were significantly more likely to endorse this complaint than were anxious 12- to 17-year-olds [58]. Nightmares were more frequently reported by anxious girls and by younger children [58,63].

When parental report of children's daytime behavior was compared with sleep complaints, those with anxiety symptoms were significantly more likely to have night-time awakenings, sleep with their lights on, require a security object for sleep, have bedtime fears, require prolonged night-time rituals, and to have nightmares. These associations were hypothesized to be a result of increased arousal and hypervigilance associated with anxiety that interrupts sleep [1]. Of note, when anxious children's self-report of sleep problems was compared with their polysomnographically recorded sleep, they exhibited a tendency to under-report problems. While they had disrupted sleep with repeated, prolonged awakenings, they did not report any greater problems with sleep maintenance than their peers. However, they did accurately report prolonged sleep onset latency [20].

Among children and adolescents with obsessive-compulsive disorder, girls and adolescents were significantly more likely to be reported by their parents as sleeping more than other children [63]. Alfano and colleagues found that higher numbers of sleep-related problems were significantly predictive of impaired

home functioning, even when the severity of anxiety was statistically controlled [58]. When the children were treated with family-based cognitive behavioral therapy, sleep problems significantly decreased, with specific reductions in nightmares, being overtired, sleeping less and more than other children, difficulty sleeping, and requiring the presence of another person to sleep [63].

Sleep characteristics in children with PTSD

Sleep complaints are a hallmark feature of PTSD. Children and adolescents with PTSD report frequent nightmares and increased nocturnal anxiety, with difficulty initiating and maintaining sleep [66–68]. Abuse frequently occurs at night, and as bedtime approaches children who have been traumatized may feel increasingly anxious and unsafe. Hypervigilance due to fear leads to persistent sleep continuity disruption [69]. Several attempts have been made to objectively characterize sleep in children with a history of abuse. Results of actigraphic monitoring indicated poorer sleep efficiency, increased nocturnal activity, and reduced quiet sleep among children who were abused compared to non-abused children or children with other psychiatric disorders [70,71]. Recurrent nightmares and flashbacks of traumatic events are frequently experienced by both children and adults with PTSD.

While acute traumatization is associated with increased arousal and reduced/fragmented sleep, longstanding significant stressors may lead to increased sleep. Type II trauma, as described by Terr, which is characterized by chronic overwhelming stress, may cause symptoms of dissociation, apathy, denial, and excessive sleepiness [69,72].

Objective sleep disturbance in anxiety disorders

Fewer polysomnographic data are available in children and adolescents with anxiety disorders than those with depression. The polysomnographic studies that have been conducted, however, generally reveal that children and adolescents with anxiety disorders have poorer sleep than depressed children and adolescents, exhibiting longer sleep onset latency, more nocturnal awakenings, and decreased SWS. Furthermore, one study demonstrated that healthy controls and depressed children and adolescents showed adaptation to the sleep laboratory with decreased REM latency from Night 1 to Night 2, whereas anxious children and adolescents did not exhibit such adaptation [20]. Children's self-report of anxiety symptoms were positively correlated with sleep onset latency and negatively correlated with stage 3 sleep and self-report of ease of waking and sleep quality [20]. Furthermore, children with obsessive-compulsive disorder exhibited reduced total sleep time as well as reduced non-REM sleep and decreased REM onset latency in comparison to healthy peers [73].

Besides polysomnographic evidence of sleep disturbance in children with anxiety disorders, the rhythmicity of the HPA axis may also be affected. Children with anxiety disorders have significantly altered nocturnal cortisol secretion with higher peri-sleep-onset cortisol secretion, an initially slower rise in cortisol secretion, followed by a quick rise later in the night [47,49]. In the middle of the night, children with anxiety disorders have lower levels of cortisol than their peers. Of note, in these studies, children with anxiety disorders initiated sleep significantly later than control children, which may have affected the timing of nocturnal cortisol secretion [47].

Predictive value of sleep problems in future anxiety

Persistent sleep disruption in children may be more strongly related to incident anxiety than depression. In a large longitudinal study of 943 children, those with ongoing sleep disturbance were significantly more likely to have internalizing problems during childhood at ages 5, 7, and 9 years. Children who had persistent sleep problems across the assessment time points were also significantly more likely to have anxiety in adulthood at the ages of 21 and 26 than those who had not experienced persistent sleep problems. This predictive value remained constant even after controlling for gender, socioeconomic status, and internalizing symptoms in childhood. However, persistent sleep problems in childhood were not predictive of adult depression in this study [74]. Furthermore, in another longitudinal study, children with sleep problems at 4 years of age were significantly more likely to have symptoms of anxiety and depression as adolescents; whereas, those with depression/anxiety in early childhood were not more likely to exhibit future sleep problems in adolescence. This overlap between sleep problems and anxious/depressed symptoms appeared to become more robust as the children aged [75].

Treatment of sleep disturbances in children with mood and anxiety disorders

Despite a high prevalence of sleep complaints among children and adolescents with psychiatric morbidities, there are currently no well-designed, large-scale systematic studies on the effective treatments of sleep disturbances associated with early-onset mood and anxiety disorders. Clinical research, however, indicates that successful treatment of primary psychiatric disorders results in significant improvement of sleep-related symptoms such as sleep initiation and maintenance insomnia, nocturnal fears, and nightmares.

Non-pharmacological treatments have been shown to be effective for both primary and co-morbid insomnias in adults [76–78] and have been used for children with symptomatic insomnia related to mood and anxiety disorders. Adult research also suggests that concurrent treatment of insomnia and depressive disorders improves outcomes and may prevent further recurrence of major depression [79–80].

Several multidisciplinary consensus groups have formulated a rational approach to pharmacological treatment of pediatric insomnia, emphasizing a non-pharmacological treatment being the first choice intervention for children and adolescents with insomnia [81–82].

Sleep hygiene education emphasizing the importance of consistent age-appropriate bedtime and night-time routine should be provided to every family seeking help for sleep-related problems in their children. Night-time fears are commonly precipitated by watching frightening movies and/or television programs. Avoiding exposure to television, computer games, and child-inappropriate websites close to bedtime and creating soothing and safe environments for the child significantly reduces nocturnal anxiety. Other therapeutic interventions with systemic desensitization to fears, exposure and response prevention with imagery exercises, and dream rehearsal techniques have been shown to be effective in treating nightmares and bedtime fears in children [83].

Pharmacological interventions may be warranted in cases when the child does not adequately respond to behavioral interventions, and/or parents are unable to implement recommended behavioral interventions. Medication may be considered for the treatment of insomnia within the context of the co-morbid psychiatric disorder. Once pharmacological treatment for insomnia is chosen, it should be short term, and clinicians should encourage regular and consistent follow-up visits with re-evaluation of target insomnia symptoms and assessment of compliance. Rational selection of pharmacological agents should be based on the presenting complaint, pharmacological properties of the drug, drug–drug interactions, safety profile of the drug, potential side-effects, and formulations available. Since a detailed description of pharmacotherapy of pediatric insomnia is beyond the scope of this chapter, the reader is referred to a recent review by Owens et al. [82] for further details.

There are no strong evidence-based treatment recommendations for insomnia associated with depression in youth. SSRIs are effectively used in the treatment of depression and anxiety disorders in pediatric patients. However, very little is known about their influence on children's subjective or objective sleep. Fluoxetine is a potent REM suppressant in adults and increases NREM sleep, frequency of arousals, periodic limb movements, and oculomotor abnormalities such as moderately fast eye movements in NREM sleep [84]. A small sample of only six children with major depression underwent nocturnal polysomnography during the course of treatment with fluoxetine [85]. These children exhibited increased stage 1 sleep, an elevated number of arousals, and oculomotor and myoclonic changes similar to adults. Interestingly, REM suppression was not seen in children treated with fluoxetine. Most children in this study reported poorer sleep quality and increased sleep fragmentation with SSRI treatment. On the other hand, when anxious children were treated with fluvoxamine, they exhibited significant reductions in both insomnia and refusal to sleep alone [58].

Concomitant use of a sedative agent and SSRI was explored in one retrospective study conducted in a group of adolescents with MDD. Patients were treated with either a combination of fluoxetine and trazodone or fluoxetine alone [86]. According to self-reports, insomnia resolved sooner in subjects treated

with combination therapy. However, the analysis of the clinical course of illness revealed that the difference between the two groups was not clinically significant.

While the use of trazodone has been observed to have therapeutic effects on symptoms of insomnia, it should be used with caution in combination with fluoxetine, as there have been reports of potential side-effects due to drug–drug interaction [87–88]. Several patients treated with a combination of fluoxetine and trazodone had to discontinue trazodone due to intolerable adverse drug reactions or because of excessive sleepiness.

In summary, sleep hygiene and cognitive behavioral therapies for insomnia should be utilized prior to considering pharmacological interventions in children and adolescents with sleep problems associated with anxiety and mood disorders. There are no FDA-approved agents for the treatment of pediatric insomnia, with very limited evidence-based research available on the effective use of medications with sedative properties in the treatment of co-morbid insomnia in children with psychiatric disorders. Choosing a pharmacological agent should be individualized based on the type of sleep problem, primary psychiatric disorder, patient's individual characteristics, family dynamics, and the pharmacological properties of currently available drugs.

Summary

Sleep disruption is a hallmark feature of both mood and anxiety disorders in children and adolescents. While the objective data is somewhat discrepant among children with mood disorders, adolescents clearly show disrupted sleep patterns, particularly in regards to REM sleep. Children and adolescents with anxiety experience significantly more disrupted sleep than their healthy peers. Interestingly, while depressed children and adolescents self-report more disrupted sleep than seen on polysomnography, anxious pediatric patients have a tendency to under-report their sleep disruption. In addition to the concurrent sleep disruption noted in children and adolescents with mood and anxiety disorders, early sleep disturbance may serve as a predictor of future mood and anxiety problems. Because sleep and mood have a bidirectional relationship, the assessment of sleep complaints among children with mood and anxiety disorders is essential.

References

1. Ivanenko A, Crabtree VM, O'Brien LM, Gozal D. Sleep complaints and psychiatric symptoms in children evaluated at a pediatric mental health clinic. *J Clin Sleep Med.* 2006;**15**:42–48.

2. Dahl RE. The development and disorders of sleep. *Adv Pediatr.* 1998;**45**:73–90.

3. Puig-Antich J, Goetz R, Hanlon C, et al. Sleep architecture and REM sleep measures in prepubertal children with major depression: A controlled study. *Arch Gen Psychiatry.* 1982;**39**:932–939.

4. Liu X, Buysse DJ, Gentzler AL, et al. Insomnia and hypersomnia associated with depressive phenomenology and comorbidity in childhood depression. *Sleep.* 2007;**30**:83–90.

5. Ryan ND, Puig-Antich J, Ambrosini P, et al. The clinical picture of major depression in children and adolescents. *Arch Gen Psychiatry.* 1987;**44**:854–861.

6. Whalen DJ, Silk JS, Semel M, et al. Caffeine consumption, sleep, and affect in the natural environments of depressed youth and healthy controls. *J Pediatr Psychol.* 2008;**33**:358–367.

7. Gregory AM, Rijsdijk FV, Dahl RE, McGuffin P, Eley TC. Associations between sleep problems, anxiety, and depression in twins at 8 years of age. *Pediatrics.* 2006;**118**:1124–1132.

8. Puig-Antich J, Goetz R, Hanlon C, et al. Sleep architecture and REM sleep measures in prepubertal major depressives: Studies during recovery from the depressive episode in a drug-free state. *Arch Gen Psychiatry.* 1983;**40**:187–192.

9. Roberts RE, Lewinsohn PM, Seeley JR. Symptoms of DSM-III-R major depression in adolescence: Evidence from an epidemiological survey. *J Am Acad Child Adolesc Psychiatry.* 1995;**34**:1608–1617.

10. Johnson EO, Chilcoat HD, Breslau N. Trouble sleeping and anxiety/depression in childhood. *Psych Res.* 2000;**94**:93–102.

11. Ong SH, Wickramaratne P, Tang M, Weissman MM. Early childhood sleep and eating problems as predictors of adolescent and adult mood and anxiety disorders. *J Affect Dis.* 2006;**96**:1–8.

12. Gregory AM, Van der Ende J, Willis TA, Verhulst FC. Parent-reported sleep problems during development and self-reported anxiety/depression, attention problems, and aggressive behavior later in life. *Arch Pediatr Adolesc Med.* 2008;**162**:330–335.

13. Roberts RE, Roberts CR, Chen IG. Impact of insomnia on future functioning of adolescents. *J Psychosom Res.* 2002;**53**:561–569.

14. Gregory AM, Rijsdijk FV, Lau JYF, Dahl RE, Eley TC. The direction of longitudinal associations between sleep problems and depression symptoms: A study of twins aged 8 and 10 years. *Sleep.* 2009;**32**:189–199.

15. Patten CA, Choi WS, Gillin JC, Pierce JP. Depressive symptoms and cigarette smoking predict development and persistence of sleep problems in US adolescents. *Pediatrics.* 2000;**106**:e23.

16. Benca RM. Mood disorders. In: Kryger MH, Roth T, Dement WC, eds. *Principles and practice of sleep medicine*, 3rd ed. Philadelphia: WB Saunders; 2000:1140–1157.

17. Ivanenko A, Crabtree VM, Gozal D. Sleep and depression in children and adolescents. *Sleep Med Rev.* 2005;**9**:115–129.

18. Young W, Knowles JB, MacLean AW, Boag L, McConville BJ. The sleep of childhood depressives: comparison with age-matched controls. *Biol Psychiatry.* 1982;**17**:1163–1168.

19. Dahl RE, Ryan ND, Birmaher B, et al. Electroencephalographic sleep measures in prepubertal depression. *Psychol Res.* 1991;**38**:201–214.

20. Forbes EE, Bertocci MA, Gregory AM, et al. Objective sleep in pediatric anxiety disorders and major depressive disorder. *J Am Acad Child Adolesc Psychiatry.* 2008;**47**:148–155.

21. Lahmeyer HW, Poznanski EO, Bellu SN. EEG sleep in depressed adolescents. *Am J Psychiatry.* 1983;**40**:1150–1153.

22. Emslie GJ, Rush AJ, Weinberg WA, Rintelmann JW, Roffwarg HP. Children with major depression show reduced rapid eye movement latencies. *Arch Gen Psychiatry.* 1990;**47**:119–124.

23. Arana-Lechuga Y, Nuñez-Ortiz R, Terán-Pérez G, et al. Sleep-EEG patterns of school children suffering from symptoms of depression compared to healthy controls. *World J Biol Psychiatry.* 2008;**9**:115–120.

24. Armitage R, Emslie GJ, Hoffmann RF, et al. Ultradian rhythms and temporal coherence in sleep EEG in depressed children and adolescents. *Biol Psychiatry.* 2000;**47**:338–350.

25. Knowles JB, MacLean AW. Age-related changes in sleep in depressed and healthy subjects. *Neuropsychopharmacology.* 1990;**3**:251–259.

26. Emslie GJ, Roffwarg HP, Rush AJ, et al. Sleep EEG findings in depressed children and adolescents. *Am J Psychiatry.* 1987;**144**:668–670.

27. Emslie GJ, Rush AJ, Weinberg WA, Rintelmann J, Roffwarg HP. Sleep EEG features of adolescents with major depression. *Biol Psychiatry.* 1994;**36**:573–581.

28. Goetz RR, Puig-Antich J, Dahl RE, et al. EEG sleep of young adults with major depression: A controlled study. *J Affect Disord*. 1991;**22**:91–100.

29. Dahl RE, Ryan ND, Matty MK, et al. Sleep onset abnormalities in depressed adolescents. *Biol Psychiatry*. 1996;**39**:400–410.

30. Rao U, Dahl RE, Ryan ND, et al. Heterogeneity in EEG sleep findings in adolescent depression: Unipolar versus bipolar clinical course. *J Affect Disord*. 2002;**70**:273–280.

31. Armitage R, Hoffmann R. Sleep electrophysiology of major depressive disorders. *Curr Rev Mood Anxiety Disord*. 1997;**1**:139–151.

32. Goetz RR, Puig-Antich J, Ryan N, et al. Electroencephalographic sleep of adolescents with major depression and normal controls. *Arch Gen Psychiatry*. 1987;**44**:61–68.

33. Williamson DE, Dahl RE, Birmaher B, et al. Stressful life events and EEG sleep in depressed and normal control adolescents. *Biol Psychiatry*. 1995;**37**:859–865.

34. Dahl RE, Puig-Antich J, Ryan ND, et al. EEG sleep in adolescents with major depression: The role of suicidality and inpatient status. *J Affect Disord*. 1990;**19**:63–75.

35. Naylor MW, Shain BN, Shipley JE. REM latency in psychotically depressed adolescents. *Biol Psychiatry*. 1990;**28**:161–164.

36. Robert JJT, Hoffman RF, Emslie GJ, et al. Sex and age differences in sleep macroarchitecture in childhood and adolescent depression. *Sleep*. 2006;**29**:351–358.

37. Bertocci MA, Dahl RE, Williamson DE, et al. Subjective sleep complaints in pediatric depression: A controlled study and comparison with EEG measures of sleep and waking. *J Am Acad Child Adolesc Psychiatry*. 2005;**44**:1158–1166.

38. Rao U, Dahl RE, Ryan ND, et al. The relationship between longitudinal clinical course and sleep and cortisol changes in adolescent depression. *Biol Psychiatry*. 1996;**40**:474–484.

39. Goetz RR, Wolk SI, Coplan JD, Ryan ND, Weissman MM. Premorbid polysomnographic signs in depressed adolescents: A reanalysis of EEG sleep after longitudinal follow-up in adulthood. *Biol Psychiatry*. 2001;**49**:930–942.

40. Emslie GJ, Armitage R, Weinberg WA, et al. Sleep polysomnography as a predictor of recurrence in children and adolescents with depressive disorder. *Int J Neuropsychopharmacol*. 2001;**4**:159–168.

41. Armitage R, Emslie GJ, Hoffman RF, Rintelmann J, Rush AJ. Delta sleep EEG in depressed adolescent females and healthy controls. *J Affect Disord*. 2001;**63**:139–148.

42. Armitage R, Hoffmann R, Emslie G, Rintelmann J, Robert J. Sleep microarchitecture in childhood and adolescent depression: Temporal coherence. *Clin EEG Neurosci*. 2006;**37**:1–9.

43. Armitage R, Hoffman RF, Emslie GJ, et al. Sleep microarchitecture as a predictor of recurrence in children and adolescents with depression. *Int J Neuropsychopharmacol*. 2002;**5**:217–228.

44. Morehouse RL, Kusumakar V, Kutcher SP, LeBlanc J, Armitage R. Temporal coherence in ultradian sleep EEG rhythms in a never-depressed, high-risk cohort of female adolescents. *Biol Psychiatry*. 2002;**51**:446–456.

45. Armitage R, Hoffmann R, Emslie G, et al. Rest-activity cycles in childhood and adolescent depression. *J Am Acad Child Adolesc Psychiatry*. 2004;**43**:761–769.

46. Kutcher S, Malkin D, Silverberg J, et al. Nocturnal cortisol, thyroid stimulating hormone, and growth hormone secretory profiles in depressed adolescents. *J Am Acad Child Adolesc Psychiatry*. 1991;**30**:407–414.

47. Feder A, Coplan JD, Goetz RR, et al. Twenty-four-hour cortisol secretion patterns in prepubertal children with anxiety or depressive disorders. *Biol Psychiatry*. 2004;**56**:198–204.

48. Dahl RE, Ryan ND, Puig-Antich J, et al. 24-hour cortisol measures in adolescents with major depression: A controlled study. *Biol Psychiatry*. 1991;**30**:25–36.

49. Forbes EE, Williamson DE, Ryan ND, et al. Peri-sleep-onset cortisol levels in children and adolescents with affective disorders. *Biol Psychiatry*. 2006;**59**:24–30.

50. NIMH Roundtable. National Institute of Mental Health Research Roundtable on Prepubertal Bipolar Disorder. *J Am Acad Child Adolesc Psychiatry*. 2001;**40**:871–878.

51. Geller B, Zimmerman B, Williams M, et al. Phenomenology of prepubertal and early adolescent bipolar disorder: Examples of elated mood, grandiose behaviors, decreased need for sleep, racing thoughts, and hypersexuality. *J Child Adolesc Psychopharmacol*. 2002;**12**:3–9.

52. Geller B, Zimmerman B, Williams M, et al. DSM-IV mania symptoms in a prepubertal and early adolescent bipolar phenotype compared to attention-deficit hyperactive and normal controls. *J Child Adolesc Psychopharmacol*. 2002;**12**:11–25.

53. Lofthouse N, Fristad, M, Splaingard M, Kelleher M. Parent and child reports of sleep problems associated with early-onset bipolar spectrum disorders. *J Fam Psychol*. 2007;**21**:114–123.

54. Kowatch RA, Youngstrom EA, Danielyan A, Findling RL. Review and meta-analysis of the phenomenology and

clinical characteristics of mania in children and adolescents. *Bipolar Disorders*. 2005;7:483–496.

55. Meyers OI, Youngstrom EA. A parent general behavior inventory subscale to measure sleep disturbance in pediatric bipolar disorder. *J Clin Psychiatry*. 2008;**69**:840–843.

56. Lofthouse N, Fristad M, Splaingard M, et al. Web survey of sleep problems associated with early-onset bipolar spectrum disorders. *J Pediatr Psychol*. 2008;**33**:349–357.

57. Dahl RE. The regulation of sleep and arousal: Development and psychopathology. *Dev Psychopathol*. 1996;**8**:3–27.

58. Alfano CA, Ginsburg GS, Kingery JN. Sleep-related problems among children and adolescents with anxiety disorders. *J Am Acad Child Adolesc Psychiatry*. 2007;**46**:224–232.

59. Muris P, Merckelbach H, Gadet B, Moulaert V. Fears, worries, and scary dreams in 4- to 12-year-old children: Their content, developmental pattern, and origins. *J Clin Child Psychol*. 2000;**29**:43–52.

60. Dollinger SJ, Molina BS, Campo Monteiro JM. Sleep and anxieties in Brazilian children: The role of cultural and environmental factors in child sleep disturbance. *Am J Orthopsychiatry*. 1996;**66**: 252–261.

61. Mindell JA, Barrett KM. Nightmares and anxiety in elementary-aged children: Is there a relationship? *Child Care Health Dev*. 2002;**28**:317–322.

62. Alfano CA, Beidel DC, Turner SM, Lewin DS. Preliminary evidence for sleep complaints among children referred for anxiety. *Sleep Med*. 2006;7:467–473.

63. Storch EA, Murphy TK, Lack CW, et al. Sleep-related problems in pediatric obsessive-compulsive disorder. *J Anxiety Disord*. 2008;**22**:877–885.

64. Pina AA, Silverman WK, Alfano CA, Saavedra LM. Diagnostic efficiency of symptoms in the diagnosis of DSM-IV: Generalized anxiety disorder in youth. *J Child Psychol Psychiatry*. 2002;**43**:959–967.

65. Masi G, Millepiedi S, Mucci M, Poli P, Bertini N, Milantoni L. Generalized anxiety disorder in referred children and adolescents. *J Am Acad Child Adolesc Psychiatry*. 2004;**43**:752–760.

66. Pynoos RS, Frederick C, Nader K, et al. Life threat and posttraumatic stress in school-age children. *Arch Gen Psychiatry*. 1987;**44**:1057–1063.

67. Ross RJ, Ball WA, Sullivan KA, Caroff SN. Sleep disturbance as the hallmark of posttraumatic stress disorder. *Am J Psychiatry*. 1989;**146**:697–707.

68. Uhde TW. Anxiety disorders. In: Kryger MH, Roth T, Dement WC, eds. *Principles and practice of sleep medicine*, 3rd ed. Philadelphia:WB Saunders; 2000:1123–1139.

69. Sadeh A. Stress, trauma and sleep in children. *Child Adolesc Clin North Am*. 1996;**5**:685–700.

70. Teicher MH, Glod CA, Harper D, et al. Locomotor activity in depressed children and adolescents: I. Circadian dysregulation. *J Am Acad Child Adolesc Psychiatry*. 1993;**32**:760–769.

71. Glod CA, Teicher MH, Hartman CR, Harakal T. Increased nocturnal activity and impaired sleep maintenance in abused children. *J Am Acad Child Adolesc Psychiatry*. 1997;**36**:1236–1243.

72. Terr LC. Childhood traumas: An outline and overview. *Am J Psychiatry*. 1991;**148**:10–19.

73. Rapoport J, Elkins R, Langer DH, et al. Childhood obsessive-compulsive disorder. *Am J Psychiatry*. 1981;**138**:1545–1554.

74. Gregory AM, Caspi A, Eley TC, et al. Prospective longitudinal associations between persistent sleep problems in childhood and anxiety and depression disorders in adulthood. *J Abnorm Child Psychol*. 2005;**33**:157–163.

75. Gregory AM, O'Connor TG. Sleep problems in childhood: A longitudinal study of developmental change and association with behavioral problems. *J Am Acad Child Adolesc Psychiatry*. 2002;**41**: 964–971.

76. Kupfer DJ, Reynolds CF 3rd. Management of insomnia. *N Engl J Med*. 1997;**336**(5):341–346.

77. Morin CM, Bootzin RR, Buysse DJ, et al. Psychological and behavioral treatment of insomnia: update of the recent evidence (1998–2004). *Sleep*. 2006;**29**(11): 1398–1414.

78. Belanger L, Vallieres A, Ivers H, et al. Meta-analysis of sleep changes in control groups of insomnia treatment trials. *J Sleep Res*. 2007;**16**(1):77–84.

79. Kupfer DJ. Pathophysiology and management of insomnia during depression. *Ann Clin Psychiatry*. 1999;**11**(4):267–276.

80. Ivanenko A. Sleep and mood disorders in children and adolescents. In: Ivanenko A, ed. *Sleep and psychiatric disorders in children and adolescents*. New York: Informa Healthcare; 2008:279–287.

81. Mindell JA, Emslie G, Blumer J, et al. Pharmacologic management of insomnia in children and adolescents: consensus statement. *Pediatrics*. 2006;**117** (6):e1223–1232.

82. Owens JA, Babcock D, Blumer J, et al. The use of pharmacotherapy in the treatment of pediatric insomnia in primary care: rational approaches. A consensus meeting summary. *J Clin Sleep Med*. 2005;**1**(1):49–59.

83. Ollendick TH, Hagopian LP, Huntzinger RM. Cognitive-behavior therapy with nighttime fearful children. *J Behav Ther Exp Psychiatry*. 1991;**22**: 113–121.

84. Dorsey CM, Lukas SE, Cunningham SL. Fluoxetine-induced sleep disturbance in depressed patients. *Neuropsychopharmacology*. 1996;**14**:437–442.

85. Armitage R, Emslie G, Rintelmann J. The effect of fluoxetine on sleep EEG in childhood depression: a preliminary report. *Neuropharmacology*. 1997;**17**:241–245.

86. Kallepalli BR, Bhatara VS, Fogas BS, et al. Trazodone is only slightly faster than fluoxetine in relieving insomnia in adolescents with depressive disorders. *J Child Adolesc Psychopharmacol*. 1997;**7**:97–107.

87. Metz A, Shader RI. Adverse interactions encountered when using trazodone to treat insomnia associated with fluoxetine. *Int Clin Psychopharmacol*. 1990;**5** (3):191–194.

88. Nierenberg AA, Cole JO, Glass L. Possible trazodone potentiation of fluoxetine: a case series. *J Clin Psychiatry*. 1992;**53**(3):83–85.

Sleep in developmental disorders

Gregory Stores

Introduction

Sleep problems are all too common in children in general but their occurrence is significantly increased in certain "high risk" subgroups, notably children with a neurodevelopmental or psychiatric disorder and those with other chronic pediatric conditions [1]. As a generalization, it can be said that collectively it is usual in children and adolescents with such conditions for their problems (and those of their families) to be compounded by sleeping difficulties and their consequences. Sad to say, advice and treatment for these difficulties is often not provided [2,3] largely because both parents and professionals often do not know what might be done to help, which, in fact, can be considerable with proper assessment and accurate diagnosis.

The term "developmental disorders" is all-embracing and needs to be defined for the special purpose of this chapter. In practice, a distinction between psychiatric developmental disorders and neurodevelopmental disorders can be misleading because of overlap between the two. Children with autism, for example, may well be seen predominantly in child psychiatric services but the condition is now acknowledged to be fundamentally of neurological origin [4]. Also, some children with unquestionably neurological conditions can be referred to psychiatric rather than neurological services because the true nature of their condition has not been recognized. Childhood-onset narcolepsy is a prime example [5].

Genuinely "primary" childhood psychiatric disorders of mood and anxiety, as well as ADHD, are considered elsewhere in this book (see Chapter 21: Sleep in attention-deficit/hyperactivity disorder (ADHD) and Chapter 22: Sleep in pediatric mood and anxiety disorders). That still leaves many disorders of development where sleep problems can loom large. For a more comprehensive coverage of various types of developmental disorder than is possible here, the reader is referred elsewhere [1].

The present selection of conditions and the relative space devoted to them is largely dictated by a combination of current topicality and the availability of information about them, including recent reports. The emphasis throughout is on clinical sleep problems and disorders rather than physiological sleep features of uncertain clinical significance.

General issues

A number of basic general points are appropriate at this stage. Some apply to children's sleep disorders as a whole; others are particularly relevant to sleep disturbance associated with developmental disorders.

1. **Treatment of a sleep disturbance should not precede diagnosis of the underlying cause**. Although in most other forms of medical practice the distinction between a health problem or complaint and its underlying cause is axiomatic, this does not always apply in the management of sleep disturbance, as there are very many medical, neurological, and psychiatric disorders that may disturb sleep. Thus, the cause of the sleep disturbance may not be identified and attempts made to treat the problem symptomatically may prove unsuccessful and further obscure the underlying issue. An example is seen in some of the claims for the use of melatonin for sleeplessness in children with multiple handicaps where imprecise accounts of the nature of the sleep disturbance add to the difficulty of evaluating the results [6].

Foundations of Psychiatric Sleep Medicine, ed. John W. Winkelman and David T. Plante. Published by Cambridge University Press.
© Cambridge University Press 2010.

There are primarily three basic sleep complaints (sleeplessness or insomnia, excessive sleepiness, and parasomnias), The 2005 *International Classification of Sleep Disorders* [7] describes nearly 100 possible causes of sleep problems, many of which are encountered in children and adolescents. Advice and treatment essentially needs to be based on the nature of the individual child's sleep disorder.

2. **Children are not simply small adults**. Regarding sleep and its disorders there are many differences to consider, not only in basic sleep physiology and sleep requirements but also in the pattern of occurrence and clinical manifestations of sleep disorders, etiological factors (especially the role of parenting factors), and the significance and prognosis for the condition. Assessment procedures and diagnostic criteria (e.g. polysomnographic evaluation) as well as the role of medications in treatment are also often different.

3. **Practicing clinicians must appreciate the myriad ways in which sleep disorders may present in children.** Misinterpretation and misdiagnosis, likely to lead to inappropriate attempts to help, are a serious risk in people with sleep problems at any age [8], but this hazard is perhaps more pronounced in young people and, even more so, in those with developmental disorders.

For example, children with narcolepsy are prone to be misjudged because of the ways in which the condition may manifest itself and the child's reaction to having such a serious disorder [5]. Sleepiness can be misjudged as laziness, disinterest, opting out of difficult situations, depression, or limited intellect; cataplexy as attention seeking. Hallucinations and/or sleep paralysis may well induce night-time fears. Also, obstructive sleep apnea (OSA) is particularly relevant to children with developmental disorders because of its association with many learning disability (mental retardation) syndromes, as discussed later. As with other causes of excessive sleepiness, the sleep disruptive effects of OSA have for long been known to possibly cause significant learning and behavior problems, including ADHD-type symptoms, which might improve following relief of the obstruction, when possible [9].

As alluded to earlier, failure to recognize that the starting point of such psychological problems has, in fact, been a sleep disorder readily leads to inappropriate referral to educational or psychiatric services alone. The possibility that disturbed sleep might lie behind any child's psychological difficulties should be considered (alongside other more conventionally acknowledged influences) with appropriate enquiries about the child's sleep pattern and associated issues. This requires more attention being paid to sleep history-taking than is usual in clinical practice [10].

4. **Persistently disrupted sleep has wide-ranging adverse effects on mood, behavior, cognition, and social (including family) relationships**. This is true across the life-span – failure to thrive is an acknowledged possible complication of early childhood sleep disturbance [11] and some of the increasingly recognized physical effects of disrupted sleep reported in adults (e.g. hypertension, obesity, endocrine/gastrointestinal disorders) [12] may well also apply to children. In children with developmental disorders, sleep disruption may also exacerbate problems such as learning difficulty and behavior problems that are secondary to the developmental disorder itself.

The important practical point is that, although the child's underlying developmental disorder may be unalterable, attention paid successfully to the sleep disorder can be expected to lessen these complications. As far as possible, a distinction needs to be made between the effects of disrupted sleep and the influence of other factors. Mothers' well-being, in particular, and parent–child relationships are examples of important aspects of the situation that can suffer [13,14] but which also can be expected to improve following successful treatment of a child's sleep disorder [15,16].

5. **Children with developmental problems do not have a separate set of sleep disorders compared with other children**. It is the relative frequency of occurrence, balance between the different sleep disorders, severity, and (if untreated) persistence of such disorders that is often different. Convincing evidence for special forms of sleep disturbance as part of a neurodevelopmental "behavioral phenotype" is sparse [1].

Needless to say, treatment issues are a basic consideration. As in any patient, appropriate advice and choice of treatment out of the many types now possible depends essentially on the nature of a child's sleep disorder. However, efficacy may be different in the presence of a developmental disorder if only because of possible compliance problems, although this is often overstated.

It needs to be more generally understood that the sleep disorders of developmentally disordered children, in some cases, may be as treatable as in other children using the same means. If parents are disabused of the idea that serious sleep problems (and their consequences for the child and also their own well-being) are inevitable, the uptake of the available treatments, which is poor [2], would be improved. Of course, this would only be possible if there was a corresponding increased awareness by professionals of the various treatment possibilities. For example, there is still undue reliance on sedative drugs in the treatment of sleeplessness in small children despite the uncertainties associated with their use and other drawbacks [17]. In contrast, much more appropriate behavioral treatments, such as setting limits on uncooperative bedtime behavior, and gradually discouraging the child's dependence on his or her parents' presence when going to sleep at bedtime or after waking during the night, are underutilized [2].

Behavioral methods for treating sleeplessness can be effective in the management of sleep disturbance in all children (Table 23.1). Nevertheless, as there is a general impression that such methods are likely to be less successful in children with developmental disorders, much thought has recently been given to the use and further development of medications for this group [18,19]. Clearly, further research is needed in this area, including evaluation of the place of melatonin, about which uncertainty remains [20].

6. The possible complexity of factors which may influence the sleep of children with a developmental disorder should not be underestimated.
Disentangling the various factors requires careful analysis in order to define an appropriate treatment program. A combination of physical and behavioral factors is common in neurodevelopmental disorders giving rise to sleep disorders of both physical and behavioral types that call for more than one treatment approach.

Learning disability (mental retardation) is the most pervasive general influence on sleep in children with developmental disorders [21]. Surveys have consistently shown that sleep problems are particularly common in learning disabled children irrespective of the cause. Sleep physiology and basic sleep–wake patterns are severely disturbed if the degree of brain abnormality is extreme. Persistent sleeplessness (especially settling and night waking problems or early morning waking) is often associated with lesser degrees of brain dysfunction.

Neurodevelopmental disorders are often complicated by the types of *psychiatric disturbances* described in Chapter 21: Sleep in attention-deficit/hyperactivity disorder (ADHD) and Chapter 22: Sleep in pediatric mood and anxiety disorders or *epilepsy*. Disturbed sleep appears to be common in children with epilepsy although this will vary with the type of epilepsy and its severity [22]. Sleep may be disrupted or "fragmented" by nocturnal seizures, but other factors again include associated psychological problems or over-permissive parenting practices. Modern *antiepilepsy medication* does not generally disturb subjective sleep, which, in fact, is likely to be consolidated by improved seizure control.

Sensory deficits may also lead to sleep disturbance, especially severe visual impairment [23], because light perception is the main cue to day or night and, therefore, the principal factor in entraining sleep–wake rhythms. Blind children often have irregular or non-24-hour sleep–wake cycle disorders but, again, parenting factors or associated psychiatric disturbance may play a part in the development of various other sleep disorders. Hearing impairment has also been linked to sleep disturbance, including that apparently caused by the distressing effect of tinnitus at night [24].

Other general factors may operate to disturb sleep. *Physical deformity* or *immobility* can cause discomfort at night and some *medications* used in pediatrics and child psychiatry (such as bronchodilators, antihistamines, and stimulant drugs) at least have the reputation of affecting sleep and wakefulness. Children needing repeated *admission to hospital* face a further risk of sleep disturbance.

It follows from many of the points just made, and also what follows, that serious attention must be paid to sleep and its possible disturbance in the assessment of children with a developmental disorder. In clinical practice in general, the topic is neglected, with insufficient attention paid to history-taking, which usually, at best, includes very limited enquiries. Medical students have been reported to be taught very little about sleep and its disorders [25] and there is little evidence that matters have improved generally since that survey.

373

Table 23.1 Behavioral prevention and treatment options for disorders of initiating and maintaining sleep in children and adolescents [26,27]

Treatment/ preventative strategy	Description
Sleep hygiene	Basic recommendations for creating internal and external environment conducive to sleep in children:
	Bedroom environment
	• dark and quiet bedroom with temperature comfortably cool
	• minimization of environmental noise (potentially utilizing white noise)
	Food and fluids
	• avoidance of hunger prior to bedtime (appropriately timed snack may be useful)
	• avoidance of methylxanthine-containing foods (e.g. caffeinated beverages, chocolate) several hours prior to bedtime
	• avoidance of alcohol and caffeine (which can be additives in over-the-counter medications) that can disrupt sleep
	• avoidance of excessive fluids before bed which may lead to nocturnal enuresis
	The following recommendations apply differently depending on developmental level:
	Sleep/wake scheduling and behaviors
	• Consistent daytime and bedtime routines from an early age are important. Both parents must be consistent with each other
	• Promote influence of infants' biological clock in establishing their circadian sleep–wake rhythm. Can be achieved by emphasizing differences between night and day, and not prolonging night-time feeds beyond age at which feeding can physiologically be confined to daytime
	• Have gradual "wind down" period as bedtime approaches with avoidance of vigorous or stimulating activity or experiences
	• Children should learn to fall asleep alone and in same circumstances as they will experience when they wake in the night. This promotes "self-soothing" (i.e. ability to get back to sleep during the night without needing their parents' presence)
	• Set limits to resistant bedtime behavior
	• Only put down to sleep when ready for sleep ("sleepy tired") avoiding association between being in bed and being awake
	• Naps should be developmentally appropriate. Excessive napping, insufficient napping causing "overtiredness" at bedtime, and last nap close to bedtime can all lead to settling problems at bedtime
Unmodified extinction	Parents/caregivers put child to bed at designated bedtime, ignoring the child until morning (except parents do monitor for illness and safety). Goal is to decrease undesired behaviors (e.g. crying) by eliminating parental attention as a reinforcer
Graduated extinction	Parents/caregivers ignore bedtime crying/tantrums for predetermined periods before briefly checking on child. A progressive (graduated) or fixed checking schedule may be used. Goal is for child to develop "self-soothing" skills and be able to fall asleep independently without undesirable sleep associations
Stimulus control techniques	Target-reduced affective and physiological arousal at bedtime

Table 23.1 (cont.)

Treatment/ preventative strategy	Description
	• *Positive routines*: parents/caregivers develop a set of bedtime routines characterized by enjoyable and quiet activities to establish a behavioral pattern leading up to sleep onset
	• *Faded bedtime*: parents/caregivers temporarily delay bedtime to coincide with child's natural sleep onset time, gradually moving it earlier as the child gains success with falling asleep
	• *Response cost*: parents/caregivers remove the child from bed for brief periods if the child does not fall asleep
Scheduled awakenings	Parents/caregivers pre-emptively awaken the child prior to usual spontaneous awakening, and provide responses as if awakening was spontaneous
Parent education	Parents/caregivers/older children and adolescents are educated (including teaching regarding behavioral strategies) to limit development or persistence of sleep problems

Autism spectrum disorders (ASD)

Recent years has seen increasing interest in sleep disturbance in children with ASD, the number of whom is now considered much greater than once supposed. Sleep disturbance in ASD has been accorded high priority in recommendations for sleep research [19]. For that reason, the condition is emphasized in this review. The cardinal features of ASD are severe impairment of social interaction with other people and of verbal and non-verbal communication, and restricted or repetitive patterns of behavior [28], all of which might make the learning of good sleep habits difficult.

Contrary to the earlier view that "autism" was of psychological origin, this group of disorders is now known to be undoubtedly neurological in nature [28]. ASD is usually considered to principally include a core syndrome of autism, Asperger syndrome or "high functioning autism," and atypical autism or pervasive developmental disorder (PDD) not otherwise specified but with autistic features. The addition of other conditions is somewhat contentious. For example, Rett syndrome is considered by some to be misplaced on the grounds that it is simply one of various medical disorders associated with autistic symptomatology [29]. Thus the term "autism" tends to refer to the core syndrome.

A main point of present relevance is that generalizations about the sleep disorders of "children with ASD" as a whole are of limited validity in view of the heterogeneous nature of this group. In fact, the heterogeneity does not stop there as there are multiple possible causes of ASD (including genetic, brain damage or dysfunction) and a range of possible co-morbid developmental, medical, and psychiatric disorders. Consequently, various factors might be contributing to an individual child's sleep disturbance, each requiring its own type of attention, as far as possible. The same can be said of other categories of developmental disorder.

Despite the recent increase in reported studies of sleep and ASD, with some exceptions [30], the role of such complicating factors has been little explored and the present literature of sleep disturbance in ASD is couched, for the most part, in terms of generalizations. However, these do not wholly undermine the conclusions drawn but do make them somewhat provisional and might explain certain inconsistencies in, for instance, responses to a given treatment.

Sleep disturbance is not a diagnostic criterion for ASD but there are now many reports which consistently describe particularly high rates of significant sleep problems in most ASD children across a wide age range [31]. This is shown clearly in comparisons made between ASD and "typically developing" children (i.e. those whose development is normal) and also between ASD and other forms of developmental delay, ASD children having the highest rates of all [32,33].

Most information has been in the form of parental reports with increasing and appropriate use of standardized and relatively informative assessments of children's sleep [34] rather than a few perhaps perfunctory items. In parallel, the diagnosis of ASD tends to have become more formalized. The sleep problems highlighted by parents of children with ASD have been mainly difficulty settling to sleep, long periods of waking during the night, and early morning waking. Some reports have emphasized additional forms of disturbed sleep [35] such as irregular sleep–wake patterns and problematic sleep routines. An unusual form of sleeplessness has also been described without any expression of discontent, yet shortening the child's overall time asleep [36].

Sleeplessness problems have been emphasized in the literature but the range of sleep disturbance may be wider in reality. For example, parasomnias have been reported to be more frequent in ASD children than in other groups [37]. The nature of these parasomnias is unclear from the little information available. This last report referred to nightmares, "disorientated awakening," and also bruxism. However, distinguishing between the various forms of dramatic parasomnias in particular is likely to be difficult in ASD children if only because of communication problems, although REM sleep behavior disorder has been confidently described in some ASD children [38].

Some investigators have used objective sleep assessment to supplement parental reports. Polysomnographic (PSG) comparisons between ASD "good sleepers" and "poor sleepers" have been reported to validate parental reports of bedtime settling difficulties and length of time their child sleeps; otherwise sleep physiology of both groups was the same as typically developing children [39]. However, another study using PSG assessment demonstrated ASD children showed some correspondence with parental reports but also subtle differences in both non-rapid eye movement (NREM) sleep and REM sleep compared with controls [40], the clinical significance of which is uncertain.

The more practical (although less detailed) objective sleep assessment of actometry (actigraphy) has also been used to give simply an overall picture of the child's sleep–wake pattern. Although the results have concurred with parental reports in some respects, disparities have also been reported. Sleep patterns measured by actigraphy do not always differ between those ASD children with or without reported sleeplessness [36]. This finding, and the fact that improvement in sleeplessness with treatment, as claimed by parents, may not be accompanied by objective change [41] raises the question of whether the beneficial treatment effect was attitudinal rather than physiological.

That parental reports of child sleep problems have been found to be associated with parental self-reports of stress may well give lie to the mechanisms involved [42]. This is likely to add to the other reasons why their own sleep suffers more than that of other parents [43,44] with the parenting and other family consequences to which reference was made earlier. Being stressed and tired, they might find it particularly difficult to cope with their children's sleep disturbance. Mothers' accounts of their children's sleep problems have been reported to be related to their own sleep difficulties and to the severity of their children's ASD symptoms [45].

Various factors (perhaps in combination) might underlie sleep problems in children with ASD [35]. Most appear to be behavioral in the sense that the child has not learned appropriate (or has developed inappropriate) ways of falling asleep and staying asleep, perhaps associated with difficult behavior or anxiety. Inappropriate bedtime routines or rituals are likely to contribute to settling problems in particular, and social and communication difficulties may well impede the process of learning good sleep habits.

Some reports suggest that physiological factors are implicated, at least in some children, such as circadian sleep–wake cycle abnormalities due to an abnormal pattern of melatonin production, and epilepsy (at least in certain forms) can have a sleep-disrupting effect where it develops. Other possibly co-morbid conditions such as OSA and mood/anxiety disorders were mentioned earlier.

Given the range of possible sleep disorders in ASD, various treatments might well be required. Most have been concerned with behavioral sleep disorders as defined earlier. A critical eye cast on the efficacy of the behavioral treatments for sleep problems that have been shown to be effective in children in the general community in children with ASD concluded that the evidence in their favor was sparse, largely because of the few reports and often their methodological limitations [46]. As already mentioned, further research is considered necessary as a priority [19].

However, more positive opinions have also been expressed [47] to the extent that a trial (conducted with conviction and with the appropriate choice of behavioral treatment in the light of parents' preference together with support and guidance for the parents) is justified.

A recent study explored the efficacy of behavioral treatment for severe bedtime and night waking sleep problems in 39 school-age children with formally diagnosed ASD [41]. The main issue was whether, given the children's social and communication difficulties, resistance to change, high levels of anxiety, and challenging behavior, this approach would be as effective as it is in normally developing children. Briefly, despite these reservations about the outcome, the parents' view was that their children's sleep had improved significantly and that this was still the case 6–8 months later. The children's behavior at home was also said to have improved. The fact that actigraphically the children's sleep had generally not changed following treatment was interpreted to suggest that a general reduction in tension and friction at home might have altered the parents' general view of the situation.

Doubts have been expressed about the enthusiastic claims for melatonin in some children with neurodevelopmental disorders because of shortcomings in the scope and design of many studies as well as the possibility of adverse effects especially in the long term [6]. In some instances, melatonin has been administered in combination with sleep hygiene advice and behavioral methods making the reason behind improved sleep difficult to ascertain. Nevertheless, melatonin continues to be used and to be the subject of positive reports [48,49], although the reported degree of improvement and the methodological sophistication of the studies have varied.

This is also true of preliminary accounts of the apparent value in the treatment of sleep disturbance of children with ASD of clonidine [50] and of iron supplements for those ASD children shown to be iron deficient [51]. The place and feasibility of other sleep treatments, such as chronotherapy and light therapy for circadian sleep–wake disorders, in children with ASD is not possible to judge in general terms because of inadequate study. Additional treatments are called for if co-morbid conditions, such as epilepsy, are present.

Asperger syndrome (AS)

Discussion continues about the classification of AS [52]. Reports of sleep problems in this condition are few and firm conclusions impossible. The small-scale studies raise questions about how far the findings can be generalized and, indeed, the findings are

very variable. In keeping with some small-scale earlier reports [35], more recent accounts have claimed that sleeplessness or insomnia is common in children with AS [53] and comparable findings have been reported in adults with this disorder [54]. There is some indication that children with AS may have a different pattern of sleep problems than those with autism and that both these groups showed a better response to medication than typically developing children [55].

The etiology of the sleeplessness problems is obscure. As the affinity between AS and the rest of the ASD subgroups is limited in a number of ways (notably the absence of significant intellectual impairment in AS), the number of influences likely to disturb sleep is less in AS. Anxiety and depression, as well as rigid adherence to routines (including at bedtime) or limited ability to appreciate social cues important in developing and maintaining satisfactory sleep–wake patterns, are some of the possible explanations that deserve further study. At present, it seems appropriate to follow the same treatment principles that apply with the core syndrome of autism.

Learning disability (mental retardation) syndromes

An important distinction throughout the range of learning disabilities is that between sleep problems of behavioral origin (for one reason or another, failure to learn good sleep habits) and those attributable to physical or medical aspects that are part of or associated with the basic condition. Often both types of sleep disorder co-exist.

Also, as mentioned before, across the spectrum of learning disability conditions, sleep disturbance is likely to add to the difficulties of the situation for both child and carer alike. An optimistic view of successful treatment prospects is appropriate with possibly beneficial effects on the child's behavior [56] and parents' sleep and emotional state, although more so in mothers compared with fathers [57]. There are preliminary indications that much can be achieved in the behavioral treatment of (at least) the settling and night waking problems of children with a learning disability by means of an instructional booklet rather than face-to-face contact with a therapist [58]. Given these treatment possibilities, it is unfortunate that parents often do not seek help for their children's sleep problem or that such help is not usually provided for other reasons [2,10].

Generalizations about "learning disability" are rarely permissible because of the range of conditions that come under that heading, their causes and severity, possible co-morbidity, and differences between individuals with the same type of disorder. Certainly this applies when considering sleep disturbance and, although some general points are relevant, there is merit in considering certain forms of learning disability separately from each other.

Down syndrome (DS)

Sleep difficulties (mainly bedtime settling and night-waking problems) are consistently reported by parents in a significantly higher proportion of children with DS compared with children in the general population [59,60]. This is in keeping with other learning disabled groups but, characteristically, the profile of sleep-related symptoms of children with DS also often contains, in addition to apparently behavioral sleep disorders, features suggesting upper airway obstruction – not only classical obstructive sleep apnea but also other types causing hypoventilation. Central sleep apnea is also reported to be common [61] as well (possibly) as fragmented sleep (reducing its restorative value) in a way that is only partly attributable to sleep-related breathing problems [62]. Epilepsy and hypothyroidism are other potentially sleep-disrupting influences in some children with this syndrome.

Studies suggest OSA may occur in 50% or more of cases of DS. This predisposition is considered to be caused by combinations of midfacial and mandibular hypoplasia, large posteriorly placed tongue, congenital narrowing of the trachea, obesity, hypotonia of the pharyngeal musculature, or laryngomalacia (Figure 23.1). In some cases of central apnea, brainstem dysfunction could be the result of atlanto-axial subluxation or instability. Tonsils and adenoids can be enlarged by upper respiratory tract infections. Congenital heart defects and pulmonary hypoplasia are further possible factors in nocturnal hypoxia, which, it has been suggested, might contribute to the high incidence of pulmonary hypertension in these children.

The likely adverse physical and psychological effects of severely disturbed sleep in children with DS indicate the need to routinely consider the possibility of a sleep disorder including OSA. PSG has been advocated for all young children with DS because of the poor correlation between parental impressions and PSG results [63]. Various treatments for OSA have been described: adenotonsillectomy (the results of which are mixed) and other more complicated surgical procedures for the correction of soft tissue or skeletal causes of obstruction. Additional treatments include prompt treatment of respiratory infections and continuous positive airway pressure in some cases.

As in other groups of children, those with DS who have sleep problems are also more likely to have psychological difficulties compared to those without such problems [64]. Although research on this point has been limited, behavioral treatments are indicated for sleep disorders of psychological origin [65]. Preliminary findings suggest that brief group instruction for parents of children with DS and behavioral sleep problems can be helpful [66].

The mucopolysaccharidoses

Mucopolysaccharidoses (MPS) refers to a group of autosomal recessive metabolic disorders characterized by lysosomal dysfunction, resulting in the inability to break down glycosaminoglycans, that can affect a wide range of organ systems. High rates of sleep disturbance are described in this group of disorders [67], severity varying from one type to another. OSA during sleep has commonly been implicated [68]. A variety of anatomical abnormalities compromise the upper airway, which (like the lower airway) may also be affected by widespread glycosaminoglycan deposits. Additional factors that contribute to high mortality rates include skeletal deformity affecting respiratory function and chronic pulmonary disease. Otherwise, bedtime settling and night waking problems of apparently behavioral origin are prominent. The Sanfilippo syndrome (MPS III) is associated with most sleep problems overall [69]. Irregular sleep patterns have been described in this type [70], possibly related to abnormal melatonin output [71]. Some unusual behaviors are reported in children with Sanfilippo syndrome, such as wandering, laughing, or singing during the night.

In general, treatments for these various sleep problems do not seem to have been evaluated in any systematic way. Reliance on melatonin is common, at least for the Sanfilippo form [72], but behavioral approaches may be effective when difficult behavior or parenting practices are thought to be responsible.

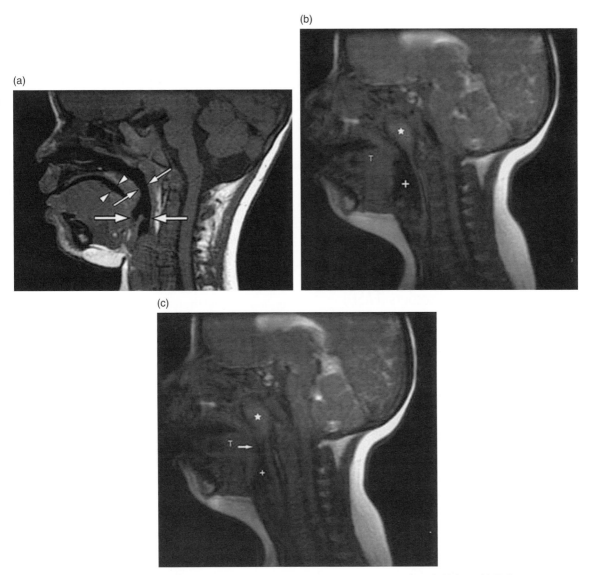

Figure 23.1 Upper airway anatomy and abnormalities associated with trisomy 21 (Down syndrome). (a) Sagittal MRI demonstrating important anatomical regions of the supraglottic airway. Hypopharynx shown as area between posterior aspect of tongue and posterior wall of pharynx (large arrows). Nasopharynx shown as area between soft palate and region of adenoid tonsils (small arrows). Oropharynx shown as region between soft palate and anterior aspect of tongue (arrowheads). (b & c) Dynamic (cine) sagittal MRI of a 7-year-old girl with trisomy 21 diagnosed with obstructive sleep apnea despite tonsillectomy and adenoidectomy at age 3. (b) demonstrates open and (c) demonstrates closed airway associated with dynamic airway motion. Notice adenoid regrowth seen in both images. (c) Also note hypopharyngeal airway decrease in size secondary to glossoptosis and hypopharyngeal collapse (*, adenoids; +, hypopharyngeal airway; T, tongue; →, glossoptosis). Adapted from Shott SR, Donnelly LF. Cine magnetic resonance imaging: evaluation of persistent airway obstruction after tonsil and adenoidectomy in children with Down syndrome. *Laryngoscope.* 2004;114(10):1724–1729. Reprinted with permission of John Wiley & Sons, Inc.

Prader-Willi syndrome (PWS)

PWS, a genetic disorder due to partial deletion of paternal chromosome 15q, is classically characterized by muscular hypotonia, polyphagia and obesity, short stature, small hands and feet, hypogonadism, and learning disability (mental retardation). Excessive daytime sleepiness, often seen in this condition, together with the characteristic obesity and noisy respiration during sleep, suggest that OSA is a usual complication. However, this appears to be so in only a minority of patients [73]. Obesity is thought to be a contributory factor but not a sufficient explanation for the sleep abnormalities. Instead, both the sleepiness and the variety of REM sleep abnormalities described in PWS are considered likely to reflect hypothalamic dysfunction resulting in persistent hypoarousal [74]. Central apnea is also said to be common [75]. Abnormal sleep is considered to be an important but often overlooked factor contributing to psychological difficulties in people with this condition [76].

These etiological uncertainties about the sleep disturbance limit treatment possibilities, although obesity and OSA should be treated as thoroughly as possible. Recently, growth hormone treatment of children with PWS is said to have produced a variety of beneficial effects (usually but not always on sleep) including improved psychological functioning [77].

Fetal alcohol spectrum disorders (FASD)

FASD refers to combinations of structural, neurocognitive, and behavioral effects of prenatal exposure to alcohol. These effects vary in severity, the most severe end of the spectrum being the fetal alcohol syndrome (FAS) in which the children suffer from severe learning disability [78].

Reference is made in some reports of sleep disturbance from infancy [79] but, despite the commonness of FASD, there appears to have been very little systematic detailed study of the sleep disorders in this group of children. Experimental animal studies of the effects of alcohol exposure in early development indicate disruption of the suprachiasmatic body clock system [80]. This can be expected to cause potentially serious sleep–wake cycle disorders.

In addition to this intrinsic predisposition to disturbed sleep, a number of other factors forming part of the FASD phenotype (although non-specific in the sense that they commonly accompany other neurodevelopmental disorders) are likely to contribute to sleep problems, in particular behavioral and psychiatric disturbance [81], including ADHD [82], the reciprocal relationship of which with sleep disturbance was mentioned earlier. To the list might be added parental and psychosocial difficulties within the family (which perhaps lay behind the mother's drinking while pregnant) and also adverse social circumstances at a later date [83].

In the absence of specific information about the nature and underlying causes of sleep problems in children with FASD, in addition to comprehensive long-term medical and psychiatric care, it is necessary to fall back on general treatment principles, as mentioned earlier, such as the possible value of behavioral treatments for sleep problems of behavioral origin as well as help for the other features of the condition as far as possible.

Other learning disability syndromes
(see [84] for additional details)
Fragile X syndrome

Fragile X syndrome is a disorder caused by a trinucleotide repeat on the X chromosome, leading to intellectual disability along with physical characteristics (elongated facies, machroorchidism, and prominent ears). Sleep problems are consistently reported by parents of children with this common cause of learning disability, but the nature of the problems is not well defined. Some children are said to have OSA for which continuous positive airway pressure might be helpful but the proportion is unclear. Marked disruption of sleep microstructure [85] and abnormal melatonin output profiles [86] have been reported. The contributions of co-morbid conditions (especially ADHD, autistic behavior, and epilepsy) need to be investigated further. Good response to behavioral treatment has been claimed [87]. It has also been reported that clonidine can improve both sleep and behavior.

Tuberous sclerosis

Tuberous sclerosis complex (TSC) is a multisystem genetic disorder with prominent signs and symptoms of CNS involvement such as learning disability (mental retardation), epilepsy, and autism. Parents of children with this disorder (of varying degrees of severity) also frequently complain of sleep disturbance, mainly settling and night waking problems [88]. Again, the origins of this disturbance are difficult to identify from published accounts. Behavioral factors (including parenting practices) may well need attention. Other likely influences include epilepsy, psychiatric disorders such as autism, and the various degrees of learning disability associated with the condition. Where children with tuberous sclerosis are reported to have responded to melatonin for their sleep disturbance, it is thought that this has been the result of its hypnotic effect rather than correction of sleep–wake rhythms [89].

Smith-Magenis syndrome

Smith-Magenis syndrome is a genetic disorder caused by a mutation of the RAI1 gene on chromosome 17, resulting in learning disability, distinctive facial features, behavioral difficulties, and sleep disturbance. The various sleep disturbances described in most children with this syndrome are generally non-specific although abnormal patterns of melatonin production, resulting in an advanced sleep phase, have been suggested as a cause, possibly reversible with treatment [90]. However, seemingly distinctive features have also been reported to occur from an early age, taking the form of early sleep onset at night, followed by sleeping in short bursts, with prolonged awakenings that terminate in very early waking with very active and possible destructive or hazardous behavior.

Angelman syndrome

Angelman syndrome, a genetic disorder due to partial deletion of maternal chromosome 15q, is typically characterized by learning disability, seizures, stereotyped movements, and a cheerful demeanor. A high rate of sleep disturbance (especially sleeplessness) has been reported in children with this rare syndrome but the details are yet to be clarified. Sleep-related breathing abnormalities and periodic limb movements have recently been reported [91]. Dramatic and destructive behavior at night has also been reported in some children with this condition, but its precise nature is unclear. The contribution of behavioral disturbance (including ADHD) and epilepsy (both common in children with this condition) is uncertain. Various treatments have been reported including low-dose melatonin, which seemed to improve sleep as judged by both parental reports and actigraphy [92].

Williams syndrome

Williams syndrome is a genetic disorder caused by a deletion on chromosome 7, resulting in characteristic "elfin" facies, learning disability, and cardiovascular problems, along with other associated symptoms. Again, the nature of the prominent sleep problems reported in many children with this syndrome appears to be non-specific and their causes ill defined. Biological factors are suggested by parental reports implying respiratory disturbance in some but more so prominent periodic limb movements in sleep, which respond to clonazepam, apparently with some improvements in both sleep and daytime behavior.

Other neurodevelopmental disorders
(see [1] for additional details)
Craniofacial syndromes

Upper airway obstruction is described in the various syndromes characterized by craniofacial deformity such as craniosynostosis syndromes (e.g. Crouzon and Apert syndrome), micrognathia syndromes (such as Pierre-Robin and Treacher Collins syndrome), Arnold-Chiari malformation, skeletal disorders such as achondroplasia, and, as already discussed, Down syndrome [93].

Not all these conditions are necessarily accompanied by learning disability, although behavioral disturbance likely to affect sleep patterns can be expected in many cases because of the impact of the conditions on the child and on the family. This is true, to some extent, of all the other disorders reviewed. The sleep-related breathing disorder usually takes the form of some degree of OSA, but central apnea is also described in the skeletal disorders and the Arnold-Chiari malformation. In central sleep apnea no breathing movements are seen and there is no air entry into the lungs because the drive to breathe, generated in the brain, is lost, or because of weakness of the respiratory muscles. In view of the complexity of the anatomical abnormalities, treatment may be difficult especially in the presence of lower airway problems.

Rett syndrome

Rett syndrome is a neurodevelopmental disorder caused by a mutation on the MECP2 gene on the X chromosome, which typically presents in girls (as male fetuses with the mutation do not survive to term) with normal development until 6–18 months, followed by regression of language and motor milestones, loss of purposeful hand movements, and deceleration in the rate of head growth. The vast majority of children with this neurodegenerative condition have been said to have sleep problems that may worsen as the condition progresses [94]. These are often multiple, taking the form of various types of sleeplessness and excessive daytime sleepiness. Laughing, crying, and screaming during the night has sometimes been reported with some evidence that this feature lessens with age, although daytime sleepiness might increase [95].

CNS dysfunction, affecting basic circadian sleep–wake rhythms, has been suggested as a cause, but behavioral factors are also likely in many cases. Epilepsy is another common complicating factor as the disease worsens. Interestingly, the abnormal daytime breathing patterns, which are common in the syndrome, do not seem to be closely related to the sleep disturbance. Only preliminary reports are available about the effectiveness of behavioral treatment or the use of melatonin.

Neurofibromatosis

Neurofibromatosis, an autosomal dominant disorder resulting in tumor growth in neural crest cells, may also be associated with sleep disturbance. Mention has been made of sleep disturbance as part of the psychosocial problems associated with neurofibromatosis in children [96] but without any details being provided. Although sleeplessness was mentioned in this report, in another preliminary parental questionnaire study only sleepwalking and sleep terrors were more often reported in children with neurofibromatosis type 1 compared with children in general [97]. In keeping with previous findings, much higher rates of behavioral disturbance were seen, including ADHD, all of which seem likely to have contributed to (or, at least, been associated with) sleep problems.

Tourette syndrome (TS)

This neuropsychiatric disorder characterized by vocal and motor tics poses intriguing questions about the origin and role of the various associated sleep abnormalities that have been described from early in the documented history of the disorder [98]. It is acknowledged that the sleep of children and adolescents with TS is markedly disturbed mainly by difficulty falling and staying asleep but also by parasomnias.

Interrupted sleep might partly be the result of the persistence of tics during sleep causing sleep fragmentation. An increased tendency to sleepwalking and sleep terrors [99] and frequent periodic limb movements during sleep [100] might have the same effect. REM sleep behavior disorder has recently been associated with TS [101]. However, common co-morbid psychiatric conditions [102], especially ADHD and obsessive-compulsive disorder, are likely to contribute their own disruptive influence.

Other conditions [1]

There have been limited accounts of sleep abnormalities in a number of other neurodevelopmental disorders, such as Lesch-Nyhan syndrome, phenylketonuria, Joubert syndrome, Rubinstein-Taybi syndrome, Smith-Lemli-Opitz syndrome, Cornelia de Lange syndrome, and Sotos syndrome. The limited information available does not permit any helpful judgment to be made about the likely nature and extent of the sleep disturbances involved.

Summary

It is all too evident that sleep disturbance is almost an inevitable accompaniment of the wide range of developmental disorders that have been reviewed. The consequences for the child's psychological development, and the well-being of the family as a whole, can be really serious. That being so, it is imperative that careful attention is routinely paid to the individual child's sleep as part of overall care, in the hope of early diagnosis of any sleep disorder and, as far as possible, treatment of the sleep disorder itself and associated conditions. Given accurate diagnosis and correct choice of treatment used with conviction, the prospects of a satisfactory outcome should be good for all concerned.

References

1. Stores G, Wiggs L. *Sleep disturbance in children and adolescents with disorders of development: its significance and management.* London: Mac Keith Press; 2001.

2. Wiggs L, Stores G. Sleep problems in children with severe intellectual disabilities: what help is being provided? *J Appl Res Intellect.* 1996;**9**:160–165.

3. Robinson AM, Richdale AL. Sleep problems in children with an intellectual disability: parental perceptions of sleep problems, and views of treatment effectiveness. *Child Care Health Dev.* 2004;**30**:139–150.

4. Courchesne E, Karns C, Davis R, et al. Unusual brain growth patterns in early life in patients with autistic disorder: an MRI study. *Neurology.* 2001;**57**:245–254.

5. Stores G. The protean manifestations of childhood narcolepsy and their misinterpretation. *Dev Med Child Neurol.* 2006;**48**:307–310.

6. Stores G. Medication for sleep–wake disorders. *Arch Dis Child.* 2003;**88**:899–903.

7. American Academy of Sleep Medicine. *International classification of sleep disorders, 2nd ed: Diagnostic and Coding Manual.* Westchester, IL: American Academy of Sleep Medicine, 2005.

8. Stores G. Clinical diagnosis and misdiagnosis of sleep disorders. *J Neurol Neurosurg Psychiatry*. 2007;**33**: 998–1009.

9. Garetz SL. Behavior, cognition, and quality of life after adenotonsillectomy for pediatric sleep-disordered breathing: summary of the literature. *Otolaryngol Head Neck Surg*. 2008;**138**(Suppl 1):S19–S26.

10. Owens JA. The practice of paediatric sleep medicine: results of a community survey. *Pediatrics*. 2001; **108**:E51.

11. Bonuck K, Parikh S, Bassila M. Growth failure and sleep disordered breathing: a review of the literature. *Int J Pediatr Otorhinolaryngol*. 2006;**70**:769–778.

12. Colton HR, Altevogt BM (eds) Committee on Sleep Medicine and Research. *Sleep disorders and sleep deprivation: an unmet public health problem*. Washington, DC: National Academies Press; 2006.

13. Meltzer LJ, Mindell JA. Relationship between child sleep disturbances and maternal sleep, mood, and parenting stress: a pilot study. *J Fam Psychol*. 2007;**21**:67–73.

14. Quine L. Severity of sleep problems in children with severe learning difficulties: description and correlates. *J Comm Appl Soc Psychol*. 1992;**2**:247–268.

15. Wolfson A, Lacks P, Futterman A. Effects of parent training on infant sleeping patterns, parents' stress and perceived parental control. *J Consult Clin Psychol*. 1992;**60**:41–48.

16. Minde K, Faucon A, Falkner S. Sleep problems in toddlers, effects of treatment on their daytime behavior. *J Am Acad Child Adolesc Psychiatry*. 1994;**33**:1114–1121.

17. Ramchandani P, Wiggs L, Webb V, Stores G. A systematic review of treatments for settling problems and night waking in young children. *BMJ*. 2000;**320**:209–213.

18. Owens J, Babcock D, Blumer J, et al. The use of pharmacotherapy in the treatment of pediatric insomnia in primary care: rational approaches. A consensus meeting summary. *J Clin Sleep Med*. 2005;**1**:49–59.

19. Mindell J, Emslie G, Blumer J, et al. Pharmacologic management of insomnia in children and adolescents: consensus statement. *Pediatrics*. 2006;**117**: e1223–e1232.

20. London New Drugs Group. *Melatonin in paediatric sleep disorders*, 2008. http://www.nelm.nhs.uk/en/ NeLM-Area/Evidence/Drug-Specific-Reviews/. Accessed 1 November, 2008.

21. Wiggs L, Stores G. General aspects of sleep and intellectual impairment. In: Stores G, Wiggs L, eds.

Sleep disturbance in children and adolescents with disorders of development: its significance and management. London: Mac Keith Press; 2001:47–52.

22. Stores G. Sleep patterns in the epilepsies. In: Stores G, Wiggs L, eds. *Sleep disturbance in children and adolescents with disorders of development: its significance and management*. London: Mac Keith Press; 2001:95–104.

23. Stores G. Visual impairment and associated sleep abnormalities. In: Stores G, Wiggs L, eds. *Sleep disturbance in children and adolescents with disorders of development: its significance and management*. London: Mac Keith Press; 2001:118–123.

24. Stores G. Disordered sleep in other neurological conditions. In: Stores G, Wiggs L, eds. *Sleep disturbance in children and adolescents with disorders of development: its significance and management*. London: Mac Keith Press; 2001:126–133.

25. Stores G, Crawford C. Medical student education in sleep and its disorders. *J R Coll Physicians Lond*. 1998;**32**:149–153.

26. Sheldon SH. Disorders of initiating and maintaining sleep. In: Sheldon SH, Ferber R, Kryger MH, eds. *Principles and practice of pediatric sleep medicine*. Philadelphia: Elsevier Saunders; 2005:127–160.

27. Morgenthaler TI, Owens J, Alessi C, et al. Practice parameters for behavioral treatment of bedtime problems and night wakings in infants and young children. *Sleep*. 2006;**29**(10):1277–1281.

28. Volkmer FR, ed. *Autism and pervasive developmental disorders*, 2nd ed. New York: Cambridge University Press; 2007.

29. Gillberg C. Autism spectrum disorders. In: Gillberg C, Harrington R, Steinhausen H-C, eds. *A clinician's handbook of child and adolescent psychiatry*. Cambridge: Cambridge University Press; 2006:447–488.

30. Liu X, Hubbard JA, Fabes RA, Adam JB. Sleep disturbances and correlates of children with autism spectrum disorders. *Child Psychiatry Hum Dev*. 2006;**37**:179–191.

31. Johnson KP, Malow BA. Sleep in children with autism spectrum disorders. *Curr Neurol Neurosci Rep*. 2008;**82**:155–161.

32. Krakowiak P, Goodlin-Jones B, Hertz-Picciotto I, Croen LA, Hansen RL. Sleep problems in children with autism spectrum disorders, developmental delays, and typical development: a population-based study. *J Sleep Res*. 2008;**17**:197–206.

33. Cotton S, Richdale A. Brief report: parental descriptions of sleep problems in children with

autism, Down syndrome, and Prader-Willi syndrome. *Res Dev Disabil.* 2006;**27**:151–161.

34. McGrew S, Malow BA, Henderson L, et al. Developmental and behavioral questionnaire for autism spectrum disorders. *Pediatr Neurol.* 2007;**37**:108–116.

35. Richdale A. Sleep in children with autism and Asperger syndrome. In: Stores G, Wiggs L, eds. *Sleep disturbance in children and adolescents with disorders of development: its significance and management.* London: Mac Keith Press; 2001:179–189.

36. Wiggs L, Stores G. Sleep patterns and sleep disorders in children with autistic spectrum disorders: insights using parent report and actigraphy. *Dev Med Child Neurol.* 2004;**46**:372–380.

37. Schreck KA, Mulick JA. Parental report of sleep problems in children with autism. *J Autism Dev Disord.* 2000;**30**:127–135.

38. Thirumalai SS, Shubin RA, Robinson R. Rapid eye movement sleep behavior disorder in children with autism. *J Child Neurol.* 2002;**17**:173–178.

39. Malow BA, Marzec ML, McGrew SG, et al. Characterizing sleep in children with autism spectrum disorders: a multidimensional approach. *Sleep.* 2006;**29**:1563–1571.

40. Miano S, Bruni O, Elia M, et al. Sleep in children with autistic spectrum disorder: a questionnaire and polysomnographic study. *Sleep Med.* 2007;**9**:64–70.

41. Wiggs L, Stores G. A randomised controlled trial of behavioural intervention for sleeplessness in children with autism spectrum disorders. *J Sleep Res.* 2006;**15** (S1):83.

42. Goodlin-Jones BL, Tang K, Liu J, Anders TF. Sleep patterns in preschool-age children with autism, developmental delay, and typical development. *J Am Acad Child Adolesc Psychiatry.* 2008;**47**:930–938.

43. Lopez-Wagner MC, Hoffman CD, Sweeney DP, Hodge D, Gilliam JE. Sleep problems of parents of typically developing children and parents of children with autism. *J Genet Psychol.* 2008;**169**:245–259.

44. Meltzer LJ. Brief report: sleep in parents of children with autism spectrum disorders. *J Pediatr Psychol.* 2008;**33**:380–386.

45. Hoffman CD, Sweeney DP, Lopez-Wagner MC, et al. Children with autism: sleep problems and mothers' stress. *Focus on Autism and other Developmental Disabilities.* 2008;**23**:155–165.

46. Schreck KA. Behavioral treatments for sleep disorders in autism: empirically supported or just universally accepted? *Behav Interventions.* 2001;**16**:265–278.

47. Richdale AL, Wiggs L. Behavioral approaches to the treatment of sleep problems in children with

developmental disorders: what is the state of the art? *Int J Behav Consult Ther.* 2005;**1**:165–189.

48. Anderson M, Kaczmarska J, McGrew SG, Malow BA. Melatonin for insomnia in children with autistic spectrum disorders. *J Child Neurol.* 2008;**23**: 482–485.

49. Wasdell MB, Jan JE, Bomben MM, et al. A randomized, controlled trial of controlled release melatonin treatment of delayed sleep phase syndrome and impaired sleep maintenance in children with neurodevelopmental disabilities. *J Pineal Res.* 2008;**44**:57–64.

50. Ming X, Gordon E, Kang N, Wagner GC. Use of clonidine in children with autistic spectrum disorders. *Brain Dev.* 2008;**30**:454–460.

51. Dosman CF, Brian JA, Drmic IE, et al. Children with autism: effect of iron supplementation on sleep and ferritin. *Pediatr Neurol.* 2007;**36**:152–158.

52. Macintosh KE, Dissanayake C. Annotation: The similarities and differences between autistic disorder and Asperger's disorder: a review of the empirical evidence. *Child Psychol Psychiatry.* 2004;**45**:421–434.

53. Allik H, Larsson JO, Smedje H. Sleep patterns in school-age children with Asperger syndrome or high-functioning autism: a follow-up study. *J Autism Dev Disord.* 2008;**38**:1625–1633.

54. Hare DJ, Jones S, Evershed K. A comparative study of circadian rhythm functioning and sleep in people with Asperger syndrome. *Autism.* 2006;**10**:565–575.

55. Polimeni MA, Richdale AL, Francis AJ. A survey of sleep problems in autism, Asperger's disorder and typically developing children. *J Intellect Disabil Res.* 2005;**9**:260–268.

56. Wiggs L, Stores G. Behavioural treatment for sleep problems in children with severe learning disabilities and challenging daytime behaviour: effect on daytime behaviour. *J Child Psychol Psychiat.* 199;**40**:627–635.

57. Wiggs L, Stores G. Behavioural treatment for sleep problems in children with severe intellectual disabilities and daytime challenging behaviour: effect on mothers and fathers. *Br J Health Psychology.* 2001;**6**:257–269.

58. Montgomery P, Stores G, Wiggs L. The relative efficacy of two brief treatments for sleep problems in young learning disabled (mentally retarded) children: a randomized controlled trial. *Arch Dis Child.* 2004;**89**:125–130.

59. Stores R. Sleep and Down syndrome. In: Stores G, Wiggs L, eds. *Sleep disturbance in children and adolescents with disorders of development: its*

significance and management. London: Mac Keith Press; 2001:53–59.

60. Carter M, McCaughey E, Annaz D, Hill CM. Sleep problems in a Down syndrome population. *Arch Dis Child*. 2009;**94**:308–310.

61. Ferri R, Curzi-Dascalova L, Del Gracco S, et al. Respiratory patterns during sleep in Down's syndrome: importance of central apnoea. *J Sleep Res*. 1997;**6**:34–141.

62. Levanon A, Tarasiuk A, Tal A. Sleep characteristics in children with Down syndrome. *J Pediatr*. 1999; **134**:755–760.

63. Schott SR, Amin R, Chini B, et al. Obstructive sleep apnoea: should all children with Down syndrome be tested? *Arch Otolaryngol Head Neck Surg*. 2006;**132**:432–436.

64. Stores R, Stores G, Fellows B, Buckley S. A factor analysis of sleep problems and their psychological associations in children with Down syndrome. *J Appl Res Intellect*. 2004;**17**:61–70.

65. Lucas P, Liabo K, Roberts H. Do behavioural treatments for sleep disorders in children with Down's syndrome work? *Arch Dis Child*. 2002;**87**:413–414.

66. Stores R, Stores G. Evaluation of brief group-administered instruction for parents to prevent or minimize sleep problems in young children with Down syndrome. *J Appl Res Intellect*. 2004; **17**:60–71.

67. Colville G, Bax M. Sleep problems in children with mucopolysaccharidosis. In: Stores G, Wiggs L, eds. *Sleep disturbance in children and adolescents with disorders of development: its significance and management*. London: Mac Keith Press; 2001:73–78.

68. Leighton SE, Papsin B, Vellodi A, Dinwiddie R, Lane R. Disordered breathing during sleep in patients with mucopolysaccharidoses. *Int J Pediatr Otolaryngol*. 2001;**58**:127–138.

69. Fraser J, Gason AA, Wraith JE, Delatychi MB. Sleep disturbance in Sanfillipo syndrome: a parental questionnaire. *Arch Dis Child*. 2005;**90**: 1239–1242.

70. Mariotti P, Della Marca G, Iuvone L, et al. Sleep disorders in Sanfilipo syndrome: a polygraphic study. *Clin Elecroencephalogr*. 2003;**34**:18–22.

71. Guerrero JM, Pozo D, Diaz-Rodriguez JL, Martinez-Cruz F, Vela-Campos F. Impairment of the melatonin rhythm in children with Sanfillipo syndrome. *J Pineal Res*. 2006;**40**:192–193.

72. Fraser J, Wraith JE, Delatycki MB. Sleep disturbance in mucopolysaccharidosis type III (Sanfillipo syndrome): a survey of managing clinicians. *Clin Genet*. 2002;**62**:418–421.

73. Vela-Bueno A, Olivan-Palacios J, Vgontzas AN. Sleep disorders and Prader-Willi syndrome. In: Stores G, Wiggs L, eds. *Sleep disturbance in children and adolescents with disorders of development: its significance and management*. London: Mac Keith Press; 2001:60–63.

74. Camfferman D, McEvoy RD, O'Donoghue F, Lushington K. Prader-Willi Syndrome and excessive daytime sleepiness. *Sleep Med Rev*. 2008;**12**:65–75.

75. Festen DA, de Weerd AW, van den Bossche RA, et al. Sleep-related breathing disorders in pre-pubertal children with Prader-Willi syndrome and effects of growth hormone treatment. *J Clin Endocrinol Metab*. 2006;**91**:4911–4915.

76. Camfferman D, Lushington K, O'Donoghue F, McEvoy RD. Obstructive sleep apnoea syndrome in Prader-Willi syndrome: an unrecognized and untreated cause of cognitive and behavioral deficits. *Neuropsychol Rev*. 2006;**16**:123–129.

77. Myers SE, Whitman BY, Carrel AL, et al. Two years of growth hormone therapy in young children with Prader-Willi syndrome: physical and neurodevelopmental benefits. *Am J Genet A*. 2007;**143**:443–448.

78. Manning MA, Hoyme HE. Fetal alcohol spectrum disorders: a practical clinical approach to diagnosis. *Neurosci Biobehav Rev*. 2007;**31**:230–238.

79. Burd L, Wilson H. Fetal, infant, and child mortality in a context of alcohol use. *Am J Med Genet C Semin Med Genet*. 2004;**127C**:51–58.

80. Spanagel R, Rosenwasser AM, Schumann G, Sarkar DK. Alcohol consumption and the body's biological clock. *Alcohol Clin Exp Res*. 2005;**29**:1550–1557.

81. Streissguth AP, O'Malley K. Neuropsychiatric implications and long-term consequences of fetal alcohol spectrum disorders. *Semin Clin Neuropsychiatry*. 2000;**5**:177–190.

82. O'Malley KD, Storoz L. Fetal alcohol spectrum disorder and ADHD: diagnostic implications and therapeutic consequences. *Exp Rev Neurotherapeutics*. 2003;**3**:477–489.

83. Streissguth AP, Bookstein FL, Barr HM, et al. Risk factors for adverse life outcomes in fetal alcohol syndrome and fetal alcohol effects. *J Dev Behav Pediatr*. 2004;**25**:228–238.

84. Stores G. Aspects of sleep in other neurodevelopmental disorders. In: Stores G, Wiggs L, eds. *Sleep disturbance in children and adolescents with disorders of development: its significance and management*. London: Mac Keith Press; 2001:87–93.

85. Miano S, Bruni O, Elia M, et al. Sleep phenotypes of intellectual disability: A polysomnographic evaluation in subjects with Down syndrome and Fragile-X syndrome. *Clin Neurophysiol*. 2008;**119**:1242–1247.

385

86. Gould El, Loesch DZ, Martin MJ, et al. Melatonin profiles and sleep characteristics in boys with fragile X syndrome: a preliminary study. *Am J Med Genet.* 2000;**95**:307–315.

87. Weiskop S, Richdale A, Matthews J. Behavioural treatment to reduce sleep problems in children with autism or fragile X syndrome. *Dev Med Child Neurol.* 2005;**47**:94–104.

88. Curatolo P, Sen S. Sleep disturbances in tuberous sclerosis complex. In: Stores G, Wiggs L, eds. *Sleep disturbance in children and adolescents with disorders of development: its significance and management.* London: Mac Keith Press; 2001:79–82.

89. Hancock E, O'Callaghan F, English J, Osborne JP. Melatonin excretion in normal children and in tuberous sclerosis complex with sleep disorder responsive to melatonin. *J Child Neurol.* 2005;**20**:21–25.

90. De Leersnyder H. Inverted rhythm of melatonin secretion in Smith-Magenis syndrome: from symptoms to treatment. *Trends Endocrinol Metab.* 2006;**17**:291–298.

91. Miano S, Bruni O, Elia M, et al. Sleep breathing and periodic leg movement pattern in Angelman syndrome: a polysomnographic study. *Clin Neurophysiol.* 2005;**116**:2685–2692.

92. Braam W, Didden R, Smits MG, Curfs LM. Melatonin for chronic insomnia in Angelman syndrome: a randomized placebo-controlled trial. *Child Neurol.* 2008;**23**:649–654.

93. Simakajornboom N, Beckman R. Sleep and craniofacial syndromes. In: Stores G, Wiggs L, eds. *Sleep disturbance in children and adolescents with disorders of development: its significance and management.* London: Mac Keith Press; 2001:64–72.

94. Roane HS, Piazza CC. Sleep disorders and Rett syndrome. In: Stores G, Wiggs L, eds. *Sleep disturbance in children and adolescents with disorders of development: its significance and management.* London: Mac Keith Press; 2001:83–86.

95. Young D, Nagarajan L, de Klerk N, et al. Sleep problems in Rett syndrome. *Brain Dev.* 2007; **29**:609–617.

96. Wadsby M, Lindehammer H, Eeg-Olofsson O. Neurofibromatosis in childhood: neuropsychological aspects. *Neurofibromatosis.* 1989;**2**:251–260.

97. Johnson H, Wiggs L, Stores G, Huson SM. Psychological disturbance and sleep disorders in children with neurofibromatosis type 1. *Dev Med Child Neurol.* 2005;**47**:237–242.

98. Kostanecka-Endress T, Banaschewski T, Kinkelbur J, et al. Disturbed sleep in children with Tourette syndrome: a polysomnographic study. *J Psychosom Res.* 2003;**55**:23–29.

99. Barabas G, Matthews WS, Ferrari M. Disorders of arousal in Gilles de la Tourette's syndrome. *Neurology.* 1984;**34**:815–817.

100. Verderholzer U, Muller N, Haag C, Riemann D, Struabe A. Periodic limb movements during sleep are a frequent finding in patients with Gilles de la Tourette syndrome. *J Neurol.* 1997;**244**:521–526.

101. Trajanovic NN, Voloh I, Shapiro, CM, Sandor P. REM sleep behaviour disorder in a child with Tourette's syndrome. *Can J Neurol Sci.* 2004;**31**:572–575.

102. Freeman RD. Tourette Syndrome International Database Consortium. *Eur Child Adolesc Psychiatry.* 2007;**16**(Suppl 1):15–23.

The future at the sleep–psychiatry interface

David T. Plante and John W. Winkelman

Introduction

The preceding chapters in this volume have discussed the development of sleep medicine and psychiatry, and detailed the current state of knowledge at the interface of these fields. This chapter will synthesize some key themes from the book and discuss future clinical and research directions in psychiatric sleep medicine. We recognize it is a daunting task to discuss the future of any field of medicine, as unforeseen scientific, economic, and social developments will undoubtedly arise, affecting any predictions made. Thus, the primary goal of this chapter will be to discuss pending developments on the horizon, promising lines of research that may or may not ultimately prove fruitful, and future questions and challenges faced by both fields.

The challenge and promise of bidirectionality

As demonstrated in numerous chapters throughout this book, sleep disturbance is far more than a mere symptom, "secondary" to psychiatric illness. Older models in which sleep complaints were assumed to be caused by an underlying psychiatric disorder are insufficient to explain the more complex interrelationships between sleep and mental illness. The new paradigm which is gaining broader acceptance is one in which sleep disturbance and psychiatric disorders share a more complicated bidirectional relationship, in which both influence the natural history of each other.

Evidence for the bidirectional model is clearly strongest for insomnia and major depressive disorder [1]. The current evidence suggests insomnia is not only a symptom of active depression, but plays an important role in the course of depression itself. There is very consistent and substantial evidence that insomnia puts individuals at risk for the development of incident depression [2–5] (as well as anxiety and substance use disorders). Furthermore, sleep disturbance is the most common residual symptom associated with treated depression, negatively affects quality of life [6,7], and increases the risk of depressive relapse in remitted patients [8,9]. On the other hand, the combination of sedative-hypnotic medications with antidepressant therapies leads to faster and more thorough antidepressant responses than can be accounted for by their amelioration of sleep disturbance alone [10,11]. Similarly, cognitive behavioral therapy for insomnia (CBT-I) may have similar effects when utilized in depressed patients [12]. All of these lines of evidence argue against the notion that insomnia is a mere epiphenomenon of psychiatric illness, and provide substantial support for the bidirectional relationship between insomnia and depression.

Despite growing appreciation for the complexities of the relationship between sleep and psychiatric disorders, much future work will be required to understand how and under what circumstances these relationships might be leveraged into meaningful advances in clinical practice. Despite data in major depression demonstrating that treatment of co-occurring insomnia may improve the psychiatric disorder in excess of direct effects on sleep, it is not clear how treating sleep disturbance will affect other functional outcomes in depression. For example, although there is evidence that sleep disturbance is associated with increased risk of suicidality [13–17], it is not clear whether treating insomnia with hypnotic medications in depressed patients affects the risk of suicide, and if it does, whether this is a positive or

Foundations of Psychiatric Sleep Medicine, ed. John W. Winkelman and David T. Plante. Published by Cambridge University Press.
© Cambridge University Press 2010.

negative effect, as clinical experience suggests sedating agents are frequently used (alone or in combination with other drugs) in intentional overdose.

Although the majority of evidence for bidirectional effects exists for major depression and insomnia, there are other psychiatric disorders for which similar relationships may exist. Unfortunately, the evidence for such relationships is oftentimes inferential or circumstantial, highlighting the need for additional work in psychiatric disorders besides depression. Such relationships are of particular interest in bipolar disorder and post-traumatic stress disorder (PTSD), where sleep disturbance is a core feature of the illness. Further research will be crucial to determine optimal treatments for sleep disturbance co-morbid with these psychiatric illnesses and whether these psychiatric disorders themselves improve with treatment of co-morbid insomnia.

Only a few studies have examined the effects of specific pharmacological and/or behavioral treatments for insomnia co-morbid with psychiatric illnesses outside of depression. Most of the recent work has focused on generalized anxiety disorder (GAD), with an open-label study (using ramelteon) and a placebo-controlled study (using zolpidem extended-release) demonstrating improvement in sleep disturbance associated with GAD [18,19]. In addition, treatment of GAD with an antidepressant (escitalopram) and a sedative-hypnotic (eszopiclone) may provide benefit for anxiety symptoms beyond the positive effects on sleep, similar to findings in recent coadministration studies in major depressive disorder [10,11,20].

There are generally fewer studies being conducted on treatment of co-morbid insomnia in psychiatric disorders beyond depression and GAD. One recent double-blind pilot study of gabapentin in the treatment of insomnia co-morbid with alcohol dependence demonstrated gabapentin significantly increased time to relapse, but did not significantly improve subjective or polysomnographic sleep measures [21]. Beyond pharmacological studies, emerging data suggests CBT-I may be valuable for insomnia co-morbid with multiple psychiatric disorders, with a recent study demonstrating its utility in a mixed population with insomnia related to multiple psychiatric disorders including depression, PTSD, and substance use [22]. However, the recent literature is certainly less developed when evaluating treatment effects on insomnia co-morbid with psychiatric disorders

beyond depression and GAD, highlighting the need for further research.

Although such studies that evaluate efficacy of insomnia treatments (either pharmacological or behavioral) in various psychiatric disorders are useful in guiding evidence-based practice, there are caveats regarding the way the evidence base is built that merit discussion. Given the current financial climate in pharmacological research, many such studies are likely to be industry sponsored and thus newer (patented) medications will undoubtedly develop a greater evidence base for use in treatment of insomnia co-morbid with psychiatric illness. We point this out not to cast industry-supported research in a pejorative light, but to point out that older agents (with proven efficacy and relatively well-understood safety profiles) may be left out of future experiments as a matter of financial reality. It is noteworthy, however, that lack of evidence is not synonymous with absence of efficacy, and it is important that clinical experience and pragmatism not be wholly forgotten. In an ideal world, there would be enough funding to test all sedative-hypnotics in all psychiatric conditions, but the reality is this will never occur with so many psychiatric illnesses being associated with insomnia and the pharmacopeia continuously expanding. Although imperfect, we would envision carefully constructed open-label protocols (potentially multisite) that track the responses of actual patients to various sedative-hypnotics as one way to help gauge the utility of medications that may not receive the same financial backing as their newer counterparts. Such strategies may allow valuable information to be obtained in a more cost-effective manner, by essentially gathering data on multitudes of individual "off-label" treatment trials that are an unavoidable reality in the practice of psychopharmacology.

Strategies for prevention

More important to the future of both fields than the evaluation of various treatments in the management of co-morbid sleep disturbance is the potential that sleep medicine has to contribute to strategies for the prevention of mental illness, which has largely proven elusive in psychiatry. Although beyond the scope of this chapter, there are certainly sociocultural factors involved, such as stigma about mental illness, which may make it difficult for patients to divulge early symptoms of mental illness, ultimately limiting the implementation of effective preventative treatments. From a biological standpoint, development of preventative strategies are hindered by numerous factors including a relative dearth of known pathophysiological mechanisms for neuropsychiatric disease, the likelihood that genetic mechanisms of mental illness are due to multiple genes of small effect as well as complicated gene-environment interactions [23], and a lack of specific biomarkers for active illness or illness susceptibility.

As discussed previously, it is well known that insomnia puts one at risk for the development of new-onset depression, anxiety, and substance use disorders. What is not known is what other factors among those with insomnia may be more likely to confer risk for incident mental illness, or whether treatment of insomnia can prevent the development of disorders such as depression in the first place. To adequately test the hypothesis that treatment of insomnia (either using pharmacotherapy or CBT-I) may ultimately prevent the development of depression (or other psychiatric disorders) requires large, longitudinal treatment studies, which are expensive and difficult to execute, but will ultimately be vital to advancing both fields. Ideally, these lines of research, particularly the use of non-pharmacological interventions, would be extended to children, as there is longitudinal data to suggest that sleep disturbance in childhood may increase the risks of anxiety disorders in adulthood [24] and neuropsychological impairment in adolescence [25]. Positive findings in such research would be a landmark accomplishment for psychiatry, could lead to preventative paradigms in the treatment of mental illness, and may dramatically alter clinical practice.

Sleep and mental illness: shared pathophysiological mechanisms?

The role of sleep as both a risk factor for, and perpetuating factor in, mental illness suggests the basic biology of sleep and its dysfunction may provide important pathophysiological insights into psychiatric disorders. In particular, current theories invoke hypothalamic-pituitary axis (HPA) activity, serotonin dysregulation, and inflammatory cytokines in the connection between depression and insomnia [1]. Additionally, alterations in GABAergic neurotransmission that are similar in depression and insomnia may reflect a shared pathophysiology [26,27].

Although it is presently not clear to what extent such lines of research will alter treatment paradigms in depression or other psychiatric illnesses, they certainly hold significant promise, and are actively under investigation.

Other lines of research are currently being developed that utilize discoveries in the burgeoning field of sleep science to explore the roots of psychiatric illness in new and exciting ways. For example, the role of orexin/hypocretin is established in narcolepsy with cataplexy [28], however, the role this neuropeptide may play in drug-seeking behavior and energy homeostasis has the potential to significantly affect the fields of addictions, eating disorders, and obesity research as there is growing evidence that orexin/hypocretin plays an important role in reward processing. Although the precise nature of cellular mechanisms involved in addiction circuits remains to be elucidated, it is thought that synaptic plasticity in the ventral tegmental area (VTA), in the form of long-term potentiation and depression (LTP and LDP, respectively), can be induced by several drugs of abuse. Interestingly, orexin/hypocretin not only plays an important role in stabilizing transitions between sleep and wakefulness, but it also plays a central role in facilitating glutamate-mediated LTP in dopaminergic VTA neurons [29–31], suggesting these neuropeptides are important moderators in the biological pathways that underlie addiction. Additionally, orexin/hypocretin has been implicated as being important in energy homeostasis, and the lateral hypothalamus (LH; the site from which orexinergic neurons originate) is an important area involved in feeding behavior [32,33]. Interestingly, in response to feeding, the amygdala may stimulate orexigenic neurons in the LH, which in turn may play a role in conditioned overeating and obesity, suggesting the orexin/hypocretin system is involved in reward processing for both food and drugs of abuse [31]. For these reasons, the orexin/hypocretin system is an attractive target for drug development with the theoretical potential to affect a broad range of neuropsychiatric diseases.

Genetics

The last few years have seen an explosion of genetics research across all fields of medicine, likely fueled by multiple factors including large collaborative efforts to characterize the genome in humans and model species, the advent of genome-wide association studies, and technological advances that increase throughput and reduce the cost of genetic analyses. Although genetic loci that confer substantial risk for the development of psychiatric disorders remain elusive, some recent findings in the field of pharmacogenetics may ultimately prove important in the clinical management of psychiatric disorders. There have been a host of candidate genes (at several levels of pharmacobiology including: serotonergic and noradrenergic neurotransmission, the cytochrome P450 system, brain-derived neurotrophic factor, and G-proteins) that may be linked with treatment response in mood and anxiety disorders [34]. Interestingly, the short allele polymorphism of serotonin transporter gene (5-HTTLPR), which has been associated with increased risk for affective disorders (particularly in response to stressors), has recently demonstrated association with primary insomnia, suggesting a genetic link between these disorders [35]. Furthermore, given that other primary sleep disorders such as obstructive sleep apnea (OSA) and restless legs syndrome (RLS) have high rates of co-morbid psychiatric disorders and often present with neurocognitive symptoms, studies that examine the association of these candidate genes with primary sleep disorders and/or how these genes may relate to therapeutic response may be a fruitful avenue of research for sleep medicine.

Just as candidate genes from psychiatric research may inform research in primary sleep disorders, genetic discoveries from sleep medicine may influence the field of psychiatry. For example, single nucleotide polymorphisms (SNPs) have recently been identified that confer the majority of population risk for idiopathic restless legs syndrome (RLS) and periodic limb movements of sleep (PLMS) [36–38]. How these genes are related to secondary forms of RLS/PLMS (e.g. due to iron deficiency, renal failure) are not well understood and are an active area of research. Notably, since RLS/PLMS is frequently induced by antidepressant treatment [39,40], these polymorphisms could conceivably be associated with increased risk of antidepressant-induced RLS/PLMS, or theoretically, be linked to treatment resistance or sleep disturbance in psychiatric patients treated with antidepressants. Beyond such theoretical links to psychiatric illness, it is noteworthy that one of the RLS/PLMS-associated SNPs (BTBD9 gene) has already been associated with Tourette syndrome (particularly without obsessive-compulsive disorder), suggesting

a common genetic predisposition among these disorders [41], strengthening the argument that these genes may be important in neuropsychiatric disease, especially those with hyperkinesia.

In addition to genes related to the risk of primary sleep disorders and their potential associations with neuropsychiatric disorders, strategies that utilize sleep and circadian endophenotypes to untangle the complicated genetic risks underlying mental illness may also prove valuable. Endophenotypes can broadly be defined as heritable, primarily state-independent biomarkers that are associated with an illness, with co-segregation of the illness and endophenotype within families [42]. An example of the potential for sleep and circadian endophenotypes in genetic research of complex psychiatric diseases is bipolar disorder, with proposed endophenotypes involving circadian rhythm instability, cholinergic sensitivity (and its effects on REM sleep), and response to sleep deprivation. These intermediate phenotypes may ultimately help parse out the underlying genetic mechanisms of this heritable psychiatric disorder, which have thus far remained elusive.

Biomarkers

Although circadian endophenotypes and their associated genes may eventually prove important in predicting the risk, presentation, treatment, course, and pathophysiological mechanisms of psychiatric illness, other sleep-related biomarkers may have similar potential to one day affect the clinical practice of both sleep medicine and psychiatry. The lack of reliable biomarkers for mental illness has limited diagnostic precision, prediction of at-risk individuals, development of preventative strategies, understanding of biological pathophysiology, and ultimately, hindered the development of successful psychiatric treatments. New technologies in sleep science, particularly the use of high-density electroencephalography (hd-EEG) and other neuroimaging modalities, offer the hope of finding biomarkers for mental illness beyond what has been typically gleaned from overnight polysomnography. Sleep recordings may be particularly advantageous when looking for psychiatric biomarkers because confounding activities that may occur during wakefulness, such as fluctuating levels of attention and motivation, and the expression of active (e.g. psychotic, depressive) symptoms, may be minimized. For example, using hd-EEG polysomnography, sleep spindle activity is significantly decreased in centroparietal regions in schizophrenia, with integrated spindle activity providing significant separation (>90%) between schizophrenic subjects and comparison groups [43]. Although these results require replication, the potential for such a sleep-related biomarker to alter our diagnostic capabilities in psychotic illness is a tantalizing prospect, and might further our understanding of the pathophysiology of the disorder. Beyond schizophrenia, hd-EEG may have other important applications in sleep medicine and psychiatry, particularly when combined with other modalities such as transcranial magnetic stimulation (TMS) and/or used to identify sensitive slow-wave parameters that may reflect changes in synaptic strength across the night [44–46]. Additionally, combining other neuroimaging modalities (e.g. functional magnetic resonance imaging (fMRI), magnetic resonance spectroscopy (MRS), etc.) with hd-EEG in the same study population may provide greater insights into the pathophysiologies of numerous sleep and psychiatric disorders.

It is not without some hesitancy that we discuss the potential of new sleep-related technologies to alter the course of psychiatry. In decades past, similar declarations were made regarding the use of sleep architecture, specifically changes in REM sleep as markers for depression. Over time, however, overt sleep architectural changes (decreased REM latency, changes in slow-wave sleep, etc.), although physiologically robust markers of depressive illness, failed to demonstrate the sensitivity and specificity sufficient to be useful in clinical psychiatric practice [47]. Still, the use of new technologies that go beyond traditional sleep staging and better characterize activity in the sleeping brain do seem to hold translational promise in distinguishing psychiatric states, biomarkers for disease susceptibility, and potentially shedding light on pathophysiological mechanisms.

Treatments on the horizon

Pharmacotherapies at the nexus of sleep medicine and psychiatry are slowly moving from agents discovered largely through serendipity to those developed using translational approaches due to an enhanced understanding of the processes involved in the regulation of sleep and the pathophysiology of sleep disorders. In this way, arousal pathways using cholinergic, adrenergic, histaminergic, orexinergic, and serotonergic neurotransmission, as well as inhibitory pathways employing γ-aminobutyric acid (GABA), have become valid targets of novel pharmacotherapies [48]. Notably, the agents we will discuss in this section are not an exhaustive list of pharmacotherapies in the pipeline; however, they are novel and have some promise to eventually expand the pharmacopeia. Additionally, we recognize that none of these agents are approved by the Food and Drug Administration (FDA), and may ultimately never be used in clinical populations. However, given the scope of this chapter, a brief discussion of these future pharmacotherapies is clearly indicated.

Agents that affect serotonergic systems in the brain have played a key role in the development of pharmacotherapies for a number of psychiatric diseases. More recently, drugs that specifically target certain subtypes of the serotonin (5-HT) receptor have moved into the pipeline as potential treatments for insomnia. Part of the rationale for targeting the 5-HT receptor system is related to its effects on slow-wave sleep (SWS). Within the seven serotonin receptor subfamilies ($5\text{-}HT_1$– $5\text{-}HT_7$), the $5\text{-}HT_2$ receptor subfamily (composed of three subtypes: $5\text{-}HT_{2A}$, $5\text{-}HT_{2B}$, and $5\text{-}HT_{2C}$) seems to play the greatest role in the modulation of SWS [49,50], with effects on SWS most likely mediated largely through the $5\text{-}HT_{2A}$ receptor subtype. In fact, it is thought that relatively higher affinities for the $5\text{-}HT_{2A}$ receptor by ziprasidone and olanzapine compared to other antipsychotics may account for the dramatic increases in SWS that can be observed with the use of these medications [51]. The use of agents that target $5\text{-}HT_2$ receptors for the treatment of insomnia is not novel, as many antipsychotics and the antidepressants mirtazapine and trazodone have $5HT_2$ receptor affinity and are used as off-label treatments for insomnia. Unfortunately, these drugs also have significant affinities for a number of other receptor types (e.g. D2, α1-adrenergic, H1) which may contribute to their other known clinical effects (e.g. neuroleptic and thymoleptic properties), but lead to unwanted side-effects (e.g. extrapyriamidal symptoms, orthostatic hypotension, and hyperphagia/weight gain) when used to treat insomnia. As a result, a number of more specific $5\text{-}HT_{2A}$ receptor antagonists or inverse agonists are currently under development for the treatment of insomnia [52]. Some of these agents have shown promise in phase II/III clinical trials, but it is unclear if or when any of these agents will come to market, as a recent 5-HT$_{2A}$ antagonist, eplivanserin, was recently removed by its parent company from consideration by the FDA and European Medicines Agency [53].

Another agent under development which has the potential to affect the sleep–psychiatry interface and also has antagonist effects on 5-HT$_2$ receptors is agomelatine. Unlike specific 5-HT$_{2A}$ antagonists, agomelatine is an agonist at melatonin (MT1 and MT2) receptors, as well as an antagonist of 5-HT$_{2C}$ receptors. The purported downstream effects of 5-HT$_{2C}$ antagonism are enhancement of dopaminergic and noradrenergic activity in frontocortical pathways [54]. As a result, agomelatine has primarily been developed as an antidepressant agent, and has shown modest promise as such [55]. However, since agomelatine is a MT1/MT2 receptor agonist, it may ultimately be a drug with clinical utility in the treatment of insomnia, either primary or co-morbid with other psychiatric disorders, particularly depression. However, it is important to note that agomelatine has not been studied specifically for insomnia, and without clinical experience with the drug, such conclusions are speculative at best. Despite this, agomelatine could theoretically have clinical utility in specific populations such as seasonal affective disorder [56]. Additionally, agomelatine may prove to be a useful treatment in bipolar depression [57] in which the use of standard antidepressants may not be effective [58] and, in some instances, may be detrimental to the course of the illness via manic switching [59–61].

One final class of investigational medications on the horizon with unique pharmacological properties is orexin receptor antagonists. Currently, an agent from this class, almorexant (an orexin 1 and 2 receptor antagonist), is in Phase III clinical trials, and has shown promise in the treatment of primary insomnia [48,62]. As previously discussed, given the potential role the orexin/hypocretin system may have in addictions, eating disorders, and obesity, pharmacotherapies which target orexinergic neurotransmission could theoretically be of value in treating insomnia co-morbid with specific psychiatric disorders (e.g. insomnia co-morbid with substance dependence) or in their effects on specific psychiatric disorders apart from sleep effects *per se*.

Beyond pharmacotherapies, there are also somatic treatments at the sleep–psychiatry interface that one day may prove valuable in the treatment of psychiatric disorders. In the case of major depression, it has long been known that sleep deprivation can paradoxically be a very effective antidepressant with a significant improvement in mood immediately following sleep deprivation in the majority of depressed patients [63]. However, use of sleep deprivation as a somatic treatment for depression has been limited due to relapse of depressive symptoms after even brief periods of recovery sleep [63], and strategies designed to extend the therapeutic effects of sleep deprivation have had limited success [64]. However, because of its potent acute effects, sleep deprivation may offer a paradigm for identifying neurobiological changes in the brain associated with relief and relapse of depression [65]. Such knowledge would be crucial for translating sleep deprivation into a pragmatic treatment for depression, and could further shed light on the pathophysiology of depression, leading to new treatment paradigms.

Nosology

One of the greatest challenges faced at the interface of psychiatry and sleep medicine is the need for communication between the fields. Without a common language to classify sleep disorders, it becomes a significant challenge to communicate findings from one field to researchers in the other. In addition, a lack of similar nomenclature between sleep medicine practitioners and psychiatrists can hinder collaborative clinical communication and treatment. Thus, nosology becomes a crucial issue around which both fields must collaborate and find common ground.

The *Diagnostic and Statistical Manual* (DSM), currently in its fourth edition [66], is the primary psychiatric nosological standard used to guide clinical and research efforts in psychiatry and psychology. Its counterpart in the field of sleep medicine, the *International Classification of Sleep Disorders* (ICSD), currently in its second edition [67], is the standard used in sleep medicine. Because sleep medicine is an interdisciplinary subspeciality, much of the detail in the ICSD-2 is beyond the scope of what is needed by the average psychiatric practitioner or researcher. However, it is clear that the current sleep disorders section of the DSM-IV does not reflect the current state of knowledge in sleep medicine, and is in need of significant revision to reflect the advances in the field of sleep science.

Presently, the next version of the DSM is under development and the DSM-V sleep–wake disorders workgroup has proposed several changes to the current schema, many of which we believe will have very positive effects [68]. Proposals to add diagnostic criteria for disorders not currently considered in the DSM-IV, including REM behavior disorder and RLS, will undoubtedly increase awareness of these illnesses among practicing mental health clinicians. Furthermore, the addition of subtypes of, and greater detail for, circadian rhythm disorders and sleep-related breathing disorders will help psychiatric practitioners better understand the presentations, pathophysiologies, and treatments of these illnesses. Perhaps most important is the inclusion of the diagnosis "insomnia disorder" with concurrent specification of co-morbid psychiatric or medical conditions, rather than primary or secondary forms of insomnia as currently described in the DSM-IV [68]. This recommendation clearly reflects the bidirectional relationship between insomnia and psychiatric disorders previously discussed, and will have significant effects on how practitioners comprehend the relationship between insomnia and mental illness.

Education and training

Although bridging the gap between the nosology of sleep medicine and psychiatry may be an important step in educating psychiatrists, psychologists, and other mental health clinicians about sleep and its disorders, it would be imprudent to assume that this alone will be sufficient. The unfortunate fact is the majority of trainees, regardless of origin of discipline, do not receive adequate training on sleep and its disorders. In psychiatric residency training, such teaching is minimal compared to the number of patients a trainee will see over the course of his/her career complaining of sleep disturbance [69]. As the chapters in this textbook have demonstrated, it is vital that a clinician take a careful history of a sleep complaint, build a differential diagnosis, and tailor treatment accordingly, including appropriate referral when primary sleep disorders (e.g. sleep apnea, REM behavior disorder, etc.) are suspected.

In order to build a differential diagnosis for a given sleep disturbance, one must first *think* of possible disorders that could cause the presenting symptoms. Second, clinicians must not only *know* the characteristic symptoms of primary sleep disorders and be cognizant that such disorders can present with predominantly psychiatric symptoms, but also have firm understanding of the sleep disturbances that can

occur in the context of mental illness. Third, clinicians must *ask* the appropriate questions to arrive at a diagnosis, which will then guide appropriate treatment. Far too often, clinicians jump directly from sleep complaint to treatment, without considering the possible underlying causes, leading to treatment failures, delays in delivering proper treatment, and ultimately, hindrance of patient care. We believe this is an important area in which we must strive to educate mental health clinicians in sleep and its disorders, through improved opportunities at all levels of training.

A significant impetus for the development of this book was to provide a textbook that was academically rigorous *and* clinically accessible for trainees and practitioners to help integrate basic skills in sleep medicine into clinical psychiatric practice, which is truly the "front line" in the management of sleep complaints among patients with mental illness. However, an additional purpose was to develop a reference which might serve as a springboard for those interested in pursuing clinical or research careers in sleep medicine. Although the vast majority of trainees will not pursue formal training in sleep medicine, some will be undoubtedly drawn into this exciting, interdisciplinary field. For them, we hope this book confirms that the community of psychiatrists and psychologists who pursue careers at the interface of sleep medicine and psychiatry is growing [70], and includes outstanding individuals with varied backgrounds spanning several continents. In addition, physicians who are interested in formal training in sleep medicine should be aware that it is now a subspecialty accredited by the American College of Medical Graduates (ACGME) and as such, fellowship programs accept trainees from a broad range of disciplines, including psychiatry, and are required to provide teaching from psychiatric and psychological perspectives as related to sleep disorders. Beyond such training in sleep as a medical subspecialty, the American Academy of Sleep Medicine (AASM) accredits training programs and a board exam in behavioral sleep medicine, open to practitioners from a wide range of backgrounds, with both doctoral and master's level certifications available [71].

Despite the growth of training opportunities, there continue to be real-world impediments faced by psychiatrists and psychologists pursuing careers in sleep medicine. Difficulties regarding reimbursement for mental health clinicians, as well as interdepartmental politics and economic forces, have at times led to unfortunate skirmishes as to the primary ownership of sleep medicine as a field as well as the locations (both physical and proprietary) of hospital and university-based sleep laboratories and clinical services. To combat such "turf wars" an increasing number of institutions have begun to develop interdisciplinary centers of sleep medicine, with some degree of autonomy beyond the traditional departmental structure. Additionally, there are pending changes to the field of sleep medicine (e.g. the use of portable monitoring studies to diagnose OSA, and auto-titrating positive airway pressure (PAP) devices to treat the disorder) that will dramatically alter the future landscape of the profession. We anticipate such changes will ultimately reduce the number of in-patient sleep laboratories and further concentrate them to academic and tertiary care centers, as in-lab polysomnography will be reserved for more complicated sleep disorders cases. Such changes would clearly affect financial aspects of sleep medicine and also would likely increase the importance of clinical acumen (beyond the interpretation of traditional polysomnography) in the evaluation and management of these disorders. Notwithstanding such issues, sleep medicine is a field with a significant potential for further development through collaboration among specialties, and as evidenced by the extraordinary contributors to this volume, one in which psychiatrists and psychologists can thrive and are valued for the clinical and research perspectives they bring to the broader sleep medicine community.

Conclusion

This text is not an attempt to recreate divisions within sleep medicine, but rather to demonstrate the growth of the field to those in the psychiatric and psychological professions. Some of the early foci of sleep researchers that initially drew psychiatrists and psychologists into the field continue to be of interest today. Moving forward, the potential for research and clinical care at the interface of sleep medicine and psychiatry is quite exciting, with new paradigms and tools available to explore the nature, functions, and pathologies of sleep and mental illness. We are hopeful that our growing understanding of the basic science of sleep may one day lead to translational advances in the treatment of psychiatric and sleep disorders. Although the future at the intersection of sleep and

psychiatry is certainly bright, the ability and motivation to communicate between fields and among researchers and clinicians of varied backgrounds remains a significant challenge. We are hopeful that this volume will inspire members of both fields to recognize how interrelated sleep and psychiatry truly are, and recognize the potential each field has to learn from the other.

References

1. Krystal AD. Sleep and psychiatric disorders: future directions. *Psychiatr Clin North Am.* 2006; **29**(4):1115–1130; abstract xi.

2. Breslau N, Roth T, Rosenthal L, Andreski P. Sleep disturbance and psychiatric disorders: a longitudinal epidemiological study of young adults. *Biol Psychiatry.* 1996;**39**(6):411–418.

3. Chang PP, Ford DE, Mead LA, Cooper-Patrick L, Klag MJ. Insomnia in young men and subsequent depression: The Johns Hopkins Precursors Study. *Am J Epidemiol.* 1997;**146**(2):105–114.

4. Ford DE, Kamerow DB. Epidemiologic study of sleep disturbances and psychiatric disorders. An opportunity for prevention? *JAMA.* 1989; **262**(11):1479–1484.

5. Szklo-Coxe M, Young T, Peppard PE, Finn LA, Benca RM. Prospective associations of insomnia markers and symptoms with depression. *Am J Epidemiol.* 2010;**171**(6):709–720.

6. Nierenberg AA, Keefe BR, Leslie VC, et al. Residual symptoms in depressed patients who respond acutely to fluoxetine. *J Clin Psychiatry.* 1999;**60**(4):221–225.

7. Carney CE, Segal ZV, Edinger JD, Krystal AD. A comparison of rates of residual insomnia symptoms following pharmacotherapy or cognitive-behavioral therapy for major depressive disorder. *J Clin Psychiatry.* 2007;**68**(2):254–260.

8. Reynolds CF 3rd, Frank E, Houck PR, et al. Which elderly patients with remitted depression remain well with continued interpersonal psychotherapy after discontinuation of antidepressant medication? *Am J Psychiatry.* 1997;**154**(7):958–962.

9. Perlis ML, Giles DE, Buysse DJ, Tu X, Kupfer DJ. Self-reported sleep disturbance as a prodromal symptom in recurrent depression. *J Affect Disord.* 1997; **42**(2–3):209–212.

10. Fava M, McCall WV, Krystal A, et al. Eszopiclone co-administered with fluoxetine in patients with insomnia coexisting with major depressive disorder. *Biol Psychiatry.* 2006;**59**(11):1052–1060.

11. Asnis GM, Chakraburtty A, DuBoff EA, et al. Zolpidem for persistent insomnia in SSRI-treated

depressed patients. *J Clin Psychiatry*. 1999;
60(10):668–676.

12. Manber R, Edinger JD, Gress JL, et al. Cognitive behavioral therapy for insomnia enhances depression outcome in patients with comorbid major depressive disorder and insomnia. *Sleep*. 2008;**31**(4):489–495.

13. Agargun MY, Kara H, Solmaz M. Sleep disturbances and suicidal behavior in patients with major depression. *J Clin Psychiatry*. 1997;**58**(6):249–251.

14. Turvey CL, Conwell Y, Jones MP, et al. Risk factors for late-life suicide: a prospective, community-based study. *Am J Geriatr Psychiatry*. 2002;**10**(4):398–406.

15. Bernert RA, Joiner TE Jr, Cukrowicz KC, Schmidt NB, Krakow B. Suicidality and sleep disturbances. *Sleep*. 2005;**28**(9):1135–1141.

16. Chellappa SL, Araujo JF. Sleep disorders and suicidal ideation in patients with depressive disorder. *Psychiatry Res*. 2007;**153**(2):131–136.

17. Wojnar M, Ilgen MA, Wojnar J, McCammon RJ, Valenstein M, Brower KJ. Sleep problems and suicidality in the National Comorbidity Survey Replication. *J Psychiatr Res*. 2009;**43**(5):526–531.

18. Gross PK, Nourse R, Wasser TE. Ramelteon for insomnia symptoms in a community sample of adults with generalized anxiety disorder: an open label study. *J Clin Sleep Med*. 2009;**5**(1):28–33.

19. Fava M, Asnis GM, Shrivastava R, et al. Zolpidem extended-release improves sleep and next-day symptoms in comorbid insomnia and generalized anxiety disorder. *J Clin Psychopharmacol*. 2009;**29**(3):222–230.

20. Pollack M, Kinrys G, Krystal A, et al. Eszopiclone coadministered with escitalopram in patients with insomnia and comorbid generalized anxiety disorder. *Arch Gen Psychiatry*. 2008;**65**(5):551–562.

21. Brower KJ, Myra Kim H, Strobbe S, et al. A randomized double-blind pilot trial of gabapentin versus placebo to treat alcohol dependence and comorbid insomnia. *Alcohol Clin Exp Res*. 2008;**32**(8):1429–1438.

22. Edinger JD, Olsen MK, Stechuchak KM, et al. Cognitive behavioral therapy for patients with primary insomnia or insomnia associated predominantly with mixed psychiatric disorders: a randomized clinical trial. *Sleep*. 2009;**32**(4):499–510.

23. Taylor L, Faraone SV, Tsuang MT. Family, twin, and adoption studies of bipolar disease. *Curr Psychiatry Rep*. 2002;**4**(2):130–133.

24. Gregory AM, Caspi A, Eley TC, et al. Prospective longitudinal associations between persistent sleep problems in childhood and anxiety and depression disorders in adulthood. *J Abnorm Child Psychol*. 2005;**33**(2):157–163.

25. Gregory AM, Caspi A, Moffitt TE, Poulton R. Sleep problems in childhood predict neuropsychological functioning in adolescence. *Pediatrics*. 2009;**123**(4):1171–1176.

26. Sanacora G. Cortical inhibition, gamma-aminobutyric acid, and major depression: there is plenty of smoke but is there fire? *Biol Psychiatry*. 2010;**67**(5):397–398.

27. Winkelman JW, Buxton OM, Jensen JE, et al. Reduced brain GABA in primary insomnia: preliminary data from 4T proton magnetic resonance spectroscopy (1H-MRS). *Sleep*. 2008;**31**(11):1499–1506.

28. Dauvilliers Y, Arnulf I, Mignot E. Narcolepsy with cataplexy. *Lancet*. 2007;**369**(9560):499–511.

29. Bonci A, Borgland S. Role of orexin/hypocretin and CRF in the formation of drug-dependent synaptic plasticity in the mesolimbic system. *Neuropharmacology*. 2009;**56**(Suppl 1):107–111.

30. Borgland SL, Ungless MA, Bonci A. Convergent actions of orexin/hypocretin and CRF on dopamine neurons: Emerging players in addiction. *Brain Res*. 2010;**1314C**:139–144.

31. Aston-Jones G, Smith RJ, Sartor GC, et al. Lateral hypothalamic orexin/hypocretin neurons: A role in reward-seeking and addiction. *Brain Res*. 2010;**1314C**:74–90.

32. Sakurai T. The neural circuit of orexin (hypocretin): maintaining sleep and wakefulness. *Nat Rev Neurosci*. 2007;**8**(3):171–181.

33. Tsujino N, Sakurai T. Orexin/Hypocretin: a neuropeptide at the interface of sleep, energy homeostasis, and reward system. *Pharmacol Rev*. 2009;**61**(2):162–176.

34. Schosser A, Kasper S. The role of pharmacogenetics in the treatment of depression and anxiety disorders. *Int Clin Psychopharmacol*. 2009;**24**(6):277–288.

35. Deuschle M, Schredl M, Schilling C, et al. Association between a serotonin transporter length polymorphism and primary insomnia. *Sleep*. 2010;**33**(3):343–347.

36. Stefansson H, Rye DB, Hicks A, et al. A genetic risk factor for periodic limb movements in sleep. *N Engl J Med*. 2007;**357**(7):639–647.

37. Winkelmann J, Schormair B, Lichtner P, et al. Genome-wide association study of restless legs syndrome identifies common variants in three genomic regions. *Nat Genet*. 2007;**39**(8):1000–1006.

38. Vilarino-Guell C, Farrer MJ, Lin SC. A genetic risk factor for periodic limb movements in sleep. *N Engl J Med*. 2008;**358**(4):425–427.

39. Yang C, White DP, Winkelman JW. Antidepressants and periodic leg movements of sleep. *Biol Psychiatry*. 2005;**58**(6):510–514.

40. Rottach KG, Schaner BM, Kirch MH, et al. Restless legs syndrome as side-effect of second generation antidepressants. *J Psychiatr Res*. 2008;**43**(1):70–75.

41. Riviere JB, Xiong L, Levchenko A, et al. Association of intronic variants of the BTBD9 gene with Tourette syndrome. *Arch Neurol*. 2009;**66**(10):1267–1272.

42. Gottesman II, Gould TD. The endophenotype concept in psychiatry: etymology and strategic intentions. *Am J Psychiatry*. 2003;**160**(4):636–645.

43. Ferrarelli F, Huber R, Peterson MJ, et al. Reduced sleep spindle activity in schizophrenia patients. *Am J Psychiatry*. 2007;**164**(3):483–492.

44. Esser SK, Hill SL, Tononi G. Sleep homeostasis and cortical synchronization: I. Modeling the effects of synaptic strength on sleep slow waves. *Sleep*. 2007;**30**(12):1617–1630.

45. Vyazovskiy VV, Riedner BA, Cirelli C, Tononi G. Sleep homeostasis and cortical synchronization: II. A local field potential study of sleep slow waves in the rat. *Sleep*. 2007;**30**(12):1631–1642.

46. Riedner BA, Vyazovskiy VV, Huber R, et al. Sleep homeostasis and cortical synchronization: III. A high-density EEG study of sleep slow waves in humans. *Sleep*. 2007;**30**(12):1643–1657.

47. Benca RM, Obermeyer WH, Thisted RA, Gillin JC. Sleep and psychiatric disorders: A meta-analysis. *Arch Gen Psychiatry*. 1992;**49**(8):651–668; discussion 669–670.

48. Sullivan SS, Guilleminault C. Emerging drugs for insomnia: new frontiers for old and novel targets. *Expert Opin Emerg Drugs*. 2009;**14**(3):411–422.

49. Sharpley AL, Solomon RA, Fernando AI, da Roza Davis JM, Cowen PJ. Dose-related effects of selective 5-HT2 receptor antagonists on slow wave sleep in humans. *Psychopharmacology (Berl)*. 1990;**101**(4): 568–569.

50. Dugovic C, Wauquier A. 5-HT2 receptors could be primarily involved in the regulation of slow-wave sleep in the rat. *Eur J Pharmacol*. 1987;**137**(1):145–146.

51. Cohrs S. Sleep disturbances in patients with schizophrenia: impact and effect of antipsychotics. *CNS Drugs*. 2008;**22**(11):939–962.

52. Teegarden BR, Al Shamma H, Xiong Y. 5-HT(2A) inverse-agonists for the treatment of insomnia. *Curr Top Med Chem*. 2008;**8**(11):969–976.

53. Withdrawal of marketing authorisation application for Sliwens (eplivanserin). http://www.ema.europa.eu/ humandocs/PDFs/EPAR/sliwens/Sliwens-H-1102-WQA.pdf. Accessed 9 February, 2010.

54. Millan MJ, Gobert A, Lejeune F, et al. The novel melatonin agonist agomelatine (S20098) is an antagonist at 5-hydroxytryptamine2C receptors, blockade of which enhances the activity of frontocortical dopaminergic and adrenergic pathways. *J Pharmacol Exp Ther*. 2003;**306**(3):954–964.

55. Howland RH. Agomelatine: a novel atypical antidepressant. *J Psychosoc Nurs Ment Health Serv*. 2007;**45**(12):13–17.

56. Pjrek E, Winkler D, Konstantinidis A, et al. Agomelatine in the treatment of seasonal affective disorder. *Psychopharmacology (Berl)*. 2007; **190**(4):575–579.

57. Calabrese JR, Guelfi JD, Perdrizet-Chevallier C, Agomelatine Bipolar Study Group. Agomelatine adjunctive therapy for acute bipolar depression: preliminary open data. *Bipolar Disord*. 2007; **9**(6):628–635.

58. Sachs GS, Nierenberg AA, Calabrese JR, et al. Effectiveness of adjunctive antidepressant treatment for bipolar depression. *N Engl J Med*. 2007; **356**(17):1711–1722.

59. Peet M. Induction of mania with selective serotonin re-uptake inhibitors and tricyclic antidepressants. *Br J Psychiatry*. 1994;**164**(4):549–550.

60. Jabeen S, Fisher CJ. Trazodone-induced transient hypomanic symptoms and their management. *Br J Psychiatry*. 1991;**158**:275–278.

61. Terao T. Comparison of manic switch onset during fluoxetine and trazodone treatment. *Biol Psychiatry*. 1993;**33**(6):477–478.

62. Neubauer DN. Almorexant, a dual orexin receptor antagonist for the treatment of insomnia. *Curr Opin Investig Drugs*. 2010;**11**(1):101–110.

63. Wu JC, Bunney WE. The biological basis of an antidepressant response to sleep deprivation and relapse: review and hypothesis. *Am J Psychiatry*. 1990;**147**(1):14–21.

64. Wirz-Justice A, Quinto C, Cajochen C, Werth E, Hock C. A rapid-cycling bipolar patient treated with long nights, bedrest, and light. *Biol Psychiatry*. 1999; **45**(8):1075–1077.

65. Benedetti F, Smeraldi E. Neuroimaging and genetics of antidepressant response to sleep deprivation: implications for drug development. *Curr Pharm Des*. 2009;**15**(22):2637–2649.

66. American Psychiatric Association. *Diagnostic and statistical manual of mental disorders*, 4th ed, Text Revision. Washington, DC: American Psychiatric Association; 2000.

67. American Academy of Sleep Medicine. *International classification of sleep disorders: diagnostic and coding*

manual, 2nd ed. Westchester, IL: American Academy of Sleep Medicine; 2005.

68. Reynolds CF 3rd, Redline S, DSM-V Sleep-Wake Disorders Workgroup and Advisors. The DSM-V sleep–wake disorders nosology: an update and an invitation to the sleep community. *Sleep*. 2010;**33** (1):10–11.

69. Krahn LE, Hansen MR, Tinsley JA. Psychiatric residents' exposure to the field of sleep medicine: a survey of program directors. *Acad Psychiatry*. 2002;**26**(4):253–256.

70. Lamberg L. More psychiatrists attracted to sleep medicine career. *Psychiatric News*. 2006; **41**(6):18.

71. Requirements for the American Board of Sleep Medicine Behavioral Sleep Medicine Certification Examinations. http://www.aasmnet.org/Resources/ PDF/BSMGuidelines.pdf. Accessed 10 February, 2010.

Index